ARTHRITIS

ARTHRITIS

PATHOPHYSIOLOGY, PREVENTION, AND THERAPEUTICS

EDITED BY

Debasis Bagchi,
Hiroyoshi Moriyama, and
Siba P. Raychaudhuri

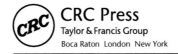

CRC Press
Taylor & Francis Group
Boca Raton London New York

CRC Press is an imprint of the
Taylor & Francis Group, an **informa** business

CRC Press
Taylor & Francis Group
6000 Broken Sound Parkway NW, Suite 300
Boca Raton, FL 33487-2742

First issued in paperback 2019

ISBN-13: 978-1-4398-1686-8 (hbk)
ISBN-13: 978-0-367-38287-2 (pbk)

Library of Congress Cataloging-in-Publication Data

Arthritis : pathophysiology, prevention, and therapeutics / editors: Debasis Bagchi, Hiroyoshi Moriyama, Siba P. Raychaudhuri.
    p. ; cm.
    Includes bibliographical references and index.
    ISBN 978-1-4398-1686-8 (hardcover : alk. paper)
    1. Arthritis. I. Bagchi, Debasis, 1954- II. Moriyama, Hiroyoshi. III. Raychaudhuri, Siba P.
    [DNLM: 1. Arthritis--physiopathology. 2. Arthritis--prevention & control. 3. Arthritis--therapy. WE 344]

RC933.A694 2011
616.7'22--dc23   2011018872

Visit the Taylor & Francis Web site at
http://www.taylorandfrancis.com

and the CRC Press Web site at
http://www.crcpress.com

To my best friend Sanjib Sengupta

—Debasis Bagchi

To my beloved mother, wife, daughter, and son

—Hiroyoshi Moriyama

To my beloved mother Bilwabasani Roychowdhury and to my father Durga Pada Roychowdhury

—Siba P. Raychaudhuri

Contents

SECTION I   Overview and Pathophysiology

SECTION II   Consequences

SECTION III Antiarthritic Drugs

SECTION IV Natural Therapeutic Interventions

SECTION VII *Commentary*

Preface

Medical science is advancing at a galloping pace. There is explosion of knowledge and information in all disciplines of medicine. In this book, we have covered cutting-edge information on arthritic diseases and their treatment. Arthritis is a debilitating disease that causes pain, inflammation, and loss of movement of the joints. The term *arthritis* literally means joint inflammation (arth = joint, ritis = inflammation). People of all ages, including children and young adults, can develop arthritis. Inflammation and inflammatory responses are key factors for causing swelling, redness, pain, and loss of movement in the affected areas. Arthritis is usually chronic and refers to more than 100 different kinds of arthritis that can affect the different parts of the body. It is important to know that in addition to the joints, some forms of arthritis are associated with diseases of other tissues and organs in the body. Also, arthritis has been shown to have direct correlations with obesity, diabetes, and cardiovascular dysfunctions.

We designed this book *Arthritis: Pathophysiology, Prevention, and Therapeutics* with a focused approach to cover the mechanistic aspects to understand the disease pathophysiology and treatment opportunities. One of the major goals and objectives of this book is to help readers understand the intricate aspects of arthritis and inflammatory responses, its consequences, the economic burden, and its huge impact on human society.

The book starts with a section on *pathophysiology*, which consists of seven chapters providing insight of rheumatoid arthritis, osteoarthritis, and psoriatic arthritis. Because arthritis has a very close relationship with other debilitating diseases including obesity, diabetes, and cardiovascular dysfunctions as well as with disability, we have dedicated the second section to *consequences* for providing a better perception of the importance of such diseases.

The third section focuses on *antiarthritic drugs*. This section starts with an overview and update on antiarthritic drug development by Dr. Micheal G. Lyon from Stanford University School of Medicine, which is followed by a chapter on nonsteroidal anti-inflammatory drugs. The third chapter highlights the diverse biologics involved in arthritic diseases. The fourth chapter discusses the topical applications for pain and arthritic diseases. The last two chapters deliver an overview on hyaluronic acid and hyaluronan in osteoarthritis and rheumatoid arthritis.

The fourth section delivers an array of *natural therapeutic interventions* in osteoarthritis and rheumatoid arthritis. This section gives an overview of glucosamine and chondroitin salts, hyaluronic acid, methylsulfonylmethane, *S*-adenosyl-L-methionine, undenatured type II collagen, curcumin, red pepper, capsaicin, *Boswellia serrata*, shark cartilage, omega-3 fatty acids, fish oil, plant-derived oils, avocado, bromelain, red ginger, *Tripterygium wilffordii,* dehydroepiandrosterone, green lipid mussel, abalone, rosmarinic acid mint, and pycnogenol.

The fifth section discusses *orthopedic approach*. This small section discusses the effect of total knee arthroplasty for osteoarthritis.

The sixth section discusses *nonpharmacological interventions*. The first chapter in this section discusses the influence of physical exercise in arthritis. This section also has an outstanding discussion on acupuncture, which is now globally used, and nonpharmacological intervention by physical exercise and rehabilitative strategy.

Finally, the seventh section is a *commentary* discussing the correlation between arthritis and the aging society and how exercise, nutrition, and preventative strategies can help the world and mankind in promoting human health.

Our sincere regards and gratitude to all the eminent scientists, researchers, doctors, and authors who contributed to complete this book. Also, my special thanks to Ms. Randy Brehm, Editor, Chemical and Life Sciences Group, Taylor and Francis Group, for her constant support, help, and cooperation.

Debasis Bagchi
University of Houston College of Pharmacy

Hiroyoshi Moriyama
Showa Pharmaceutical University

Siba P. Raychaudhuri
University of Davis

Editors

Debasis Bagchi, PhD, MACN, CNS, MAIChE, received his PhD degree in Medicinal Chemistry in 1982. He is a professor in the Department of Pharmacological and Pharmaceutical Sciences at University of Houston, Houston, TX. Dr. Bagchi is the Senior Vice President of Research and Development of InterHealth Nutraceuticals, Inc., in Benicia, CA. He is the immediate past President of American College of Nutrition, Clearwater, FL, and also serves as a distinguished advisor on the Japanese Institute for Health Food Standards, Tokyo, Japan, and immediate past chairman of the Nutraceuticals and Functional Foods Division of the Institutes of Food Technologists, Chicago, IL. Dr. Bagchi received the prestigious "Master of American College of Nutrition" (MACN) award in October 2010. His research interests include free radicals, human diseases, carcinogenesis, pathophysiology, mechanistic aspects of cytoprotection by antioxidants, regulatory pathways in obesity, and gene expression.

Dr. Bagchi has 275 articles in peer-reviewed journals, 9 books, and 14 patents. He has delivered invited lectures in various national and international scientific conferences, organized workshops, and group discussion sessions. Dr. Bagchi is a fellow of the American College of Nutrition, a member of the Society of Toxicology, a member of the New York Academy of Sciences, a fellow of the Nutrition Research Academy, and a member of the TCE stakeholder Committee of the Wright Patterson Air Force Base, OH. He is a member of the Study Section and Peer Review Committee of the National Institutes of Health, Bethesda, MD. He is also the associate editor of the *Journal of Functional Foods* and the *Journal of the American College of Nutrition* and also serves as an editorial board member of numerous peer-reviewed journals, including *Antioxidants and Redox Signaling*, *Cancer Letters*, *Toxicology Mechanisms and Methods*, and other scientific and medical journals. He is also the consulting editor of CRC Press/Taylor & Francis.

Dr. Bagchi received funding from various institutions and agencies, including the U.S. Air Force Office of Scientific Research, the Nebraska State Department of Health, the Biomedical Research Support Grant from the National Institutes of Health, the National Cancer Institute, the Health Future Foundation, The Procter & Gamble Company, and the Abbott Laboratories.

Hiroyoshi Moriyama, PhD, is a marketing and technical consultant at Moriyama Technical Institute, which he founded in 1992 to promote environmentally friendly products first and then cosmetic and nutraceutical ingredients in Japan. He is also a research fellow at the Laboratory of Pharmacotherapeutics at Showa Pharmaceutical University in Tokyo, Japan. He obtained his BS and MS degrees in Chemistry from the University of San Francisco and San Jose State University in 1978 and 1979, respectively. Dr. Moriyama received his PhD degree in pharmacognosy from Hoshi University of Pharmaceutical Sciences in Tokyo, Japan. He worked for various multinational companies in the fields of pharmaceuticals, cosmetics, and functional foods as a product and marketing manager before becoming independent. He has published a number of articles, patents, abstracts, and book chapters.

Dr. Moriyama is currently a board member of the Japanese Institute for Health Food Standards. He has been a member of American Chemical Society since 1982. He is also a member of Japanese Association for Food Immunology (JAFI). He was the special invited speaker of the Ministry of Research and Technology of the Republic of Indonesia to lecture on "Developing Market Oriented Research Culture on Natural Medicines" at LAPTIAB and Indonesia University in May 2009. His wide array of research interests include Japanese traditional medicine, functional foods and cosmetics, food immunology, drug delivery system, and regulatory system surrounding cosmetics and health foods in Japan.

Siba P. Raychaudhuri, MD, received his MD in 1987. He received his rheumatology training at Stanford University. In his early research career, he directed one of the most successful psoriasis research program at the Psoriasis Research Institute, Palo Alto, and worked on cutting-edge immune-based therapy for autoimmune disease at the Stanford University School of Medicine. The long-term goal of his research group is to explore the inflammatory cascades in inflammatory diseases and to develop safe and effective therapies by targeting the critical molecular events specific for these groups of diseases.

Currently, he is the chief of the Rheumatology Division at the VA Sacramento Medical Center and an assistant professor at the Division of Rheumatology, Allergy, and Clinical Immunology of University of California, Davis. He is also the director of the Psoriasis Clinic at the VA Sacramento Medical Center. His research group works on arthritis, inflammation, human autoimmune diseases, and animal models of inflammation.

Dr. Raychaudhuri is a fellow of the American College of Rheumatology, American Academy of Dermatology, and a member of the American College of Physicians.

Contributors

Michele Abate
Department of Clinical Sciences and Bioimaging
Institute of Advanced Biomedical Technologies
  (ITAB)
University "G. d' Annunzio"
Chieti-Pescara, Italy

Bharat B. Aggarwal
Cytokine Research Laboratory
Department of Experimental Therapeutics
University of Texas MD Anderson Cancer Center
Houston, Texas

Kwang Seok Ahn
Cytokine Research Laboratory
Department of Experimental Therapeutics
University of Texas MD Anderson Cancer Center
Houston, Texas

Akhtar Afshan Ali
Division of Hepatotoxicity
Department of Systems Biology
National Center for Toxicological Research
Jefferson, Arkansas

Allen P. Anandarajah
Division of Allergy, Immunology, and
  Rheumatology
University of Rochester Medical Center
Rochester, New York

Akira Asari
Hyaluronan Research Institute, Inc.
Tokyo, Japan

Debasis Bagchi
Research and Development
InterHealth Research Center
Benicia, California

Department of Pharmacological and
  Pharmaceutical Sciences
University of Houston College of Pharmacy
Houston, Texas

Manashi Bagchi
Research and Development
InterHealth Research Center
Benicia, California

Hai-li-Cai
Department of Orthopaedics
Tongde Hospital of Zhejiang Province
Health Bureau of Zhejiang Province
Hangzhou, China

Pooi-See Chan
Department of Animal Science
Michigan State University
East Lansing, Michigan

Shampa Chatterjee
Institute for Environmental Medicine
University of Pennsylvania Medical Center
Philadelphia, Pennsylvania

Maripat Corr
Division of Rheumatology, Allergy, and
  Immunology
University of California San Diego
La Jolla, California

Christine Dawczynski
Institute of Nutrition
Friedrich Schiller University
Jena, Germany

Dilip Ghosh
Neptune Bio-Innovation Pty Ltd.
Sydney, Australia

Om P. Gulati
Horphag Research Management Ltd.
Geneva, Switzerland

Qiao-feng Guo
Department of Orthopedic Surgery
Tongde Hospital of Zhejiang Province
Health Bureau of Zhejiang Province
Hangzhou, China

Rajiva Gupta
Clinical Immunology and Rheumatology
    Services
Department of Medicine
All India Institute of Medical Sciences
New Delhi, India

Ramesh C. Gupta
Toxicology Department
Murray State University
Hopkinsville, Kentucky

Xiaojuan He
Institute of Basic Research in Clinical
    Medicine
Beijing, China

Ayako Honmura
Maruha Nichiro Holdings, Inc.
Ibaraki, Japan

Kai Huang
Department of Orthopedic Surgery
Tongde Hospital of Zhejiang Province
Health Bureau of Zhejiang Province
Hangzhou, China

Muneaki Ishijima
Department of Medicine for Motor Organ,
    Department of Orthopaedics, and
    Sportology Center
Juntendo University School of Medicine
Tokyo, Japan

Yukihide Iwamoto
Department of Orthopaedic Surgery
Kyushu University
Fukuoka, Japan

Gerhard Jahreis
Institute of Nutrition
Friedrich Schiller University
Jena, Germany

Miao Jiang
Institute of Basic Research in Clinical
    Medicine
Beijing, China

Haruka Kaneko
Department of Medicine for Motor Organ and
    Department of Orthopaedics
Juntendo University School of Medicine
Tokyo, Japan

Kazuo Kaneko
Department of Medicine for Motor Organ,
    Department of Orthopaedics, and
    Sportology Center
Juntendo University School of Medicine
Tokyo, Japan

Tomoyuki Kanemitsu
Health and Function R&D Center
Kewpie Corporation R&D Division
Tokyo, Japan

Fumihito Kasai
Department of Rehabilitation Medicine
Showa University School of Medicine
Tokyo, Japan

Nobuyuki Kawate
Department of Rehabilitation Medicine
Showa University School of Medicine
Tokyo, Japan

Toshiaki Kogure
Department of Integrated Japanese Oriental
    Medicine
School of Medicine
Gunma University
Maebashi Gunma, Japan

Tatsuya Konishi
Maruha Nichiro Holdings, Inc.
Ibaraki, Japan

Alluri Venkata Krishnaraju
Laila Impex R&D Centre
Vijayawada, India

Daiki Kubomura
R&D of Functional Food Division
Yaizu Suisankagaku Industry Co., Ltd.
Shizuoka, Japan

S. Kumar
Clinical Immunology and Rheumatology
    Services
Department of Medicine
All India Institute of Medical Sciences
New Delhi, India

Shisei Kuninaga
Maruha Nichiro Holdings, Inc.
Ibaraki, Japan

Ajaikumar B. Kunnumakkara
Cytokine Research Laboratory
Department of Experimental Therapeutics
University of Texas MD Anderson Cancer
    Center
Houston, Texas

Hisashi Kurosawa
Juntendo Tokyo Koto Geriatric
    Medical Center
Juntendo University School of Medicine
Tokyo, Japan

Anand Lal
Department of Rheumatology
The Permanente Medical Group
Roseville, California

Francis C. Lau
Research and Development
InterHealth Research Center
Benicia, California

Julian E. Leakey
Office of Scientific Coordination
National Center for Toxicological Research
Jefferson, Arkansas

Hyangsook Lee
Studies of Translational Acupuncture Research
    (STAR)
Acupuncture and Meridian Science Research
    Center (AMSRC)
Kyung Hee University
Seoul, South Korea

Na Lin
Institute of Basic Research in Clinical
    Medicine
Beijing, China

Michael I. Lindinger
Department of Human Health and Nutritional
    Sciences
University of Guelph
Ontario, Canada

Aiping Lu
Institute of Basic Research in Clinical
    Medicine
Beijing, China

Michael G. Lyon
VA Palo Alto Health Care System
Palo Alto, California

Stanford University School of Medicine
Stanford, California

Kotaro Maekawa
Hisamitsu Pharmaceutical Co., Inc.
Ibaraki, Japan

Yoshiharu Matahira
R&D of Functional Food Division
Yaizu Suisankagaku Industry Co., Ltd.
Shizuoka, Japan

Shuichi Matsuda
Department of Orthopaedic Surgery
Kyushu University
Fukuoka, Japan

Hiromasa Miura
Department of Orthopaedic Surgery
Kyushu University
Fukuoka, Japan

Masazumi Mizuma
Department of Rehabilitation Medicine
Showa University School of Medicine
Tokyo, Japan

Hiroyoshi Moriyama
Laboratory of Pharmacotherapeutics
Showa Pharmaceutical University
Tokyo, Japan

Stanley Naguwa
Department of Rheumatology
UC Davis School of Medicine
Sacramento, California

Masaru Nakanishi
Hisamitsu Pharmaceutical Co., Inc.
Ibaraki, Japan

Toshiaki Nakano
Medical Science Division
Denkikagaku Kogyo Co., Ltd
Tokyo, Japan

Uzuka Naoaki
R&D of Functional Food Division
Yaizu Suisankagaku Industry Co., Ltd.
Shizuoka, Japan

Hiroshi Oda
Maruha Nichiro Holdings, Inc.
Ibaraki, Japan

Tsuyoshi Okada
Maruha Nichiro Foods, Inc.
Tokyo, Japan

Kazuo Okamoto
Department of Cell Signaling
Graduate School of Medical and Dental
    Sciences
Tokyo Medical and Dental University
Tokyo, Japan

Michael W. Orth
Department of Animal Science
Michigan State University
East Lansing, Michigan

Manoj K. Pandey
Cytokine Research Laboratory
Department of Experimental Therapeutics
University of Texas MD Anderson Cancer
    Center
Houston, Texas

Hi-Joon Park
Studies of Translational Acupuncture Research
    (STAR)
Acupuncture and Meridian Science Research
    Center (AMSRC)
Kyung Hee University
Seoul, South Korea

Wendy Pearson
Department of Plant Agriculture
University of Guelph
Ontario, Canada

Smriti K. Raychaudhuri
Immunology and Rheumatology Section
VA Medical Center
Sacramento, California

Graduate Group Immunology and School of
    Medicine
University of California Davis
Davis, California

Siba P. Raychaudhuri
Division of Rheumatology, Allergy and
    Immunology
Department of Medicine
School of Medicine
University of California Davis
Davis, California

Chief Rheumatologist
Department of Rheumatology
VA Medical Center Sacramento
Mather, California

Cathy Creger Rosenbaum
Rx Integrative Solutions, Inc.
Loveland, Ohio

Bethesda North Hospital Pharmacy
Cincinnati, Ohio

Akinori Sakamoto
Maruha Nichiro Foods, Inc.
Tokyo, Japan

William Salminen
Division of Hepatotoxicity
Department of Systems Toxicology
National Center for Toxicological Research
Jefferson, Arkansas

Ankit Saxena
UC Davis School of Medicine and VA
    Sacramento Medical Center
Sacramento, California

Gabriela Schmajuk
Stanford University School of Medicine
Stanford, California

Krishanu Sengupta
Laila Impex R&D Centre
Vijayawada, India

Gautam Sethi
Cytokine Research Laboratory
Department of Experimental Therapeutics
University of Texas MD Anderson Cancer
    Center
Houston, Texas

Arathi R. Setty
Department of Rheumatology
Mount Auburn Hospital, Harvard Medical School
Boston, Massachusetts

Seeta Sharma
Division of Allergy, Immunology, and
    Rheumatology
University of Rochester Medical Center
Rochester, New York

Department of Rheumatology
VA Sacramento Medical Center
Sacramento, California

Li-feng Shen
Department of Orthopedic Surgery
Tongde Hospital of Zhejiang Province
Health Bureau of Zhejiang Province
Hangzhou, China

Hiroshi Shimoda
Research and Development Division
Oryza Oil & Fat Chemical Co., Ltd.
Aichi, Japan

Bokyung Sung
Cytokine Research Laboratory
Department of Experimental Therapeutics
University of Texas MD Anderson Cancer Center
Houston, Texas

Yasufumi Takahashi
Medical Science Division
Denkikagaku Kogyo Co., Ltd
Tokyo, Japan

Hiroshi Takayanagi
Department of Cell Signaling
Graduate School of Medical and Dental
    Sciences
Tokyo Medical and Dental University
Tokyo, Japan

Hiroyuki Takeuchi
Department of Food and Nutrition
Toyama College
Toyama, Japan

Tadakazu Tamai
Maruha Nichiro Holdings, Inc.
Ibaraki, Japan

Norifumi Tanida
Hisamitsu Pharmaceutical Co., Inc.
Ibaraki, Japan

Golakoti Trimurtulu
Laila Impex R&D Centre, Unit-I, Phase-III
Vijayawada, India

Li-dong Wu
Department of Orthopedic Surgery
The Second Hospital of Medical College
Zhejiang University
Zhejiang Province, China

Shaohua Xu
Institute of Basic Research in Clinical
    Medicine
Beijing, China

Mitsumasa Yoda
Department of Rehabilitation Medicine
Showa University School of Medicine
Tokyo, Japan

Hisashi Yoshioka
Maruha Nichiro Holdings, Inc.
Ibaraki, Japan

Naomi Yoshioka
Department of Rehabilitation Medicine
Showa University School of Medicine
Tokyo, Japan

Chun Zhang
Department of Orthopedic Surgery
Tongde Hospital of Zhejiang Province
Health Bureau of Zhejiang Province
Hangzhou, China

Xiao-wen Zhang
Department of Orthopedic Surgery
Tongde Hospital of Zhejiang Province
Health Bureau of Zhejiang Province
Hangzhou, China

Section I

Overview and Pathophysiology

1 An Overview on Rheumatologic Disorders

S. Kumar and Rajiva Gupta

CONTENTS

INTRODUCTION

One of the earliest descriptions of rheumatologic diseases came from the classical Indian medicine text *Charaka Samhita*, which described a condition with painful and swollen joints. Paleopathological studies have shown evidence of rheumatoid arthritis (RA) in the remains of native North American skeletons in Tennessee and Kansas as early as 4500 BC. The first modern scientific description was given in 1951 by a French physician, Guillaume de Baillou. He used the term "rheumatism" to describe an ailment with inflammation, joint pain, and stiffness in the muscles. Work done in the last 50 years has resulted in an explosion of knowledge of the epidemiology, pathogenesis, and surgical techniques translating into the better and early use of disease-modifying agents, potent therapies like biological agents, and widespread use of joint replacement surgeries limiting the morbidity of rheumatic diseases.

Musculoskeletal problems encompass a range of illness, from those of inflammatory origin, like RA and ankylosing spondylitis (AS), to mechanical degenerative illness, like osteoarthritis (OA). There are many studies that have reflected on the high prevalence of rheumatic diseases in the world. The National Health Interview Survey (NHIS) has provided very reliable estimates of musculoskeletal diseases in the United States. NHIS is an annual questionnaire-based survey of a representative U.S. noninstitutionalized population. NHIS (2005) showed that 21% of the population reported being told by a health care professional of having some form of musculoskeletal disease. Also, stiffness or pain related to a joint within last 3 months was reported by 27% individuals. The prevalence was higher among women (24.4%) than among men (17.9%). Asians and Hispanics showed the lowest prevalence, whereas native Alaskans and Americans the showed the highest prevalence [1]. Similar estimates have come from the European population, which has shown that almost 100 million Europeans suffer from some form of inflammatory or degenerative rheumatic disease leading to a significant burden of rheumatic diseases on the society. In persons 65 years or older, rheumatic diseases account for half of all chronic conditions. The quality of life (QOL) of approximately 7.5% of the European population is severely and permanently reduced by pain and functional impairment caused by rheumatic diseases [2]. Data available from the COPCORD survey have shown a similar higher prevalence in developing countries. The prevalence of rheumatic musculoskeletal diseases from developing world has varied from 12% to 47% in urban surveys and from 12% to 55% in rural surveys. In all the surveys, there was a female predominance [3]. The prevalence of some of these illnesses increases markedly with age, and some are also affected by lifestyle factors, like obesity and lack of physical activity. This has led to a substantial increase in the socioeconomic burden of musculoskeletal diseases throughout the world. Previously, the major costs of treatment were indirectly related to sickness absenteeism, disability, and rehabilitation. Also, some of these illnesses start in the younger age group, with a chronic course continuing throughout the working life, posing considerable limitation of activities and also requiring long-term health care. Now with advancement of management of these conditions related to use of biologicals and more common use of arthroplasties, the direct costs have also increased substantially. Other drug-related side effects, such as chronic analgesic use–related gastropathy, a common problem in musculoskeletal illnesses, also has a significant effect on treatment costs. The magnitude of the burden of musculoskeletal disorders and their potential implications for health and social spending has been recognized by the World Health Organization (WHO), with their endorsement of Bone and Joint Decade (2000–2010). The aim of the Bone and Joint Decade is to increase the awareness of the society about the burden of musculoskeletal disease and to emphasize this before national and international institutions to increase resources devoted to its management. Its aim is to promote partnership between patients, health care professionals, scientific organizations, and various governmental and nongovernmental institutions all over the world. Four diseases including trauma, joint diseases, spinal disorders, and osteoporosis have been particularly emphasized.

In this chapter, we will discuss the epidemiology, health outcome, and economic burden associated with the important rheumatologic diseases such as RA, OA, juvenile inflammatory arthritis (JIA), AS, osteoporosis, gout, and fibromyalgia.

RHEUMATOID ARTHRITIS

EPIDEMIOLOGY OF RA

RA is a chronic inflammatory polyarthritis. The course of RA in individual patients is highly variable, but most patients with RA develop chronic progressive disease with significant functional limitation and physical disability. RA is also associated with decreased survival when compared with the general population [4]. The slow and variable onset and a variable disease course are the major limiting factors in conducting the epidemiological studies of rheumatologic diseases. The standardization of diagnoses of RA patients using the American College of Rheumatology (ACR) criteria is of significant help in epidemiological studies. The 1987 revised ACR criteria have now been accepted internationally for RA diagnosis and classification. By using these criteria, individuals can be classified as having RA if they fulfill four of seven criteria.

Most of the incidence studies are from developed countries. There are no incidence studies from developing countries. Prevalence studies were from many countries, both from the developed and developing world. The overall incidence of RA is 20–300 per 10^5 persons [5], although incidence and prevalence studies of RA conducted during the last two decades suggest a considerable heterogeneity in the disease frequency among different population groups (Tables 1.1 and 1.2). The prevalence was shown to be almost nil in Australian Aboriginal [6] and West African population [7] compared with a very high prevalence in North American Indian population [8]. Epidemiological studies from European countries suggest a significantly lower incidence and prevalence in south European countries compared with north European and North American countries. The median annual incidence of RA in south European countries is 16.5 cases per 10^5 [9–24] compared with 29 cases per 10^5 [24–36] in north European countries and 38 per 10^5 [31–45] in North American countries. Similarly, prevalence estimate of RA in south European countries is 0.3% compared with 0.5% in north European countries and 1% in North American countries [9].

TABLE 1.1
Incidence Rates of RA in Studies Based on ACR Criteria

	Country	Study Period	Incidence (1/100,000)		
			Overall	Male	Female
Doran et al. [10]	Rochester (United States)	1955–2000	50	30	60
Savolainen et al. [12]	Finland	2000	40	30	50
Soderlin et al. [13]	Sweden	1999–2000	24	18	29
Kaipiainen-Seppanen et al. [14]	Finland	2001	30	20	40
Uhlig et al. [15]	Norway	1988–1993	26	14	37
Symmons et al. [16]	United Kingdom	1990–1991		14	36
Drosos et al. [17]	Greece	1987–1995	24	12	36

TABLE 1.2
Prevalence Rates of RA in Studies Based on ACR Criteria

	Country	Study Period	Incidence (%)		
			Overall	Male	Female
Symmons et al. [18]	United Kingdom	2002	0.85	0.44	1.1
Andrianakos et al. [19]	Greece	2003	0.7		1.9
Dai et al. [20]	China	2003	0.28	0.14	0.41
Kvien et al. [21]	Norway	1997	0.44	0.19	0.67
Gabriel et al. [22]	United States	1999	1.07	0.74	1.37
Stojanovic et al. [23]	Yugoslavia	1998	0.18	0.09	0.2

There are only few retrospective long-term studies that have followed the secular trend from the same area and on the basis of similar criteria for diagnosis. Doran et al. [10] estimated the time trend of RA incidence in Rochester, Minnesota, during a 40-year period. During the study period, incidence rate fell from 61.2 per 10^5 in 1955–1964 to 32.7 per 10^5 in 1985–1994. Similarly, in the study of Kaipiainen-Seppanen and Aho [11] performed in Finland, the annual incidence of RA in the adult population was estimated during 3 years: 1980, 1985, and 1990. In 1990, there was a decline in incidence of approximately 15% compared with previous study years.

QOL MEASURES IN RA

RA is a disabling disease in which the disability starts early in the course of disease and progresses thereafter resulting in mild-to-moderate disability in two-thirds of patients with 10% of patients having severe disability [24, 25]. Around 25% of RA patients at 6.4 years and 50% at 20.9 years after disease onset are unable to continue a full time employment. These individuals have more pain, global severity, Health Assessment Questionnaire (HAQ) disability, anxiety, and depression [26]. In the recent past, there has been an increasing interest in the assessment of QOL. In chronic debilitating diseases such as RA in which the effect on mortality is limited, the health status is mainly assessed in functional terms: disability, restriction of activities, and also their emotional response to it. This makes QOL assessments especially important. Studies have shown that the Health-Related Quality of Life (HRQOL) assessment in RA is an accurate monitoring tool in clinical practice as well as in trials. There are validated generic and disease-specific patient-reported QOL instruments, such as the HAQ Disability Index and the 36-item Short-Form Health Survey (SF-36), which have shown to be sensitive for the assessment of changes in QOL.

The QOL instruments most widely used in RA are HAQ and the MHAQ. The HAQ Disability Index includes 20 items on daily functioning during the previous week. These cover eight areas: dressing and grooming, arising, eating, walking, hygiene, reach, grip, and outdoor activities. The scale is easy to perform and can be either self-reported by patient or applied in a personal or telephonic interview. Each response is scored on a four-point scale of ability: without any difficulty, with some difficulty, with much difficulty, and unable to do. There are also a number of generic scales, but the SF-36 and its derivatives are predominately used in the clinical trials and health resource allocation studies. It has 36 questions that measure eight dimensions: physical functioning, social functioning, physical limitations, social limitations, pain, mental health, vitality, and general health perception. It uses a 4-week recall period. It can also be either self-reported by the patient or used in personal or telephonic interviews. The score has two components, the physical component summary score and the mental component summary scores. These have been shown to be among the most valid SF-36 scales for measuring physical and mental health, respectively [27]. These scales are easier to administer and can be self-administered. Among adults with inflammatory rheumatic diseases, the self-reported health status (SF-36) was poorest as compared with those without arthritis in physical component summary score. Also, RA had the worst HRQOL for physical dimensions of SF-36 [28].

COST OF TREATMENT

RA has a substantial economic impact on patients, their families, and on the society overall. Majority of the cost of treatment for RA patients are indirect as a consequence of disability or unemployment. Early retirement because of the disease is frequent, with up to 50% of patients of RA having to leave the workforce and apply for a disability pension within 20 years of disease onset. The direct costs associated with RA include hospital care, physician visits, drug costs, rehabilitation, surgical treatments like arthroplasty, and loss of disability-adjusted life years (DALYs). Finally, there are intangible costs related to impairment in QOL, although not easily estimated because of difficulties in estimating this.

The annual cost of RA has been estimated to be \$2 billion in England in 1992 [29] and \$8.7 billion in the United States in 1991 [30], out of which the direct cost was half of the total cost and the other half was related to loss of productivity among working-age group patients. In a study from Spain, cost per RA patient was approximately US\$11,341 in 2001 [31]. The direct costs represented almost 70% of the total cost of the disease. This distribution of costs differs from other studies in which direct costs represented no more than 50% of total costs [29, 30]. The costs were higher initially although stabilized later until when surgery was required because of progression of joint damage. Joint surgeries were a major contributor to the direct cost of RA accounting to 17% of the total direct cost [31]. In a 10-year follow-up of patients with early RA, 17% had to undergo joint replacements in Sweden [32]. In Germany, the mean total direct costs of RA treatment calculated from the German Collaborative Arthritis Centres database was €4727 mainly attributed to drug costs and inpatient treatments [33]. The medical consultations required are also an important contributor to the direct cost. In the United States, annual number of visits to physician averages 11–12 [34, 35].

The indirect costs are typically between 50% and 75% of the total in developed countries. Days lost from work vary in studies from 2.7 to 30 days per year. In the United States, patients with RA lost their jobs, were unable to get employed, or retired early because of their illness, leading to a loss of productivity and income [36]. Sick leave is the predominant cost in the initial phase, but in the long term, disability benefits become more important. RA also has a considerable impact on all aspects of QOL. The morbidity and the mortality associated with the side effects of analgesics and steroids also are included in the cost of treatment. It is expected now that the economic burden of the disease is going to rise because of the widespread use of anti–tumor necrosis factor therapy. But because it is a chronic disabling disease, the indirect costs from disability associated with RA would be substantial. This argument may arise that only direct costs being included is inappropriate in such diseases, although inclusion of these costs in pharmacoeconomic analyses is contentious. In a study from the United States, when infliximab plus methotrexate was compared with methotrexate alone, 54 weeks infliximab plus methotrexate decreased the likelihood of severe disability from 23% to 11% at 54 weeks, which resulted in a lifetime marginal cost-effectiveness ratio of \$30,500 per discounted quality-adjusted life year (QALY) gained, when only direct medical costs were considered. When indirect costs were also included, the marginal cost-effectiveness ratio for infliximab was \$9100 per discounted QALY gained [37].

OSTEOARTHRITIS

EPIDEMIOLOGY

OA is a condition characterized by focal areas of loss of articular cartilage within the synovial joints, associated with hypertrophy of the bone (osteophytes and subchondral bone sclerosis) and thickening of the joint capsule, which is thought as a reaction of the synovial joints to injury. It most commonly involves joints of the hand, spine, knee, foot, and hip. OA is the most common form of arthritis, affecting almost every population and ethnic group. Murphy et al. [38] reported the lifetime risk for symptomatic knee OA to be 44.7%. The main risk factors for OA are older age, family history, obesity, and joint trauma. Trauma predisposing to OA may be related to some repetitive activity leading to an association between involvement of specific joint and certain occupations, that is, OA of the knee being more common in persons in occupations involving heavy lifting and knee-bending activities. There are also racial differences in the prevalence and involvement of OA at different joint sites. Despite being the commonest form of arthritis, the prevalence estimates of OA are not very accurate and have certain limitations. The diagnosis of OA is based on radiographic evidence in many studies. However, prevalence rates on the basis of radiographic imaging can vary considerably depending on whether only moderate and severe radiologic changes are accounted or even mild changes are included. Also, not all individuals with these radiographic changes have joint symptoms, like pain, stiffness, and loss of function. Whether such persons should be considered as having OA is not clear, as joint damage is not the only predictor of symptoms [39]. An ACR committee has suggested definitions of clinical OA for each joint that include the presence of symptoms and radiographic changes suggestive of OA, although these criteria are rarely used in epidemiologic studies as they have not been properly validated [40–42]. It is now thought that estimates of the prevalence of OA involving any joints must be based on symptoms and not just imaging. Thus, the reported prevalence rates in the literature have a wide range because they depend on the joints involved (e.g., knee, hip, or hand) as well as the method of diagnosis used in the study, whether radiographic or clinical. Estimation of incidence of OA is difficult because its symptoms are nonspecific and also the radiological changes do not correlate well with the disease process; hence, onset cannot be well defined, although it may be obtained from estimating the progression from a lower to higher radiographic severity score. A study from Australia used the DISMOD software to determine the incidence of OA in Australia. It used the available data of prevalence, remission, case fatality rates, and background mortality to estimate the incidence of OA [43]. The study showed that women had a higher incidence rate of 2.95 per 1000 population compared with 1.71 per 1000 population in men. The highest incidence of OA in women was among those aged 65–74 years, 13.5 per 1000 population per year, and in men among those 75 years or older, 9 per 1000 population per year. The prevalence estimates of OA are mostly based on radiographic surveys, which may be inaccurate as they do not take into account patients' symptoms and also as they may be present in almost everyone older than 70 years. The studies estimating the prevalence on the basis of significant clinical symptoms are few, and also the clinical criteria for establishing the diagnosis of OA have not been properly validated, although these studies do suggest that almost 10% of the world population older than 60 years suffer from clinical symptoms of OA [44].

DISEASE BURDEN AND ECONOMIC COST

OA has been estimated to be the eighth leading nonfatal burden of disease in the world in 1990, accounting for 2.8% out of all years of living with disability [45]. It was the sixth leading cause of years of living with disability internationally, accounting for 3% of the total global years of living with disability [46]. OA has a major effect on the burden of disability among the ageing population. OA causes more dependency in walking, climbing stairs, and other lower extremity tasks compared with any other disease because of high prevalence of knee and hip OA [47]. As this disease mostly affects the elderly, its impact is confounded by the presence and severity of comorbidities that may exaggerate the disability. This may also apparently magnify the socioeconomic burden of the disease. Still the economic impact of OA in terms of both direct medical costs and loss of employment is significant. A study from France showed that OA accounted from 0.1% of 1991 gross national product, which was equivalent to US$51.4 billion (in 2000) out of which two-thirds of the total was attributable to direct medical costs [48]. Similar studies from the United States have attributed two-thirds of the total cost related to OA to direct costs [49]. In a study from Canada, the average annual cost attributed to individual patients with hip and/or knee OA the cost was estimated at $12,200 [50]. In the United States, annual physician visits average 9 per person, and noninstitutionalized people with OA have an average of 0.3 hospitalizations lasting 8–9 days [46]. Joint replacement surgery for advanced OA is responsible for significant burden on health care resources. Hip replacement rates in Organization for Economic Cooperation and Development countries vary between 50 and 140 procedures per 100,000 [51]. In the United Kingdom, 47,932 total hip replacements were performed in 2000 [52]. The estimated cost was £4076 per patient at the 2000 National Health Service prices [53]. The indirect costs related to OA are difficult to estimate, still it is estimated that more than half of the individuals with symptomatic OA reported work disability [54]. As many patients are already retired, the work loss is still not very significant. The costs of treatment of arthritic conditions, primarily OA, are expected to increase as the population ages and may eventually exceed that because of conditions like cardiovascular diseases. This was reflected in a study from the United States, which showed that cost of hospital admissions for musculoskeletal procedures, mainly hip replacements and knee arthroplasties, totaled $31.5 billion, which 10 years earlier was estimated at $15.5 billion (in 1994). This highlights the dramatic increase in costs and burden of OA [55, 56].

JUVENILE INFLAMMATORY ARTHRITIS

JIA represents a heterogeneous group of chronic inflammatory arthritides in children and is very variable in its presentation and course. By definition, JIA begins before age 16 years. The most commonly affected are children between 1 and 3 years old and with a male-to-female ratio of 1:2, although systemic-onset JIA is an exception with a 1:1 female-to-male ratio [57]. Most epidemiological studies in the literature are from populations of northern European descent. In a study to determine the incidence and prevalence of JIA, the data from the Rochester Epidemiology Project, which included the medical records of all Rochester residents with any potential diagnoses of JIA from 1978 to 1993 and another cohort, were combined. The overall age- and sex-adjusted incidence rate was 11.7 per 100,000. The incidence rate per 100,000 population was 15.0, 14.1, and 7.8 for the time periods 1960–1969, 1970–1979, and 1980–1993, respectively [58]. An overall decrease in the incidence rate over the last decade was observed, most marked in the pauciarticular and systemic-onset subtypes. In a Norwegian study, the estimated prevalence of childhood chronic arthritis was 148/100,000 children [59]. In another study where all children were examined by a pediatric rheumatologist, the prevalence was 400/100,000 children, a relatively higher prevalence estimate [60]. The studies from other population groups suggest that JIA is less frequent in children of Asian and African descent [61].

HEALTH OUTCOME

Recent studies have shown that adult JIA patients have significant limitation of functions and restricted activity, causing a considerable impact on the patient's ability to function. A study from Denmark reported that 37% of patients had active juvenile chronic arthritis 26 years after onset, 11% were in functional class III or IV, and 22% had undergone surgery related to their juvenile chronic arthritis [62]. Similar studies have suggested that the fraction of patients with active disease was approximately 30%–50% and that the fraction of patients with significant residual disability increased with the follow-up time [63, 64], also because this disease involves children at an age that interferes with their becoming a productive member of the society. It was found that patients with JIA, on an average, had missed more days of school per year compared with controls; 7.15 days versus 5.03 days [65]. Also, 56.7% of children with JIA had missed at least one school day per year compared with 29.6% of controls.

ECONOMIC BURDEN

The average direct annual cost of JIA as determined by Minden et al. [65] was 1925 euros per year ($3136 in 2005 Canadian dollars). Similar estimates of direct annual health costs had come from a pediatric population from Canada. The direct annual cost of treatment was $3002 (95% confidence interval = $2330–$3672) [66]. These findings were in contrast to a previous a study of around two decades earlier showing a very high direct cost. Allaire et al. [67] estimated a mean annual direct health care cost of approximately US$5700 in 1989 ($10,801 in 2005 Canadian dollars). This was due to a very high inpatient care rate (mean annual inpatient costs were one-third of direct medical costs). This practice has declined in the current era. The indirect costs in JIA are lower than the direct costs because this patient cohort is composed of adolescents and young adults who are usually not working. However, as a significant proportion of these patients remain in active disease during adulthood, they may be considered. Indirect costs were highest in patients with seropositive polyarthritis and extended oligoarthritis who experienced more severe functional impairment. Indirect cost also includes the cost sustained by caregivers, which in this condition is the burden over the parent in the form of out-of-pocket expense or parental salary loss because of loss of days of work. The estimated parental salary loss in a study was $1241 in JIA patients compared with $404 in the control group [65]. The current practice of increasing use of biologicals has resulted in more children being treated with biologic agents such as etanercept. These are more expensive drugs, although they may reduce the overall cost of management by achieving remission in JIA and reducing the disability while improving the productivity.

ANKYLOSING SPONDYLITIS

AS commonly starts in early adulthood and has a chronic, progressive course leading to severe disability and limitation of function. The incidence and the prevalence of AS reflect the prevalence of HLA-B27 positivity in the population. HLA-B27 is present throughout Eurasia but is virtually absent among the genetically unmixed native populations of South America, Australia, and in certain regions of equatorial and southern Africa. The disease is also more common in HLA-B27-positive first-degree relatives of HLA-B27-positive AS patients, with around 10%–30% of them having signs or symptoms of AS. A positive family history of AS is considered a strong risk factor for the disease.

Two major population-based studies have provided the estimate of incidence and prevalence of AS. Carbone et al. [68] determined the incidence of AS using the data from the Rochester Epidemiology Project. The overall age- and sex-adjusted incidence was 7.3 per 100,000 person years, and there was a decline in the incidence rate over the decades. Similarly, a population-based study from Finland by Kaipiainen-Seppanen et al. [69] determined the annual incidence of AS to be 6.9 per 100,000 adults. The incidence of AS in northern Norway was shown to be 7.26 per 100,000 population [70]. The incidence has been found to be relatively low in Greece [71]. AS and HLA-B27 are nearly absent (prevalence of B27 < 1%) in Africans and Japanese [72]. The estimated prevalence of AS in the Netherlands and the United States as per the modified New York criteria was shown to be 68 and 197 per 100,000 persons older than 20 years, respectively [73, 74]. Similarly, the prevalence of the disease in Finland was also 150 per 100,000 people [69].

HEALTH BURDEN AND ECONOMIC COST

AS has multiple extra-articular manifestations, such as anterior uveitis, enthesitis, spinal osteoporosis leading to vertebral fractures, and thoracic kyphosis and comorbidities like inflammatory bowel disease (IBD) and psoriasis. These features result in a decreased QOL and restricted physical functioning. In a systematic literature review of original studies published after 1980 in which work status in AS was an outcome, it was found that employment rates varied from 34% to 96% after 45 and 5 years disease duration, respectively, and work disability from 3% to 50% after 18 and 45 years disease duration, respectively [75]. There is usually a long delay in the diagnosis and specialist management of AS. As the burden of illness increases with duration of disease, early diagnosis and treatment become necessary to prevent unnecessary morbidity and reduce functional decline. AS has a substantial impact on utilization of health care and non–health care resources. The direct costs are variable depending on the management pattern prevalent in the country. In a study from Europe including patients from France, Belgium, and the Netherlands, the average annual direct costs were €2640 (median, €1242) per patient, and direct health care costs accounted for 82% of total whereas the direct health costs were only 26% of the total annual costs in the United States, with average direct costs of $1775 [76, 77]. This difference between Europe and the United States was explained by the prevailing medical practices there; for example, physiotherapy is not covered by health insurance, and inpatient care in AS is uncommon. The indirect costs of AS are also substantial as the disease affects the younger productive age group with a chronic and progressive disease course. In a German study, indirect costs were mostly due to sickness absenteeism, early retirement, and lost productivity and were estimated at €7204, accounting for 49% of the total cost of illness [78]. Anti-tumor necrosis factor α is now being used widely and has been shown to be very efficacious in the treatment of AS. The average cost of infliximab treatment, including an outpatient visit for drug infusion, is estimated at around £12,500 per year (infusions of 5 mg/kg every 6 weeks). This is expected to increase the direct costs of AS substantially. In a study from Europe, to determine the cost-effectiveness of inflix-imab in the treatment of AS, there was a documented reduction of 31% in total costs in patients being treated with infliximab. The savings in other resources exceeded the treatment cost by £7888, leaving an incremental cost of £6214. Treatment also increased the number of QALYs [79].

GOUT

Gout is an inflammatory arthritis, which is mediated by the deposition of crystals of uric acid in the joints. It is primarily a male disease. Gout is the most common form of inflammatory arthritis affecting men. There are both nonmodifiable and modifiable risk factors for hyperuricemia and gout. Nonmodifiable risk factors are age and sex, whereas modifiable risk factors are obesity, use of certain medications, high purine intake, and consumption of purine-rich alcoholic beverages.

EPIDEMIOLOGY

Gout prevalence increases with age. Increasing prevalence of gout has also been attributed to changes in diet and lifestyle, aging-related conditions like metabolic syndrome and hypertension, and treatments with thiazide diuretics. In a study using the Framingham data, prevalence of gout was shown to be at 1.5% (2.8% in men and 0.4% in women). The estimates available from the UK General Practice Research Database show a similar prevalence of gout, approximately 2% among men and approximately 1% among men and women combined [80]. It has been proposed that because of increasing obesity and life style–related diseases in the population and the increasingly aging population, the prevalence of gout and hyperuricemia would also increase. In a population-based study in Rochester, Minnesota, the incidence of gout was shown to have increased markedly from 1977–1978 to 1995–1996 [81]. The incidence in 1977–1978 was 45 per 100,000 persons, which increased to 62.3 per 100,000 during the 1995–1996 time period. In a study by Wallace et al. [82], the incidence of gout in individuals older than 75 years showed an increase from 21/1000 persons in 1990 to 41/1000 persons in 1999 and in the 65- to 74-year age group from 21/1000 to 24/1000 persons from 1990 to 1992 to more than 31/1000 from 1997 to 1999. In contrast, prevalence rates in persons younger than 65 years remained consistently low throughout the study. In a multicenter study from the United Kingdom in 1991, the prevalence of gout was shown to have increased three times compared with estimates from the 1970s [83]. It is now estimated that approximately 2 million people are affected from gout according to the NHIS [84].

HEALTH OUTCOME

Chronic tophaceous gout may develop with inadequate treatment after 10–20 years of onset. Currently, with better management, this has become less common. This was reflected in a retrospective study in which the percentage of patients who developed tophaceous gout declined from 14% in 1949 to 3% in 1972. Patients with gout often exhibit poor performance in various health parameters. As gout often presents as an intermittent, progressive chronic disease assessment of QOL measures in this disease becomes especially challenging. Despite this limitation, studies have shown that patients with gout exhibited worse score than those with hypertension, angina, diabetes, or lower urinary tract symptoms in the QOL measures like SF-36 in all domains: physical functioning, general health perception, vitality, role limitations due to emotional problems, and mental health [85]. Recent studies suggest that a significant proportion of gout patients are not adequately managed with currently available antigout therapy, and it is expected that even with the very best of conditions, between 100,000 and 300,000 in the United States are expected to be classified as "treatment-failure gout" cases with presently available antigout therapies [86]. This "treatment-failure gout" has a significant effect on the patient's QOL as the symptoms do not respond to the treatment.

ECONOMIC BURDEN

Gout is associated with a decline in productivity and a significant burden on the health resources. The annual direct burden of illness for new cases of acute gout among men in the United States is estimated at $27.4 million [87]. This study by Kim et al. did not include women because the data on women are lacking, so this cost might be an underestimate. Gout accounted for approximately 37 million days of restricted activity from 1979 to 1981 in the United States, with 9.2% of all men with gout reporting limitations in performing major activities. In a study by Brook et al. [88], gout was associated with approximately $1800 in incremental medical and prescription drug costs per person per year in an employed population. In a recent study analyzing the claims database of the Integrated Healthcare Information Services (1999–2005), which includes approximately 40 private health plans in the United States for approximately 13 million beneficiaries, approximately 4% of whom are 65 years or older showed that the difference in total 12-month all-cause health care costs between gout patients and those without gout was $3038 [89]. Gout-related costs represent approximately 6% of total health care costs in elderly patients with gout.

OSTEOPOROSIS

Osteoporosis is a skeletal disorder, characterized by low bone mass and microarchitectural deterioration of bone tissue, resulting in an increase in bone fragility and susceptibility to fracture [90]. Fractures related to osteoporosis are found at bony areas rich in trabecular bone, which includes proximal femur, vertebrae, and distal radius. The risk factors for fragility fracture are female gender, Asian or white race, premature menopause, primary or secondary amenorrhea, primary and secondary hypogonadism in men, prolonged immobilization, vitamin D and calcium deficiency, high bone turnover, poor visual acuity, glucocorticoid therapy, and family history of hip fracture. The main clinical consequence of osteoporosis is the occurrence of characteristic low-trauma fractures, the most common among these are hip, vertebral, and distal forearm fractures.

A WHO expert panel in 1994 [91] defined the diagnostic criteria for osteoporosis on the basis of measurement of bone mineral density (BMD), relating it to the mean BMD of young adult women of same race (T score):

- Osteoporosis: BMD more than 2.5 standard deviations below the mean BMD of young adult women (T score < -2.5)
- Osteopenia: BMD value between 1 and 2.5 standard deviations below the mean BMD of young adult women ($-2.5 < T$ score < -1)

EPIDEMIOLOGY

Because of the increasing life expectancy, the burden of osteoporosis is increasing substantially not only in the developed countries but also in the developing countries. On the basis of the WHO definition, 54% of postmenopausal white women in northern parts of the United States are estimated to have osteopenia and a further 30% to have osteoporosis in at least one skeletal site. Similarly in the United Kingdom, around 23% of women older than 50 years are estimated to have osteoporosis as defined by WHO [92].

INCIDENCE

The incidence of osteoporosis is best measured as the incidence of osteoporotic fractures. A recent British study estimated the lifetime risk for fracture to be 53.2% at age 50 years among women, or in other words almost 50% of women older than 50 years are expected to suffer an osteoporotic fracture. The rate of fractures at the same age among men was shown to be 20.7% [93]. Site-specific lifetime risks at age 50 years are shown in Table 1.3. Among women, the 10-year risk for any fracture increased from 9.8% at age 50 years to 21.7% at age 80 years, whereas among men, the 10-year risk remained stable with advancing age at 7%–8% [94].

HIP FRACTURE

The incidence of hip fractures in western population increases exponentially with age, with rates of 2 per 100,000 person years in women 35 years or younger to 3032 per 100,000 person years in women older than 85 years [95]; the rates in men are 4 and 1909, respectively. The incidence ratio of women and men older than 50 years is approximately 2:1. Globally, 1.66 million hip fractures were estimated to have occurred in 1990, out of which 1.19 million occurred in women and 463,000 in men [96]. Overall, approximately 98% of hip fractures occur among people 35 years and older and 80% occur in women [97]. Fracture rates are highest in North America and Europe [98, 99], whereas it is much lower in Africa and Asia, but future projections suggest that it will increase markedly in the future even in the low incidence areas [100, 101].

VERTEBRAL FRACTURES

Most of the vertebral fractures are incidental, and only one-third of vertebral fractures present clinically [102]. Most vertebral fractures are the result of compressive loading associated with activities, such as lifting or changing positions. The incidence rate of vertebral fractures in the European Prospective Osteoporosis Study per year among men and women aged 50–79 years were 0.6% and 1% per year, respectively [103], which was obtained using lateral thoracolumbar x-rays. Overall, approximately one in eight women and men 50 years and older had evidence of vertebral deformity. Similar incidence estimates in the United States have been reported from the Framingham Study.

TABLE 1.3
Site-Specific Lifetime Risks at Age 50 Years

Lifetime Risk	Women (%)	Men (%)
Radius/ulna	16.6	2.9
Femur/hip	11.4	3.1
Vertebral body	3.1	1.2

Source: Adapted from Dennison, E., Mohhamad, A.M., and Cooper, C. *Rheum. Dis. Clin. N. Am.*, 32, 617–629, 2006.

DISTAL FOREARM FRACTURE

Most distal forearm fractures occur in women with a female-to-male ratio of 4:1. The incidence of distal forearm fractures in women shows a typical pattern of incidence with a linear increase among women between the age of 40 and 65 years, plateauing thereafter, whereas the incidence rate in men remains constant between the age of 20 and 80 years. A multicentre study in the United Kingdom found annual incidences of 9 and 37 per 10,000 men and women older than 35 years, respectively [104].

HEALTH OUTCOME OF OSTEOPOROTIC FRACTURE

All osteoporotic fractures are associated with significant morbidity, especially hip and vertebral fractures, which are also associated with excess mortality. In the United States, approximately 7% of survivors of all types of osteoporotic fractures have some degree of permanent disability and 8% require long-term nursing home care. Hip fracture results in marked morbidity with loss of mobility, pain, and excess mortality with almost all patients requiring hospitalization and most of them undergoing surgical intervention. A recent study estimated that there were 1.31 million new hip fractures in 1990, and the prevalence of hip fractures with disability was 4.48 million. It was estimated that there were 740,000 deaths related to hip fracture and 1.75 million DALYs lost, representing 0.1% of the global burden of disease worldwide and 1.4% of the burden among women in developed countries [105]. Hip fracture is associated with 20% mortality within the first year along with significant loss of function [106]. The degree of functional dependence after hip fracture is age dependent, with around 14% of patients in the 50- to 55-year age group getting discharged to nursing homes compared with 55% of those older than 90 years [107]. The vertebral fractures are usually clinically silent, but multiple fractures may cause significant morbidity because of progressive loss of height and kyphosis along with back pain. The loss of mobility resulting from it can also aggravate underlying osteoporosis [108]. The vertebral fracture also affects QOL by restricting activities. Also, a significant proportion of patients get hospitalized and require long-term care. Pain and disability worsen with each new vertebral fracture [109]. Vertebral fractures also lead to an increased mortality. In a study from the United States, there was a 1.23-fold greater age-adjusted mortality rate in women with one or more vertebral fractures compared with those who did not have a vertebral fracture [110]. Among the patients with distal forearm fracture, the hospitalization rates are found to be 23% among men and 19% among women [104], with around 50% of patients having a good functional outcome at 6 months although not associated with an increased mortality [111].

ECONOMIC COST

In a recent study from the United States, the estimated number of fractures and total cost attributed to osteoporotic fractures were 2.0 million and $16.9 billion, respectively [112]. The total cost distribution by fracture type is skewed toward hip fractures, which accounted for 72% of total costs. The overall distribution of fracture costs was 57% for inpatient care, 13% for outpatient care, and 30% for long-term care. By 2025, the burden in the United States is projected to grow by almost 50% to >3 million fractures and $25.3 billion. Estimates from Europe are considerably lower though at $17.9 billion for whole of Europe but are projected to increase substantially, which is a matter of concern for health policy makers.

FIBROMYALGIA

Fibromyalgia (FM) is a chronic pain condition that is characterized by chronic widespread pain, fatigue, sleep disturbance, morning stiffness, paresthesias, headache, and concurrent medical and psychiatric disorders. The cause of FM pain is not known, although it is generally agreed that patients with FM have a dysregulation of central sensory processing [113, 114].

EPIDEMIOLOGY

The prevalence of FM in the adult general population is generally similar across the world, ranging from 2% to 3% [115, 116]. FM is predominantly seen in women with a female-to-male ratio of 9:1 [117]. The studies from the United States have estimated an overall prevalence of fibromyalgia at 2% (females—3.4%, males—0.5%) [118]. The most recent estimates from the United States suggest that FM affects approximately 5% of all women and is the third most common rheumatic disorder after low back pain and OA [119]. Similarly, in a recent study from Europe, the estimated overall prevalence of FM was 4.7% for chronic widespread pain and was 2.9% when stronger pain and fatigue criteria were simultaneously used [120]. The estimates available from other countries have also shown a similar prevalence. The prevalence of FM is greater in clinic settings compared with population-based studies. It was reported to be 5.7% [121] in general medical clinics and 2.1% in family practice [122], whereas in specialized clinic setting fibromyalgia prevalence was expectedly higher ranging from 12% [123].

HEALTH OUTCOME

FM, as has been shown in various studies, is associated with substantial impairments in both physical and mental health status. Assessment of the health status in FM patients is complicated because there are no clinical markers, and it is mainly based on patients' self-reported symptoms. Also, assessment of tender points in fibromyalgia is inherently accurate. A recent review of 37 studies that measured health status with the SF-36 or the 12-item Short-Form Health Survey showed that FM patients were significantly more impaired than people in the general population in multiple health status domains assessed, including physical problems, bodily pain, general health, vitality, emotional problems, and mental health [124]. Also, when compared to those with RA, OA, osteoporosis, systemic lupus erythematosus, myofacial pain syndrome, primary Sjogren's syndrome, and others, FM groups had similar or significantly lower physical and mental health status scores. Other similar studies have also reported that FM patients consistently rate their HRQOL significantly below the general population and comparably with or lower than patients with other chronic conditions [125–128]. However, it is suggested that the long-term outcome is essentially benign in FM.

ECONOMIC COST

The increasing cost related to FM has been suggested by many, but adequate evidence supporting this is not available. There are very few studies on the economic cost of FM. The studies from North America have suggested that utilization of health services by fibromyalgia patients was significantly higher compared with the control population without widespread pain. In a multicenter study, the direct annual costs of FM treatment were $2274 per patient in 1996 dollars, and the cost of care was independently associated with the severity of functional disability [129]. Similarly, Sicras-Mainar et al. [130] showed that the utilization of health care and non-health care resources in the FM patients exceeded the reference population, with an increase in the cost by more than €5000. FM resulted in more medical visits and showed a higher average of work days missed. In a survey from the Netherlands, the average annual disease-related total costs were estimated at €7813 per patient [131]. On the basis of these data, it can be suggested that FM has a significant impact on the daily lives of the patients and the health care cost.

REPETITIVE STRAIN INJURY

Repetitive strain injury (RSI), also known as cumulative trauma disorder, is as an umbrella term used for conditions associated with activity-related arm pain such as carpal tunnel syndrome, cubital tunnel syndrome, thoracic outlet syndrome, DeQuervain's syndrome, trigger finger, golfer's elbow, and tennis elbow. These disorders supposedly develop as a result of overuse, repetitive movements, awkward postures, and sustained force although a clear-cut correlation is not there. This term is most commonly used for patients in whom there is no discrete pathophysiology that can correspond with the pain complaints. As the etiology is uncertain work-related musculoskeletal disorders (WRMSDs) is a better acceptable term to describe this condition. The WRMSDs are among the most widespread occupational health disorder particularly in the developed world. These disorders accounted for 48% of all reported workplace illnesses in 1990, up from 18% in 1980 [132]. The data available from Bureau of Labor and Statistics had shown that WRMSDs accounted for more than 60% of all newly reported occupational disorders (332,000 cases per year) in 1994 [133]. The Bureau of Labor and Statistics identified 92,576 cases of alleged RSI of the upper extremity that resulted in significant loss of DALYs. A diagnosis of carpal tunnel syndrome was made in 37,804 (41%) of these cases [134]. Certain professions and industrial settings have an especially high prevalence of RSI. In jobs such as tailors, dressmakers, construction workers, typists, and people who load, unload, or pack goods, a very high prevalence is noted. There has been a lot of focus in the recent past on keyboard operators because of a slew of litigations against computer manufacturers under the products liability theories of defective design and failure to warn, on the pretext that typing on computer keyboards caused repetitive stress injuries. One of the common consequences of typing is presumed to be carpal tunnel syndrome. However, its association with carpal tunnel syndrome is not well established, and recent evidence suggests that typing may in fact be protective [135]. The morbidity associated with repetitive injuries is significant. The impact of these conditions is variable extending from minor annoying pain to loss of function because of severe disability. In individuals such as musicians, performing artists, and craftsmen, loss of function at even a minor level can result in a significant loss of livelihood. The economic burden of RSI is large, especially because of the high costs associated with absence from work. Also, in this era of litigations, such publicized occupational conditions may become a major burden on health resources as well as the industry. Expectedly, the mean costs of a worker's compensation claim for this disorder ranges from $5000 to $8000, and the total is $6.5 billion every year in the United States [136].

REFERENCES

1. Pleis JR, Lethbrige-Cezku M. Summary health statistics of US adults: National Health Interview Survey, 2005. Vital Health Stats 2006;10:232.
2. Badley EM, Tennant A. Impact of disablement due to rheumatic disorders in a British population: estimates of severity and prevalence from the Calderdale Rheumatic Disablement Survey. Ann Rheum Dis 1993;52:6–13.
3. Chopra A, Naseer Abdel A. Epidemiology of rheumatic musculoskeletal disorders in the developing world. Best Pract Res Clin Rheumatol 2008;22:583–604.
4. Pincus T. Is mortality increased in patients with rheumatoid arthritis? J Musculoskelet Med 1988;5:27–46.
5. WHO Scientific Group. The burden of musculoskeletal conditions at the start of the new millennium. World Health Organ Technical Rep Ser 2003;919:i-x, 1–218.
6. Minaur N, Sawyers S, Parker J, Darmawan J. Rheumatic disease in an Australian Aboriginal community in North Queensland, Australia. A WHO-ILAR COPCORD survey. J Rheumatol 2004;31:965–972.
7. Silman AJ, Ollier W, Holligan S, Birrell F, Adebajo A, Asuzu MC, Thomson W, Pepper L. Absence of rheumatoid arthritis in a rural Nigerian population. J Rheumatol 1993;20:618–622.
8. Del Puente A, Knowler WC, Pettitt DJ, Bennett PH. High incidence and prevalence of rheumatoid arthritis in Pima Indians. Am J Epidemiol 1989;129:1170–1178.
9. Alamanos Y, Voulgari PV, Drosos AA. Incidence and prevalence of rheumatoid arthritis, based on the 1987 American College of Rheumatology criteria: a systematic review. Semin Arthritis Rheum 2006;36:182–188.

10. Doran MF, Pond GR, Crowson CS, O'Fallon WM, Gabriel SE. Trends in incidence and mortality in rheumatoid arthritis in Rochester, Minnesota, over a forty-year period. Arthritis Rheum 2002; 46:625–631.

11. Kaipiainen-Seppanen O, Aho K. Incidence of chronic inflammatory joint diseases in Finland in 1995. J Rheumatol 2000;27:94–100.

12. Savolainen E, Kaipiainen-Seppanen O, Kroger L, Luosujarvi R. Total incidence and distribution of inflammatory joint diseases in a defined population: results from the Kuopio 2000 arthritis survey. J Rheumatol 2003;30:2460–2468.

13. Soderlin MK, Borjeson O, Kautiainen H, Skogh T, Leirisalo-Repo M. Annual incidence of inflammatory joint diseases in a population based study in southern Sweden. Ann Rheum Dis 2002;61:911–915.

14. Kaipiainen-Seppanen O, Aho K, Nikkarinen M. Regional differences in the incidence of rheumatoid arthritis in Finland in 1995. Ann Rheum Dis 2001;60:128–132.

15. Uhlig T, Kvien TK, Glennas A, Smedstad LM, Forre O. The incidence and severity of rheumatoid arthritis, results from a county register in Oslo, Norway. J Rheumatol 1998;25:1078–1084.

16. Symmons DP, Barrett EM, Bankhead CR, Scott DG, Silman AJ. The incidence of rheumatoid arthritis in the United Kingdom: results of the Norfolk Arthritis Register. Br J Rheumatol 1994;33:735–739.

17. Drosos AA, Alamanos I, Voulgari PV, Psychos DN, Katsaraki A, Papadopoulos I, Dimou G, Siozos C. Epidemiology of adult rheumatoid arthritis in northwest Greece 1987–1995. J Rheumatol 1997;24:2129–2133.

18. Symmons D, Turner G, Webb R, Asten P, Barrett E, Lunt M, et al. The prevalence of rheumatoid arthritis in the United Kingdom: new estimates for a new century. Rheumatology 2002;41:793–800.

19. Andrianakos A, Trontzas P, Christoyannis F, Dantis P, Voudouris C, Georgountzos A, Kaiolas G, et al. Prevalence of rheumatic diseases in Greece: a cross-sectional population based epidemiological study (The ESORDIG Study). J Rheumatol 2003;30:1589–1601.

20. Dai SM, Han XH, Zhao DB, Shi YQ, Liu Y, Meng JM. Prevalence of rheumatic symptoms, rheumatoid arthritis, ankylosing spondylitis, and gout in Shanghai, China: a COPCORD study. J Rheumatol 2003;30:2245–2251.

21. Kvien TK, Glennas A, Knudsrod OG, Smedstad LM, Mowinckel P, Forre O. The prevalence and severity of rheumatoid arthritis in Oslo. Results from a county register and a population survey. Scand J Rheumatol 1997;26:412–418.

22. Gabriel SE, Crowson CS, O'Fallon WM. The epidemiology of rheumatoid arthritis in Rochester, Minnesota, 1955–1985. Arthritis Rheum 1999;42:415–420.

23. Stojanovic R, Vlajinac H, Palic-Obradovic D, Janosevic S, Adanja B. Prevalence of RA in Belgrade, Yugoslavia. Br J Rheumatol 1998;37:729–732.

24. Hakala M, Nieminen P, Koivisto O. More evidence from a community based series of better outcome in rheumatoid arthritis. Data on the effect of multidisciplinary care on the retention of functional ability. J Rheumatol 1994;21:1432–1437.

25. Hochberg MC, Chang RW, Dwosh I, Lindsey S, Pincus T, Wolfe F. The American College of Rheumatology 1991 revised criteria for the classification of global functional status in rheumatoid arthritis. Arthritis Rheum 1992;35:498–502.

26. Wolfe F, Hawley DJ. Longterm outcomes of rheumatoid arthritis: work disability: a prospective 18 year study of 823 patients. J Rheumatol 1998;25:2108–2117.

27. Ware JE. SF-36 health survey update. Spine 2000;25:3130–3139.

28. Salaffi F, Carotti M, Gasparin S, Intorcia M, Grassi W. The health-related quality of life in rheumatoid arthritis, ankylosing spondylitis, and psoriatic arthritis: a comparison with a selected sample of healthy people. Health Qual Life Outcomes 2009;7:25–29.

29. McIntosh E. The costs of rheumatoid arthritis. Br J Rheumatol 1996;35:781–790.

30. Yelin EK. The cost of rheumatoid arthritis: absolute, incremental and marginal estimates. J Rheumatol 1996;23:47–51.

31. Lajas C, Abasolo L, Bellajdel B, Hernández-García C, Carmona L, Vargas E, Lázaro P, Jover JA. Costs and predictors of costs in rheumatoid arthritis: a prevalence-based study. Arthritis Rheum 2003; 49:64–70.

32. Kuper IH, Prevoo M, van Leeuwen MA. Disease-associated time consumption in early rheumatoid arthritis. J Rheumatol 2000;27:1183–1189.

33. Huscher D, Merkesdal S, Thiele K. Cost of illness in rheumatoid arthritis, ankylosing spondylitis, psoriatic arthritis and systemic lupus erythematosus in Germany. Ann Rheum Dis 2006;65:1175–1183.

34. Felts W, Yelin E. The economic impact of the rheumatic diseases in the United States. J Rheumatol 1989;16:867–884.

35. Kramer JS, Yelin EH, Epstein WV. Social and economic impacts of four musculoskeletal conditions: a study using national community-based data. Arthritis Rheum 1983;26:901–907.

36. Gabriel SE, Crowson CS, Campion ME, O'Fallon WM. Indirect and nonmedical costs among people with rheumatoid arthritis and osteoarthritis compared with nonarthritic controls. J Rheumatol 1997;24:43–48.

37. Wong JB, Singh G, Kavanaugh A. Estimating the cost-effectiveness of 54 weeks of infliximab for rheumatoid arthritis. Am J Med 2002;113:400–408.

38. Murphy L, Schwartz TA, Helmick CG, Renner JB, Tudor G, Koch G, Dragomir A, Kalsbeek WD, Luta G, Jordan JM. Lifetime risk of symptomatic knee osteoarthritis. Arthritis Rheum 2008;59:1207–1213.

39. Dieppe P. What is the relationship between pain and osteoarthritis? Rheumatol Eur 1998;27:55–56.

40. Altman R, Alarcón G, Appelrouth D, Bloch D, Borenstein D, Brandt K, Brown C, et al. The ACR criteria for the classification and reporting of osteoarthritis of the hand. Arthritis Rheum 1990;33:1601–1610.

41. Altman R, Alarcón G, Appelrouth D, Bloch D, Borenstein D, Brandt K, Brown C, et al. The ACR criteria for the classification and reporting of osteoarthritis of the hip. Arthritis Rheum 1991;34:505–514.

42. Altman R, Asch E, Bloch D, Bole G, Borenstein D, Brandt K, Christy W, et al. Development of criteria for the classification and reporting of osteoarthritis: classification of osteoarthritis of the knee. Arthritis Rheum 1986;29:1039.

43. Mathers C, Vos T, Stevenson C. The burden of disease and injury in Australia. Australian Institute of Health and Welfare; 1999. AIHW Catalogue No. PHE 17.

44. World Health Organization. The burden of musculoskeletal conditions at the start of the new millennium. World Health Organ Technical Rep Ser 2003; 919.

45. Murray CJL, Lopez AD. The global burden of disease. A comprehensive assessment of mortality and disability from diseases, injuries, and risk factors in 1990 and projected to 2020. Cambridge, MA: Harvard School of Public Health on behalf of the World Health Organization and The World Bank; 1996.

46. Symmons D, Mathers C, Pfleger B. Global burden of osteoarthritis in the year 2000. Geneva: World Health Organization; 2003.

47. Felson DT, Zhang Y. An update on the epidemiology of knee and hip osteoarthritis with a view to prevention. Arthritis Rheum 1998;41:1343–1355.

48. Levy E, Ferme A, Perocheau D, Bono I. Socioeconomic costs of osteoarthritis in France. Rev Rhum Ed Fr 1993;60:63–67.

49. Dunlop DD, Manheim LM, Yelin EH, Song J, Chang RW. The costs of arthritis. Arthritis Rheum 2003;49:101–113.

50. Gupta S, Hawker GA, Laporte A, Croxford R, Coyte PC. The economic burden of disabling hip and knee osteoarthritis (OA) from the perspective of individuals living with this condition. Rheumatology 2005;44:1531–1537.

51. Merx H, Dreinhöfer K, Schräder P, Stürmer T, Puhl W, Günther KP, Brenner H. International variation in hip replacement rates. Ann Rheum Dis 2003;62:222–226.

52. Dixon T, Shaw M, Ebrahim S, Dieppe P. Trends in hip and knee joint replacement: socioeconomic inequalities and projections of need. Ann Rheum Dis 2004;63:825–830.

53. Vale L, Wyness L, McCormack K, McKenzie L, Brazzelli M, Stearns SC. A systematic review of the effectiveness and cost-effectiveness of metal-on-metal hip resurfacing arthroplasty for treatment of hip disease. Health Technol Assess 2002;6:100–109.

54. Pincus T, Mitchell JM, Burkhauser RV. Substantial work disability and earnings losses in individuals less than age 65 with osteoarthritis: comparisons with rheumatoid arthritis. J Clin Epidemiol 1989;42:449–457.

55. Agency for Healthcare Research and Quality National and regional statistics in the national inpatient sample. http://www.hcup-us.ahrq.gov/reports/statbriefs/sb34.jsp. Accessed April 25, 2009.

56. Yelin E. The economics of osteoarthritis. In: Brandt K, Doherty M, Lohmander LS, eds. Osteoarthritis. New York: Oxford University Press; 1998:23–30.

57. Woo P. Systemic juvenile idiopathic arthritis: diagnosis, management, and outcome. Nat Clin Pract Rheumatol 2006;2:28–34.

58. Peterson LS, Mason T, Nelson AM, O'Fallon WM, Gabriel SE. Juvenile rheumatoid arthritis in Rochester, Minnesota 1960–1993. Is the epidemiology changing? Arthritis Rheum 1996;39:1385–1390.

59. Moe N, Rygg M. Epidemiology of juvenile chronic arthritis in northern Norway: a ten year retrospective study. Clin Exp Rheumatol 1998;16:99–101.

60. Manners PJ, Diepeveen DA. Prevalence of juvenile chronic arthritis in a population of 12-year-old children in urban Australia. Pediatrics 1996;98:84–90.

61. Saurenmann RK, Rose JB, Tyrrell P, Feldman BM, Laxer RM, Schneider R, Silverman ED. Epidemiology of juvenile idiopathic arthritis in a multiethnic cohort: ethnicity as a risk factor. Arthritis Rheum 2007;56:1974–1984.

62. Zak M, Pedersen FK. Juvenile chronic arthritis into adulthood: a long-term follow-up study. Rheumatology (Oxford) 2000;39:198–204.

63. Calabro JJ, Marchesano JM, Parrino GR. Juvenile rheumatoid arthritis: long-term management and prognosis. J Musculoskelet Med 1989;6:17–32.

64. Levinson JE, Wallace CA. Dismantling the pyramid. J Rheumatol 1992;19:6–10.

65. Minden K, Niewerth M, Listing J, Biedermann T, Schontube M, Zink A. Burden and cost of illness in patients with juvenile idiopathic arthritis. Ann Rheum Dis 2004;63:836–842.

66. Bernatsky S, Duffy C, Malleson P, Feldman DE, Pierre YS, Clarke AE. Economic impact of juvenile idiopathic arthritis. Arthritis Rheum (Arth Care Res) 2007;57:44–48.

67. Allaire SH, DeNardo BS, Szer IS, Meenan RF, Schaller JG. The economic impacts of juvenile rheumatoid arthritis. J Rheumatol 1992;19:952–955.

68. Carbone LD, Cooper C, Michet CJ, Atkinson EJ, O'Fallon WM, Melton LJD. Ankylosing spondylitis in Rochester, Minnesota, 1935–1989. Is the epidemiology changing? Arthritis Rheum 1992;35:1476–1482.

69. Kaipiainen-Seppanen O, Aho K, Heliovaara M. Incidence and prevalence of ankylosing spondylitis in Finland. J Rheumatol 1997;24:496–499.

70. Bakland G, Nossent HC, Gran JT. Incidence and prevalence of ankylosing spondylitis in Northern Norway. Arthritis Rheum 2005;53:850–855.

71. Alamanos Y, Papadopoulos N, Voulgari P, Karakatsanis A, Siozos C, Drosos A. Epidemiology of ankylosing spondylitis in Northwest Greece, 1983–2002. Rheumatology (Oxford) 2002;43:615–618.

72. Hukuda S, Minami M, Saito T, Mitsui H, Matsui N, Komatsubara Y, Makino H, et al. Spondyloarthropathies in Japan: nationwide questionnaire survey performed by the Japan Ankylosing Spondylitis Society. J Rheumatol 2001;28:554–559.

73. Van der Linden SM, Valkenburg HA, de Jongh BM, Cats A. The risk of developing ankylosing spondylitis in HLA-B27 positive individuals: a comparison of relatives of spondylitis patients with the general population. Arthritis Rheum 1984;27:241–249.

74. Ahearn JM, Hochberg MC. Epidemiology and genetics of ankylosing spondylitis. J Rheumatol 1988;16:22–28.

75. Boonen A, de Vet H, van der Heijde D, van der Linden S. Work-status and its determinants among patients with ankylosing spondylitis. A systematic literature review. J Rheumatol 2001;28:1056–1062.

76. Boonen A, van der Heijde D, Landewe R, Guillemin F, Rutten-van Mölken M, Dougados M, Mielants H, et al. Direct costs of ankylosing spondylitis and its determinants: an analysis among three European countries. Ann Rheum Dis 2003;62:732–740.

77. Ward MM. Functional disability predicts total costs in patients with ankylosing spondylitis. Arthritis Rheum 2002;46:223–231.

78. Huscher D, Merkesdal S, Thiele K, Zeidler H, Schneider M, Zink A, et al. Cost of illness in rheumatoid arthritis, ankylosing spondylitis, psoriatic arthritis and systemic lupus erythematosus in Germany. Ann Rheum Dis 2006;65:1175–1183.

79. Kobelt G, Sobocki PA, Brophy S, Jönsson L, Calin A, Braun J. The burden of ankylosing spondylitis and the cost-effectiveness of treatment with infliximab. Rheumatology 2004;43:1158–1166.

80. Mikuls T, Farrar J, Bilker W, Fernandes S, Saag K. Suboptimal physician adherence to quality indicators for the management of gout and asymptomatic hyperuricaemia: results from the UK General Practice Research Database (GPRD). Rheumatology 2005;44:1038–1042.

81. Arromdee E, Michet CJ, Crowson CS, O'Fallon WM, Gabriel SE. Epidemiology of gout: is incidence rising? J Rheumatol 2002;11:2403–2406.

82. Wallace KL, Riedel AA, Joseph-Ridge N, Wortmann R. Increasing prevalence of gout and hyperuricemia over 10years among older adults in a managed care population. J Rheumatol 2004;31:1582–1587.

83. Harris CM, Lloyd DC, Lewis J. The prevalence and prophylaxis of gout in England. J Clin Epidemiol 1995;48:1153–1158.

84. Adams PF, Hendershot GE, Marano MA, Centers for Disease Control and Prevention/National Center for Health Statistics: current estimates from the National Health Interview Survey, 1996. Vital Health Stat 1999;10:1–203.

85. Welch G, Weinger K, Barry MJ. Quality-of-life impact of lower urinary tract symptom severity: results from the health professionals follow-up study. Urology 2002;59:245–250.

86. Edwards N. Treatment-failure gout: a moving target. Arthritis Rheum 2008;58:2587–2590.

87. Kim KY, Ralph SH, Hunsche E, Wertheimer AI, Kong SX. A literature review of the epidemiology and treatment of acute gout. Clin Ther 2003;25:1593–1617.

88. Brook RA, Kleinman NL, Patel PA, Melkonian AK, Brizee T, Smeeding JE, Joseph-Ridge N, et al. The economic burden of gout on an employed population. Curr Med Res Opin 2006;22:1381–1389.

89. Wu EQ, Patel PA, Yu AP, Mody RR, Cahill KE, Tang J, et al. Disease-related and all-cause health care costs of elderly patients with gout. J Manag Care Pharm 2008;14:164–175.

90. Consensus Development Conference. Prophylaxis and treatment of osteoporosis. Osteoporos Int 1991;1:114–117.

91. World Health Organization. Assessment of fracture risk and its application to screening for postmenopausal osteoporosis. World Health Organ Technical Rep Ser; 1994:843.

92. Kanis JA, Johnell O, Oden A, Jonsson B, De Laet C, Dawson A. Risk of hip fracture according to the World Health Organization criteria for osteopenia and osteoporosis. Bone 2000;27:585–590.

93. Van Staa TP, Dennison EM, Leufkens HGM, Cooper C. Epidemiology of fractures in England and Wales. Bone 2001;29:517–522.

94. Dennison E, Mohhamad AM, Cooper C. Epidemiology of osteoporosis. Rheum Dis Clin North Am 2006;32:617–629.

95. Cooper C, Melton LJ III. Epidemiology of osteoporosis. Trends Endocrinol Metab 1992;314:224–229.

96. Carmona L, Laffon A. EPISER Study Group. The prevalence of 6 rheumatic diseases in the Spanish population. Ann Rheum Dis 2000;59:67–72.

97. Valkenburg HA. Clinical versus radiological osteoarthrosis in the general population. In: Peyron JG, ed. Epidemiology of osteoarthritis. Paris: Geigy; 1980:53–58.

98. Bacon WE, Maggi S, Looker A, Harris T, Nair CR, Giaconi J, Hankanen R, International comparison of hip fracture rates in 1988–89. Osteoporos Int 1996;6:69–75.

99. Johnell O, Gullberg B, Allander E, Kanis JA. The apparent incidence of hip fracture in Europe: a study of national register sources. MEDOS Study Group. Osteoporos Int 1992;2:298–302.

100. Cooper C, Campion G, Melton LJ III. Hip fractures in the elderly: a worldwide projection. Osteoporos Int 1992;2:285–289.

101. Gullberg B, Johnell O, Kanis JA. World-wide projections for hip fracture. Osteoporos Int 1997;7:407–413.

102. Cooper C, Melton LJ III. Vertebral fracture: how large is the silent epidemic? Br Med J 1992;304:793–794.

103. The European Prospective Osteoporosis Study Group. Incidence of vertebral fractures in Europe: results from the European Prospective Osteoporosis Study (EPOS). J Bone Miner Res 2002;17:716–724.

104. O'Neill TW, Cooper C, Finn JD, Lunt M, Purdie D, Reid DM, Woolf AD, Wallace WA, and on behalf of the UK Colles' Fracture Study Group. Incidence of distal forearm fracture in British men and women. Osteoporos Int 2001;12:555–558.

105. Johnell O, Kanis JA. An estimate of the worldwide prevalence, mortality and disability associated with hip fracture. Osteoporos Int 2004;15:897–902.

106. Sernbo I, Johnell O. Consequences of a hip fracture: a prospective study over 1 year. Osteoporos Int 1993;3:148–153.

107. Baudoin C, Fardellone P, Bean K, Ostertag-Ezembe A, Hervy F. Clinical outcomes and mortality after hip fracture: a 2-year follow-up study. Bone 1996;18 :149–157.

108. Gold DT. The clinical impact of vertebral fractures: quality of life in women with osteoporosis. Bone 1996;18:185–189.

109. O'Neill TW, Cockerill W, Matthis C, Raspe HH, Lunt M, Cooper C, Banzer D, et al. Back pain, disability, and radiographic vertebral fracture in European women: a prospective study. Osteoporos Int 2004;15:760–765.

110. Kado DM, Browner WS, Palermo L, Nevitt MC, Genant HK, Cummings SR. Vertebral fractures and mortality in older women: a prospective study. Arch Intern Med 1999;159:1215–1220.

111. Kaukonen JP, Karaharju EO, Porras M, Luthje P, Jakobsson A. Functional recovery after fractures of the distal forearm. Analysis of radiographic and other factors affecting the outcome. Ann Chir Gynaecol 1988;77:27–31.

112. Burge R, Solomon D, Tosteson A, Wong J, Dawson-Hughes B. Incidence and economic burden of osteoporosis related fractures in the United States, 2005–2025. J Bone Miner Res 2007;22:465–475

113. Bennett RM. Emerging concepts in the neurobiology of chronic pain: evidence of abnormal sensory processing in fibromyalgia. Mayo Clin Proc 1999;19:385–398.

114. Staud R, Domingo M. Evidence for abnormal pain processing in fibromyalgia syndrome. Pain Med 2001;2:208–215.

115. Carmona L, Ballina J, Gabriel R, Laffon A. The burden of musculoskeletal diseases in the general population of Spain: results from a national survey. Ann Rheum Dis 2001;60:1040–1045.
116. White K, Speechley M, Harth M, Ostbye T, et al. The London Fibromyalgia Epidemiology Study: the prevalence of fibromyalgia syndrome in London, Ontario. J Rheumatol 1999;26:19–28.
117. Wolfe F. The epidemiology of fibromyalgia. J Musculoskelet Pain 1993;1:137–148.
118. Wolfe F, Ross K, Anderson J, Russel IJ, Herbert L. The prevalence and characteristics of fibromyalgia in the general population. Arthritis Rheum 1995;38:19–28.
119. Lawrence RC, Felson DT, Helmick CG, Arnold LM, Choi H, Deyo RA, Gabriel S, et al. National Arthritis Work Group: estimates of the prevalence of arthritis and other rheumatic conditions in the United States. Part II. Arthritis Rheum 2008;58:26–35.
120. Branco JC, Bannwarth B, Failde I, Abello Carbonell J, Blotman F, Spaeth M, et al. Prevalence of fibromyalgia: a survey in five European countries. Semin Arthritis Rheum 2010;39:448–453.
121. Campbell SM, Clark S, Tindall EA, Forehand ME, Benenett RM. Clinical characteristics of fibrositis: I. A "blinded," controlled study of symptoms and tender points. Arthritis Rheum 1983;26:817–824.
122. Hartz A, Kirchdoerfer E. Undetected fibrositis in primary care practice. J Fam Pract 1987;25:365–369.
123. Wolfe F, Cathey MA. Prevalence of primary and secondary fibrositis. J Rheumatol 1983;10:965–968.
124. Hoffman DL, Dukes EM. The health status burden of people with fibromyalgia: a review of studies that assessed health status with the SF-36 or the SF-12. Int J Clin Pract 2008;62:115–126.
125. Burckhardt CS, Clark SR, Bennett RM. FM and quality of life: a comparative analysis. J Rheumatol 1993;20:475–479.
126. White KP, Speechley M, Harth M, Ostbye T. Comparing self-reported function and work disability in 100 community cases of fibromyalgia syndrome versus controls in London, Ontario: the London Fibromyalgia Epidemiology Study. Arthritis Rheum 1999;42:76–83.
127. Kaplan RM, Schmidt SM, Cronan TA. Quality of well being in patients with fibromyalgia. J Rheumatol 2000;27:785–789.
128. Wolfe F, Hawley DJ, Goldenberg DL, Russell IJ, Buskila D, Neumann L. The assessment of functional impairment in fibromyalgia (FM): Rasch analyses of 5 functional scales and the development of the FM Health Assessment Questionnaire. J Rheumatol 2000;27:1989–1999.
129. Wolfe F, Anderson J, Harkness D, Bennett RM, Caro XJ, Goldenberg DL, Russel IJ, Yunus MB. A prospective, longitudinal, multicenter study of service utilization and costs in fibromyalgia. Arthritis Rheum 1997;40:1560–1570.
130. Sicras-Mainar A, Rejas J, Navarro R, Blanca M, Morcillo A, Larios R, Velasco S, Villarroya C. Treating patients with fibromyalgia in primary care settings under routine medical practice: a claim database cost and burden of illness study. Arthritis Res Ther 2009;11:R54.
131. Boonen A, van den Heuvel R, van Tubergen A, Goossens M, Severens JL, van der Heijde D, van der Linden S. Large differences in cost of illness and wellbeing between patients with fibromyalgia, chronic low back pain, or ankylosing spondylitis. Ann Rheum Dis 2005;64:396–402.
132. Siebenaler MJ, McGovern P. Carpal tunnel syndrome. Priorities for prevention. AAOHN J 1992;40:62–71.
133. United States Government Bureau of Labor Statistics. Occupational Injuries and Illnesses in the United States, 1992. Washington, DC: United States Government Bureau of Labor Statistics, United States Department of Labor; 1994:97–188.
134. Mackinnon SE, Novak CB. Repetitive strain in the workplace. J Hand Surg 1997;22:2–18.
135. Atroshi I, Gummesson C, Ornstein E, Johnsson R, Ranstam J. Carpal tunnel syndrome and keyboard use at work: a population-based study. Arthritis Rheum 2007;56:3620–3625.
136. Baldwin ML, Butler RJ. Upper extremity disorders in the workplace: costs and outcomes beyond the first return to work. J Occup Rehabil 2006;16:303–323.

2 Pathogenesis of Osteoarthritis

Allen P. Anandarajah

CONTENTS

INTRODUCTION

Osteoarthritis (OA), also known as degenerative joint disease or osteoarthrosis, is the most common type of arthritis. OA is a functional disorder of the joint, characterized by a change in joint shape secondary to a loss of articular cartilage, osteophyte formation, subchondral sclerosis, bone marrow lesions, and synovial proliferation, with consequent alteration of mechanical properties that result in decreased stability, movement, and loading [1, 2]. It is estimated to affect more than 27 million people in the United States and is the leading cause of physical disability and impaired quality of life in the industrialized countries. OA is strongly related to but not caused by aging, with most affected persons being older than 50 years. The higher life expectancy, the aging population, and the increase in number of overweight persons in the United States have led to an increase in prevalence of OA [3]. The resulting disability, comorbid disease, and expense of treatment are associated with an extremely high economic burden. The increase in prevalence will contribute to an even larger economic and social burden in the future.

OA most commonly occurs in the weight-bearing joints of the hips, knees, and spine but can also affect the fingers and the toes (Figures 2.1a through d). Clinical presentation is often with pain, mild stiffness, crepitus, restriction in range of movement, and loss of function and in severe cases with evident joint deformity and disability. Radiographically, OA is characterized by the formation of osteophytes and joint space narrowing. Traditionally, OA was described as a joint disease consequent of the wear and tear of the cartilage from aging. Histopathological studies along with newer imaging modalities have however shown that OA is not exclusively a disease of articular cartilage. Current concepts support the notion that OA is due to multiple risk factors and that joint damage is secondary to varying contributions from systemic and local mechanical causes that result in damage to cartilage, bone, and synovium. Recent studies have also highlighted the role of proteases and inflammatory cytokines in the pathogenesis of OA. This chapter will review recent advances made toward understanding the pathogenesis of OA and highlight the recent shift in paradigm from an emphasis on cartilage damage to a concept of "disease of the whole joint."

RISK FACTORS FOR OA

While no single definite cause for OA is known, several risk factors have been well identified. These are shown in Table 2.1 and can be broadly divided into local and systemic risk factors and include

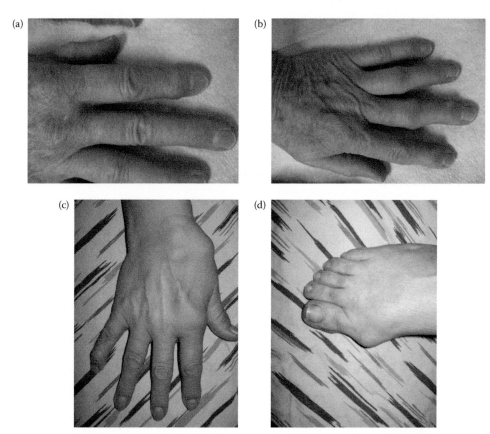

FIGURE 2.1 (a) Image shows nodal OA of the hands with Heberden's nodes—second and third distal interphalangeal joints. (b) Image shows nodal OA of the hands with Bouchard's nodes—third and fourth proximal interphalangeal joints. (c) Image shows OA of the carpometacarpal joint (base of thumb). (d) Image shows metatarsophalangeal OA.

TABLE 2.1
Risk Factors Associated with Etiology of OA

Systemic	Local
Age	Previous damage (trauma, surgery)
Gender	Occupational trigger
Race	Nonoccupational physical activity
Genetics	Muscle weakness
Congenital abnormalities	Malalignment
Nutrition	Proprioceptive defects
Obesity/excess body weight	Biomechanics
Infection	
Metabolic disorders	
Bone mineral density	
Postmenopausal hormone replacement therapy	

age, gender, genetics, congenital abnormalities, trauma, overuse, obesity, and abnormal biomechanics. Research in the past decade has led to a better understanding for the role of age, gender, obesity, trauma, joint overuse, malalignment, inflammation, and genetics in the pathogenesis of OA.

AGE

Age is the risk factor most strongly correlated with development of OA. Changes in the constituents of extracellular matrix, with an increase in water and hyaluronan content and a decrease in the amount of aggrecan, lead to cartilage degeneration. In addition, there is mechanical stress on the joints secondary to muscle weakness, changes in proprioception, and altered gait.

GENDER

The overall prevalence of OA is higher in women compared with men [4]. Men appear to have a significantly reduced risk for OA of the hip and hands, but are at higher risk for OA of the hips and cervical spine. A role for estrogen in the pathogenesis has been proposed on the basis of some studies that suggest a decreased risk for OA with estrogen replacement therapy [5].

GENETIC PREDISPOSITION

Epidemiological and twin studies have indicated a strong role for genetics in the pathogenesis of OA. A significantly higher concordance for OA between monozygotic twins compared with dizygotic twins has been reported [6]. Multiple genetic factors are know to contribute to the incidence and severity of OA, and its effects may vary according to joint or gender [7, 8]. Clinical evidence is provided by observations that the presence of Heberden's nodes confers a sixfold increased risk for progression of knee OA [9]. The influence of genetic factors of OA may approach 70% for some joints [10]. Genetic factors can cause OA in one of several ways. For example, mutations of genes expressed in the cartilage and of the latent transforming growth factor (TGF) binding protein-3 can affect structure and consistency of the cartilage and bone, respectively [2, 11, 12]. Heritable systemic diseases such as ochronosis are also risk factors for premature OA. Meanwhile, the function of inflammatory pathways in OA have demonstrated a role for the genes for interleukin-1α (IL-1α), IL-1β, IL receptor antagonist, and cyclooxygenase-2 (COX-2) in OA pathogenesis [13].

OBESITY

Obesity is an important risk factor for OA of the knee and hip [14]. Recent studies implicate a role for adipokines, a product of adipocytes, in the inflammatory changes seen in OA. Leptin is an adipose derived hormone that plays a role in regulation of body weight and metabolism. Leptin expression is increased in the cartilage, and osteophytes of subjects with OA and may help explain the association between obesity and risk for onset and progression of OA [15].

JOINT MALALIGNMENT

Joint malalignment in the form of varus or valgus deformity may be one of the most important risk factors in knee OA [16, 17]. Obesity, age, and muscle weakness may cause joint damage in OA as a result of malalignment [18]. An interesting observation of a recent study was that new bone marrow lesions occurred more in malaligned limbs [19].

INJURY

Joint injuries are the most common risk factor for development of OA in young adults. Studies have shown that the majority of patients between age 35 and 44 years with OA of knees had a history of knee injury [20, 21]. These injuries may be in the form of a sports injury resulting in damage to the anterior cruciate ligament or after surgical procedures such as meniscectomy [22, 23]. Similarly, OA of the spine may follow a severe back injury.

STRUCTURAL PATHOLOGY IN OA

The joint is a specialized structure whose design allows for stability, loading, and movement. The human joints do not typically wear out despite completing more than a million movements a year and undergoing frequent situations with extreme loading. A typical synovial joint is comprised of bone, articular cartilage, joint capsule, menisci, muscles, tendons, ligaments, and bursa. Traditionally, OA was heralded as a disease primarily of the articular cartilage. Recent evidence however supports the theory that synovium and bone also play crucial roles in the pathogenesis of OA. It is now generally accepted that damage to any of the joint structures can lead to an alteration of the delicate balance of joint function and consequently lead to joint damage.

CARTILAGE

Joint surfaces are covered by a thin layer of cartilage. Articular cartilage is a specialized form of hyaline cartilage that is characterized by its fibrous architecture and does not have nerves, blood vessels, or lymphatic flow. The avascular nature of cartilage is important in allowing for its mechanical properties. It is composed of four regions: (1) the superficial tangential zone composed of thin collagen fibril, (2) the middle zone with radial bundles of thicker collagen fibrils, (3) the deep zone where the collagen bundles are thickest, and (4) the calcified cartilage located just above the subchondral bone [24]. Approximately 75% of the cartilage is composed of water, with collagen and proteoglycans accounting for the rest. The biochemical composition and the geometric distribution of water and organic matrix within the articular cartilage allow for the conformational changes associated with weight bearing.

The articular cartilage is constructed to withstand the compressive stresses, to decrease friction during movement, and to help distribute the functional forces to other components of the joint. This is made possible because of the fact that the cartilage is both flexible and strong. Proteoglycans, especially aggrecan, impart the flexibility and elasticity to cartilage. The flexibility of the cartilage aids its ability to absorb the forces associated with loading. Tensile strength is due to collagen, which also provides a framework in which proteoglycans and chondrocytes are embedded. Cartilage is comprised of several types of collagen, but type II collagen contributes to approximately 90% of the fibrin network.

The organic matrix of cartilage is synthesized and maintained by the chondrocytes. The chondrocytes are highly specialized cells, which live singly or in small clusters, and secrete glycoproteins, including proteases and their inhibitors, collagenases, proteinases, cathepsins, and cytokines, in response to mechanical stimuli as well as to cytokines and growth factors such as insulin-like growth factor-1 (IGF-1), TGF-β, and βFGF. Chondrocytes stimulate matrix production through the synthesis of growth factors such as bone morphogenetic protein 2, cartilage derived morphogenetic proteins, IGF-1, and TGF-β [25]. In combination with the synovial cells, the chondrocytes are also responsible for the secretion of matrix metalloproteinases (MMPs), nitric oxide (NO), NO synthase, and inflammatory cytokines such as tumor necrosis factor-α (TNF-α), interleukin-1β (IL-1β), IL-6, IL-8, and prostaglandin E2 [26]. These cytokines and proteolytic enzymes are responsible for the catabolic activity of chondrocytes. In addition, the chondrocytes synthesize inhibitors of angiogenesis. In summary, the chondrocytes respond to mechanical stresses, joint instability, and cytokines and growth factors and thereby contribute to structural changes in the surrounding cartilage matrix.

The loss of cartilage is a central feature in OA. Under normal circumstances, damage to the matrix would be associated with an increased activity of chondrocytes to replace the lost matrix along with a decrease in the catabolic activity of these cells. In OA, the dynamic equilibrium between the synthesis and the degradation of the matrix is lost. Instead, there appears to be an imbalance in the process of remodeling with an exaggerated attempt to remove the damaged cartilage and insufficient anabolic activity.

Inflammation and Molecular Mechanisms of Cartilage Destruction

The absence of the typical clinical signs of inflammation and the paucity of inflammatory cells in the synovial fluid in OA led to the traditional description of OA as a "noninflammatory" or degenerative joint disease. There is however mounting evidence to support a role for inflammation in the pathogenesis of OA. Furthermore, there is emerging evidence to suggest that inflammation is a predecessor to cartilage destruction [26, 27]. The avascular and aneural nature of cartilage may be the reason for the absence of the classic signs of inflammation. It is postulated that the inflammatory mediators act within the cartilage in an autocrine or paracrine manner to cause progressive cartilage damage in OA [28]. Indeed, the cartilage in OA has been shown to have signs of fibrillation, vascularization, and local calcification [3].

The inflammatory process is mediated by the chondrocytes, which are activated by cytokines produced by the synovium that diffuse into cartilage from the synovial fluid.

The activated chondrocytes and the synovium release several inflammatory cytokines and chemokines such as the ILs and monocyte chemoattractant protein-1 as well as members of reactive oxygen species (ROS) such as NO in response to mechanical stimuli. See Table 2.2 for a list of these inflammatory mediators. These inflammatory mediators in turn upregulate release of cartilage-degrading proteinases including aggrecanases and MMPs that then cause destruction of the collagen network and cartilage matrix. In addition, these inflammatory mediators promote apoptosis of the chondrocytes and inhibit matrix synthesis. IL-1β and TNF-α play a particularly important role in cartilage destruction and stimulate the production of other cytokines such as IL-6, IL-8, leukocyte inhibitory factor, proteases, and prostaglandins, in addition to stimulating their own production [29].

The role of IL-1 in OA is substantiated by studies that have shown an upregulation of the IL-1β-converting enzyme, a protease that plays a crucial role in the in the generation of IL-1β, in the OA cartilage [30]. Type I IL-1 receptor has also been shown to be significantly increased in OA chondrocytes and synovial fibroblasts, thereby making these cells more sensitive to IL-1β stimulation [31]. Similarly, an increase in expression of TNF-α-converting enzyme and TNF receptor 55 has been demonstrated in OA [32, 33]. The actions of both IL-1 and TNF-α are mediated by nuclear

TABLE 2.2
Inflammatory Mediators Associated
with Pathogenesis of OA

Cytokines and chemokines
IL-1β
IL-6
IL-8
IL-17
IL-18
TNF-α
Monocyte chemoattractant protein-1
Leukemia inhibitory factor
Regulated on activation, normal T cell expressed and secreted
Growth-related oncogene
Oncostatin M

Prostaglandins
Prostaglandin E2
ROS
NO
Superoxide anion
Hydrogen peroxide
Hydroxyl radicals

Others
Peroxynitrite
Leukotrienes

factor kappa-activated B cells (NFκB), which in addition to increasing their own expression also increases expression of the inducible form of NO synthase and COX-2, thereby creating an autocatalytic cascade that promotes cartilage destruction [34].

MMPs and aggrecanases are among the more important proteinases that degrade cartilage collagens and proteoglycans [35]. Several MMPs, including MMP-1, MMP-8, MMP-13, MMP-2, MMP-9, MMP-3, and MMP-14, are known to play an important role in cartilage catabolism. Of the three major MMPs (MMP-1, MMP-8, and MMP-13), MMP-13 may be most important as it preferentially degrades type II collagen [36]. Aggrecanases, which belong to a family of proteases known as a disintegrin and metalloprotease with thrombospondin motifs (ADAMTS), play an important role in the pathogenesis of OA, with ADAMTS-4 and ADAMTS-5 known to be especially involved in cartilage degradation [36].

NO also plays an essential role in cartilage catabolism. An increase in the inducible form of NO synthase causes an excessive production of NO by the cartilage [37, 38]. NO inhibits the synthesis of cartilage matrix components such as aggrecans and collagen, enhances activity of MMPs, reduces IL-1Rα synthesis by chondrocytes, increases susceptibility to injury by other oxidants, and increases apoptosis of chondrocytes [26]. Excess production of NO has also been associated with apoptosis of OA chondrocytes [39]. In addition, increased NO levels leads to increased expression of the inducible COX-2 in OA chondrocytes [40]. COX-2 appears to mediate the increased production of prostaglandins by inflammatory cytokines. Prostaglandin E2 produced by OA cartilage has been shown to decrease proteoglycan synthesis and enhance the degradation of aggrecan and type II collagen [41]. These effects are associated with an upregulation of MMP-13 and ADAMTS-5. Other members of the ROS, such as superoxide anion, hydrogen peroxide, and hydroxyl radicals, appear to contribute to OA pathology by the promotion of chondrocyte apoptosis [42].

Age and Cartilage Loss

Increased age is associated with a decrease in the tensile strength and stiffness of the articular matrix. These changes in turn are due to changes in the content, composition, and structural properties of the extracellular matrix [25]. There is an increase in the hyaluronan content and a decrease in the amount and molecular size of aggrecan. A degradation and loss of type II collagen and an increase in the prevalence of cartilage calcification have also been reported. In addition, an accumulation in the extent of advanced glycation end products leads to enhanced collagen cross linking and contribute to altered cartilage function [43, 44]. The alteration in the matrix content may also be secondary to age-related changes in the chondrocytes that have a reduced synthetic capacity and exhibit decreased responsiveness to anabolic growth factors. The chondrocytes have been demonstrated to have a reduced anabolic response to IGF-1 stimulation [45–47]. Recent studies have demonstrated that an increase in endogenous ROS might also contribute to a decreased responsiveness to growth factor [48]. These changes in chondrocytes function result in a decreased capacity to repair the damaged articular matrix [49, 50]. In addition to a reduced function, there is also a modest decline in chondrocyte numbers. This may be related to a decrease in proliferative capacity of chondrocytes with increased age and to an increase in chondrocytes apoptosis [51].

Obesity and Cartilage Loss

As discussed earlier, adipocytes are known to contribute toward the inflammatory effects in joint tissues. Leptin expression is increased in the cartilage and osteophytes of subjects with OA and stimulates IGF-1 and TGF-β1 synthesis in chondrocytes [15]. Leptin in conjunction with IL-1 also increases NO production by chondrocytes [52]. Furthermore, it has been proposed that that the dysregulated balance between leptin and other adipokines promotes destructive inflammatory processes [53]. Other adipocyte-derived factors such as IL-6 and C-reactive protein also appear to have a procatabolic effect on chondrocytes.

Mechanical Stress and Cartilage Loss

Mechanical stress from trauma is an important cause of OA in young individuals. Recent reports have described the presence of osmosensors and mechanosensors in chondrocytes [54]. These receptors respond to mechanical stimuli, with changes in gene expression and increase in production of inflammatory cytokines and matrix-degrading enzymes that lead to changes in quantity, distribution, and composition of cartilage matrix proteins [10]. In the early stages of OA, there is an increase in chondrocyte proliferation and metabolic activity, which results in localized loss of proteoglycans, cleavage of type II collagen, and increase in water content that in turn result in decreased tensile strength of the matrix [55, 56]. Trauma also results in increased expression of inflammatory mediators, cartilage-degrading proteinases, and stress response factors [57]. Several signaling cascades including the NFκB cascade are activated [58]. Mechanical stress can also induce abnormal production of ROS that eventually leads to oxidative stress, which then impairs growth factor responses [10]. COX-2 also appears to play a role in chondrocytes response to mechanical stress, with a reduction in antioxidant capacity and an increase in apoptosis [59].

Genetics and Cartilage Loss

The relationship between genetic disorder and OA has been discussed earlier. These disorders often result in abnormalities in cartilage structure. For example, mutations of genes that encode the synthesis or remodeling of extracellular matrix can result in congenital cartilage dysplasias [60, 61]. Point mutations in type II collagen as well as in other genes expressed in cartilage are associated with early development of OA [62, 63]. For example, chondrodysplasia is a condition that is associated with point mutations in type II collagen that results in abnormal collagen production and often leads to premature cartilage failure. Gene defects can also affect patterning of skeletal elements and thereby cause joint malalignment [60, 61].

Gender and Cartilage Loss

There is a marked increase in prevalence of OA of the hip in women after the age of 50 years. The realization that articular chondrocytes possess functional estrogen receptors and that estrogen can upregulate proteoglycan synthesis suggests a role for estrogen deficiency in pathogenesis of OA [41].

In summary, cartilage loss is an important and a common finding in OA. Cytokines and other inflammatory mediators produced by chondrocytes and synovial cells result in an increase in cartilage catabolism and at the same time decrease cartilage synthesis. Although there are several risk factors, their effect on cartilage are interrelated and appear to cause joint damage through the activation of common cytokine cascades. For example, it is hypothesized that traumatic injury leads to global gene expression activation that results in an increased expression of inflammatory mediators, cartilage-degrading proteinases, and stress response factors [57]. The discovery that there is a twofold increase in NFκB levels, a signaling transcription factor, in OA as compared with normal cartilage, raises speculation that NFκB may be a common factor for the inflammatory, biochemical, and mechanical pathways [27].

BONE

In addition to the progressive loss of articular cartilage, OA is characterized by progressive changes in the structure and function of periarticular bone. Several studies have helped establish that these changes in bone occur early in the course of OA and may manifest before changes in cartilage are detected [64]. The changes in bone include osteophyte formation (formation of new bone at the joint margins), sclerosis of subchondral bone (increased subchondral plate thickness), and the development of bone marrow edema (BME) lesions (Figure 2.2a).

Role of Remodeling and Modeling of Bone in Pathogenesis of OA

The process of modeling and remodeling contributes to the changes in structure and function of the bone. Bone remodeling is a process that under physiologic conditions permits for adaptation to and repair of damage from mechanical stress and thereby helps maintain the integrity and function of bone. The remodeling process comprises a process of bone resorption mediated by osteoclasts coupled with a process of bone formation mediated by osteoblasts [65]. In OA, there is a failure of the remodeling process with consequent progressive loss of function. In contrast to remodeling, modeling involves bone formation or resorption that is not coupled, leading to addition of bone or bone loss [66]. This process can result in an increase in bone mass and can also be associated with alteration of bone shape. Remodeling and modeling therefore help modify the properties of subchondral cortical and trabecular bone and thereby help with the adaptation process to mechanical stresses. Endochondral ossification, is yet another mechanism responsible for periarticular bone changes and involves new bone formation by replacement of the cartilaginous matrix [67]. Endochondral ossification is postulated to be one possible mechanism for the formation of osteophytes. A similar mechanism, characterized by vascular invasion of calcified cartilage, followed by chondrocyte hypertrophy and eventual replacement with bone, occurs at the tidemark [68]. This leads to an extension of calcified cartilage into the deep zones of articular cartilage and at the same time a thinning of the articular cartilage.

Osteophytes

The formation of osteophytes represents one of the radiographic hallmarks of OA. They are skeletal outgrowths that are localized to the joint margins. Osteophytes can be a source of pain and

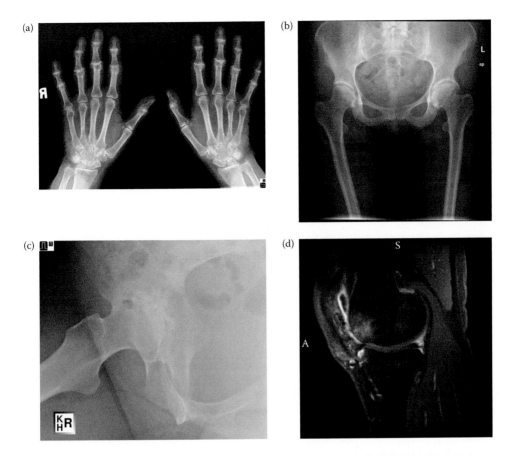

FIGURE 2.2   (a) Erosive OA of the hands. X-ray of hands shows new bone formation and bone sclerosis as well as joint space narrowing and erosions at the proximal interphalangeal and distal interphalangeal joints of both hands. (b) X-ray of pelvis showing moderate to severe OA of the hip. This x-ray shows severe joint space narrowing bilaterally; new bone formation and flattening of articular surfaces are noted at the right hip; early distortion of the articular surface is seen at the left hip. (c) Severe OA of the hip. This x-ray shows the distortion of the articular surface and collapse of the cancellous bone resulting in severe joint deformity. (d) BME-like lesions. This MRI of knee in a patient with OA demonstrates the presence of BME-like lesions and shows presence of periarticular soft tissue swelling.

loss of function [69]. There is ample evidence to suggest that osteophyte formation represents a skeletal adaptation to local mechanical factors. It is a reflection of the adaptive response to stabilize an already damaged joint in an attempt to maintain joint function and stability to deal with load and strain [70]. These changes, however, may adversely affect the capacity of the joint to adapt to mechanical stress. Other studies, however, have shown that mechanical stimuli are not indispensable to formation of osteophytes. Animal studies have led to speculation that osteophyte formation may occur as a result of penetration of blood vessels into the degenerating cartilage [71]. The development of these bony outgrowths appears to be associated with but does not completely correlate with cartilage loss. The formation of osteophyte starts with proliferation of periosteal cells at the joint margin. These cells then undergo differentiation into chondrocytes along with deposition of matrix molecules such as aggrecan at the joint margins. This is followed by hypertrophy of chondrocytes and the process of endochondral calcification to create an enlarging skeletal outgrowth at the joint margin. Local production of growth factors appears to be implicated in the formation of osteophytes [72]. TGF-β, IGF-1, and leptin are some of the growth factors that have been shown to be associated with osteophyte formation [73].

Subchondral Sclerosis

Subchondral bone changes are an important part of progressive bone destruction in OA. A significantly greater thickness of subchondral cortical plate has been described in patients with OA of the hands compared with subjects without arthritis [74]. For example, an increase in subchondral bone thickness of femur and tibia has been reported in subjects with OA knees [75]. Several studies have demonstrated these bone changes to be present in very early OA [74]. Interestingly, an increase in vascularity at the subchondral sites with sclerosis has been described [76]. The subchondral thickening is due to increased turnover and reactivation of the secondary center of ossification which in turn results from a change in joint mechanics [77]. The subchondral bone from OA patients is however less dense and therefore mechanically weaker [78]. Radiographically, the weakening may be seen as a flattening of the articular surfaces in OA of the hip and knee [79] (Figure 2.2b). In advanced disease, the articular surface becomes distorted and deformed with the collapse of the cancellous bone in the subarticular region, leading to joint malalignment and deformity (Figure 2.2c). The formation of bone in the region of subchondral sclerosis appears to be an attempt at repair but results in increased stress within the thinned cartilage and also leads to an increase in surface area of contact between the articular elements [79].

BME-like Lesions

The use of magnetic resonance imaging (MRI) in imaging studies of OA patients led to the descriptions of BME lesions (Figure 2.2d). These lesions were first described in OA, but since then there have been several reports of BME in OA as well in inflammatory arthritides [80–82]. The presence and the extent of BME-like lesions appear to correlate with pain in knee OA [82, 83]. These lesions are also a potent risk factor for progression of structural deterioration [84]. Histologically, BME represents sites with bone marrow necrosis, bone marrow fibrosis, trabecular abnormalities evidence of microdamage, and bone repair [80]. The sites with BME also appear to correlate with areas of most severe cartilage loss. The association of BME lesions with regions of skeletal and cartilage damage as well as the histological findings described earlier strongly supports a primary role for mechanical and traumatic etiology as the cause for the BME-like lesions.

Synovium

The use of ultrasound and MRI in rheumatology practice has led to several reports that describe the presence of synovitis in OA, and recent studies suggest that synovitis is more common in OA than previously appreciated [85–87]. Furthermore, these studies have demonstrated that synovitis can occur early in OA (Figures 2.3a and b). Other studies have reported the presence of extensive synovial tissue in end-stage OA, noted at time of joint replacement [88]. Synovitis is often localized to areas adjacent to pathologically damaged cartilage and bone and can be asymptomatic. However, recent studies have shown that synovial thickening is more common in patients with knee OA who have pain compared with OA patients who do not have pain. These findings suggest an association between the presence of synovitis and pain [89, 90]. Synovial volumes have also been correlated to the extent of bone marrow lesions [87]. Interestingly, no relationship is reported between the degree of synovitis and cartilage loss [90].

Under normal physiological conditions, the synovium is a thin tissue that consists of a pseudoepithelial lining layer with synovial fibroblasts, macrophages, and loose connective tissue in the sublining zone. Histological studies in OA show the presence of synovial hypertrophy and hyperplasia with an increase in the number of lining cells. Reports also indicate that in some cases, the synovium

(a)   (b)

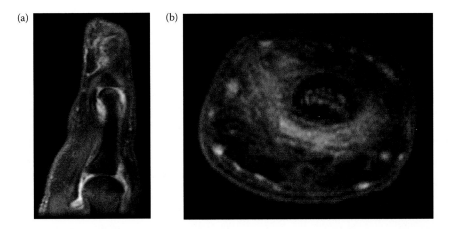

FIGURE 2.3   Synovitis in OA. A 1.5-T MRI of index finger shows the presence of synovitis and soft tissue swelling in a patient with early OA of the hands. (a) Sagittal T1 post-gadolinium image; and (b) same joint in an axial T1 post-gadolinium view.

is infiltrated with subsynovial inflammatory cells. Activated B and T cells and overexpression of proinflammatory mediators are relatively common in early and established OA [91]. Evidence has emerged to show that the release of proteins from cartilage and bone triggers the nonspecific inflammation of the synovium in OA. The synovium when activated secretes excess synovial fluid, resulting in joint swelling. Synovial tissue, when activated, also produces proteases and cytokines that may accelerate cartilage breakdown. Studies of synovial fluid in OA have revealed the presence of prostaglandins, NO, IL-1β, and TNF-α [25]. Indeed, it is now hypothesized that synovial inflammation may play a key role in stimulating chondrocyte dysregulation. Cartilage breakdown products in turn lead to the release collagenase and other hydrolytic enzymes by the synovium and contribute to vascular hyperplasia. Angiogenesis, a key component of chronic inflammation, therefore appears to be facilitated by these cartilage breakdown products, which then further potentiate inflammatory changes in synovium and accelerate progression of disease. The role of angiogenesis in synovial tissue of patients with OA has been highlighted in recent literature [92, 93]. Angiogenesis therefore maybe facilitated by inflammation but then perpetuates the inflammatory response by providing access for the inflammatory cells and nutrients to the sites of inflammation. Despite the increased reports of the presence of synovitis in OA, the relevance to pathogenesis of OA is still not clear. It also remains to be established whether synovitis is only present during flares of OA or if it is an ongoing process.

MUSCLES, LIGAMENTS, AND NERVES

The role of muscle weakness and ligamentous disease as a cause of OA has also been established in recent years. Earlier reports assumed muscle weakness and associated joint instability as a consequence of joint damage, but there is mounting evidence to suggest that muscle weakness is often the cause of joint damage [77, 94]. Ligament damage can result in joint laxity and thereby cause joint malalignment and lead to OA. Ligamentous laxity as well as its association with OA is seen in patients with hypermobility syndrome. A role for collateral ligaments injury in OA pathogenesis of the interphalangeal joints has been described [95]. Similarly, injury to collateral ligaments in knee can increase risk for knee OA [96, 97]. Neuropathy can be another factor that can be associated with joint laxity and OA. Charcot's joint is an example of arthritis that follows a decrease in peripheral sensation and proprioception. A possible relationship between impaired proprioception and knee OA has also been studied [98].

CONCLUSIONS

The aging of the Western population of has made OA an increasingly important public health issue. Although, initially described as solely a disease of cartilage, OA is now widely accepted as a disease that involves all tissues of the articular joint. Bone and synovial tissue in particular are thought to play crucial roles in joint pathology. In addition to mechanical factors, OA is associated with several other risk factors, but they all appear to cause joint damage through their effect on cytokines and proteases. OA can hence be described as a mechanically induced disorder in which the consequences of abnormal joint mechanics provoke effects that are mediated biochemically. There is mounting evidence in current scientific literature to suggest that inflammation, notably involving the synovium and bone, is an important part of OA, but the specific role of inflammation in the pathogenesis of OA is yet to be fully elucidated. Recent findings especially over the past decade have led to a better understanding of pathogenesis of OA and hopefully will facilitate the development of disease modifying agents for this disabling arthritis.

REFERENCES

1. Dieppe PA, Lohmander LS. Pathogenesis and management of pain in osteoarthritis. Lancet 2005;365:965–973.
2. Klippel JH, Dieppe PA. Rheumatology. Mosby; 1998.
3. Bos SD, Slagboon PE, Meulenbelt I. New insights into osteoarthritis: early developmental features of an ageing-related disease. Curr Opin Rheumatol 2008;20:553–559.
4. Peyron JG, Altman RD. The epidemiology of osteoarthritis. In: Moskowitz RW, Howell DS, Goldberg VM, et al., eds. Osteoarthritis: diagnosis and medical/ surgical management (2nd ed.). Philadelphia: Saunders; 1992:15–37.
5. Nevitt MC, Cummungs SR, Lane NE, Hochberg MC, Scott JC, Pressman AR, Genant HK, Cauley JA. Association of estrogen replacement therapy with the risk of osteoarthritis of the hip in elderly white women. Study of osteoporotic fractures research group. Arch Intern Med 1996;156:2073–2080.
6. Zhai G, Hart DJ, Kato BS, MacGregor A, Spector D. Genetic influence on the progression of radiographic knee osteoarthritis: a longitudinal twin study. Osteoarthritis Cartilage 2007;15:222–225.
7. Bukulmez H, Matthews AL, Sullivan CM, Chen C. Hip joint replacement surgery for idiopathic osteoarthritis aggregates in families. Arthritis Res Ther 2006;8:R25.
8. Valdes AM, Loughlin J, Oene MV, Chapman K, Surdulescu GL, Doherty M, Spector TD. Sex and ethnic differences in the association of ASPN, CALM1, COL2A1, COMP and FRZB with genetic susceptibility to osteoarthritis of the knee. Arthritis Rheum 2007;56:137–146.
9. Schousten JS, van den Ouweland FA, Valkenburg HA. A 12-year follow-up study in the general population on prognostic factors of cartilage loss in osteoarthritis of the knee. Ann Rheum Dis 1992;51:932–937.
10. Goldring MB, Marcu KB. Cartilage homeostasis in health and rheumatic diseases. Arthritis Res Ther 2009;11:224.
11. Reginato AM, Olsen BR. The role of structural genes in the pathogenesis of osteoarthritic disorders. Arthritis Res 2002;4:337–345.
12. Dabovic B, Chen Y, Colarossi C, Zambuto L, Obata H, Rifkin DB. Bone defects in latent TGF-beta binding protein (Ltbp)-3 null mice: a role for Ltbp in TGF- beta presentation. J Endocrinol 2002;175:129–141.
13. Valdes AM, Spector TD. The contribution of genes to osteoarthritis. Rheum Dis Clin North Am 2008;34:581–603.
14. Anderson JJ, Felson DT. Factors associated with osteoarthritis of the knee in the first national Health and Nutrition Examination Survey (HANES I). Evidence for an association with overweight, race and physical demands of work. Am J Epidemiol 1988;128:179–189.
15. Dumond H, Presie N, Terlain B, Mainard D, Loeuille D, Netter P, Pottie P. Evidence for a key role of leptin in osteoarthritis. Arthritis Rheum 2003;48:3118–3129.
16. Sharma L. Song J, Felson DR, Cahue S, Shamiyeh E, Dunlop DD. The role of knee alignment in disease progression and functional decline in knee osteoarthritis. JAMA 2001;286:188–195.
17. Sharma L. The role of varus and valgus alignment in knee osteoarthritis. Arthritis Rheum 2007;56:1044–1047.
18. Sharma L, Lou C, Cahue S, Dunlop DD. The mechanism of the effect of obesity on knee osteoarthritis: the mediating role of malalignment. Arthritis Rheum 2000;43:568–575.

19. Hunter DJ, Zhang Y, Niu J, Goggins J, Amin S, LaValley MP, Guermazi A, Genant H, Gale D, Felson DT. Increase in bone marrow lesions associated with cartilage loss: a longitudinal study of knee osteoarthritis. Arthritis Rheum 2006;54:1529–1535.

20. Petersson IF, Boegard T, Saxne T, Silman AJ, Svensson B. Radiographic osteoarthritis of the knee classified by the Ahlback and Kellgren & Lawrence systems for the tibiofemoral joint in people aged 35–54 years with chronic knee pain. Ann Rheum Dis 1997;56:493–496.

21. Roos EM. Joint injury causes knee osteoarthritis in young adults. Curr Opin Rheumatol 2005;17:195–200.

22. Lohmander LS, Ostenberg A, Englund M, Roos EM. High prevalence of knee osteoarthritis, pain and functional limitations in female soccer players twelve years after anterior cruciate ligament injury. Arthritis Rheum 2004;50:3145–3152.

23. Roos H, Lauren M, Adalberth T, Roos EM, Jonsson K, Lohmander LS. Knee osteoarthritis after meniscectomy: prevalence of radiographic changes after twenty-one years, compared with matched control. Arthritis Rheum 1998; 41:687–693.

24. Goldring MB, Marcu KB. Cartilage homeostasis in health and rheumatic diseases. Arthritis Res Ther 2009;11:224.

25. Loeser RF. Molecular mechanisms of cartilage destruction: mechanics, inflammatory mediators and aging collide. Arthritis Rheum 2006;54:1357–1360.

26. Pelletier JP, Pelletier JM, Abramson SB. Osteoarthritis, an inflammatory disease: potential implications for the selection of new therapeutic targets. Arthritis Rheum 2001;44:1237–1247.

27. Attur MG, Dave M, Akamatsu M, Katoh M, Amin AR. Osteoarthritis or osteoarthroses: the definition of inflammation becomes a semantic issue in the genomic era of molecular medicine. Osteoarthritis Cartilage 2002;10:1–4.

28. Attur MG, Patel IR, Patel RN, Abramson SB, Amin AR. Autocrine production of IL-1 beta by human osteoarthritis-affected cartilage and differential regulation of endogenous nitric oxide, IL-6, prostaglandin E2 and IL-8. Proc Assoc Am Physicians 1998;110:65–72.

29. Van de Loo FAJ, Joosten LAB, van Lent PLEM, Arntz OJ, ven den Berg WB. Role of interleukin-1, tumor necrosis factor-α and interleukin-6 in cartilage proteoglycan metabolism and destruction: effect of in-situ blocking in murine antigen and zymosan-induced arthritis. Arthritis Rheum 1995;38:164–172.

30. Saha N, Moldovan F, Tardif G, Pelletier JP, Cloutier JM, Martel-Pelletier J. Interluekin-1 b-converting enzyme/caspase-1 in human osteoarthritic tissues: localization and role in the maturation of interleukin-1β and interleukin-18. Arthritis Rheum 1999;42:1577–1587.

31. Martel-Pelletier J, McCollum R, Di Barrista J, Faure MP, Chin JA, Fournier S, Sarfati M, Pelletier JP. The interleukin-1-receptor in normal and osteoarthritic human articular chondrocytes: identification as the type I receptor and analyses of binding, kinetics and biologic function. Arthritis Rheum 1992;35:530–540.

32. Amin AR. Regulation of tumor necrosis factor-alpha and tumor necrosis factor converting enzyme in human osteoarthritis. Osteoarthritis Cartilage 1999;7:392–394.

33. Alaaeddine N, di Battista JA, Pelletier JP, Cloutier JM, Klansa K, Dupuis M, Martel-Pelletier J. Osteoarthritic synovial fibroblasts possess an increased level of tumor necrosis factor-receptor 55 (TNF-R55) that mediates biological activation by TNF-alpha. J Rheumatol 1997;24:1985–1994.

34. Lianxu C, Hongti J, Changlong Y. NF-kappaBp65-specific siRNA inhibits expression of genes of COX-2, NOS-2 and MMP-9 in rat and IL-1 beta-induced and TNF-alpha induced chondrocytes. Osteoarthritis Cartilage 2006;14:367–376.

35. Rengel Y, Ospelt C, Gay S. Proteinases in the joint: clinical relevance of proteinases in joint destruction. Arthritis Res Ther 2007;9:221.

36. Tetlow LC, Adlam DJ, Woolley DE. Matrix metalloproteinase and proinflammatory cytokine production by chondrocytes of human osteoarthritic cartilage; associations with degenerative changes. Arthritis Rheum 2001;44:585–594.

37. Grabowski PS, Wright PK, Van't Hot RJ, Helfrich MH, Ohshima H, Ralston SH. Immunolocalization of inducible nitric oxide synthase in synovium and cartilage in rheumatoid arthritis and osteoarthritis. Br J Rheumatol 1997;36:651–655.

38. Pelletier JP, Minea F, Ranger P, Tardif G, Martel-Pelletier J. The increased synthesis of inducible nitric oxide inhibits IL-1Ra synthesis by human articular chondrocytes: possible role in osteoarthritic cartilage degradation. Osteoarthritis Cartilage 1996;4:77–84.

39. Hashimoto S, Takahashi K, Amiel D, Coutts RD, Lotz M. Chondrocyte apoptosis and nitric oxide production during experimentally induced osteoarthritis. Arthritis Rheum 1998;41:1266–1274.

40. Amin AR, Attur MG, Patel RN, Thakker GD, Marshall PJ, Rediske J, Stuchin SA, Patel IR, Abramson SB. Superinduction of cycloozygenase-2 activity in human osteoarthritis-affected cartilage: influence of nitric oxide. J Clin Invest 1997;99:1231–1237.
41. Abramson SB, Attur M. Developments in the scientific understanding of osteoarthritis. Arthritis Res Ther 2009;11:227.
42. Afonso V, Champy R, Mitrovic D, Collin P, Lomri A. Reactive oxygen species and superoxide dismutases: role in joint disease. Joint Bone Spine 2007;74:324–329.
43. Verziji N, DeGroot J, Ben Zaken C, Brau-Benjamin O, Maroudas A, Bank RA, Mizrahi J, Schalkwijk VG, Thorpe SR, Baynes JW, et al. Crosslinking by advanced glycation end products increases the stiffness of the collagen network in human articular cartilage: a possible mechanism through which age is a risk factor for osteoarthritis. Arthritis Rheum 2002;46:114–123.
44. Verziji N, Bank RA, TeKoppele JM, DeGroot J. AGEing and osteoarthritis. A different perspective. Curr Opin Rheumatol 2003;15:616–622.
45. Dore S, Duchossoy Y, Khatib A, et al. Articular chondrocytes posses an increased number of insulin-like growth factor 1 binding sites but are unresponsive to its stimulation. Possible role of IGF-1 binding proteins. Arthritis Rheum 1994;37:253–263.
46. Loeser RF, Shanker G, Carlson CS, Gardin JF, Shelton BJ, Sonntag WE. Reduction in the chondrocytes response to insulin like growth factor 1 in aging and osteoarthritis: studies in a non-human primate model of naturally occurring disease. Arthritis Rheum 2000;43:2110–2120.
47. Guerne PA, Blanco F, Kaelin A, Desgeorges A. Growth factor responsiveness of human articular chondrocytes in aging and development. Arthritis Rheum 1995;38:960–968.
48. Finkel T, Holbrook NJ. Oxidants, oxidative stress and the biology of ageing. Nature 2000;408:239–247.
49. Aigner T, Haag J, Martin J, Buckwalter J. Osteoarthritis. Aging of matrix and cells—going for a remedy. Curr Drug Targets 2007;8:325–331.
50. Horton WE Jr, Yagi R, Laverty D, Weiner S. Overview of studies comparing human normal cartilage with minimal and advanced osteoarthritic cartilage. Clin Exp Rheumatol 2005;23:103–112.
51. Loeser RF, Shakoor N. Aging or osteoarthritis: which is the problem? Rheum Dis Clin North Am 2003;46:114–123.
52. Otero M, Lago R, Lago F, Reino JJ, Gualillo O. Signaling pathway involved in nitric oxide synthase type II activation in chondrocytes: synergistic effect of leptin with interleukin-1. Arthritis Res Ther 2005;7:R581-R591.
53. Lago F, Dieguez C, Gomez-Reino J, Gualillo O. The emerging role of adipokines as mediators of inflammation and immune responses. Cytokine Growth Factor Rev 2007;18:313–325.
54. Abramson SB, Attur M. Developments in the scientific understanding of osteoarthritis. Arthritis Res Ther 2009;11:227.
55. Lee JH, Fitzgerald JB, Dimicco MA, Grodzinsky AJ. Mechanical injury of cartilage explants causes specific time-dependent changes in chondrocytes gene expression. Arthritis Rheum 2005;52:2386–2395.
56. Roach HI, Aigner T, Soder S, Haag J, Welkerling H. Pathobiology of osteoarthritis: pathomechanisms and potential therapeutic targets. Curr Drug Targets 2007;8:271–282.
57. Kurz B, Lemke AK, Fay J, Pufe T, Grodzinsky AJ, Schunke M. Pathomechanisms of cartilage destruction by mechanical injury. Ann Anat 2005;187:473–485.
58. Fan Z, Soder S, Oehler S, Fundel K, Aigner T. Activation of interleukin-1 signaling cascades in normal and osteoarthritic cartilage. Am J Pathol 2007;171:938–946.
59. Healy ZR, Lee NH, Gao X, Goldring MB, Talalay P, Kensler TW, Konstantopoulos K. Divergent responses of chondrocytes and endothelial cells to shear stress: cross-talk among COX-2, the phase 2 response and apoptosis. Proc Natl Acad Sci U S A 2005;102:14010–14015.
60. Valdes AM, Van Oene M, Hart DJ, Surdulescu GL, Loughlin J, Doherty M, Spector TD. Reproducible genetic associations between candidate genes and clinical knee osteoarthritis in men and women. Arthritis Rheum 2006;54:533–539.
61. Li Y, Xu L, Olsen BR. Lessons from genetic forms of osteoarthritis for the pathogenesis of the disease. Osteoarthritis Cartilage 2007;15:1101–1105.
62. Mier RJ, Holderbaum D, Ferguson R, Moskowitz R. Osteoarthritis in children associated with a mutation in the type II procollagen gene (COL2A). Mol Genet Metab 2001;74:338–341.
63. Reginato AM, Olsen BR. The role of structural genes in the pathogenesis of osteoarthritic disorders. Arthritis Res 2002;4:337–345.

64. Goldring SR. The role of bone in osteoarthritis pathogenesis. Rheum Dis Clin North Am 2008;34:561–571.
65. Anandarajah AP. Role of RANKL in bone disease. Trends Endocrinol Metab 2009;20:88–94.
66. Burr DB. Anatomy and physiology of the mineralized tissues: role in the pathogenesis of osteoarthritis. Osteoarthritis Cartilage 2004;12:S20–S30.
67. van der Kraan PM, van den Berg WB. Osteophytes: relevance and biology. Osteoarthritis Cartilage 2007;15:237–244.
68. Patel N, Buckland-Wright C. Advancement in the zone of calcified cartilage in osteoarthritic hands of patients detected by high definition macroradiography. Osteoarthritis Cartilage 1999;7:520–525.
69. van der Kraan PM, van den Berg WB. Osteophytes: relevance and biology. Osteoarthritis Cartilage 2007;15:237–244.
70. Pottenger LA, Phillips FM, Draganich LF. The effect of marginal osteophytes on reduction of varus–valgus instability in osteoarthritic knees. Arthritis Rheum 1990;33:853–858.
71. Gilbertson EM. Development of periarticular osteophytes in experimentally induced osteoarthritis in the dog. A study using microradiographic, microangiographic and fluorescent bone-labelling techniques. Ann Rheum Dis 1975;34:12–25.
72. Blaney Davidson EN, van der Kraan PM, van der Berg QB. TGF-beta and osteoarthritis. Osteoarthritis Cartilage 2007;15:597–604.
73. Uchino M, Izumi T, Tominaga T, Wakita R, Minehara H, Sekiguchi M, Itoman M. Growth factor expression in the osteophytes of the human femoral head in osteoarthritis. Clin Orthop Relat Res 2000;377:119–125.
74. Buckland-Wright C, Macfarlane D, Lynch J. Relationship between joint space width and subchondral sclerosis in the osteoarthritic hand: a quantitative microfocal study. J Rheumatol 1992;19:788–795.
75. Buckland-Wright C, Macfarlane DG, Jasani MK, Lynch JA. Quantitative microfocal radiographic assessment of osteoarthritis of the knee from weight bearing tunnel and semiflexed standing views. J Rheumatol 1994;21:1734–1741.
76. Imhof H, Breitenseher M, Kainberger F, Tratting S. Degenerative joint disease: cartilage or vascular disease? Skeletal Radiol 1997;26:398–403.
77. Brandt KD, Radin EL, Dieppe PA, van de Putte L. Yet more evidence that osteoarthritis is not a cartilage disease. Ann Rheum Dis 2006;65:1261–1264.
78. Li A, Aspden R. Mechanical and material properties of the subchondral bone plate form the femoral head of patients with osteoarthritis or osteoporosis. Ann Rheum Dis 1997;56:247–254.
79. Buckland-Wright C. Subchondral bone changes in hand and knee osteoarthritis detected by radiography. Osteoarthritis Cartilage 2004;12:S10-S19.
80. Zanetti M, Bruder E, Romero J, Hodler J. Bone marrow edema pattern in osteoarthritic knees: correlation between MR imaging and histologic findings. Radiology 2000;215:835–840.
81. Wilson AJ, Murphy WA, Hardy DC, Totty WG. Transient osteoporosis: transient bone marrow edema? Radiology 1988;167:757–760.
82. Felson DT, Chaisson CE, Hill CL, Totterman SM, Gale ME, Skinner KM, Kazis L, Gale DR. The association of bone marrow lesions with pain in knee osteoarthritis. Ann Intern Med 2001;134:541–549.
83. Felson DT, Niu J, Guermazi A, Roemer F, Aliabadi P, Clancy M, Torner J, Lewis CE, Nevitt MC. Correlation of the development of knee pain with enlarging bone marrow lesions on magnetic resonance imaging. Arthritis Rheum 2007;56:2986–2992.
84. Felson DT, McLaughlin S, Goggins J, LaValley MP, Gale ME, Totterman S, Li W, Hill C, Gale D. Bone marrow edema and its relation to progression of knee osteoarthritis. Ann Intern Med 2003;139:330–336.
85. Ayral X, Pickering EH, Woodworth TG, Mackillop N, Dougados M. Synovitis: a potential predictive factor of structural progression of medial tibiofemoral knee osteoarthritis—results of a 1 year longitudinal arthroscopic study in 422 patients. Osteoarthritis Cartilage 2005;13:361–367.
86. Ayral X, Dougados M, Listrat V, Bonvarlet JP, Simonnet J, Amor B. Arthroscopic evaluation of chondropathy in osteoarthritis of the knee. J Rheumatol 1996;23:698–706.
87. Krasnokutsky S, Samuels J, Attur M, et al. Synovial but not cartilage volumes on MRI predict radiographic severity of knee OA. Osteoarthritis Cartilage 2007;15:C29–C30.
88. Shibakawa A, Aoki H, Mauko-Hongo K, Kato T, Tanaka M, Nishioka K, Nakamura H. Presence of pannus-like tissue on osteoarthritic cartilage and its histological character. Osteoarthritis Cartilage 2003;11(2):133–140.

89. Hill CL, Gale DG, Chaisson CE, Skinner K, Kazis L, Gale ME, Felson DT. Knee effusions, popliteal cysts and synovial thickening: association with knee pain in those with and without osteoarthritis. J Rheumatol 2001;28:1330–1337.

90. Hill CL, Hunter DJ, Niu J, Clancy M, Geurmazi A, Genant H, Gale D, Grainger A, Conaghan P, Felson DT. Synovitis detected on magnetic resonance imaging and its relation to pain and cartilage loss in knee osteoarthritis. Ann Rheum Dis 2007;66:1599–1603.

91. Benito MJ, Veale DJ, Fitzgerald O, van den Berg WB, Bresnihan B. Synovial tissue inflammation in early and late osteoarthritis. Ann Rheum Dis 2005;64:1263–1267.

92. Walsh DA, Boneet CS, Turner EL, Wilson D. Angiogenesis in the synovium and at the osteochondral junction in osteoarthritis. Osteoarthritis Cartilage 2007;15:743–751.

93. Bonnet CS, Walsh DA, Osteoarthritis, angiogenesis and inflammation. Rheumatology 2005;44:7–16.

94. Slemenda C, Heilman DK, Brandt KD, Katz BP, Mazzuca SA, Braunstein EM, Byrd D. Reduced quadriceps strength relative to body weight: a risk factor for knee osteoarthritis in women? Arthritis Rheum 1998;41:1951–1959.

95. Tan AL, Grainger AJ, Tanner SF, Shelley DM, Pease C, Emery P, McGonagle D. High-resolution magnetic resonance imaging for the assessment of hand osteoarthritis. Arthritis Rheum 2005;52:2355–2365.

96. Kannus P. Nonoperative treatment of grade II and grade III sprains of the lateral ligament compartment of the knee. Am J Sports Med 1989;17:83–88.

97. Bird HA, Tribe CR, Bacon PA. Joint hypermobility leading to osteoarthrosis and chondrocalcinosis. Ann Rheum Dis 1978;37:203–211.

98. Sharma L, Pai Y-C, Holtkamp K, Rymer WZ. Is knee joint proprioception worse in the arthritic knee versus the unaffected knee in unilateral knee osteoarthritis? Arthritis Rheum 1997;40:1518–1525.

3 Biomarkers in Osteoarthritis

Muneaki Ishijima, Hisashi Kurosawa,
Haruka Kaneko, and Kazuo Kaneko

CONTENTS

INTRODUCTION

OSTEOARTHRITIS

Osteoarthritis (OA) is an age-related progressive joint disease. The symptoms of OA are often associated with significant functional impairment, symptoms of inflammation, including pain, stiffness, and loss of mobility, disability and diminished activity in daily life, and diminished overall quality of life for OA patients (Felson, 2003; Felson, 2006; Goldring and Goldring, 2007). There are no current interventions proven to restore cartilage or curtail the disease processes, and OA ultimately results in joint destruction, chronic pain, disability, and other associated conditions such as depression and social isolation (Krasnokutsky et al., 2008). As the prevalence of this disease is gradually increasing because of the increasing longevity of the population, OA is therefore an increasingly important public health concern (Dieppe and Lohmander, 2005). However, the only current sensitive diagnostic technique is classical radiography, and we cannot inhibit the progression of disease by any methods, such as medication. Furthermore, we are unable to predict who will progress to OA. Therefore, it is essential to establish a better overall management system for OA (Dove, 2002).

PATHOPHYSIOLOGY OF OA

The etiology and the pathophysiology of OA are still poorly understood and are speculated to vary between individuals (Pollard et al., 2008). OA is primarily induced by the degeneration and destruction of the articular cartilage. The subchondral bone and the synovium, in addition to articular cartilage, are also involved in this aspect of OA progression, although the changes of these tissues are considered to be a secondary phenomenon that is induced by primary changes (Abramson and Attur, 2009). In comparison with rheumatoid arthritis, the changes that occur in the affected joints are local adjustments to the changes in articular cartilage (Ayral et al., 2005). The molecular- and cytokine-based events that drive joint damage in inflammatory arthritis have gradually been recognized as pathogenic paradigms in OA and will be highly relevant to the development of future OA therapeutics. With the increasing appreciation of the contribution of all three joint compartments (cartilage, bone, and synovium) to disease progression, current research and understanding of OA pathogenesis, biomarker identification, and treatment have immensely broadened in recent years (Krasnokutsky et al., 2008).

CLINICAL MANIFESTATIONS OF OA

OA is clinically characterized by joint pain, limitation of movement, crepitus, occasional effusion, and variable degrees of local inflammation, but without systemic effects (Flores and Hochberg, 2003). Osteoarthritic joint damage may be associated with clinical problems, but the severity of joint disease is only weakly related to the clinical problem. For this reason, the associations and pathogenesis of pain must be investigated in addition to examining joint damage. The subchondral bone and synovium may be responsible for nociceptive stimuli, and peripheral neuronal sensitization is an important feature that may cause pain during normal activities, such as walking.

The treatment of symptomatic knee OA is focused on controlling the pain, maintaining patients' functional independence and improving patients' quality of life, in addition to preventing structural deterioration and thereby delaying the need for a total knee arthroplasty (Hochberg, 2006). The guidelines for the medical management of symptomatic knee OA emphasize a multidisciplinary approach that includes nonpharmacologic measures (patient education, physical and occupational therapy, aerobic and muscle-strengthening exercises, weight control, and use of assistive devices) as well as pharmacologic agents (oral and topical analgesic agents, nonsteroidal anti-inflammatory drugs including cyclooxygenase-2-selective inhibitors, and intra-articular therapies such as corticosteroids and hyaluronan preparations) (Zhang et al., 2007, 2008; Conaghan et al., 2008). Dietary and nutritional supplements, including glucosamine and chondroitin sulfate, are frequently used by patients and are increasingly recommended by practitioners (Clegg et al., 2006; Hochberg et al., 2008; Kahan et al., 2009).

PROBLEMS TO BE OVERCOME FOR THE MANAGEMENT OF OA

Although symptomatic OA is very common in the community, much of it is mild, and progression to severe disease is fairly uncommon (Dieppe and Lohmander, 2005). Many patients never seek medical advice. We believe that it is important not to overtreat those who do seek physician advice and that it is unnecessary to administer medicine for most of those patients displaying mild OA. Given the huge economic and personal burdens of OA and the fact that it is the main cause of the increasing need for joint replacements (Kim, 2008), we must consider preventive measures. However, it is impossible to predict the disease of individuals, although many candidate markers have been reported that may predict a high risk for the progression of disease (Belo et al., 2007).

The radiographic analysis of patients has been the traditional means of diagnosing and monitoring the progression of OA, and the measurements of changes in joint space width as assessed by radiography remain the standard protocol. However, it is difficult to detect early joint tissue damage for the purpose of preventing joint destruction because of the poor sensitivity and relatively large precision errors of radiography (Garnero et al., 2000). In addition to the detection of early joint tissue damage and early prognosis of the disease, the development of tools to evaluate the efficacy of new drugs is necessary. Although various disease-modifying treatments have been studied for OA, no drugs have achieved approval of the U.S. Food and Drug Administration as disease-modifying osteoarthritis drugs (DMOADs) (Abramson and Krasnokutsky, 2006). At present, the development of DMOADs requires the slowing of radiographic joint space narrowing that is clinically meaningful and that will be associated with improvement in symptoms or function. Given the slow rate of progression of joint space narrowing in many patients, the lack of specificity and sensitivity of standard radiography, and the fact that candidate DMOADs may slow joint space narrowing but not ameliorate patient symptoms, the development of DMOADs has been a very difficult task. Therefore, there is a need for more effective techniques than radiography alone, and there is an urgent necessity for reliable, quantitative, and dynamic tests that will detect early OA damage and allow the response of treatments targeted at joint destruction to be measured (Young-Min et al., 2001).

There are many problems that must be overcome for significant progression in this field. First, the disease mechanisms of OA will have to be better understood to identify the best targets for initiating treatments in preclinical and clinical trials. The heterogeneous etiology of OA and the pathophysiological events that may be stage and perhaps site specific may slow our advancement toward this knowledge. Second, patients have variable progression of disease, so we must be able to predict which patients will progress to OA over time and whether these patients have distinguishing features on the basis of clinical, radiological, or laboratory assessments. Third, once potentially disease-modifying treatments are available, determining the efficacy of intervention will be important. Therefore, it is widely agreed that the validation of improved imaging and chemical biomarkers will circumvent these problems.

Candidates: Magnetic Resonance Imaging and Biomarkers

The interest in developing another therapy has stimulated the search for more sensitive indicators of OA for use in conjunction with or possibly as a substitute for the traditional radiographic outcomes. Preliminary studies suggest that both biomarkers and magnetic resonance imaging (MRI) measurements are sensitive to changes in OA (Bauer et al., 2006).

Magnetic Resonance Imaging

MRI is currently being optimized for OA imaging. MRI is more sensitive than radiography to detect bone and soft tissue changes, which are features of OA (Felson et al., 2007). In early knee OA, before the appearance of radiographic features, MRI detection of structural abnormalities provides clues to the subsequent disease course. Identifying the prognostic structural characteristics would aid decision making for both the individual and the treating physician as well as highlight potential pathological mechanisms for the research community (Javaid et al., 2009).

Bone marrow abnormalities (BMAs) are known to be associated with clinical outcomes (Garnero et al., 2005). An increase in the size of BMAs observed on knee MRI is related to the concurrent onset of knee pain (Felson et al., 2007). These MRI findings were predictive of incident knee symptoms in patients with normal knees as later evaluated by radiograph (Javaid et al., 2009).

Biomarkers

The ultimate biomarkers for clinical research, in general, purpose a surrogate end point and substitute for a clinical outcome of a patient (De Gruttola et al., 2001). They are defined as objective indicators of normal biologic processes, pathogenic processes, or pharmacologic responses to therapeutic interventions (De Gruttola et al., 2001) and have the potential to decrease the length and cost of trials and to enrich our understanding of the pathogenesis of the disease. The identification of biomarkers in OA, in addition to MRI, will help identify patients who have a risk for disease progression or make it possible to evaluate the patient responses to treatment (Abramson and Krasnokutsky, 2006).

BIOMARKERS IN OA

VALIDITY OF BIOMARKERS: LESSONS FROM THE MANAGEMENT OF OSTEOPOROSIS

The effectiveness of treatment for osteoporosis is determined by the reduction of bone fractures. However, bone mineral density is often used as surrogate marker for the effectiveness of treatment for osteoporosis. Acute changes in bone are difficult to monitor by bone mineral density because changes are below the detection limit (Glover et al., 2009). Because biomarkers of bone turnover change more rapidly, they are sufficiently sensitive to allow the effective monitoring of acute changes in bone turnover. A suitable combination of bone turnover markers may be used to monitor the pharmacologic effect and potential efficacy of treatment for osteoporosis (Nishizawa et al., 2005).

Changes in biochemical markers of bone formation after 1 month of anabolic therapy were correlated with improvements in bone structure after 22 months of therapy (Dobnig et al., 2005). Greater decreases in bone resorption markers were associated with a lower incidence of vertebral fractures (Eastell et al., 2003). It is thus believed that maintaining the optimal levels of bone metabolism within the reference ranges is necessary to maintain bone strength in premenopausal women (Weinstein, 2000).

Therefore, the development of the biomarkers related to bone metabolism for osteoporosis stimulated the development of new drugs, particularly the bisphosphonates, which reduce the loss of body height and bone mass, fracture risk, reduction of patients' activity of daily life, and, as a result, patients mortality (Black et al., 2007; Garnero, 2009), thus leading to a better management system for osteoporosis.

A CLASSIFICATION OF OA BIOMARKERS: BIPED

Recently, the Osteoarthritis Biomarkers Network, funded by the National Institutes of Health (NIH)/National Institute of Arthritis and Musculoskeletal and Skin Disease (NIAMs), proposed a classification of OA biomarkers to develop and characterize new biomarkers and to refine existing OA biomarkers (Bauer et al., 2006). This classification scheme includes five categories: evaluation of the disease burden, investigative degree, prediction of prognosis, treatment efficacy, and disease diagnosis (BIPED). This classification was developed to assist OA researchers with ongoing biomarker work and in most instances will be achieved in a progressive validation strategy.

CANDIDATES FOR BIOMARKERS IN OA

The structure of molecules or their fragments derived from cartilage, bone, and the synovium, which are affected by OA, are good candidate biological markers for OA (Rousseau and Delmas, 2007) (Table 3.1).

TABLE 3.1
Potential Biomarkers of Cartilage, Bone, and Synovium Turnover for the Management of OA

Tissue	Molecule		Markers	References and BIPED Classification
Cartilage	Type II collagen	Synthesis marker	CPII or PIICP	Shinmei et al., 1993 (D)
				Sugiyama et al., 2003 (P)
				Cahue et al., 2007 (P)
			PIIANP	Rousseau et al., 2004 (D)
				Sharif et al., 2007 (P)
		Degradation marker	CTX-II	Christgau et al., 2001 (D)
				Reijman et al., 2004 (B, P)
				Jung et al., 2004 (D)
				Gineyts et al., 2004 (E)
				Christgau et al., 2004 (E)
				Garnero et al., 2005 (P)
				Bingham et al., 2006 (E)
				Meulenbelt et al., 2006 (B)
				Mazieres et al., 2006 (P)
				Bruyere et al., 2006 (P)
				Sharif et al., 2007 (P)
				Garnero et al., 2008 (E)
				Petersen et al., 2010 (E)
			C2C	King et al., 2004 (D)
				Cibere et al., 2005 (E)
				Cahue et al., 2007 (P)
			C1,2C	Cibere et al., 2005 (E)
				Cahue et al., 2007 (P)
	Noncollagenous proteins	Synthesis marker	Epitopes 3-B-3 and 846 (Aggrecan)	Rizkalla et al., 1992 (B)
		Degradation marker	COMP	Vilim et al., 2001 (D)
				Vilim et al., 2002 (P)
				Sharif et al., 2004 (P)
				Petersen et al., 2010 (E)
	Proteases and their inhibitors	Synthesis marker		
		Degradation marker	MMP3	Lohmander et al., 2005 (P)
Bone	Type I collagen	Synthesis marker		
		Degradation marker	NTX-I	Bettica et al., 2002 (D)
			CTX-I	Bettica et al., 2002 (D, P)
	Noncollagenous proteins	Synthesis marker	Osteocalcin	Sowers et al., 1999 (D)
				Bruyere et al., 2003 (P)
		Degradation marker		
Synovium	Type III collagen	Synthesis marker		
		Degradation marker	Glc-Gal-PYD	Garnero et al., 2001 (D, P)
				Jordan et al., 2006 (D)

continued

TABLE 3.1 (continued)
Potential Biomarkers of Cartilage, Bone, and Synovium Turnover for the Management of OA

Tissue	Molecule	Markers	References and BIPED Classification
	Noncollagenous proteins	Synthesis marker	HA	Sharif et al., 1995 (D, P)
				Sharma et al., 1998 (D)
				Sharif et al., 2000 (P)
				Garnero et al., 2001 (D)
				Bruyere et al., 2003 (P)
				Elliott et al., 2005 (B)
				Mazieres et al., 2006 (P)
				Bruyere et al., 2006 (P)
				Turan et al., 2007 (D)
				Belo et al., 2007 (P)
		Degradation marker		

BIPED classification: B, burden of disease; D, diagnostic; E, efficacy of intervention; I, investigative; P, prognostic. C1,2C, types I and II collagen cleavage neoepitopes; C2C, type II collagen cleavage neoepitopes; COMP, cartilage oligomeric matrix protein; CPII, C-propeptide of type II procollagen; CTX-I, C-terminal cross-linked telopeptides of type I collagen; CTX-II, C-telopeptide fragments of type II collagen; Glc-Gal-PYD, glucosyl-galactosyl-pyridinoline; HA, hyaluronic acid; MMP-3, matrix metalloprotease-3; NTX-I, N-terminal cross-linked telopeptides of type I collagen; PIIANP, N-propeptide of collagen type IIA; PIICP, procollagen type II C-terminal propeptide.

Markers of Cartilage Metabolism

The majority of the OA biomarkers to date are derived from the matrix of the articular cartilage (Wieland et al., 2005).

Type II Collagen

Type II collagen is the predominant collagen type in articular cartilage, which is cartilage specific and forms the basic fibrillar structure of the extracellular matrix (Garnero, 2007). The synthesis and degradation of type II collagen can be assessed by several markers. Type II collagen is degraded by proteolytic enzymes such as the matrix metalloproteinases (MMPs) and cysteine proteases, which are secreted by chondrocytes and synovial cells.

The urinary concentration of C-telopeptide fragments of type II collagen (CTX-II) has been used as one of the markers for type II collagen degradation (Christgau et al., 2001; Jung et al., 2004; Reijman et al., 2004; Garnero et al., 2005, 2008; Bingham et al., 2006; Meulenbelt et al., 2006; Sharif et al., 2007). These levels were elevated in patients with knee and hip OA in comparison with control subjects (Christgau et al., 2001; Jung et al., 2004; Reijman et al., 2004). There was a significant association between the total radiographic OA score and the urinary levels of CTX-II (Meulenbelt et al., 2006). Increased levels of urinary CTX-II were associated with a high risk of progression in patients with knee OA (Reijman et al., 2004; Sharif et al., 2007). The BMA on MRI significantly correlated with the levels of urinary CTX-II. In addition, patients with the highest baseline urinary CTX-II levels were likely to have worsening BMAs at 3 months after diagnosis (Garnero et al., 2005). The urinary levels of CTX-II, together with decreases on bone turnover marker levels, were dramatically decreased by resedronate treatment (Bingham et al., 2006). However, neither knee joint structure as monitored by standard radiography nor patient symptoms were affected by resedronate treatment over 2 years. Garnero et al. reported that although urinary levels of CTX-II decreased with resedronate treatment in patients with knee OA, the levels after 6 months were associated with radiological progression at 24 months, suggesting CTX-II as a marker for intervention efficacy (Garnero et al., 2008).

The urinary levels of type II and types I and II collagen cleavage neoepitopes (C2C and C1,2C) were also reported as markers of cartilage destruction (King et al., 2004).

Type II collagen synthesis can also be assessed by a biomarker. The serum levels of C-propeptide of type II procollagen (CPII), which are also called procollagen type II C-terminal propeptide (PIICP), increased in the early stages of OA (Shinmei et al., 1993; Nelson et al., 1998; Birmingham et al., 2007). This is released from the newly synthesized molecule, which is directly related to the synthesis of type II collagen. Although serum CPII (PIICP) levels were not associated with either the severity of disease at baseline or the progression of the disease, a greater C2C:CPII (PIICP) ratio and C1,2C:CPII (PIICP) ratio were each associated with increased progression of the disease (Cahue et al., 2007).

Aggrecan

Aggrecan, in addition to type II collagen, is one of the most abundant proteins of the cartilage matrix. It is a proteoglycan composed of a core protein and glycosaminoglycan chains that are covalently attached to the core protein (Garnero, 2007).

Markers for aggrecan synthesis include epitopes located on the chondroitin sulfate chains of the aggrecan such as the 3-B-3 and the 846 epitopes. In the cartilage, the concentrations of these aggrecan synthesis epitopes were age and disease dependent (Rizkalla et al., 1992).

Cartilage Oligomeric Matrix Protein

The cartilage oligomeric matrix protein (COMP) is a member of the thrombospondin family of glycoproteins among noncollagenous proteins in cartilage. Although COMP was thought to be secreted only in cartilage, it has also been observed in the ligaments, meniscus, tendons, and synovium (Di Cesare et al., 1996; Muller et al., 1998). COMP is present in the intact molecule form and in several fragments (Di Cesare et al., 1996).

The serum levels of COMP in patients with knee OA with synovitis were significantly increased in comparison with those without synovitis (Vilim et al., 2001). When serum levels of baseline COMP were elevated, there was an association with loss of join space narrowing over 3 years in patients with knee OA (Vilim et al., 2002).

Proteolytic Enzymes

Proteolytic enzymes were also reported to be useful biomarkers of OA. Although baseline serum levels of MMP-3, which degrade cartilage matrix molecules, were not correlated to knee pain, these were significant predictor values for joint space narrowing (Lohmander et al., 2005).

Markers of Bone Metabolism

Bone turnover is determined on the basis of the balance between bone formation by osteoblasts and bone resorption by osteoclasts. In OA, loss of articular cartilage and subchondral bone activity are increased. However, whether these changes occur independently or are linked still remain unclear (Westacott, 2003).

Type I Collagen

The urinary levels of N-terminal and C-terminal cross-linked telopeptides of type I collagen (NTX-I and CTX-I), which are markers for bone resorption, were higher in patients with progressive OA than in patients with nonprogressive OA (Bettica et al., 2002).

Osteocalcin

The serum levels of osteocalcin, a noncollagenous protein and a marker for bone formation, in patients with knee OA were lower than in patients without OA (Sowers et al., 1999).

Markers of Synovial Metabolism

Little attention has been paid to the examination of synovial tissue metabolism in OA. However, there is increasing evidence showing that alterations in synovial tissue metabolism are involved in the progression of joint destruction, leading to an interest in this phenomenon (Garnero, 2007). Abnormalities of the medial perimeniscal synovium are a common feature of painful medial knee OA (Pelletier et al., 2001). Moreover, synovitis may be considered a predictive factor for the progression of OA (Ayral et al., 2005).

It was speculated that the enhancement of systemic inflammation in OA is detectable by the measurement of C-reactive protein (CRP). Patients whose knee OA progressed over 4 years had higher baseline serum CRP concentrations compared with patients who did not progress (Sharif et al., 2000). However, CRP is not joint specific and can be affected by other chronic medical conditions, suggesting that CRP is unlikely to be a useful marker in OA. On the basis of these findings, several biomarkers have been proposed to assess synovitis, including serum hyaluronic acid (HA) or hyaluronan, glucosyl-galactosyl-pyridinoline (Glc-Gal-PYD), and other noncollagenous proteins in the synovium (Garnero and Delmas, 2003). The activity of the synovial membrane can be specifically assessed by monitoring these molecules (Garnero, 2007).

Type III Collagen

Because serum levels of HA are not specific to synovial tissue, Garnero et al. have characterized the glycosylated pyridinoline derivative Glc-Gal-PYD, which is a glycosylated analogue of pyridinoline that is a trivalent structure that forms the mature cross-links of type III fibrillar collagen, and it is found in large amounts in the human synovium, but only in very low levels in the cartilage and other soft tissues (Gineyts et al., 2001).

Urinary Glc-Gal-PYD is significantly increased in patients with knee OA (Garnero et al., 2001; Jordan et al., 2006). In addition, increased levels of urinary Glc-Gal-PYD were associated with both the reduction of the joint space width and worsening of clinical symptoms (Garnero et al., 2001).

Hyaluronic Acid

The synovial lining cells secrete HA, which is a component of the synovial fluid. The lymphatic vessels in the sublining layer regulate synovial fluid by draining excess fluid from the joint cavity and by removing macromolecules such as degraded cartilage, plasma protein, and HA, maintaining pressure in the joint. Therefore, HA enters the circulation, and serum levels of HA are increased as a result of cartilage degradation and synovial inflammation (Konttinen et al., 1990; Nishida et al., 2000). Because serum HA is rapidly taken up by the liver, HA serum levels are increased in patients with liver disease (Laurent et al., 1986, 1996).

Serum levels of HA are increased in patients with OA in comparison with subjects without OA (Sharif et al., 1995; Sharma et al., 1998; Garnero et al., 2001; Elliott et al., 2005; Turan et al., 2007). Moreover, the serum levels of HA are a potential prognostic marker of joint destruction in OA (Sharif et al., 1995; Sharif et al., 2000; Bruyere et al., 2003, 2006).

POTENTIAL USAGE OF BIOMARKERS FOR THE MANAGEMENT OF OA

The potential clinical usage of the biomarkers is introduced on the basis of the BIPED classification, as described previously (Bauer et al., 2006) (Table 3.1).

Diagnostic Markers

Diagnostic markers are defined by an ability to classify individuals into those with disease and those without disease (Bauer et al., 2006). Diagnostic tests with the candidate biomarkers must be compared with the established gold standard in an appropriate spectrum of subjects. In OA, the accepted standard diagnostic test is radiography, in which a Kellgren–Lawrence grade of greater than or equal to 2 is required for the diagnosis of OA (Altman et al., 1986). In addition, individuals with and without OA must be included in the studies of OA diagnostic biomarkers. It is almost impossible to establish diagnostic tests that have an accuracy of 100%, as false-positives and false-negatives will occur. A test is valid if it shows high sensitivity and high specificity. Such a test will detect most people with the target disorder and will exclude the majority of people without the disorder. One of the useful diagnostic test parameters derived from the receiver operator curve analyses is the area under the curve, which quantifies the overall ability of a diagnostic test to correctly classify diseased and nondiseased individuals (McNeil and Hanley, 1984).

When urinary levels of CTX-II were used, the optical cutoff value for the subgroup of hip OA was at 308 ng/mmol creatinine with 94% specificity and 80% sensitivity, whereas that of knee OA was 266 ng/mmol creatinine with 88% specificity and 76% sensitivity (Jung et al., 2004).

Burden of Disease Markers

A burden of disease marker assesses the severity or extent of OA among affected individuals with OA at a single time point (Bauer et al., 2006). The establishment of such a marker classification is often based on cross-sectional data of individuals with OA from cohorts from the community or from baseline assessment of subjects enrolled in a clinical trial. The parameters used to assess burden of disease markers are similar to those described for diagnostic markers. The burden of disease markers can be used only for clinical studies because individual values obtained in groups of patients with different degrees of OA burden overlap considerably (Rousseau and Delmas, 2007).

A risk ratio and an odds ratio (OR) are often reported in studies of burden of disease markers. Baseline urinary CTX-II concentrations were higher in subjects with baseline radiographic knee OA than in those without baseline radiographic knee OA. The OR adjusted by age, sex, and body mass index in the fourth quartile of the subjects with CTX-II levels was 4.2 (95% confidence interval [CI] = 2.5–7.0) in comparison with the first quartile of the subjects (Reijman et al., 2004). There was a significant association between the total radiographic signs of OA and the CTX-II levels in the GARP (Genetics, Arthrosis, and Progression) study (Meulenbelt et al., 2006). The serum levels of HA were positively associated with the severity of knee OA (Elliott et al., 2005).

Prognostic Markers

The key feature of a prognostic marker is the ability to predict the future of OA among those without OA at baseline times or to predict the progression of OA among those with existing disease. The evaluation of prognostic markers requires longitudinal studies that show an association of the marker at baseline with the risk of development of new OA or progression (Bauer et al., 2006).

In the subjects of the Rotterdam study (1235 subjects), those with a CTX-II level in the highest quartile at baseline had a 6.0-fold increased risk for progression of radiographic OA at the knee (95% CI = 1.2–30.8) (Reijman et al., 2004). An increase in CTX-II after 3 months was significantly correlated with a 1-year decrease in mean thickness of medial and lateral tibial cartilage (Bruyere et al., 2006). In a 5-year study, urinary CTX-II concentrations at baseline were higher in progressive subjects in comparison with those in the nonprogressing group (Sharif et al., 2007). Increases in the levels of urinary CTX-II were associated with a higher risk of progression with a relative risk (RR) of 3.4 (95% CI = 1.2–9.4) in patients with 5-year levels above the median (Sharif et al., 2007).

In a 4-year prospective study of female subjects, the radiographic joint space narrowing of the knee joint in patients with tibiofemoral joint OA over 4 years was directly and positively correlated with baseline CPII (PIICP) levels of synovial fluid after adjusting for age and body mass index ($r = 0.395$, 95% CI = 0.23–0.53, $p < 0.001$) (Sugiyama et al., 2003).

Several markers for noncollagenous proteins in the cartilage and synovium have also been reported to be potential candidates for predicting the progression of knee OA. The baseline level of serum MMP-3 was significantly higher in patients with a progression of knee OA as assessed by radiographic joint space narrowing than in patients with nonprogressive knee OA (Lohmander et al., 2005). The serum levels of baseline COMP in a study of 115 patients with knee OA were significantly higher in the patients whose disease progressed than in those whose disease did not (Sharif et al., 2004).

A clinical study, which followed 94 patients with knee OA for 5 years, revealed that the patients whose disease had progressed were significantly higher levels of serum HA at baseline in comparison with those whose disease had not progressed (Sharif et al., 1995). Changes in serum HA after 1 year were significantly correlated with 3-year progression in mean joint space width (Bruyere et al., 2003). A prospective 1-year study showed that high baseline levels of HA in subjects with knee OA are predictive of a worsening of the whole organ MRI score of the knee (Bruyere et al., 2006). On the basis of these data, a systematic review of observational studies for the prognostic factors of progression of knee OA, in which 37 studies were included from the 1004 studies listed, reported that serum HA is predictive for the progression of knee OA in addition to generalized OA (Belo et al., 2007).

In addition to cartilage and synovium metabolism, bone turnover markers also reflect a progression of knee OA. The progression of knee OA as assessed by radiographic joint space narrowing over 3 years was associated with changes after 1 year in serum osteocalcin (Bruyere et al., 2003). The urinary levels of CTX-I were higher in the patients with progressive knee OA than in those with nonprogressive OA (Bettica et al., 2002).

Efficacy of Intervention

An efficacy of intervention marker provides information about the efficacy of treatment among those with OA or in those at a high risk of developing OA (Bauer et al., 2006). The efficacy of intervention markers may be measured before therapy to predict treatment efficacy or may be measured several times to assess short-term changes that occur as a result of pharmacologic or other interventions. The efficacy of candidate for intervention marker must be tested in a clinical trial with appropriate OA end points, such as patient symptoms and/or function, or OA progression by imaging studies. The efficacy of intervention markers must demonstrate a statistically significant relationship between treatment-related changes in a biomarker and the relevant clinical or radiographic OA outcomes. However, as there are no current medications that have a disease-modifying effect, the assessment of the potential role of biomarkers for the monitoring of patient response to the treatment for OA is limited (Rousseau and Delmas, 2007). At the same time, the lack of appropriate biomarkers that accurately monitor and assess the effects of candidates for disease-modifying agents may delay the development of these medications. The CTX-II and the COMP have been reported to be useful as intervention markers. The efficacies of the candidate medications, which have been evaluated by biomarkers, are herein introduced.

Bisphosphonate

The bisphosphonates can decrease the urinary levels of CTX-II, although they are considered to inhibit bone resorption and are effective for the treatment of osteoporosis.

Patients who received risedronate and whose CTX-II levels returned to low levels (<150 ng/mmol creatinine) at 6 months had a lower risk of radiographic progression at 24 months than patients whose CTX-II levels were increased both at baseline and at 6 months (OR = 0.57, 95% CI = 0.39–0.85) after adjusting for demographics and joint space width (Garnero et al., 2008).

Risedronate treatment did not significantly reduce radiographic progression, which was measured by a reduction in joint space width, although a dose-dependent reduction in the levels of CTX-II associated with progressive OA was observed in patients who received risedronate (Bingham et al., 2006).

Nonsteroidal anti-inflammatory drugs

In addition to bisphosphonates, nonsteroidal anti-inflammatory drugs are also reported to modulate cartilage metabolism in OA patients. When patients with knee OA were treated with ibuprofen, their urinary CTX-II levels were not increased after 4–6 weeks (+2%, NS), whereas those with the placebo group significantly increased in comparison with the baseline (+17%, $p = 0.023$) (Gineyts et al., 2004).

Glucosamines

In the search for disease-modifying treatments for OA, the dietary supplements glucosamine and chondroitin sulfate have been advocated as safe and effective options for the management of OA symptoms (Cibere et al., 2005; Clegg et al., 2006). Some of the studies examining glucosamine effects have reported positive effects on OA symptoms. In 1583 patients with symptomatic knee OA, the rate of response for patients with moderate-to-severe pain at baseline was significantly higher with combined therapy (1500 mg of glucosamine daily and 1200 mg of chondroitin sulfate daily) than those with placebo treatment (Clegg et al., 2006). An international, randomized, double-blind, placebo-controlled trial, in which 622 patients with knee OA were randomly assigned to receive either 800 mg of chondroitin sulfate or a placebo once daily for 2 years, revealed the long-term combined structure- and symptom-modifying effects of chondroitin sulfate in patients with knee OA (Kahan et al., 2009). The meta-analysis of randomized double-blind placebo-controlled clinical trials to assess the efficacy of chondroitin sulfate as a structure-modifying drug for knee OA reported that chondroitin sulfate is effective for reducing the rate of decline in minimum joint space width in patients with knee OA, thus suggesting that chondroitin sulfate is a structure-modifying treatment for knee OA (Hochberg et al., 2008).

However, no significant differences in urinary CTX-II levels were observed between placebo- and glucosamine-sulfate-treated groups in a study of 121 patients with knee OA, although patients with CTX-II levels in the highest quartile at baseline showed the greatest decrease in CTX-II over a 3-year period in response to glucosamine-sulfate treatment (Christgau et al., 2004). No significant differences were observed between patients in the placebo- or glucosamine-sulfate-treated groups with respect to the ratio of collagen type II breakdown markers (Cibere et al., 2005). When 36 elderly patients with knee OA were randomly assigned to groups treated with glucosamine ($n = 12$), ibuprofen ($n = 12$), or placebo ($n = 12$), the serum levels of COMP were significantly reduced in the glucosamine group in comparison with those in the placebo and ibuprofen groups, whereas urinary CTX-II levels were not significantly changed in any of the three experimental groups (Petersen et al., 2010).

Investigative Marker

As Bauer et al. (2006) described, an investigative marker is one for which there is insufficient information to allow inclusion of this marker into category as described above. A genotype assessment or an assay of molecules or fragments released into the joint or systemic circulation may be candidate markers in this category. These promising genetic and metabolic approaches are anticipated and will add new information concerning the pathogenesis of OA and will facilitate and encourage identification of potential OA biomarkers (Bauer et al., 2006; Rousseau and Delmas, 2007).

Combination of Biomarkers

It is difficult for a single biomarker to adequately represent a complex interaction of several tissues and different pathophysiological pathways for the progression of joint destruction in OA. Therefore, a combination of biochemical markers will be more useful for identifying OA patients at increased risk for disease progression (Garnero, 2007).

Assessing two biomarkers for type II collagen synthesis and breakdown was shown to be more effective in predicting OA progression than a single biomarker alone. In a 5-year observational study with 84 patients with knee OA, the patients with serum N-propeptide of collagen type IIA, which is a splice variant form in N-propeptide of type II procollagen (Rousseau et al., 2004), in the highest quartile had a significantly higher risk of progression than the other patients (RR = 3.2, 95% CI = 1.1–9.2). Increased levels of urinary CTX-II were also associated with a higher risk of progression with an RR of 3.4 (95% CI = 1.2–9.4) in patients with 5-year levels of urinary CTX-II above median levels. The risk of progression was highest in patients with 5-year levels of N-propeptide of collagen type IIA in the highest quartile and/or CTX-II in the two highest quartiles with an RR of progression, 11.8 (95% CI = 2.5–64.0) (Sharif et al., 2007). A multicenter prospective double-blind 3-year follow-up trial of the patients with hip OA showed that patients in whom urinary levels of CTX-II and serum levels of HA were in the upper tertile had an RR of progression of 3.73 (95% CI = 2.5–5.6) compared with patients with markers in the two lower tertiles. Therefore, the combination of urinary levels of CTX-II with serum levels of HA was thus found to be more predictive than either of these markers alone (Mazieres et al., 2006).

THE CONFRONTING LIMITATIONS AND THEIR SOLUTIONS FOR THE DEVELOPMENT OF BIOMARKERS FOR OA

Despite our present understanding of cartilage, bone, and synovial tissue metabolism, as described above, biomarkers in OA have not yet emerged as accepted tools for characterizing the status of the disease or its prognosis, nor as measures of treatment response, because there are confronting limitations to be overcome in this field. Numerous limitations have been pointed out, including (1) the unavailability for the clinical use of these biomarkers in the management of individual patients, (2) the inherently slow rate of disease development, (3) the lack of a standard for the presence or absence of disease, (4) the lack of standardized disease models, and (5) the absence of methods to predictably modify the disease in these models (Lohmander and Eyre, 2008; Felson and Lohmander, 2009).

The additional limitations in reporting the results of biomarker studies and in conceptualizing the role of biomarkers in OA might also inhibit the ability to make advances in this field (Felson and Lohmander, 2009). Kraus compared the validation process for OA biomarkers with "a blindfolded individual seeking his reflection in a broken mirror" (Kraus, 2006). Because such conventional approaches as radiographic examinations may not be sufficiently sensitive to detect any changes that are detectable by new biomarkers and the radiographic outcomes are relatively late-stage determinants of the OA disease status, the OA biomarkers have little chance of seeking its reflection in the mirror until a precise and reliable standard outcome biomarker measure can become available (Kraus, 2006).

On the basis of these limitations, it was proposed that the development of biomarker science in OA will have to circumvent the existing limitations in the morphological assessment of the joint, in contrast to the situation in some other diseases (Felson and Lohmander, 2009).

CONCLUSIONS

An effective disease-modifying treatment for OA remains to be developed, although OA is by far the most common type of arthritis encountered worldwide. Current goals that must be achieved include understanding how the numerous multifactorial forces converge to manifest the OA phenotype and the identification of patients at risk of clinically meaningful progression by using the epidemiological, genetic, biochemical, and imaging findings, perhaps in a combinational manner (Krasnokutsky et al., 2008). The advent of a disease-specific biomarker has the potential to create a paradigm shift in the diagnosis, prognosis, and treatment monitoring of a disease (Kraus, 2006). Development of OA biomarkers that can monitor the current metabolic status of the joint is currently required not only to assess the efficacy of supplements and DMOADs but also for the development of a better OA management system. These biomarkers will play a crucial role in changing OA to a controllable disease and also in improving the activity of daily life and quality of life of patients with OA.

ACKNOWLEDGMENTS

The authors thank Dr. Ippei Futami for his valuable help in data collection. They also express deep appreciation to Dr. Tokuhide Doi and Dr. Eri Arikawa-Hirasawa for their helpful comments and suggestions.

This study was partially supported by a High Technology Research Center Grant from the Ministry of Education, Culture, Sports, Science and Technology of Japan and by the Takeda Science Foundation.

REFERENCES

Abramson SB, Attur M. Developments in the scientific understanding of osteoarthritis. Arthritis Res Ther 2009;11(3):227.

Abramson S, Krasnokutsky S. Biomarkers in osteoarthritis. Bull NYU Hosp Jt Dis 2006;64(1–2):77–81.

Altman R, Asch E, Bloch D, Bole G, Borenstein D, Brandt K, Christy W, et al. Development of criteria for the classification and reporting of osteoarthritis. Classification of osteoarthritis of the knee. Diagnostic and Therapeutic Criteria Committee of the American Rheumatism Association. Arthritis Rheum 1986;29(8):1039–1049.

Ayral X, Pickering EH, Woodworth TG, Mackillop N, Dougados M. Synovitis: a potential predictive factor of structural progression of medial tibiofemoral knee osteoarthritis—results of a 1 year longitudinal arthroscopic study in 422 patients. Osteoarthritis Cartilage 2005;13(5):361–367.

Bauer DC, Hunter DJ, Abramson SB, Attur M, Corr M, Felson D, Heinegard D, et al. Classification of osteoarthritis biomarkers: a proposed approach. Osteoarthritis Cartilage 2006;14(8):723–727.

Belo JN, Berger MY, Reijman M, Koes BW, Bierma-Zeinstra SM. Prognostic factors of progression of osteoarthritis of the knee: a systematic review of observational studies. Arthritis Rheum 2007;57(1):13–26.

Bettica P, Cline G, Hart DJ, Meyer J, Spector TD. Evidence for increased bone resorption in patients with progressive knee osteoarthritis: longitudinal results from the Chingford study. Arthritis Rheum 2002;46(12):3178–3184.

Bingham CO 3rd, Buckland-Wright JC, Garnero P, Cohen SB, Dougados M, Adami S, Clauw DJ, et al. Risedronate decreases biochemical markers of cartilage degradation but does not decrease symptoms or slow radiographic progression in patients with medial compartment osteoarthritis of the knee: results of the two-year multinational knee osteoarthritis structural arthritis study. Arthritis Rheum 2006;54(11):3494–3507.

Birmingham JD, Vilim V, Kraus VB. Collagen biomarkers for arthritis applications. Biomark Insights 2007;1:61–76.

Black DM, Delmas PD, Eastell R, Reid IR, Boonen S, Cauley JA, Cosman F, et al. Once-yearly zoledronic acid for treatment of postmenopausal osteoporosis. N Engl J Med 2007;356(18):1809–1822.

Bruyere O, Collette JH, Ethgen O, Rovati LC, Giacovelli G, Henrotin YE, Seidel L, Reginster JY. Biochemical markers of bone and cartilage remodeling in prediction of longterm progression of knee osteoarthritis. J Rheumatol 2003;30(5):1043–1050.

Bruyere O, Collette J, Kothari M, Zaim S, White D, Genant H, Peterfy C, et al. Osteoarthritis, magnetic resonance imaging, and biochemical markers: a one year prospective study. Ann Rheum Dis 2006; 65(8):1050–1054.

Cahue S, Sharma L, Dunlop D, Ionescu M, Song J, Lobanok T, King L, Poole AR. The ratio of type II collagen breakdown to synthesis and its relationship with the progression of knee osteoarthritis. Osteoarthritis Cartilage 2007;15(7):819–823.

Christgau S, Garnero P, Fledelius C, Moniz C, Ensig M, Gineyts E, Rosenquist C, Qvist P. Collagen type II C-telopeptide fragments as an index of cartilage degradation. Bone 2001;29(3):209–215.

Christgau S, Henrotin Y, Tanko LB, Rovati LC, Collette J, Bruyere O, Deroisy R, Reginster JY. Osteoarthritic patients with high cartilage turnover show increased responsiveness to the cartilage protecting effects of glucosamine sulphate. Clin Exp Rheumatol 2004;22(1):36–42.

Cibere J, Thorne A, Kopec JA, Singer J, Canvin J, Robinson DB, Pope J, et al. Glucosamine sulfate and cartilage type II collagen degradation in patients with knee osteoarthritis: randomized discontinuation trial results employing biomarkers. J Rheumatol 2005;32(5):896–902.

Clegg DO, Reda DJ, Harris CL, Klein MA, O'Dell JR, Hooper MM, Bradley JD, et al. Glucosamine, chondroitin sulfate, and the two in combination for painful knee osteoarthritis. N Engl J Med 2006;354(8):795–808.

Conaghan PG, Dickson J, Grant RL. Care and management of osteoarthritis in adults: summary of NICE guidance. BMJ 2008;336(7642):502–503.

De Gruttola VG, Clax P, DeMets DL, Downing GJ, Ellenberg SS, Friedman L, Gail MH, Prentice R, Wittes J, Zeger. Considerations in the evaluation of surrogate endpoints in clinical trials. Summary of a National Institutes of Health workshop. Control Clin Trials 2001;22(5):485–502.

Di Cesare PE, Carlson CS, Stolerman ES, Hauser N, Tulli H, Paulsson M. Increased degradation and altered tissue distribution of cartilage oligomeric matrix protein in human rheumatoid and osteoarthritic cartilage. J Orthop Res 1996;14(6):946–955.

Dieppe PA, Lohmander LS. Pathogenesis and management of pain in osteoarthritis. Lancet 2005; 365(9463):965–973.

Dobnig H, Sipos A, Jiang Y, Fahrleitner-Pammer A, Ste-Marie LG, Gallagher JC, Pavo I, Wang J, Eriksen EF. Early changes in biochemical markers of bone formation correlate with improvements in bone structure during teriparatide therapy. J Clin Endocrinol Metab 2005;90(7):3970–3977.

Dove A. Biomarker database may yield blockbuster drug. Nat Med 2002;8(10):1049–1050.

Eastell R, Barton I, Hannon RA, Chines A, Garnero P, Delmas PD. Relationship of early changes in bone resorption to the reduction in fracture risk with risedronate. J Bone Miner Res 2003;18(6):1051–1056.

Elliott AL, Kraus VB, Luta G, Stabler T, Renner JB, Woodard J, Dragomir AD, Helmick CG, Hochberg MC, Jordan JM. Serum hyaluronan levels and radiographic knee and hip osteoarthritis in African Americans and Caucasians in the Johnston County Osteoarthritis Project. Arthritis Rheum 2005;52(1):105–111.

Felson DT. Clinical practice. Osteoarthritis of the knee. N Engl J Med 2006;354(8):841–848.

Felson DT. Epidemiology of osteoarthritis. In: Brandt KD, Doherty M, Lohmander LS, eds. Osteoarthritis. New York: Oxford University Press; 2003.

Felson DT, Lohmander LS. Whither osteoarthritis biomarkers? Osteoarthritis Cartilage 2009; 17(4):419–422.

Felson DT, Niu J, Guermazi A, Roemer F, Aliabadi P, Clancy M, Torner J, Lewis CE, Nevitt MC. Correlation of the development of knee pain with enlarging bone marrow lesions on magnetic resonance imaging. Arthritis Rheum 2007;56(9):2986–2992.

Flores RH, Hochberg MC. Definition and classification of osteoarthritis. In: Brandt KD, Doherty M, Lohmander LS, eds. Osteoarthritis (2nd ed.). New York: Oxford University Press; 2003.

Garnero P. Noninvasive biochemical markers in osteoarthritis. In: Moskowitz RW, Altman RD, Hochberg MC, Buckwalter JA, Goldberg VM, eds. Osteoarthritis (4th ed.). Philadelphia: Lippincott Williams & Wilkins; 2007.

Garnero P. Bone markers in osteoporosis. Curr Osteoporos Rep 2009;7(3):84–90.

Garnero P, Aronstein WS, Cohen SB, Conaghan PG, Cline GA, Christiansen C, Beary JF, Meyer JM, Bingham CO 3rd. Relationships between biochemical markers of bone and cartilage degradation with radiological progression in patients with knee osteoarthritis receiving risedronate: the Knee Osteoarthritis Structural Arthritis randomized clinical trial. Osteoarthritis Cartilage 2008;16(6):660–666.

Garnero P, Delmas PD. Biomarkers in osteoarthritis. Curr Opin Rheumatol 2003;15(5):641–646.

Garnero P, Peterfy C, Zaim S, Schoenharting M. Bone marrow abnormalities on magnetic resonance imaging are associated with type II collagen degradation in knee osteoarthritis: a three-month longitudinal study. Arthritis Rheum 2005;52(9):2822–2829.

Garnero P, Piperno M, Gineyts E, Christgau S, Delmas PD, Vignon E. Cross sectional evaluation of biochemical markers of bone, cartilage, and synovial tissue metabolism in patients with knee osteoarthritis: relations with disease activity and joint damage. Ann Rheum Dis 2001;60(6):619–626.

Garnero P, Rousseau JC, Delmas PD. Molecular basis and clinical use of biochemical markers of bone, cartilage, and synovium in joint diseases. Arthritis Rheum 2000;43(5):953–968.

Gineyts E, Garnero P, Delmas PD. Urinary excretion of glucosyl-galactosyl pyridinoline: a specific biochemical marker of synovium degradation. Rheumatology (Oxford) 2001;40(3):315–323.

Gineyts E, Mo JA, Ko A, Henriksen DB, Curtis SP, Gertz BJ, Garnero P, Delmas PD. Effects of ibuprofen on molecular markers of cartilage and synovium turnover in patients with knee osteoarthritis. Ann Rheum Dis 2004;63(7):857–861.

Glover SJ, Gall M, Schoenborn-Kellenberger O, Wagener M, Garnero P, Boonen S, Cauley JA, Black DM, Delmas PD, Eastell R. Establishing a reference interval for bone turnover markers in 637 healthy, young, premenopausal women from the United Kingdom, France, Belgium, and the United States. J Bone Miner Res 2009;24(3):389–397.

Goldring MB, Goldring SR. Osteoarthritis. J Cell Physiol 2007;213(3):626–634.

Hochberg MC. Nutritional supplements for knee osteoarthritis—still no resolution. N Engl J Med 2006;354(8): 858–860.

Hochberg MC, Zhan M, Langenberg P. The rate of decline of joint space width in patients with osteoarthritis of the knee: a systematic review and meta-analysis of randomized placebo-controlled trials of chondroitin sulfate. Curr Med Res Opin 2008;4(11):3029–3035.

Javaid MK, Lynch JA, Tolstykh I, Guermazi A, Roemer F, Aliabadi P, McCulloch C, et al. Pre-radiographic MRI findings are associated with onset of knee symptoms: the most study. Osteoarthritis Cartilage 2010; 18(3):323–328.

Jordan KM, Syddall HE, Garnero P, Gineyts E, Dennison EM, Sayer v, Delmas PD, Cooper C, Arden NK. Urinary CTX-II and glucosyl-galactosyl-pyridinoline are associated with the presence and severity of radiographic knee osteoarthritis in men. Ann Rheum Dis 2006;65(7):871–877.

Jung M, Christgau S, Lukoschek M, Henriksen D, Richter W. Increased urinary concentration of collagen type II C-telopeptide fragments in patients with osteoarthritis. Pathobiology 2004;71(2):70–76.

Kahan A, Uebelhart D, De Vathaire F, Delmas PD, Reginster JY. Long-term effects of chondroitins 4 and 6 sulfate on knee osteoarthritis: the study on osteoarthritis progression prevention, a two-year, randomized, double-blind, placebo-controlled trial. Arthritis Rheum 2009;60(2):524–533.

Kim S. Changes in surgical loads and economic burden of hip and knee replacements in the US: 1997–2004. Arthritis Rheum 2008;59(4):481–488.

King KB, Lindsey CT, Dunn TC, Ries MD, Steinbach LS, Majumdar S. A study of the relationship between molecular biomarkers of joint degeneration and the magnetic resonance-measured characteristics of cartilage in 16 symptomatic knees. Magn Reson Imaging 2004;22(8):1117–1123.

Konttinen YT, Saari H, Honkanen VE, Szocsik K, Mussalo-Rauhamaa H, Tulensalo R, Friman C. Serum baseline hyaluronate and disease activity in rheumatoid arthritis. Clin Chim Acta 1990;193(1–2):39–47.

Krasnokutsky S, Attur M, Palmer G, Samuels J, Abramson SB. Current concepts in the pathogenesis of osteoarthritis. Osteoarthritis Cartilage 2008;16(Suppl 3):S1-S3.

Kraus VB. Do biochemical markers have a role in osteoarthritis diagnosis and treatment? Best Pract Res Clin Rheumatol 2006;20(1):69–80.

Laurent TC, Dahl IM, Dahl LB, Engstrom-Laurent A, Eriksson S, Fraser JR, Granath KA, et al. The catabolic fate of hyaluronic acid. Connect Tissue Res 1986;15(1–2):33–41.

Laurent TC, Laurent UB, Fraser JR. Serum hyaluronan as a disease marker. Ann Med 1996;28(3):241–253.

Lohmander LS, Brandt KD, Mazzuca SA, Katz BP, Larsson S, Struglics A, Lane KA. Use of the plasma stromelysin (matrix metalloproteinase 3) concentration to predict joint space narrowing in knee osteoarthritis. Arthritis Rheum 2005;52(10):3160–3167.

Lohmander LS, Eyre D. Biochemical markers as surrogate endpoints of joint disease. In: Reid DM, Miller CG, eds. Clinical Trials in Rheumatoid Arthritis and Osteoarthritis. London: Springer Verlag; 2008.

Mazieres B, Garnero P, Gueguen A, Abbal M, Berdah L, Lequesne M, Nguyen M, Salles JP, Vignon E, Dougados M. Molecular markers of cartilage breakdown and synovitis at baseline as predictors of structural progression of hip osteoarthritis. The ECHODIAH Cohort. Ann Rheum Dis 2006;65(3):354–359.

McNeil BJ, Hanley JA. Statistical approaches to the analysis of receiver operating characteristic (ROC) curves. Med Decis Making 1984;4(2):137–150.

Meulenbelt I, Kloppenburg M, Kroon HM, Houwing-Duistermaat JJ, Garnero P, Hellio Le Graverand MP, Degroot J, Slagboom PE. Urinary CTX-II levels are associated with radiographic subtypes of osteoarthritis in hip, knee, hand, and facet joints in subject with familial osteoarthritis at multiple sites: the GARP study. Ann Rheum Dis 2006;65(3):360–365.

Muller G, Michel A, Altenburg E. COMP (cartilage oligomeric matrix protein) is synthesized in ligament, tendon, meniscus, and articular cartilage. Connect Tissue Res 1998;39(4):233–244.

Nelson F, Dahlberg L, Laverty S, Reiner A, Pidoux I, Ionescu M, Fraser GL, et al. Evidence for altered synthesis of type II collagen in patients with osteoarthritis. J Clin Invest 1998;102(12):2115–2125.

Nishida Y, D'Souza AL, Thonar EJ, Knudson W. Stimulation of hyaluronan metabolism by interleukin-1alpha in human articular cartilage. Arthritis Rheum 2000;43(6):1315–1326.

Nishizawa Y, Nakamura T, Ohta H, Kushida K, Gorai I, Shiraki M, Fukunaga M, et al. Guidelines for the use of biochemical markers of bone turnover in osteoporosis (2004). J Bone Miner Metab 2005;23(2):97–104.

Pelletier JP, Martel-Pelletier J, Abramson SB. Osteoarthritis, an inflammatory disease: potential implication for the selection of new therapeutic targets. Arthritis Rheum 2001;44(6):1237–1247.

Petersen SG, Saxne T, Heinegard D, Hansen M, Holm L, Koskinen S, Stordal C, Christensen H, Aagaard P, Kjaer M. Glucosamine but not ibuprofen alters cartilage turnover in osteoarthritis patients in response to physical training. Osteoarthritis Cartilage 2010;18(1):34–40.

Pollard TC, Gwilym SE, Carr AJ. The assessment of early osteoarthritis. J Bone Joint Surg Br 2008; 90(4):411–421.

Reijman M, Hazes JM, Bierma-Zeinstra SM, Koes BW, Christgau S, Christiansen C, Uitterlinden AG, Pols HA. A new marker for osteoarthritis: cross-sectional and longitudinal approach. Arthritis Rheum 2004;50(8):2471–2478.

Rizkalla G, Reiner A, Bogoch E, Poole AR. Studies of the articular cartilage proteoglycan aggrecan in health and osteoarthritis. Evidence for molecular heterogeneity and extensive molecular changes in disease. J Clin Invest 1992;90(6):2268–2277.

Rousseau JC, Delmas PD. Biological markers in osteoarthritis. Nat Clin Pract Rheumatol 2007;3(6):346–356.

Rousseau JC, Zhu Y, Miossec P, Vignon E, Sandell LJ, Garnero P, Delmas PD. Serum levels of type IIA procollagen amino terminal propeptide (PIIANP) are decreased in patients with knee osteoarthritis and rheumatoid arthritis. Osteoarthritis Cartilage 2004;12(6):440–447.

Sharif M, George E, Shepstone L, Knudson W, Thonar EJ, Cushnaghan J, Dieppe P. Serum hyaluronic acid level as a predictor of disease progression in osteoarthritis of the knee. Arthritis Rheum 1995;38(6):760–767.

Sharif M, Kirwan J, Charni N, Sandell LJ, Whittles C, Garnero P. A 5-yr longitudinal study of type IIA collagen synthesis and total type II collagen degradation in patients with knee osteoarthritis—association with disease progression. Rheumatology (Oxford) 2007;46(6):938–943.

Sharif M, Kirwan JR, Elson CJ, Granell R, Clarke S. Suggestion of nonlinear or phasic progression of knee osteoarthritis based on measurements of serum cartilage oligomeric matrix protein levels over five years. Arthritis Rheum 2004;50(8):2479–2488.

Sharif M, Shepstone L, Elson CJ, Dieppe PA, Kirwan JR. Increased serum C reactive protein may reflect events that precede radiographic progression in osteoarthritis of the knee. Ann Rheum Dis 2000;59(1):71–74.

Sharma L, Hurwitz DE, Thonar EJ, Sum JA, Lenz ME, Dunlop DD, Schnitzer TJ, Kirwan-Mellis G, Andriacchi TP. Knee adduction moment, serum hyaluronan level, and disease severity in medial tibiofemoral osteoarthritis. Arthritis Rheum 1998;41(7):1233–1240.

Shinmei M, Ito K, Matsuyama S, Yoshihara Y, Matsuzawa K. Joint fluid carboxy-terminal type II procollagen peptide as a marker of cartilage collagen biosynthesis. Osteoarthritis Cartilage 1993;1(2):121–128.

Sowers M, Lachance L, Jamadar D, Hochberg MC, Hollis B, Crutchfield M, Jannausch ML. The associations of bone mineral density and bone turnover markers with osteoarthritis of the hand and knee in pre- and perimenopausal women. Arthritis Rheum 1999;42(3):483–489.

Sugiyama S, Itokazu M, Suzuki Y, Shimizu K. Procollagen II C propeptide level in the synovial fluid as a predictor of radiographic progression in early knee osteoarthritis. Ann Rheum Dis 2003;62(1):27–32.

Turan Y, Bal S, Gurgan A, Topac H, Koseoglu M. Serum hyaluronan levels in patients with knee osteoarthritis. Clin Rheumatol 2007;26(8):1293–1298.

Vilim V, Olejarova M, Machacek S, Gatterova J, Kraus VB, Pavelka K. Serum levels of cartilage oligomeric matrix protein (COMP) correlate with radiographic progression of knee osteoarthritis. Osteoarthritis Cartilage 2002;10(9):707–713.

Vilim V, Vytasek R, Olejarova M, Machacek S, Gatterova J, Prochazka B, Kraus VB, Pavelka K. Serum cartilage oligomeric matrix protein reflects the presence of clinically diagnosed synovitis in patients with knee osteoarthritis. Osteoarthritis Cartilage 2001;9(7):612–618.

Weinstein RS. True strength. J Bone Miner Res 2000;15(4):621–625.

Westacott CI. Subchondral bone in the pathogenesis of osteoarthritis. Biological effects. In: Brandt KD, Doherty M, Lohmander LS, eds. Osteoarthritis. New York: Oxford University Press; 2003.

Wieland HA, Michaelis M, Kirschbaum BJ, Rudolphi KA. Osteoarthritis—an untreatable disease? Nat Rev Drug Discov 2005;4(4):331–344.

Young-Min SA, Cawston TE, Griffiths ID. Markers of joint destruction: principles, problems, and potential. Ann Rheum Dis 2001;60(6):545–548.

Zhang W, Moskowitz RW, Nuki G, Abramson S, Altman RD, Arden N, Bierma-Zeinstra S, et al. OARSI recommendations for the management of hip and knee osteoarthritis. Part I: critical appraisal of existing treatment guidelines and systematic review of current research evidence. Osteoarthritis Cartilage 2007;15(9):981–1000.

Zhang W, Moskowitz RW, Nuki G, Abramson S, Altman RD, Arden N, Bierma-Zeinstra S, et al. OARSI recommendations for the management of hip and knee osteoarthritis, Part II: OARSI evidence-based, expert consensus guidelines. Osteoarthritis Cartilage 2008;16(2):137–162.

4 Rheumatoid Arthritis
Disease Pathophysiology

Ankit Saxena, Smriti K. Raychaudhuri, and Siba P. Raychaudhuri

CONTENTS

INTRODUCTION

Rheumatoid arthritis (RA) is a systemic, chronic inflammatory disease that is manifested as a destructive polyarthritis in association with serological evidence of autoreactivity. It is characterized by chronic pain and joint destruction, premature mortality, and elevated risk of disability, with high costs for those suffering from this disease and for the society. It affects up to 0.5%–1% of the world's population, with a male-to-female ratio of 3:1, and is the most common inflammatory joint disease. The onset of disease can occur at any age; however, the prevalence increases with age and the peak incidence is between the fourth and the sixth decade (Abdel-Nasser et al., 1997). Clinically, RA is symmetrical polyarticular arthritis marked by chronic systemic inflammation, synovial infiltrates, and progressive cell-mediated destruction of the joints and their adjacent chronic inflammation of the synovium along with various clinical features of a systemic disease. The disease is characterized by persistent and progressive synovitis of peripheral joints, leading to destruction of cartilage and subchondral bone. The pathogenic basis of RA is a sustained specific immune response against yet unknown self-antigens. It is believed that in RA, the persistent autoimmune response mediates local synovial inflammation and cellular infiltration, which ultimately result in tissue damage. The two main pathophysiologic events leading to RA are (1) hyperplastic synovial lining cells, the layer in direct contact with the intra-articular cavity, and (2) mononuclear cell infiltration in the subintimal layer. The hyperplastic lining is composed of macrophage-like type I synoviocyte and fibroblast-like type II synoviocyte. Many cell groups exist in the infiltrate of the subintimal synovial layer, including T cells, B cells, dendritic cells (DCs), macrophages, fibroblasts, granulocytes, and mast cells. Another major pathological phenomenon in RA is the formation of a destructive type of tissue that invades at the interface between cartilage and bone and is known as pannus. Pannus formation is one of the distinctive characteristic features of RA, which makes it distinct from other inflammatory arthropathies. Eventually, the chronic synovitis can progress to destruction of adjacent bone and cartilage, leading to joint deformity and disability.

Recent advancements in the field of immunology and rheumatology have helped in development of better understanding of the immune dysfunction in RA. Treatment has evolved from nonspecific immunosuppressive therapy to specific molecule-targeted biologics such as anticytokine agents, T-cell costimulator blocking agents, and anti-B-cell agents and signal kinase inhibitors (Cohen, 2002). More drug targets on the basis of immune mechanisms are on the horizon. However, in daily practice, the use of recently developed therapeutic agents as well as traditional disease modifying antirheumatic drugs (DMARDs) is based on the clinical course and response to previous therapy rather than the individual features of immune dysfunction.

The search for disease markers to predict outcome and therapeutic response in individual patients is of great interest. Here we will describe current understandings of immune dysfunction in RA and lessons learned from animal models of autoimmune arthritis.

T CELLS IN RA

Patients with RA frequently carry clonal T-cell populations. These clones give rise to several percent of circulating lymphocytes, suggesting that the clonal sizes are in the order of 1×10^9–1×10^{10} lymphocytes. Large clonal expansions of CD8 T cells in the circulation as well as the synovial tissue of patients with RA that shared the usage of the T-cell receptor (TCR)-AV12 gene segment has been reported (DerSimonian et al., 1993). Such CD8 clones can also be found in healthy elderly individuals, but they appear to be more frequent in patients with RA. A clonal expansion of CD4 T cells is rarely observed in healthy individuals but is a common finding in patients with RA (Goronzy et al., 1994). These clones may possibly arise in response to chronic stimulation with antigen; however, comparing the expanded clones in paired samples of synovial tissue and peripheral blood of patients with RA, it was observed that the clones are present in the synovial tissue but are not selectively enriched, suggesting that the antigen is not selectively expressed in the joint (Gonzalez-Quintial et al., 1996; Rittner et al., 1997). CD4 T-cell clones from the peripheral blood of patients with RA have been isolated and clonally expanded for similar studies (Schmidt et al., 1996). These clones characteristically lacked the expression of the CD28 molecule and proliferated to autologous monocytes. CD8 T-cell clones in patients with RA also appear to recognize autoantigens; at least for one of these clones, the antigen could be identified (Behar et al., 1998). Taken together, these data provide evidence that patients with RA clonally expand CD4 and CD8 T cells and that at least some of these clones recognize autoantigens that are not specific for the synovium, such as peptides derived from self–major histocompatibility complex (MHC) molecules. The clonal expansion of such autoreactive T cells could indeed indicate a defect in thymic selection.

CD4+ T cells comprise almost 50% of the total cellular infiltrates in RA synovium. Activated CD4+ T cells infiltrates, found in the inflammatory rheumatoid synovium, propel local inflammation via their effector functions. Transfer of CD4+ T cells from sick animals into healthy syngeneic recipients can initiate tissue damaging autoimmunity (Banerjee et al., 1992). The association of aggressive forms of the disease with particular MHC II alleles, such as subtypes of HLA-DR4 that contain similar amino acid motifs in the CDR3 region of the DRβ-chain (Calin et al., 1989), remains as the most compelling evidence implying a central role for CD4 T cells in propagating rheumatoid inflammation. Inheritance of these genes increases risks for RA and predicts severity of disease in North Americans (Young et al., 1984). Individual alleles have been found in several subsets in the HLA-DR4 family, which codes for the β-chain of HLA class II antigen. The presence of HLA-DRB1 increases relative risk from 1.5- to 6-fold in different populations. These genotypes have a strong association with susceptibility, severity, and response to treatment (O'Dell et al., 1998). The common sequence was found in the third hypervariable region of HLA-DR β-chain, which is particularly amino acids 70–74 (QKRAA or QRRAA) (Nepom et al., 1989). This common sequence led to the shared epitope hypothesis and has been found not only in the DR4 family but also in DR1, DR6, and DR10 genes with increased risk of RA in different ethnic groups (Willkens et al., 1991; De Vries et al., 1993; Yelamos et al., 1993). The mechanism by which the shared epitope predisposes or causes RA is unknown. Several potential mechanisms have been suggested to explain how this sequence may influence the interaction between the TCR, a peptide (antigen), and the MHC molecule. The shared epitope may bind to arthritogenic peptides, foreign or self, that can be presented to T cells. Alternatively, it can influence the direct recognition of the MHC–peptide complex by T cells, or a combination of these events could be at play. This could result in peptide-specific TCR recognition, selection of autoreactive T cells, or both. Genetic typing adds to early identification of patients with poor prognosis. Although the exact meaning of this association has not been resolved, all interpretations imply that CD4 T cells orchestrate local inflammation and cellular infiltration, following which a large number of subsequent inflammatory events are unleashed. Thus, T cells and in particular CD4+ T cells are central for both the induction and the effector phases of specific immune responses in RA and therefore represent an ideal target for immunotherapy. Although the antigen(s) involved in the initiation of synovitis in RA remains elusive, several candidate antigens have been found to trigger antigen-specific T-cell proliferation in animal models of arthritis.

In vitro T-cell proliferation assays have revealed autoreactive T-cell clones against type II collagen (CII), proteoglycan, and heat shock proteins (HSP) in animal model studies. The collagen-induced arthritis (CIA) model is similar to human RA in many aspects (Brand et al., 2003). Peripheral arthritis is induced in susceptible strains of mice with CII emulsified in complete or incomplete Freund adjuvant. The development of arthritis against collagen is linked to MHC class II (H-2^r, H-2^q) in mice. Susceptible strains carry H-2^q and H-2^r, but there is no distinctive sequence similarities, suggesting a role for a shared epitope in CIA. HLA-DR transgenic mice develop arthritis with bovine or human CII in nonsusceptible strains. There is a Th1 cytokine (interleukin-2 [IL-2], interferon-gamma [IFN-γ]) activation pattern with development of arthritis. A B-cell response with anti-CII antibody is critical to develop arthritis. Passive transfer of arthritis can be induced with serum (Stuart and Dixon, 1983) but not with CII-specific T cells. CII-specific T cells are necessary but not sufficient for the development of CIA. In humans, anti-CII antibody is detected, but it is neither sensitive nor specific to RA. The CIA model has been a valuable asset for the design and testing of new treatments in RA.

In the adjuvant arthritis model, polyarthritis is produced in rats with a single intradermal injection of complete Freund's adjuvant (Prakken et al., 2003). The animals may develop not only arthritis but also systemic inflammation such as uveitis or GI tract inflammation. The presence of mycobacteria in complete Freund's adjuvant suggests a link between infection and arthritis. Arthritis can be transferred with a single T-cell clone. T-cell epitope mapping shows a sequence derived from a mycobacterial hsp65. Immunization with whole mycobacterial HSP65 protects the rats from arthritis. HSPs are highly conserved cellular proteins for stabilizing the structure and function of proteins against environmental insults such as heat, infection, or oxidative injury. Expression of HSP is increased at sites of inflammation. Bacterial HSP are strong immunogens that could cause cross-recognition of self-HSP, suggesting a link between infection and autoimmunity.

Human cartilage glycoprotein-39 (HCgp-39) is a secretory product of both synovial fibroblast and chondrocyte. It is expressed in synovial joint during inflammation. Of patients with RA, 40%–50% have recall-type proliferative T-cell responses to HCgp-39. Very little humoral response to HCgp-39 has been observed. Transgenic mice have been generated with HCgp-39 and DR0401, in the hope that this antigen can be presented with shared epitope to T cells. However, these transgenic mice did not develop arthritis (Sonderstrup, 2003).

SKG mice spontaneously develop T-cell-mediated chronic autoimmune arthritis as a consequence of a mutation of the gene encoding ZAP-70, which is a key signal transduction molecule in T cells (Sakaguchi et al., 2003). This mutation impairs positive and negative selection of T cells in the thymus, leading to thymic production of arthritogenic T cells. SKG mice develop severe arthritis spontaneously and also extra-articular manifestations, such as interstitial pneumonitis, vasculitis, and subcutaneous nodules. High titers of rheumatoid factor (RF) and anti-CII antibody are found in these mice. CD4+ T cells can adoptively transfer arthritis from SKG mice to T-cell-deficient BALB/c nude mice.

The concepts of T-cell subpopulations and the understanding of how T cells function in RA are also evolving (Figure 4.1). Cytokine/chemokine profiles of T-helper 1 (Th1), Th2, and Th17 cells are described in Table 4.1. Classic T-helper 1 (Th1) versus Th2 paradigms for T-cell activation fit poorly in models of RA pathogenesis. Very little, if any, Th1 (e.g., IFN-γ) or Th2 (e.g., IL-4) cytokines were identified in synovial tissues or fluid (Van der Graaff et al., 1999). Recent characterization of a Th17 cell subset, characterized by secretion of IL-17, provides new insight into how T cells may function in RA. Unlike IFN-γ or IL-4, IL-17 is abundantly produced by RA synovium and is a potent stimulus of the synovial lining layer. Blockade of IL-17 has been shown to treat several animals of arthritis while local overexpression exacerbates disease, suggesting a critical role for this T-cell cytokine in RA (Li et al., 2010). Th17-driven inflammation during host defense markedly resembles the inflamed synovial tissue in RA and other forms of autoimmune arthritis. The RA synovium is characterized by elevated levels of IL-6, TNF-α, and IL-1β along with nitric oxide and prostaglandin E2 (PGE2) (Afzali et al., 2007). Th17 cells and IL-17 in particular have been shown to synergize with or upregulate each of these proinflammatory factors. IL-17 mediates the induction of IL-6 and IL-8 in both adult RA and juvenile idiopathic arthritis (Bertazzolo et al., 1994; Hwang et al., 2004; Saxena et al., 2005; Agarwal et al., 2008); these cytokines are associated with inflammation in synovial fluid and activate fibroblast-like synoviocytes through the phosphatidylinositol 3-kinase/Akt and nuclear factor κB (NF-κB) pathways (Georganas et al., 2000). In addition, IL-17 induces the expression of cyclooxygenase-2 (COX-2) in synoviocytes, a stress response molecule conducive to the high levels of PGE2 observed during inflammation (Stamp et al., 2004). Although *in vitro* cultures have suggested a regulatory role for PGE2 (Stamp et al., 2004; Lemos et al., 2009), experimental models of arthritis demonstrate that deficiency in COX-2 or the major inducible PGE2 synthetase attenuates acute and chronic inflammation (Strassmann et al., 1994; Myers et al., 2000; Shinomiya et al., 2001; Trebino et al., 2003). Furthermore, PGE2 favors the expansion of the Th17 lineage by shifting the DC phenotype away from the IL-12 axis in favor of IL-23 (Sheibanie et al.,

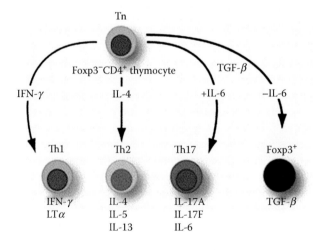

FIGURE 4.1   T-cell subsets in RA: Fate of naive T cells is determined by the cytokine milieu in which they develop. Development of effector T cells-Th1, Th2, and Th17 is facilitated by cytokines like IFN-γ, IL-4, IL-6, and IL-23, whereas development of regulatory T cells occurs in the presence of TGF-β without IL-6. Breach of this balance may lead to the autoimmune activation of T cells.

TABLE 4.1
Cytokine and Chemokine Profiles of Th1, Th2, and Th17 Cells

	Th1	Th2	Th17
IL-2	+	–	+
IL-4	–	+	–
IFN-γ	+	–	–
IL-10	–	+	–
TGF-β	–	+	+
IL-5	–	+	–
IL-17A	–	–	+
IL-17F	–	–	+
IL-6	–	–	+
TNF	+	–	+
IL-22	–	–	+
IL-12Rb2	+	–	–
IL-23R	–	–	+
Granzyme	+	–	–
Fas ligand	+	–	–
TRAIL	+	–	–
CCL5	+	–	–
CCL6	–	–	+
α3 Integrin	–	–	+

Abbreviation: TRAIL, tumor necrosis factor-related apoptosis-inducing ligand.

2007; Khayrullina et al., 2008). Through synergy with TNF, IL-17 has also been proposed to induce the alternative complement pathway proteins C3 and factor B, both of which are upregulated in RA synovial tissue (Katz et al., 2000). Abnormalities in the activation of the alternative complement pathway have been observed in RA synovium (Mollnes et al., 1986) and have been implicated in pathogenesis in autoimmune arthritis models (Banda et al., 2006; Katschke et al., 2007). In addition, IL-17 activates RA synovial fibroblasts through the PI2K/Akt, p38 MAPK, and NF-κB signaling pathways, inducing the IL-23-specific subunit, IL-23p19, in a probable positive feedback loop (Kim et al., 2007). Two other members of the IL-17 cytokine family, IL-17B and IL-17C, have also been implicated in chronic inflammation in an experimental model of arthritis; CD4+ T cells transduced with IL-17B or IL-17C exacerbated murine CIA to the same degree as IL-17, and both cytokines stimulated the expression of proinflammatory IL-1β, IL-6, TNF, and IL-23 (Yamaguchi et al., 2007). Although comparatively few studies have examined the relationship between IL-17 and the autoantibodies characteristic of RA, recently the B-cell-activating factor, associated with autoantibody production, and an associated family member TNFSF13 (or APRIL) have been demonstrated to regulate the production of IL-17 in CIA (Pers et al., 2005; Lai Kwan Lam et al., 2008; Swaidani et al., 2009). Taken together, these data are consistent with the localization of CD4+ T cells to the inflammatory pannus tissue formed during CIA (Ju et al., 2008; Xiao et al., 2008). However, qualifying these reports, a recent animal study suggests that IL-17 can only augment the inflammatory reaction rather than initiate it (Maione et al., 2009).

Analysis of the frequency of peripheral blood CD4+ CD25+ regulatory T cells (Tregs) in patients with RA has yielded contradictory results (Leipe et al., 2005). Although some papers have reported an increased frequency of peripheral blood Tregs (Van Amelsfort et al., 2004), others have demonstrated either no difference in the frequency of Tregs compared with healthy donors or a decreased level of peripheral blood Tregs (Cao et al., 2004; Ehrenstein et al., 2004; Mottonen et al., 2005; Benito-Miguel et al., 2009). These conflicting results might be in part due to the different methodologies used to analyze the Treg populations. In contrast, however, there is clear evidence that the frequency of CD4+ CD25+ Tregs is higher in the synovial fluid than that in peripheral blood of patients with RA (Lawson et al., 2006). These results are consistent with those observed in other arthropathies such as JIA and spondylarthropathies (Cao et al., 2003). The reasons for the increased frequencies of Tregs in inflamed synovia are not known. In addition to preferential homing to synovia from peripheral blood, it is possible that Treg population expands within the synovia. However, the persistence of inflammation in the rheumatoid joints despite the increased number of Tregs indicates that these cells are ineffective in controlling the inflammatory response. One possible explanation is that Tregs in the joint are defective in mediating their suppressive, anti-inflammatory activity.

Consistent with the general features described for these cells, CD4+ CD25+ Tregs isolated from patients with active RA show the expression of FoxP3, an anergic phenotype upon TCR stimulation, and an ability to suppress the proliferation of effector T cells from synovia and from peripheral blood *in vitro* (Sakaguchi, 2005). However, these Tregs are able to neither suppress proinflammatory cytokine secretion from activated T cells and monocytes nor confer a suppressive phenotype on "conventional" T cells (de Kleer et al., 2004). A recent study by demonstrated that TNF-α, one of the major inflammatory cytokines in the inflamed joint, inhibits the suppressive function of naturally occurring CD4+ CD25+ Tregs and transforming growth factor β1 (TGF-β1)–induced CD4+ CD25+ Tregs (Valencia et al., 2006). The mechanism of this inhibition was shown to involve signaling through TNFRII, which is constitutively expressed on unstimulated Tregs, and the expression of which is upregulated by TNF-α. TNF-α-mediated inhibition of suppressive function was associated with a decrease in the expression of FoxP3 mRNA and protein by CD4+ CD25 high Tregs isolated from patients with active RA (Valencia et al., 2006). The results suggest an interaction between the innate and the adaptive immune systems, in which TNF-α, a product of the innate immune compartment, could promote immune reactivity by limiting the action of Tregs.

There has been progress in targeting T cells for the treatment of RA. Early efforts involving anti-CD4, anti-CD5, and anti-CD52 (alemtuzumab [CAMPATH-1H/CamPath; Berlex Oncology, Richmond CA, USA]) monoclonal antibodies failed to provide consistent or sustained clinical benefit. T-cell costimulatory molecules are new targets for RA (Genovese et al., 2005). Once antigen presentation by MHC molecule activates naive T cells, they require additional signals from interactions between T-cell costimulatory ligands and their receptors for activation, clonal expansion, and survival as effector T cells (Kremer et al., 2005). Of the several costimulatory receptors in the T-cell surface, CD28 is critical to activate naive T cells; otherwise, T cells become anergic. CD80/86 is the ligand for CD28, which is expressed on the surface of antigen-presenting cells. Cytotoxic T-lymphocyte-associated antigen-4 (CTLA4) is one of the costimulatory receptors that can bind to CD80/86 and suppress T-cell activation. Because CTLA4 has higher affinity to CD80/86, a fusion protein of CTLA4 and immunoglobulin (CTLA4–Ig) can suppress T-cell activation by blocking the CD28-mediated costimulation. Clinical trials using CTLA4–Ig with methotrexate showed 60% of ACR20 response (Kremer et al., 2003). This T-cell-targeting therapeutic may be released for clinical use in the near future.

B CELLS AND AUTOANTIBODY

Since the discovery of RF in 1939, numerous antibodies have been identified in the serum of patients with RA, including antibodies against CII, HSPs, cyclic citrullinated peptide (CCP), glucose 6-phosphate isomerase (GPI), BiP (immunoglobulin heavy gene binding protein), and hnRNP-33 (RA33). Those self-reactive antibodies strongly suggest B-cell involvement in pathogenesis of RA. Although the serum transfer from active patients with RA to healthy subjects did not trigger any joint inflammation (Harris and Vaughan, 1961), arthritis can be induced with serum transfer in some animal models.

The major evidence of B-cell activation is the presence of RF. RF is an antibody that binds the Fc portion of aggregated immunoglobulin G and is present in 60%–70% of patients with RA. Naturally occurring RF is produced by CD5+ B cells, and almost every healthy individual has a low level of RF of immunoglobulin M isotype. RF is found in 75%–80% of patients with RA and is associated with a more aggressive and destructive course. This suggested that RA could be a disease mediated by autoantibodies. However, RF can be found in the normal population ranging from 3% to 25%, and the incidence increases with aging. It can be induced during several chronic infections such as tuberculosis, hepatitis C, endocarditis, and parasite infection.

A serum transfer model of arthritis, the K/BxN transgenic mouse model, is a new murine model of spontaneous arthritis. These transgenic mice express TCR reactive against bovine ribonuclease in the background of NOD (I-A^{g7}) mice. In this model, B cells secrete autoantibody to GPI. Arthritis in normal mice can be induced by transferring serum from this arthritic mouse to normal mice. Interestingly, anti-GPI immunoglobulin G found in human RA is not specific. Anti-GPI antibodies were frequently observed in patients with RA with the extra-articular manifestations such as rheumatoid nodules, vasculitis, and Felty's syndrome (Van Gaalen et al., 2004). GPI is glycolytic enzyme expressed by all cells. It is unclear how an antibody to such a ubiquitous antigen could cause joint-specific immune response. However, the local environment of the joint may provide some clues to understand the mechanism (Matsumoto et al., 2002). There is a lack of several complement regulatory proteins such as membrane cofactor of proteolysis and decay-accelerating factor on the surface of cartilage. Complement activation is more likely in this environment by the alternative pathway interacting with anti-GPI antibody. In addition, accumulation of extracellular GPI has been found in the cartilage surface. GPI can diffuse into the joint from the circulation, facilitated by the absence of basal membrane in the joint vasculature and might be trapped. These findings suggest that the target antigen does not need to be of articular origin.

Anti-CCP antibody is highly specific in patients with RA. Initially, it was reported as anti-perinuclear factor in buccal mucosa cell substrate and antikeratin antibody in rat esophagus samples. It was determined that these autoantibodies recognize epidermal filaggrin containing citrulline residues. There was a great interest in determining why an autoantibody from arthritis patients reacts with an antigen of epithelial origin. It turned out that all of these antibodies react with citrulline-containing peptides. Anti-Sa antibody has been known to be highly specific for RA, and its reactivity has been reported to unknown antigen in the placenta and spleen (Despres et al., 1994). Recently, the target antigen to anti-Sa antibody has been also found to be citrullinated vimentin (Vossenaar et al., 2004). Candidate citrullinated autoantigens are filaggrin, fibrin, vimentin, keratin, and histone, and their role in the development of RA needs to be evaluated further.

The currently available anti-CCP ELISA test uses as a substrate a synthetic cyclic peptide variant that contains citrulline (Schellekens et al., 2000). Anti-CCP antibody has several interesting clinical associations in RA. Anti-CCP antibody is found in 60%–80% of patients with RA, and its specificity is up to 98%. Anti-CCP antibody is detectable in the early stages of RA even before clinical synovitis is apparent (Rantapaa-Dahlqvist et al., 2003). The presence of anti-CCP antibody may help predict disease outcome. Patients with anti-CCP antibody develop more severe radiologic changes (Kroot et al., 2000). The role of anti-CCP antibody in RA is still unclear. Is it merely an epiphenomenon in RA, or is it related to the development of the disease? Citrullination is the posttranslational deamination of arginine residues to citrulline by peptidyl arginine deiminases. Citrullination is not specific to RA and has been found in other types of inflammatory arthritis (Vossenaar et al., 2004). However, immune response to citrullinated protein might be specific to RA with certain genetic background. For example, peptidyl arginine deiminase type IV polymorphisms are associated with RA in Japanese population (Suzuki et al., 2003). There is a close relationship of anti-CCP antibody reactivity with HLA class II genes. Especially with two copies of the shared epitope, there is an increased risk for more severe disease (Van Gaalen et al., 2004). It is unknown how citrullination of protein can induce B-cell autoimmunity. Citrullination may contribute to the generation of neoepitopes by altering the character of original protein.

Epitope spreading is a diversification of B- and/or T-cell responses to a particular antigen or group of antigens over time. This is a common feature of the natural immune response to compete against some pathogens, which can rapidly develop mutations to escape host immunity. Autoantibodies can recognize more than one self-antigen through cross-reactivity of shared determinants present in autoantigens. Numerous autoantibodies have been found in RA. With the progression of arthritis, more autoantibodies are found in the peripheral blood of patients with RA and CIA animal model, consistent with epitope spreading. This could be facilitated with the exposure of cryptic epitopes through inflammation or tissue destruction.

Recently, there have been reignited interests in the therapeutic manipulation of B cells in RA with the reports of efficacy of rituximab, an anti-CD20 monoclonal antibody (Edwards et al., 2004). CD20 is a cell surface marker found on early B cells through mature B cells but not in early pre B cells or plasma cells. Anti-CD20 monoclonal antibody treatment showed significant improvement in patients with RA who failed methotrexate treatment. There is substantial decrease in RF level after rituximab treatment without change in total immunoglobulin level. The production of total immunoglobulin by plasma cells is not affected by rituximab treatment.

CYTOKINES IN RA

Cytokines act as local messengers in almost all important biologic processes, including cell growth, repair, inflammation, and immunity. Many cytokines are involved in the regulation of inflammatory reactions but are also central to the progression of RA, a disease in which excess or dysregulation of proinflammatory cytokines mediates the pathological process (Table 4.1), although RA is considered as a Th1-type immune response–driven disease with significant synovial infiltration of T cells. However, low concentration of Th1 cytokines (IL-2 and IFN-γ) in synovial fluid has been found, which is called the T-cell paradox. In contrast, there is a high concentration of macrophage and fibroblast cytokines (IL-1, IL-6, IL-15, IL-18, TNF-α, and GM-CSF) in the synovial fluid. Targeting Th1 cytokines has not shown any benefit in RA, but treatment against inflammatory cytokines like TNF-α or IL-1 has shown dramatic suppression of synovitis.

PROINFLAMMATORY CYTOKINES

The important role of TNF in the proinflammatory cascade of RA has been demonstrated in the TNF-α transgenic mouse model showing overexpression of TNF-α along with development of RA-like features (Keffer et al., 1991). Multiple lines of TNF transgenic mice were generated with different constructs, and there is 100% penetration of arthritis. Transgenic mice have erosive arthritis with pannus formation, and cartilage destruction closely resembling human RA (Li and Schwarz, 2003). They have a chronic progressive course, and no joints are spared, including the temporomandibular joint. The development of arthritis is independent of T or B cells. When they are backcrossed with RAG-1 knockout mice, which do not have immunoglobulin or TCR, they still develop erosive arthritis but with less severity. Similarly, when they have a background of CIA-resistant MHC haplotypes, such as H-2^k and H-2^b, they also develop arthritis. These findings support the notion that TNF-α, once produced, is sufficient to provoke erosive arthritis. The key role of TNF in inflammatory arthritis led to the development of anti-TNF agents for the treatment of RA. Three anti-TNF agents are available. Etanercept is a fusion protein of soluble TNF receptor and immunoglobulin Fc portion. Infliximab and adalimumab are monoclonal antibodies to TNF. Anti-TNF agents have been shown to be superior to methotrexate, but the combination of these agents with methotrexate results in further improvement. Interestingly, TNF-α is not essential to develop arthritis because TNF knockout mice can develop severe CIA (Campbell et al., 2001). This may partially explain the limited response to anti-TNF agents in 20%–30% of patients with RA.

IL-1 is involved in the pathogenesis of RA by activation of T cells and stimulation of matrix metalloproteinases (MMPs) from fibroblast and chondrocytes. Studies of arthritis in animals have strongly implicated IL-1 in joint damage. Injection of IL-1 into the knee joints of rabbits results in the degradation of cartilage (Pettipher et al., 1986), whereas the injection of antibodies against IL-1 ameliorates CIA in mice and decreases the damage to cartilage (Joosten et al., 1996). Inhibition of IL-1 activity can be achieved with soluble forms of receptors and IL-1 Ra (receptor antagonist), which is naturally occurring antagonist. IL-1 Ra competes with IL-1 for its receptor but does not allow engagement of IL-1 receptor accessory protein (IL-1RacP), thereby blocking activation of signal transduction mechanisms. Anakinra is a recombinant IL-1Ra (Bresnihan et al., 1998). It has an inferior efficacy compared with anti-TNF, probably because IL-1 Ra is a competitive inhibitor for the receptor requiring a high concentration for optimal inhibition. Several clinical trials are ongoing to provide better blocking of the IL-1 signal with IL-1 neutralizing antibodies and IL-1 trap, a recombinant fusion protein of type I IL-1 receptor and IL-1RacP coupled to Fc fraction of human immunoglobulin G protein (Braddock and Quinn, 2004).

IL-6 has several distinct features including stimulations for both B- and T-cell functions as well as the production of acute phase reactants (Van Snick, 1990). It can be produced by Th2 cells for B-cell differentiation and antibody production enhancement and also by macrophages with proinflammatory action. IL-6 is present at very high levels in serum and synovial fluids of RA and of juvenile patients with RA (Guerne et al., 1989). It has a synergistic effect with IL-1 or with TNF-α to induce vascular endothelial growth factor by RA synoviocytes. IL-6-deficient mice were protected from the development of arthritis when they were backcrossed into CIA mice (Alonzi et al., 1998). An anti-IL-6 receptor blocking antibody has also been shown to be effective in human RA (Choy et al., 2002).

IL-15 is produced by macrophages and induces TNF-α with activation of T cells in an autocrine- and antigen-independent fashion. Expression of IL-15 RNA is increased in early RA synovium. Blocking IL-15 receptor has been reported to be effective in preclinical studies of CIA mice (Ferrari-Lacraz et al., 2004).

IL-17 is produced by T cells and enhances induction of proinflammatory cytokines. It is involved in the induction of COX-2 in chondrocytes and in the induction of osteoclast differentiation factor expression in osteoblasts. The association of IL-17 and IL-1 was studied using IL-1Ra-deficient mice, which can develop arthritis because of excess IL-1 signaling. The spontaneous development of arthritis did not occur in IL-1Ra$^{-/-}$ mice also deficient in IL-17. This suggests that IL-17 plays a crucial role in T-cell activation, downstream of IL-1, causing the development of autoimmune arthritis (Nakae et al., 2003). IL-17 drives neutrophil differentiation, maturation, activation, and cytokine release; monocyte activation and cytokine release; and synovial fibroblast activation, cytokine and chemokine release, prostaglandin production, and MMP synthesis (Weaver et al., 2007). The activation of DCs in the joint by IL-17 together with TNF is also likely. A synergistic effect has also been observed with low concentrations of IL-17, IL-1β, and TNF, which together leads to synovial fibroblast activation and cytokine production, indicating a pathogenic role for these inflammatory cascades (Miossec, 2003). A potent role for IL-17 in joint damage has also been proposed (Lubberts et al., 2005; Steinman, 2007). That TH17 cells may mediate their effects via other cytokines is also now becoming clear. For example, the IL-10 family member IL-22 is also produced by TH17 cells in response to IL-6 or IL-23 stimulation and has recently been shown to promote inflammation in the skin and to modulate cutaneous acanthosis (Zheng et al., 2007). The expression of IL-22 and its receptor has been detected in rheumatoid synovial membranes, but rather than being associated with T cells, they were mainly associated respectively with CD68+ or vimentin+ cells, which are indicative of macro phages or synovial fibroblasts (Ikeuchi et al., 2005).

IL-18 is a proinflammatory cytokine, which can activate T cells, NK cells, macrophages, neutrophils, and nonlymphoid cells and induce production of several proinflammatory and cytotoxic mediators. Also, it inhibits osteoclast formation. There are structural similarities between IL-1β and IL-18. It was originally described as IFN-γ-inducing factor because it induces a Th1 phenotype such IFN-γ production in combination with IL-12. Injection of IL-18 into mouse footpad leads to the local accumulation of inflammatory cells (Komai-Koma et al., 2003). IL-18 deficiency ameliorates the development of arthritis in CIA mice (Wei et al., 2001).

ANTI-INFLAMMATORY CYTOKINES

IL-10 is produced by monocytes, macrophages, and Th2 lymphocytes. It inhibits proliferation of Th1 lymphocytes, activated macrophages, and DCs (Isomäki and Punnonen, 1997). IL-10 showed inhibition of proinflammatory cytokine production of stimulated RA mononuclear cells with an additive effect of IL-4 (Van Roon et al., 1996). *In vitro*, IL-4 inhibits the activation of type I helper T cells, and this in turn decreases the production of IL-1 and TNF-α and inhibits cartilage damage (Van Roon et al., 1995). IL-4 also inhibits the production of IL-6 and IL-8 (Sugiyama et al., 1995). In cultures of synovium samples from patients with RA, IL-4 inhibited the production of IL-1 and increased the expression of IL-1-receptor antagonist, both of which actions should decrease inflammation (Chomarat et al., 1995). However, recombinant human IL-10 and IL-4 clinical trials in patients with RA did not reveal significant clinical benefits despite efficacy in experimental models (Smolen and Steiner, 2003).

CHEMOKINES (CHEMOTACTIC CYTOKINES)

Chemokine is a large family of cytokines that regulates the migration of neutrophils, lymphocytes, and monocytes from the blood to tissues such as synovium. Chemokines are produced by a variety of cell types either constitutively or in response to inflammatory stimuli. The chemokine binds to its receptor on the target cell surface for recruitment and positioning in the inflammatory tissue. For example, IL-8 (CXCL8) recruits neutrophils and Eotaxin (CCL11) recruits eosinophils. Although there is some target cell specificity, multiple chemokines can bind the same receptor. So far, 50 chemokines and 20 chemokine receptors have been found in the human chemokine system. Depending on the spacing of cysteine residues in the N-terminal region, chemokines are divided into four structural families, for example, CXC, CC, CX3C, and C.

Chemokines play an important role in synovitis and tissue destruction. In the RA synovium, macrophages are the main producers of chemokines. The expression pattern of chemokine receptors on monocytes in the RA synovium is different from that of peripheral blood monocytes, which may be related to recruitment or retaining of cells (Szekanecz et al., 2003). RA synovium is typified by infiltration of Th1 cells. Cells expressing CXCR3 and CCR5 accumulate in RA synovial fluid (Qin et al., 1998; Suzuki et al., 1999). Memory T cells in the RA synovium express CCR5, CXCR3, and CXCR4 (Nanki et al., 2000). B cells in RA synovium express CXCR5, which is important in the development of ectopic germinal center (Hjelmstrom, 2001). Endothelial cells express receptors for angiogenic chemokines, which is important in angiogenesis in RA (Szekanecz and Koch, 2001). IP-10, Mig, Mip-1a, and Mip-1b are preferentially expressed in inflamed RA compared with control (traumatic or osteoarthritis [OA]) synovial fluids and tissues. In RA, there was a chemotactic gradient between the serum and the synovium for IP-10, Mig, Mip-1a, and Mip-1b, and it favored migration into the tissue. In OA, the gradient was the opposite for IP-10, Mig, and Mip-1b, favoring retention of receptor-expressing cells in the blood (Patel et al., 2001).

Inhibiting the actions of specific chemokines or chemokine receptors could provide new therapeutic opportunities (Shadidi, 2004).

INNATE IMMUNITY AND TOLL-LIKE RECEPTORS

Toll-like receptors (TLRs) are a family of receptors that can respond to pathogens. They are ubiquitously expressed and have also been detected on cells found in the RA synovial joint in particular antigen-presenting cells and synovial fibroblast–like cells (Seibl et al., 2003; Iwahashi et al., 2004; Radstake et al., 2004). Microbial triggers have been long suspected to be involved in the pathogenesis of RA. TLRs recognize not only pathogen-associated molecular patterns (e.g., lipoproteins, lipopolysaccharide, unmethylated CpG, flagellin, dsRNA, etc.) but also endogenous proteins and other molecules released during inflammation and cell death, such as HSP70 and fibronectin. There are already examples of endogenous molecules signaling through TLR2, TLR3, TLR4, and TLR9. HSPs are recognized by TLR2 and TLR4, in particular HSP60 (Vabulas et al., 2001), HSP70 (Vabulas et al., 2002a, b), and gp96 (Arnold-Schild et al., 1999), which are released by cells undergoing necrosis. HSP–peptide complexes are able to elicit peptide-specific CD8+ T-cell responses without adjuvants (Binder et al., 2000; Castellino et al., 2000) as well as delivering an endogenous maturation signal to antigen-presenting DCs (Arnold-Schild et al., 1999). Another endogenous ligand that can activate TLR4 is cellular fibronectin, produced in response to tissue damage (Jarnagin et al., 1994; Hino et al., 1995; Saito et al., 1999; George et al., 2000).

It has been hypothesized that genomic DNA may promote host survival by improving immune recognition of pathogens at sites of tissue damage or infection. However, it is still unclear through which receptor this signal is transmitted. One candidate is TLR9, which recognizes CpG DNA. Endogenous DNA on its own is normally inert (Richardson et al., 1990). However, activation of the antigen receptor on B cells primes the cells so that TLR9 is able to be stimulated by endogenous DNA. The defining difference between bacterial and endogenous DNA is bacterial DNA, which is unmethylated whereas endogenous DNA has 70%–80% of its CpGs methylated. Interestingly, cells from autoimmune mice and humans show a decrease in this methylation, but elimination of methylation from murine DNA does not enable it to stimulate B cells (Krieg et al., 1995; Sun et al., 1997). So the mechanism by which bacterial and endogenous DNA activates TLR9 appears to be more complex than simply methylation.

Reports of bacterial components and endogenous TLR ligands in the synovium of patients with RA have supported the idea of TLRs having a role in the initiation or progression of the disease. Peptidoglycan and bacterial DNA, recognized by TLR2 and TLR9, have been reported in the human RA synovium (Van der Heijden et al., 2000), although the presence of DNA is debatable. Interestingly, bacterial components have also been reported in normal synovial tissue without any excessive inflammation (Schumacher et al., 1999) as observed in RA. Endogenous TLR ligands such as hyaluronan oligosaccharides, fibronectin fragments, HSPs, necrotic cells, and antibody–DNA complexes are present in the RA joint (Scott et al., 1981; Yu et al., 1997; Schett et al., 1998). Bacterial components have been used to induce experimental arthritis in animal models. Rats injected with a streptococcal cell wall preparation develop a chronic arthritis similar to human RA (Cromartie et al., 1977). Mice given an intra-articular injection with bacterial peptidoglycan develop severe destructive arthritis (Liu et al., 2001). Animal models suggest that TLRs may play a part in disease pathogenesis, although their direct relevance to human disease is unclear. Another approach to investigating the role of TLRs in RA has been through examination of naturally occurring TLR polymorphisms. Recent studies of gene polymorphisms of TLR2 and TLR4 have shown no association with susceptibility to RA. A single nucleotide polymorphism (+896A→G), resulting in the amino acid substitution Asp299Gly within the TLR4 gene disrupting TLR4 signaling, was not associated with susceptibility to RA (Kilding et al., 2003; Lamb et al., 2005). Another group investigated two polymorphisms of TLR2 (Arg677Trp and Arg753Gln) and two of TLR4 (Asp299Gly and Thr399Ile) and also found no association of these polymorphisms with the disease (Sanchez et al., 2004).

In the last few years, data providing evidence of TLR expression and/or up-regulation in the synovium of patients with RA have been published, although no functional consequences of their presence in the synovium have yet been demonstrated. More encouraging evidence comes from animal models that demonstrate pathogen-initiated models of arthritis, but these data are in contrast with the absence of significant polymorphisms in patients. Overall, TLRs are attractive candidates for the receptors involved in early inflammatory mechanisms of RA, but much more work needs to be done to determine if there is a functional link and to evaluate the exact role and extent to which they influence disease.

GROWTH FACTORS

The precise mechanism of hyperproliferation of synovial tissues in RA is still unclear. The trigger for hyperproliferation of fibroblast like synovial cells (FLS) is presumed to be a resultant of cellular immune response mediated by T cell and other infiltrating immune cells along with the cytokines and growth factor. Endothelial growth factor, TGF-β, platelet-derived growth factor (PDGF), and nerve growth factor (NGF) have been observed to be constitutively produced by synoviocytes (FLS) of human and animal inflammatory arthritis, and these growth factors have myriad of autocrine effects including proliferation/survival of FLS and up-regulation of inflammatory mediators (Brinckerhoff, 1983; Bucala et al., 1991; Satoh et al., 2001; Bonnet and Walsh, 2005; Raychaudhuri and Raychaudhuri, 2009; Rosengren, 2010). Also, angiogenic growth factors, including PDGF, vascular endothelial growth factor, and angiopoietins, are markedly increased in RA synovial tissues (Maruotti et al., 2006; Hunzelmann et al., 2007).

We have been working on the role of growth factors in inflammatory disease more so focused on NGF and its high-affinity receptor in the inflammatory and proliferative cascades of psoriasis, psoriatic arthritis (PsA), and RA. A growing number of studies on inflammatory diseases have demonstrated that the inflammatory state is characterized by up-regulation of NGF synthesis (Aloe, 2001; Raychaudhuri et al., 2004; Abe et al., 2007; Raychaudhuri and Raychaudhuri, 2009). Numerous cytokines such as IL-1, TNF-α, and IL-6 can induce NGF production in fibroblasts, endothelial cells, and glial cells (Otten et al., 2000; Raychaudhuri and Raychaudhuri, 2009). These observations have led to the development of the current concept that either de novo synthesis of NGF or NGF induced by proinflammatory cytokines such as TNF, IL-1, and IL-6 plays a critical role in initiation, maintenance, and perpetuation of a chronic inflammatory process (Raychaudhuri and Raychaudhuri, 2001). Our hypothesis is that NGF and other growth factors induce mammalian target of rapamycin (m-TOR) signaling proteins and regulate the critical biologic events such as T-cell activation, angiogenesis, and hyperproliferation of epidermis and synovial tissue.

In a recent publication, we observed similarly that NGF levels in SF were significantly higher in patients with PsA (365.5 ± 85.2 pg/mL) or RA (120 ± 35 pg/mL) than that in patients with OA (30 ± 6 pg/mL) (Raychaudhuri and Raychaudhuri et al., 2009). Furthermore, we observed that NGF induces proliferation of FLS. A fully formed pannus is characterized by proliferation of FLSs, inflammatory infiltrates, and marked angiogenesis. NGF and its receptor system are known to influence angiogenesis and cell trafficking (Raychaudhuri and Raychaudhuri 2001, 2008). In patients with RA or PsA, pannus tissue adheres to the surface of articular cartilage; proliferating FLSs produce proteinases that degrade cartilage and underlying cortical bone (Wernicke et al., 2002). These observations suggest that dysregulated production of NGF has the potential to influence the inflammatory and proliferative cascades of PsA and RA.

CARTILAGE/BONE DESTRUCTION

RA is distinguished by invasive synovial tissue that results in neoangiogenesis and local destruction of cartilage and bone. Prevention of cartilage/bone destruction is one of the major goals of treatment. RA has many characteristics of a locally invasive tumor. The RA synoviocyte can grow under anchorage-independent conditions and have defective contact inhibition. There is oligoclonality in the synoviocyte population (Imamura et al., 1998). There are mutations in key genes in synoviocytes such as p53 (Firestein et al., 1997). Microsatellite instability occurs in RA synovium, which is an indicator of DNA damage (Lee et al., 2003). It is postulated that DNA damage and mutation can happen because of persistent oxidative stress in a hostile environment (Yamanishi et al., 2005).

MMP mediates irreversible destruction of cartilage matrix, which consists largely of CII and proteoglycans. The MMP family consists of 25 proteinases and can be classified into five main groups (collagenase, gelatinases, stromelysins, matrilysins, and membrane-bound MMPs) on the basis of their substrate specificity and structure. However, they share substrates with redundant activities. Stromelysin (MMP-3) degrades cartilage proteoglycans, fibronectin, and type IV collagen in basement membrane. Collagenase-1 and collagenase-13 (MMP-1 and MMP-13) can degrade CII and aggrecan. Collagenase activity may be a rate-limiting step in cartilage destruction (Mengshol et al., 2002). These enzymes are produced by the proliferating synovial cells and induced by proinflammatory cytokines (TNF-α and IL-1). MMP-3 knockout mice are not resistant to arthritis (Mudgett et al., 1998). This animal model suggests that MMP-3 activity can be compensated for by other MMPs because of redundancy of enzyme activities. Tissue inhibitors of metalloproteinases are naturally occurring inhibitors for MMP. MMPs pose interesting therapeutic targets in arthritis as well as in cancer. However, doxycycline with its MMP inhibiting activities did not show any therapeutic benefits in RA (St Clair et al., 2001).

Bony erosion is associated with activation of osteoclasts. In RA synovial tissue, cells of monocyte/macrophage lineage can differentiate into functional osteoclasts by the action of several proinflammatory cytokines (M-CSF, TNF-α, and IL-1). Receptor activator of NF-κB ligand (RANKL) is also an essential factor for osteoclast differentiation and augments T-cell–DC interactions (Gravallese, 2002). RANKL is produced by synovial fibroblasts and T cells in RA synovium and is upregulated by TNF-α, IL-1, and IL-17. Osteoprotegerin (OPG) is a naturally occurring decoy receptor for RANKL (Simonet et al., 1997; Kong et al., 1999). OPG prevents the binding of RANKL to RANK. In the adjuvant arthritis animal model, RANKL blockade with OPG treatment at the onset of disease prevents bone and cartilage destruction but not inflammation. RANKL knockout mice in the K/BxN background mouse model can develop arthritis after serum transfer but are protected from bone erosion (Pettit et al., 2001).

The bisphosphonates, a popular treatment for osteoporosis, inhibit osteoclast formation, function, and survival. Interestingly, bisphosphonates diminished histologic scores of focal bone erosion by up to 80% in CIA, although synovitis scores were unchanged (Pettit et al., 2001; Sims 2004).

CONCLUSIONS

RA is a multifactorial disease involving genetic, immunologic, and environmental factors. Animal model studies have shown diverse immune dysfunctions and different clinical features in RA disease process. These animal models have provided valuable information to understand the pathogenesis of inflammatory arthritis and have contributed to develop new therapeutic targets. On the other hand, none of these animal models reproduce human RA in its entirety, and several new lines of agents showing therapeutic efficacy in animal models failed in human trials. Nonetheless, many innovative drugs have been developed on the basis of advances of our understanding of the immune dysfunction in RA. Significant therapeutic responses (ACR70) are typically achieved and sustained only in some of the patients with currently available drugs. No single drug has yet been shown to be effective for a majority of patients with RA. These observations suggest that RA is a heterogeneous disease comprising of several subsets of patients with variations in disease pathogenesis. Defining these differences in pathogenic mechanisms may lead to improved therapeutic modalities.

REFERENCES

Abdel-Nasser AM, Rasker JJ, Valkenburg HA. Epidemiological and clinical aspects relating to the variability of rheumatoid arthritis. Semin Arthritis Rheum 1997;27:123–140.

Abe Y, Akeda K, An HS, et al. Proinflammatory cytokines stimulate the expression of nerve growth factor by human intervertebral disc cells. Spine 2007;32(6):635–642.

Afzali B, Lombardi G, Lechler RI, Lord GM. The role of T helper 17 (Th17) and regulatory T cells (Treg) in human organ transplantation and autoimmune disease. Clin Exp Immunol 2007;148:32–46.

Agarwal S, Misra R, Aggarwal A. Interleukin 17 levels are increased in juvenile idiopathic arthritis synovial fluid and induce synovial fibroblasts to produce proinflammatory cytokines and matrix metalloproteinases. J Rheumatol 2008;35:515–519.

Aloe L. Nerve growth factor and neuroimmune responses: basic and clinical observations. Arch Physiol Biochem 2001;109(4):354–356.

Alonzi T, Fattori E, Lazzaro D, et al. Interleukin 6 is required for the development of collagen-induced arthritis. J Exp Med 1998;187:461.

Arnold-Schild D, Hanau D, Spehner D, et al. Cutting edge: receptor-mediated endocytosis of heat shock proteins by professional antigen-presenting cells. J Immunol 1999;162:3757–3760.

Banda NK, Thurman JM, Kraus D, et al. Alternative complement pathway activation is essential for inflammation and joint destruction in the passive transfer model of collagen-induced arthritis. J Immunol 2006;177:1904–1912.

Banerjee S, Webber C, Poole AR. The induction of arthritis in mice by the cartilage proteoglycan aggrecan: roles of CD4+ and CD8+ T cells. Cell Immunol 1992;144:347–357.

Behar SM, Roy C, Lederer J, et al. Clonally expanded Valpha12+ (AV12S1), CD8+ T cells from a patient with rheumatoid arthritis are autoreactive. Arthritis Rheum 1998;41:498–506.

Benito-Miguel M, García-Carmona Y, Balsa A, et al. A dual action of rheumatoid arthritis synovial fibroblast IL-15 expression on the equilibrium between CD4+CD25+ regulatory T cells and CD4+CD25- responder T cells. J Immunol 2009;15, 183(12):8268–8279.

Bertazzolo N, Punzi L, Stefani MP, et al. Interrelationships between interleukin (IL)-1, IL-6 and IL-8 in synovial fluid of various arthropathies. Inflamm Res 1994;41:90–92.

Binder RJ, Harris ML, Menoret A, et al. Saturation, competition, and specificity in interaction of heat shock proteins (hsp) gp96, hsp90, and hsp70 with CD11b+ cells. J Immunol 2000;165:2582–2587.

Bonnet CS, Walsh DA. Osteoarthritis, angiogenesis and inflammation. Rheumatology 2005;44:7–16.

Braddock M, Quinn A. Targeting IL-1 in inflammatory disease: new opportunities for therapeutic intervention. Nat Rev Drug Discov 2004;3:330.

Brand DD, Kang AH, Rosloniec EF. Immunopathogenesis of collagen arthritis. Springer dSemin Immunopathol 2003;25(1):3–18.

Bresnihan B, Alvaro-Gracia JM, Cobby M, et al. Treatment of rheumatoid arthritis with recombinant human interleukin-1 receptor antagonist. Arthritis Rheum 1998;41:2196.

Brinckerhoff CE. Morphologic and mitogenic responses of rabbit synovial fibroblasts to transforming growth factor beta require transforming growth factor alpha or epidermal growth factor. Arthritis Rheum 1983;26:1370–1379.

Bucala R, Ritchlin C, Winchester R, et al. Constitutive production of inflammatory and mitogenic cytokines by rheumatoid synovial fibroblasts. J Exp Med 1991;173:569–574.

Calin A, Elswood J, Klouda PT. Destructive arthritis, rheumatoid factor, and HLA-DR4: susceptibility versus severity, a case-control study. Arthritis Rheum 1989;32:1221–1225.

Campbell IK, O'Donnell K, Lawlor KE, et al. Severe inflammatory arthritis and lymphadenopathy in the absence of TNF. J Clin Invest 2001;107:1519.

Cao D, et al. Isolation and functional characterization of regulatory CD25bright CD4+ T cells from the target organ of patients with rheumatoid arthritis. Eur J Immunol 2003;33:215–223.

Cao D, van Vollenhoven R, Klareskog L, et al. CD25brightCD4+ regulatory T cells are enriched in inflamed joints of patients with chronic rheumatic disease. Arthritis Res Ther 2004;6:R335–R346.

Castellino F, Boucher PE, Eichelberg K, et al. Receptor-mediated uptake of antigen/heat shock protein complexes results in major histocompatibility complex class I antigen presentation via two distinct processing pathways. J Exp Med 2000;191:1957–1964.

Chomarat P, Vannier E, Dechanet J, et al. Balance of IL-1 receptor antagonist/IL-1b in rheumatoid synovium and its regulation by IL-4 and IL-10. J Immunol 1995;154:1432–1439.

Choy EH, Isenberg DA, Garrood T, et al. Therapeutic benefit of blocking interleukin-6 activity with an anti-interleukin-6 receptor monoclonal antibody in rheumatoid arthritis: a randomized, double-blind, placebo-controlled, dose-escalation trial. Arthritis Rheum 2002;46:3143.

Cohen P. Protein kinases—the major drug targets of the twenty-first century. Nat Rev Drug Discov 2002;1:309.

Cromartie WJ, Craddock JG, Schwab JH, et al. Arthritis in rats after systemic injection of streptococcal cells or cell walls. J Exp Med 1977;146:1585–1602.

de Kleer IM, Wedderburn LR, Taams LS, et al. CD4+CD25bright regulatory T cells actively regulate inflammation in the joints of patients with the remitting form of juvenile idiopathic arthritis. J Immunol 2004;172:6435–6443.

De Vries N, Ronningen KS, Tilanus MG, et al. HLA-DR1 and rheumatoid arthritis in Israeli Jews: sequencing reveals that DRB1*0102 is the predominant HLA-DR1 subtype. Tissue Antigens 1993;41:26.

DerSimonian H, Sugita M, Glass DN, et al. Clonal V alpha 12.1+ T cell expansions in the peripheral blood of rheumatoid arthritis patients. J Exp Med 1993;177:1623–1631.

Despres N, Boire G, Lopez-Longo, et al. The Sa system: a novel antigen–antibody system specific for rheumatoid arthritis. J Rheumatol 1994;21:1027.

Edwards JC, Szczepanski L, Szechinski J, et al. Efficacy of B-cell-targeted therapy with rituximab in patients with rheumatoid arthritis. N Engl J Med 2004;350:2572.

Ehrenstein MR, et al. Compromised function of regulatory T cells in rheumatoid arthritis and reversal by anti-TNF-α therapy. J Exp Med 2004;200:277–285.

Ferrari-Lacraz S, Zanelli E, Neuberg M, et al. Targeting IL-15 receptor-bearing cells with an antagonist mutant IL-15/Fc protein prevent disease development and progression in murine collagen-induced arthritis. J Immunol 2004;173:5818.

Firestein GS, Echeverri F, Yeo M, et al. Somatic mutations in the p53 tumor suppressor gene in rheumatoid arthritis synovium. Proc Natl Acad Sci U S A 1997;94:10895.

Genovese MC, et al. Abatacept for rheumatoid arthritis refractory to tumor necrosis factor α inhibition. N Engl J Med 2005;353:1114–1123.

Georganas C, Liu H, Perlman H, et al. Regulation of IL-6 and IL-8 expression in rheumatoid arthritis synovial fibroblasts: the dominant role for NFkB but not C/EBP-beta or c-Jun. J Immunol 2000; 165:7199–7206.

George J, Wang SS, Sevcsik AM, et al. Transforming growth factor-beta initiates wound repair in rat liver through induction of the EIIIA-fibronectin splice isoform. Am J Pathol 2000;156:115–124.

Gonzalez-Quintial R, Baccala R, Pope RM, et al. Identification of clonally expanded T cells in rheumatoid arthritis using a sequence enrichment nuclease assay. J Clin Invest 1996;97:1335–1343.

Goronzy JJ, Bartz-Bazzanella P, Hu W, et al. Dominant clonotypes in the repertoire of peripheral CD4+ T cells in rheumatoid arthritis. J Clin Invest 1994;94:2068–2076.

Gravallese EM. Bone destruction in arthritis. Ann Rheum Dis 2002;61(Suppl II):II-84.

Guerne PA, Zuraw BL, Vaughan JH, et al. Synovium as a source of interleukin 6 in vitro. Contribution to local and systemic manifestations of arthritis. J Clin Invest 1989;83:585.

Harris J, Vaughan JH. Transfusion studies in rheumatoid arthritis. Arthritis Rheum 1961;4:47.

Hino K, Shiozawa S, Kuroki Y, et al. EDA-containing fibronectin is synthesized from rheumatoid synovial fibroblast-like cells. Arthritis Rheum 1995;38:678–683.

Hjelmstrom P. Lymphoid neogenesis: de novo formation of lymphoid tissue in chronic inflammation through expression of homing chemokines. J Leukoc Biol 2001;69:331.

Hunzelmann N, Eming S, Rosenkranz S. Growth factors. J Rheumatol 2007;66(4):290,292–296.

Hwang SY, Kim JY, Kim KW, et al. IL-17 induces production of IL-6 and IL-8 in rheumatoid arthritis synovial fibroblasts via NFkB- and PI3- kinase/Akt-dependent pathways. Arthritis Res Ther 2004;6:R120-R128.

Ikeuchi H, et al. Expression of interleukin-22 in rheumatoid arthritis: potential role as a proinflammatory cytokine. Arthritis Rheum 2005;52:1037–1046.

Imamura F, Aono H, Hasunuma T, et al. Monoclonal expansion of synoviocytes in rheumatoid arthritis. Arthritis Rheum 1998;41:1979.

Isomäki P, Punnonen J. Pro- and anti-inflammatory cytokines in rheumatoid arthritis. Ann Med 1997;29:499.

Iwahashi M, Yamamura M, Aita T, et al. Expression of toll-like receptor 2 on CD16+ blood monocytes and synovial tissue macrophages in rheumatoid arthritis. Arthritis Rheum 2004;50:1457–1467.

Jarnagin WR, Rockey DC, Koteliansky VE, et al. Expression of variant fibronectins in wound healing: cellular source and biological activity of the EIIIA segment in rat hepatic fibrogenesis. J Cell Biol 1994;127:2037–2048.

Joosten LAB, Helsen MMA, van de Loo FAJ, et al. van den Berg WB. Anticytokine treatment of established type II collagen-induced arthritis in DBA/1 mice: a comparative study using anti-TNFα, anti-IL-1a/b, and IL-1Ra. Arthritis Rheum 1996;39:797–809.

Ju JH, Cho ML, Jhun JY, et al. Oral administration of type-II collagen suppresses IL-17-associated RANKL expression of CD4+ T cells in collagen-induced arthritis. Immunol Lett 2008;117:16–25.

Katschke KJ Jr, Helmy KY, Steffek M, et al. A novel inhibitor of the alternative pathway of complement reverses inflammation and bone destruction in experimental arthritis. J Exp Med 2007;204:1319–1325.

Katz Y, Nadiv O, Rapoport MJ. IL-17 regulates gene expression and protein synthesis of the complement system, C3 and factor B, in skin fibroblasts. Clin Exp Immunol 2000;120:22–29.

Keffer J, Probert L, Cazlaris H, et al. Transgenic mice expressing human tumour necrosis factor: a predictive genetic model of arthritis. EMBO J 1991;10:4025.

Khayrullina T, Yen JH, Jing H, et al. In vitro differentiation of dendritic cells in the presence of prostaglandin E2 alters the IL-12/IL-23 balance and promotes differentiation of Th17 cells. J Immunol 2008;181:721–735.

Kilding R, Akil M, Till S, et al. A biologically important single nucleotide polymorphism within the toll-like receptor-4 gene is not associated with rheumatoid arthritis. Clin Exp Rheumatol 2003;21:340–342.

Kim HR, Cho ML, Kim KW, et al. Up-regulation of IL-23p19 expression in rheumatoid arthritis synovial fibroblasts by IL-17 through PI3-kinase-, NFkB- and p38 MAPK-dependent signalling pathways. Rheumatology 2007;46:57–64.

Komai-Koma M, Gracie JA, Wei XQ, et al. Chemoattraction of human T cells by IL-18. J Immunol 2003;15:1084.

Kong YY, Feige U, Sarosi I, et al. Activated T cells regulate bone loss and joint destruction in adjuvant arthritis through osteoprotegerin ligand. Nature 1999;265:144.

Kremer JM, et al. Treatment of rheumatoid arthritis with the selective costimulation modulator abatacept: twelve-month results of a phase iib, double-blind, randomized, placebo-controlled trial. Arthritis Rheum 2005;52:2263–2271.

Kremer JM, Westhovens R, Leon M, et al. Treatment of rheumatoid arthritis by selective inhibition of T-cell activation with fusion protein CTLA4Ig. N Engl J Med 2003;349:1907.

Krieg AM, Yi AK, Matson S, et al. CpG motifs in bacterial DNA trigger direct B-cell activation. Nature 1995;374:546–549.

Kroot EJ, de Jong BA, van Leeuwen MA, et al. The prognostic value of anti-cyclic citrullinated peptide antibody in patients with recent-onset rheumatoid arthritis. Arthritis Rheum 2000;43:1831.

Lai Kwan Lam Q, King Hung Ko O, Zheng BJ, et al. Local BAFF gene silencing suppresses Th17-cell generation and ameliorates autoimmune arthritis. Proc Natl Acad Sci U S A 2008;105:14993–14998.

Lamb RM, Zeggini E, Thomson W. Toll-like receptor 4 gene polymorphisms and susceptibility to juvenile idiopathic arthritis. Ann Rheum Dis 2005;64:767–769.

Lawson CA, et al. Early rheumatoid arthritis is associated with a deficit in the CD4+CD25high regulatory T cell population in peripheral blood. Rheumatology (Oxford) 2006;45:1210–1217.

Lee SH, Chang DK, Goel A, et al. Microsatellite instability and suppressed DNA repair enzyme expression in rheumatoid arthritis. J Immunol 2003;170:2214.

Leipe J, et al. Regulatory T cells in rheumatoid arthritis. Arthritis Res Ther 2005;7:93–99.

Lemos HP, Grespan R, Vieira SM, et al. Prostaglandin mediates IL-23/IL-17-induced neutrophils migration in inflammation by inhibiting IL-12 and IFN-production. Proc Natl Acad Sci U S A 2009;106: 5954–5959.

Li P, Schwarz EM. The TNF-alpha transgenic mouse model of inflammatory arthritis. Springer Semin Immunopathol 2003;25:19.

Li X, Yuan FL, Lu WG, et al. The role of interleukin-17 in mediating joint destruction in rheumatoid arthritis. Biochem Biophys Res Commun 2010;397(2):131–135.

Liu ZQ, Deng GM, Foster S, et al. Staphylococcal peptidoglycans induce arthritis. Arthritis Res 2001;3:375–380.

Lubberts E, Koenders MI, et al. The role of T-cell interleukin-17 in conducting destructive arthritis: lessons from animal models. Arthritis Res Ther 2005;7:29–37.

Maione F, Paschalidis N, Mascolo N, et al. Interleukin 17 sustains rather than induces inflammation. Biochem Pharmacol 2009;77(5):878–887.

Maruotti N, Cantatore FP, Crivellato E, et al. Angiogenesis in rheumatoid arthritis. Histol Histopathol 2006;21(5):557–566.

Matsumoto I, Maccioni M, Lee D, et al. How antibodies to a ubiquitous cytoplasmic enzyme may provoke joint-specific autoimmune disease. Nat Immunol 2002;3:360.

Mengshol JA, Mix KS, Brinckerhoff CE. Matrix metalloproteinases as therapeutic targets in arthritic diseases: bull's-eye or missing the mark? Arthritis Rheum 2002;46:13.

Miossec P. Interleukin-17 in rheumatoid arthritis: if T cells were to contribute to inflammation and destruction through synergy. Arthritis Rheum 2003;48:594–601.

Mollnes TE, Lea T, Mellbye OJ, et al. Complement activation in rheumatoid arthritis evaluated by C3dg and the terminal complement complex. Arthritis Rheum 1986;29:715–721.

Mottonen M, et al. CD4+ CD25+ T cells with the phenotypic and functional characteristics of regulatory T cells are enriched in the synovial fluid of patients with rheumatoid arthritis. Clin Exp Immunol 2005;140:360–367.

Mudgett JS, Hutchinson NI, Chartrain NA, et al. Susceptibility of stromelysin 1-deficient mice to collagen-induced arthritis and cartilage destruction. Arthritis Rheum 1998;41:110.

Myers LK, Kang AH, Postlethwaite AE, et al. The genetic ablation of cyclooxygenase 2 prevents the development of autoimmune arthritis. Arthritis Rheum 2000;43:2687–2693.

Nakae S, Saijo S, Horai R, et al. IL-17 production from activated T cells is required for the spontaneous development of destructive arthritis in mice deficient in IL-1 receptor antagonist. Proc Natl Acad Sci U S A 2003;100:5986.

Nanki T, Hayashida K, El-Gabalawy HS, et al. Stromal cell-derived factor-1-CXC chemokine receptor 4 interactions play a central role in CD4+ T cell accumulation in rheumatoid arthritis synovium. J Immunol, 2000;165:6590.

Nepom GT, Byers P, Seyfried C, et al. HLA genes associated with rheumatoid arthritis. Identification of susceptibility alleles using specific oligonucleotide probes. Arthritis Rheum 1989;32:15.

O'Dell JR, Nepom BS, Haire C, et al. A HLA-DRB1 typing in rheumatoid arthritis: predicting response to specific treatments. Ann Rheum Dis 1998;57:209.

Otten U, März P, Heese K, et al. Cytokines and neurotrophins interact in normal and diseased states. Ann N Y Acad Sci 2000;917:322–330.

Patel DD, Zachariah JP, Whichard LP. CXCR3 and CCR5 ligands in rheumatoid arthritis synovium. Clin Immunol 2001;98:39–45.

Pers JO, Daridon C, Devauchelle V, et al. BAFF overexpression is associated with autoantibody production in autoimmune diseases. Ann N Y Acad Sci 2005;1050:34–39.

Pettipher ER, Higgs GA, Henderson B. Interleukin 1 induces leukocyte infiltration and cartilage proteoglycan degradation in the synovial joint. Proc Natl Acad Sci U S A 1986;83:8749–8753.

Pettit AR, Ji H, von Stechow D, et al. TRANCE/RANKL knockout mice are protected from bone erosion in a serum transfer model of arthritis. Am J Pathol 2001;159:1689.

Prakken BJ, Roord S, Ronaghy A, et al. Heat shock protein 60 and adjuvant arthritis: a model for T cell regulation in human arthritis. Springer Semin Immunopathol 2003;25:47.

Qin S, Rottman JB, Myers P, et al. The chemokine receptors CXCR3 and CCR5 mark subsets of T cells associated with certain inflammatory reactions. J Clin Invest 1998;101:746–754.

Radstake TR, Roelofs MF, Jenniskens YM, et al. Expression of toll-like receptors 2 and 4 in rheumatoid synovial tissue and regulation by proinflammatory cytokines interleukin-12 and interleukin-18 via interferon-gamma. Arthritis Rheum 2004;50:3856–3865.

Rantapaa-Dahlqvist S, de Jong BA, Berglin E, et al. Antibodies against cyclic citrullinated peptide and IgA rheumatoid factor predict the development of rheumatoid arthritis. Arthritis Rheum 2003;48:2741.

Raychaudhuri SK, Raychaudhuri SP, Weltman H, et al. Effect of nerve growth factor on endothelial cell biology: proliferation and adherence molecule expression on human dermal microvascular endothelial cells. Arch Dermatol Res 2001;293:291–295.

Raychaudhuri SK, Raychaudhuri SP. NGF and its receptor system: a new dimension in the pathogenesis of psoriasis and psoriatic arthritis. Ann N Y Acad Sci 2009;1173:470–477.

Raychaudhuri SP, Jiang WY, Raychaudhuri SK. Revisiting the Koebner Phenomenon: role of NGF and its receptor system in the pathogenesis of psoriasis. Am J Pathol 2008;172(4):961–971.

Raychaudhuri SP, Raychaudhuri SK. The regulatory role of nerve growth factor and its receptor system in fibroblast-like synovial cells. Scand J Rheumatol 2009a;38(3):207–215.

Raychaudhuri SP, Sanyal M, Weltman H, et al. K252a, a high affinity NGF receptor blocker improves psoriasis: an in vivo study using the SCID mouse-human skin model. J Invest Dermatol 2004;122(3):812–819.

Richardson B, Scheinbart L, Strahler J, et al. Evidence for impaired T cell DNA methylation in systemic lupus erythematosus and rheumatoid arthritis. Arthritis Rheum 1990;33:1665–1673.

Rittner HL Zettl A, Jendro MC, et al. Multiple mechanisms support oligoclonal T cell expansion in rheumatoid synovitis. Mol Med 1997;3:452–465.

Rosengren S, Corr M, Boyle DL. Platelet-derived growth factor and transforming growth factor beta synergistically potentiate inflammatory mediator synthesis by fibroblast-like synoviocytes. Arthritis Res Ther 2010;12(2):R65.

Saito S, Yamaji N, Yasunaga K, et al. The fibronectin extra domain A activates matrix metalloproteinase gene expression by an interleukin-1-dependent mechanism. J Biol Chem 1999;274:30756–30763.

Sakaguchi N, Takahashi T, Hata H, et al. Altered thymic T-cell selection due to a mutation of the ZAP-70 gene causes autoimmune arthritis in mice. Nature 2003;426:454.

Sakaguchi S. Naturally arising Foxp3-expressing CD25+CD4+ regulatory T cells in immunological tolerance to self and non-self. Nat Immunol 2005;6:345–352.

Sanchez E, Orozco G, Lopez-Nevot MA, et al. Polymorphisms of toll-like receptor 2 and 4 genes in rheumatoid arthritis and systemic lupus erythematosus. Tissue Antigens 2004;63:54–57.

Satoh K, Kikuchi S, Sekimata M, et al. Involvement of ErbB-2 in rheumatoid synovial cell growth. Arthritis Rheum 2001;44:260–265.

Saxena N, Aggarwal A, Misra R. Elevated concentrations of monocyte derived cytokines in synovial fluid of children with enthesitis related arthritis and polyarticular types of juvenile idiopathic arthritis. J Rheumatol 2005;32(7):1349–1353.

Schellekens GA, Visser H, de Jong BA, et al. The diagnostic properties of rheumatoid arthritis antibodies recognizing a cyclic citrullinated peptide. Arthritis Rheum 2000;43:155.

Schett G, Redlich K, Xu Q, et al. Enhanced expression of heat shock protein 70 (hsp70) and heat shock factor 1 (HSF1) activation in rheumatoid arthritis synovial tissue. Differential regulation of hsp70 expression and hsf1 activation in synovial fibroblasts by proinflammatory cytokines, shear stress, and antiinflammatory drugs. J Clin Invest 1998;102:302–311.

Schmidt D, Goronzy JJ, Weyand CM. CD4+ CD7– CD28– T cells are expanded in rheumatoid arthritis and are characterized by autoreactivity. J Clin Invest 1996;97:2027–2037.

Schumacher HR Jr, Arayssi T, Crane M, et al. Chlamydia trachomatis nucleic acids can be found in the synovium of some asymptomatic subjects. Arthritis Rheum 1999;42:1281–1284.

Scott DL, Delamere JP, Walton KW. The distribution of fibronectin in the pannus in rheumatoid arthritis. Br J Exp Pathol 1981;62:362–368.

Seibl R, Birchler T, Loeliger S, et al. Expression and regulation of toll-like receptor 2 in rheumatoid arthritis synovium. Am J Pathol 2003;162:1221–1227.

Shadidi KR. New drug targets in rheumatoid arthritis: focus on chemokines. BioDrugs 2004;18:181.

Sheibanie AF, Khayrullina T, Safadi FF, et al. Prostaglandin E2 exacerbates collagen-induced arthritis in mice through the inflammatory interleukin-23/interleukin-17 axis. Arthritis Rheum 2007;56:2608–2619.

Shinomiya S, Naraba H, Ueno A, et al. Regulation of TNF-alpha and interleukin-10 production by prostaglandins I2 and E2: studies with prostaglandin receptor-deficient mice and prostaglandin E-receptor subtype-selective synthetic agonists. Biochem Pharmacol 2001;61:1153–1160.

Simonet WS, Lacey DL, Dunstan CR, et al. Osteoprotegerin: a novel secreted protein involved in the regulation of bone density. Cell 1997;89:309.

Sims NA, Green JR, Glatt M, et al. Targeting osteoclasts with zoledronic acid prevents bone destruction in collagen-induced arthritis. Arthritis Rheum 2004;50:2338.

Smolen JS, Steiner G. Therapeutic strategies for rheumatoid arthritis. Nat Rev 2003;2:473.

Sonderstrup, G. Development of humanized mice as a model of inflammatory arthritis. Springer Semin Immunopathol 2003;25:35.

St Clair EW, Wilkinson WE, Pisetsky DS, et al. The effects of intravenous doxycycline therapy for rheumatoid arthritis: a randomized, double-blind, placebo-controlled trial. Arthritis Rheum 2001;44:1043.

Stamp LK, Cleland LG, James MJ. Upregulation of synoviocytes COX-2 through interactions with T lymphocytes: role of interleukin 17 and tumor necrosis factor-alpha, J Rheumatol 2004;31: 1246–1254.

Steinman L. A brief history of TH17, the first major revision in the TH1/TH2 hypothesis of T cell-mediated tissue damage. Nature Med 2007;13:139–145.

Strassmann G, Patil-Koota V, Finkelman F, et al. Evidence for the involvement of interleukin 10 in the differential deactivation of murine peritoneal macrophages by prostaglandin E2. J Exp Med 1994;180:2365–2370.

Stuart JM, Dixon FJ. Serum transfer of collagen-induced arthritis in mice. J Exp Med 1983;158:378.

Sugiyama E, Kuroda A, Taki H, et al. Interleukin 10 cooperates with interleukin 4 to suppress inflammatory cytokine production by freshly prepared adherent rheumatoid synovial cells. J Rheumatol 1995;22:2020–2026.

Sun S, Beard C, Jaenisch R, et al. Mitogenicity of DNA from different organisms for murine B cells. J Immunol 1997;159:3119–3125.

Suzuki A, Yamada R, Chang X, et al. An intronic SNP in a RUNX1 binding site of SLC22A4, encoding an organic cation transporter, is associated with rheumatoid arthritis. Nat Genet 2003;34:395.

Suzuki N, Nakajima A, Yoshino S, et al. Selective accumulation of CCR51 T lymphocytes into inflamed joints of rheumatoid arthritis. Int Immunol 1999;11:553–559.

Swaidani S, Bulek K, Kang Z, et al. The critical role of epithelial-derived Act1 in IL-17- and IL-25-mediated pulmonary inflammation. J Immunol 2009;182(3):1631–1640.

Szekanecz Z, Koch AE. Chemokines and angiogenesis. Curr Opin Rheumatol 2001;13:202.

Szekanecz Z, Kim J, Koch AE. Chemokines and chemokine receptors in rheumatoid arthritis. Semin Immunol 2003;15:15.

Trebino CE, Stock JL, Gibbons CP, et al. Impaired inflammatory and pain responses in mice lacking an inducible prostaglandin E synthase. Proc Natl Acad Sci U S A 2003;100:9044–9049.

Vabulas RM, Ahmad-Nejad P, da Costa C, et al. Endocytosed HSP60s use toll-like receptor 2 (TLR2) and TLR4 to activate the toll/interleukin-1 receptor signaling pathway in innate immune cells. J Biol Chem 2001;276:31332–31339.

Vabulas RM, Ahmad-Nejad P, Ghose S, et al. HSP70 as endogenous stimulus of the toll/interleukin-1 receptor signal pathway. J Biol Chem 2002a;277:15107–15112.

Vabulas RM, Braedel S, Hilf N, et al. The endoplasmic reticulum-resident heat shock protein Gp96 activates dendritic cells via the toll-like receptor 2/4 pathway. J Biol Chem 2002b;277:20847–20853.

Valencia X, et al. TNF downmodulates the function of human CD4+CD25high T-regulatory cells. Blood 2006;108:253–261.

Van Amelsfort JM, Jacobs KM, Bijlsma JW, et al. CD4 (+) CD25 (+) regulatory T cells in rheumatoid arthritis: differences in the presence, phenotype, and function between peripheral blood and synovial fluid. Arthritis Rheum 2004;50:2775–2785.

Van der Graaff WL, Prins AP, Niers TM, et al. Quantitation of interferon gamma- and interleukin-4-producing T cells in synovial fluid and peripheral blood of arthritis patients. Rheumatology (Oxford) 1999;38(3):214–220.

Van der Heijden IM, Wilbrink B, Tchetverikov I, et al. Presence of bacterial DNA and bacterial peptidoglycans in joints of patients with rheumatoid arthritis and other arthritides. Arthritis Rheum 2000;43:593–598.

Van Gaalen FA, Toes RE, Ditzel HJ, et al. Association of autoantibodies to glucose-6-phosphate isomerase with extraarticular complications in rheumatoid arthritis. Arthritis Rheum 2004a;50:395.

Van Gaalen FA, van Aken J, Huizinga TW, et al. Association between HLA class II genes and autoantibodies to cyclic citrullinated peptides (CCPs) influences the severity of rheumatoid arthritis. Arthritis Rheum 2004b;50:2113.

Van Roon JA, van Roy JL, Gmelig-Meyling FH, Lafeber FP, Bijlsma JW. Prevention and reversal of cartilage degradation in rheumatoid arthritis by interleukin-10 and interleukin-4. Arthritis Rheum 1996; 39:829.

Van Roon JAG, van Roy JLAM, Duits A, et al. Proinflammatory cytokine production and cartilage damage due to rheumatoid synovial T helper-1 activation is inhibited by interleukin-4. Ann Rheum Dis 1995;54:836–840.

Van Snick J. Interleukin-6: an overview. Annu Rev Immunol 1990;8:253.

Vossenaar ER, Deprés N, Lapointe E, et al. Rheumatoid arthritis specific anti-Sa antibodies target citrullinated vimentin. Arthritis Res Ther 2004a;6:R142.

Vossenaar ER, Smeets TJ, Kraan MC, et al. The presence of citrullinated proteins is not specific for rheumatoid synovial tissue. Arthritis Rheum 2004b;50:3485.

Weaver CT, Hatton RD, Mangan PR, et al. IL-17 family cytokines and the expanding diversity of effector T cell lineages. Annu Rev Immunol 2007;25:821–852.

Wei XQ, Leung BP, Arthur HM, et al. Reduced incidence and severity of collagen-induced arthritis in mice lacking IL-18. J Immunol 2001;166:517.

Wernicke D, Schulze-Westhoff C, Brauer R, et al. Stimulation of collagenase 3 expression in synovial fibroblasts of patients with rheumatoid arthritis by contact with a three dimensional collagen matrix or with normal cartilage when co-implanted in NOD/SCID mice. Arthritis Rheum 2002;46:64–74.

Willkens RF, Nepom GT, Marks CR, et al. Association of HLA-Dw16 with rheumatoid arthritis in Yakima Indians. Further evidence for the "shared epitope" hypothesis. Arthritis Rheum 1991;34:43.

Xiao Y, Motomura S, Podack ER. APRIL (TNFSF13) regulates collagen-induced arthritis, IL-17 production and Th2 response. Eur J Immunol 2008;38:3450–3458.

Yamaguchi Y, Fujio K, Shoda H, et al. IL-17B and IL-17C are associated with TNF-alpha production and contribute to the exacerbation of inflammatory arthritis. J Immunol 2007;179:7128–7136.

Yamanishi Y, Boyle DL, Green DR, et al. P53 tumor suppressor gene mutations in fibroblast-like synoviocytes from erosion synovium and non-erosion synovium in rheumatoid arthritis. Arthritis Res Ther 2005;7:R12.

Yelamos J, Garcia-Lozano JR, Moreno I, et al. Association of HLA-DR4-Dw15 (DRB1*0405) and DR10 with rheumatoid arthritis in a Spanish population. Arthritis Rheum 1993;36:811.

Young A, Jaraquemada D, Awad J. Association of HLA-DR4/Dw4 and DR2/Dw2 with radiologic changes in a prospective study of patients with rheumatoid arthritis. Preferential relationship with HLA-Dw rather than HLA-DR specificities. Arthritis Rheum 1984;27:20.

Yu D, Rumore PM, Liu Q, Steinman CR. Soluble oligonucleosomal complexes in synovial fluid from inflamed joints. Arthritis Rheum 1997;40:648–654.

Zheng Y, et al. Interleukin-22, a TH17 cytokine, mediates IL-23-induced dermal inflammation and acanthosis. Nature 2007;445:648–651.

5 Osteoclasts and Interleukin-17-Producing Helper T Cells in Rheumatoid Arthritis

Kazuo Okamoto and Hiroshi Takayanagi

CONTENTS

INTRODUCTION

The bony skeleton, an essential component of the skeletal system, enables locomotive activity, the storage of calcium, and the harboring of hematopoietic stem cells. This multifunctional organ is characterized by the calcified hard tissue composed of type I collagen and highly organized deposits of calcium phosphate (hydroxyapatite) (Seeman and Delmas, 2006). Although bone seems to be metabolically inert, it is restructured at such a high speed that approximately 10% of the total bone content is replaced per year in adult vertebrates. This process, called bone remodeling, is dependent on the dynamic balance of bone formation and resorption, which are mediated by osteoblasts and osteoclasts, respectively. A delicate regulation of this process is a prerequisite for normal bone homeostasis, and an imbalance is often related to metabolic bone diseases in humans (Takayanagi, 2007).

Rheumatoid arthritis (RA) is an autoimmune disease that primarily affects the joints, but the pathogenesis of tissue destruction is different from that of typical autoimmune diseases.

Matrix-degrading enzymes, such as matrix metalloproteinases, were initially proposed to have a fundamental role in bone and cartilage destruction (Okada et al., 1987), but attention has been turned toward osteoclast-mediated mechanism. It is critically important to understand the pathogenesis of bone destruction in arthritis to develop effective therapeutic strategies that specifically target the pathway(s) involved in this destructive process. Here, we summarize recent progress in the understanding of the cellular and molecular mechanisms of bone destruction in arthritis by focusing on osteoclasts and osteoclastogenic helper T (Th) cells, Th17 cells.

OSTEOCLASTS AND BONE DESTRUCTION

The identification of osteoclast-like giant cells at the interface between the synovium and the bone in rheumatoid joints dates back to the early 1980s (Bromley and Woolley, 1984). These multinucleated giant cells were further characterized as being positive for the expression of tartrate-resistant acid phosphatase (TRAP) and the calcitonin receptor; this expression is characteristic of authentic osteoclasts (Gravallese et al., 1998). Notably, TRAP-positive multinucleated cells were frequently observed in the synovium, which is not in direct contact with bone. These pathological findings stimulated researchers to hypothesize that osteoclasts formed in the synovium have an important role in bone resorption in arthritis (Takayanagi et al., 1997; Gravallese et al., 1998). Subsequent efforts were made to answer the question of whether osteoclasts could be generated from synovial cells *in vitro*. Ultimately, osteoclast formation from cultured synovial cells was successfully performed without adding any other cells, thus demonstrating that rheumatoid synovial cells contain both osteoclast precursor cells and osteoclastogenesis-supporting cells (Takayanagi et al., 1997). Further studies indicated that synovial fibroblasts express membrane-bound factors that stimulate osteoclastogenesis and induce the differentiation of synovial macrophages into osteoclasts; however, it was not until receptor activator of nuclear factor-κB ligand (RANKL) was cloned that the membrane-bound factor on the synovial cells was identified (Takayanagi et al., 2000a).

THE ROLE OF RANKL/RANK IN OSTEOCLASTOGENESIS

In the late 1980s, an *in vitro* osteoclast formation system was established by culturing bone marrow-derived cells of monocyte/macrophage lineage with osteoclastogenesis-supporting cells, such as osteoblasts (Takahashi et al., 1988a, b). These supporting mesenchymal cells provide factors that are necessary for osteoclast differentiation (Suda et al., 1999). Analysis of *op/op* mice with osteopetrosis revealed one of the essential factors to be macrophage colony-stimulating factor (M-CSF) (Yoshida et al., 1990). M-CSF stimulation alone, however, does not induce the differentiation of osteoclasts. Forced expression of antiapoptotic molecule Bcl-2 partially rescues the osteopetrotic phenotype of the *op/op* mice (Lagasse and Weissman, 1997), suggesting that M-CSF is a survival factor for osteoclast precursor cells.

Yasuda et al. and Lacey et al. ultimately did clone the long-sought ligand mediating an essential signal for osteoclast differentiation in 1998 as osteoclast differentiation factor (ODF) and osteoprotegerin (OPG) ligand, respectively (Lacey et al., 1998; Yasuda et al., 1998). Interestingly, this cytokine, which belongs to the tumor necrosis factor (TNF) family, was shown to be identical to RANKL and TNF-related activation-induced cytokine, which had been cloned in the immune system (Anderson et al., 1997; Wong et al., 1997). The cloning of ODF (RANKL, hereafter) enabled investigation of the differentiation process in a sophisticated culture system using recombinant RANKL and M-CSF (Theill et al., 2002).

The receptor for RANKL is RANK, a type I transmembrane protein, sharing high homology with CD40. RANK is expressed on osteoclast precursor cells and mature osteoclasts, and the binding of RANKL to RANK is inhibited by the decoy receptor OPG (Simonet et al., 1997; Tsuda et al., 1997). In bone, RANKL is expressed by osteoclastogenesis-supporting cells including osteoblasts, in response to osteoclastogenic factors, such as 1,25-dihydroxyvitamin D_3, prostaglandin E_2, and parathyroid hormone, and is a crucial determinant of the level of bone resorption *in vivo* (Suda et al., 1999; Theill et al., 2002). Mice with a disruption of *Rank* or *Rankl* exhibit severe osteopetrosis accompanied by a defect in tooth eruption caused by a complete lack of osteoclasts (Dougall et al., 1999; Kong et al., 1999b; Li et al., 2000). In contrast, mice lacking *Opg* exhibit severe osteoporosis caused by both an increased number and an enhanced activity of osteoclasts (Bucay et al., 1998; Mizuno et al., 1998). These genetic findings clearly demonstrated that RANK/RANKL signaling is essential for osteoclastogenesis *in vivo*. Furthermore, mutations in RANK, RANKL, and OPG were identified in human patients with bone disorders such as familial expansile osteolysis, autosomal recessive osteopetrosis, and juvenile Paget's disease of bone, respectively (Hughes et al., 2000; Whyte et al., 2002; Sobacchi et al., 2007; Guerrini et al., 2008).

RANKL SIGNALING

The ligation of RANK with RANKL results in trimerization of RANK and recruitment of adaptor molecules such as the TNF receptor-associated factor (TRAF) family of proteins, among which TRAF6 has been revealed to be the major adaptor molecule (Lomaga et al., 1999; Naito et al., 1999). TRAF6 also trimerizes upon RANK stimulation and activates nuclear factor-κB (NF-κB) and mitogen-activated protein kinases (MAPKs) including Jun N-terminal kinase and p38. The essential role of NF-κB in osteoclastogenesis was demonstrated genetically (Franzoso et al., 1997; Iotsova et al., 1997). Although it has been recently reported that the specific deletion of the p38α gene in osteoclast lineages results in the partial blockade of osteoclastogenesis *in vivo* (Bohm et al., 2009), the *in vivo* functions of the other MAPKs are largely unknown. The lysine 63-linked polyubiquitination mediated by the really interesting new gene (RING)-finger motif of TRAF6 was shown to be important for NF-κB activation in other cell types, but deletion analysis indicated that the RING-finger domain of TRAF6 is dispensable for the formation of osteoclasts (Kobayashi et al., 2001). Therefore, the importance of the ubiquitin-ligase activity of TRAF6 in osteoclastogenesis needs to be tested *in vivo*. TRAF6 is activated by many receptors including CD40, Toll-like receptors (TLRs), and interleukin (IL)-1 receptor, but RANK alone is able to strongly stimulate osteoclastogenesis. It is likely that additional RANK-specific adaptor molecule(s) exists and enhances TRAF6 signaling (Gohda et al., 2005). For example, the molecular scaffold Grb2-associated binding protein 2 and/or four-and-a-half LIM domain 2 were reported to be associated with RANK and to have an important role in its signal transduction (Bai et al., 2005; Wada et al., 2005). The RANK signaling cascades during osteoclastogenesis is summarized in Figure 5.1.

NUCLEAR FACTOR OF ACTIVATED T CELLS CYTOPLASMIC 1: THE MASTER TRANSCRIPTION FACTOR FOR OSTEOCLASTOGENESIS

RANK also activates the transcription-factor complex, activator protein 1 (AP-1), through the induction of its component c-Fos (Wagner and Eferl, 2005). The induction mechanism of c-Fos is dependent on the activation of Ca^{2+}/calmodulin-dependent protein kinase IV (CaMKIV) and the cyclic adenosine monophosphate response element-binding protein (CREB) (Sato et al., 2006a) as well as the activation of NF-κB (Yamashita et al., 2007). Importantly, RANKL specifically and potently induces nuclear factor of activated T cells cytoplasmic 1 (NFATc1), the master regulator of osteoclast differentiation, and this induction is dependent on both the TRAF6 and the c-Fos pathways (Takayanagi et al., 2002a). The activation of NFAT is mediated by a specific phosphatase, calcineurin, which is activated by calcium-calmodulin signaling. The *NFATc1* promoter contains NFAT binding sites, and NFATc1 specifically autoregulates its own promoter during osteoclastogenesis and enables the robust induction of NFATc1 (Asagiri et al., 2005). The essential role of NFATc1 has been proven by genetic experiments (Asagiri et al., 2005; Winslow et al., 2006; Aliprantis et al., 2008). NFATc1 regulates a number of osteoclast-specific genes such

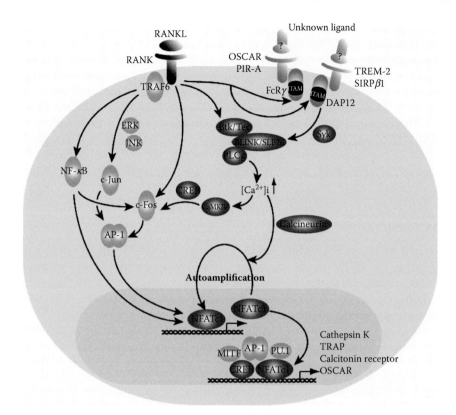

FIGURE 5.1 **(See color insert.)** Signal transduction in osteoclast differentiation. RANKL–RANK binding results in the recruitment of TRAF6, which activates NF-κB and MAPKs. RANKL also stimulates the induction of c-Fos through NF-κB and CaMKIV. NF-κB and c-Fos are important for the robust induction of NFATc1. Several costimulatory receptors associate with the ITAM-harboring adaptors, FcRγ subunit, and DAP12: OSCAR and TREM-2 associate with FcRγ, and SIRPβ1 and PIR-A associate with DAP12. RANK and ITAM signaling cooperate to phosphorylate PLCγ and activate calcium signaling, which is critical for the activation and autoamplification of NFATc1. Tec family tyrosine kinases (Tec and Btk) activated by RANK are important for the formation of the osteoclastogenic signaling complex composed of Tec kinases, B-cell linker (BLNK)/SH2 domain containing leukocyte protein of 76 kDa (SLP76) (activated by ITAM-Syk), and PLCγ, which are essential for the efficient phosphorylation of PLCγ.

as cathepsin K, TRAP, calcitonin receptor, osteoclast-associated receptor (OSCAR), and β3 integrin, in cooperation with other transcription factors such as AP-1, PU.1, microphthalmia-associated transcription factor (MITF), and CREB (Takayanagi, 2007). NFATc1 was originally discovered in T cells, but this transcription factor was subsequently revealed to play a crucial role in osteoclastogenesis. It is worthy to note that calcium signaling and its downstream effector molecules are shared by osteoclasts and T cells.

CALCIUM SIGNALING AND IMMUNORECEPTORS IN OSTEOCLASTOGENESIS

During osteoclastogenesis, activation of calcium signaling is dependent on the immunoglobulin-like receptors associated with immunoreceptor tyrosine-based activation motif (ITAM)–harboring adaptors, Fc receptor common γ subunit (FcRγ), and DNAX-activating protein 12 (DAP12) (Negishi-Koga and Takayanagi, 2009). Importantly, mice doubly deficient in FcRγ and DAP12 exhibit severe osteopetrosis owing to a differentiation blockade of osteoclasts, demonstrating that the immunoglobulin-like receptors associated with FcRγ and DAP12 are essential for osteoclastogenesis (Koga et al., 2004; Mocsai et al., 2004). These receptors include OSCAR, triggering receptor expressed in myeloid cells-2 (TREM-2), signal-regulatory protein β1 (SIRPβ), and paired immunoglobulin-like receptor-A (PIR-A), although the ligand and the exact function of each of these receptors remain to be determined. ITAM-mediated signals cooperate with RANK to stimulate calcium signaling through ITAM phosphorylation and the resulting activation of spleen tyrosine kinase (Syk) and phospholipase Cγ(PLCγ) (Figure 5.1). Because this pathway is crucial for the robust induction of NFATc1 that leads to osteoclastogenesis but ITAM signals alone cannot induce osteoclastogenesis, these signals should be considered costimulatory signals for RANK. Initially characterized in natural killer and myeloid cells, the immunoglobulin-like receptors associated with FcRγ or DAP12 are thus identified as previously unexpected but nevertheless essential partners of RANK during osteoclastogenesis.

It is conceivable that RANK activates an as yet unknown pathway that specifically synergizes with or upregulates ITAM signaling. We have shown that Tec family tyrosine kinases (Tec and Btk) activated by RANK cooperate with Syk to induce efficient phosphorylation of PLCγ(Shinohara et al., 2008). An osteopetrotic phenotype in Tec and Btk double-deficient mice revealed that these two kinases play an essential role in the regulation of osteoclastogenesis. Tec and Btk had been known to play a key role in proximal B-cell receptor signaling, but this study established their crucial role in linking the RANK and ITAM signals (Figure 5.1).

CROSSTALK BETWEEN RANKL AND OTHER CYTOKINE SIGNALING

Osteoclasts are derived from the monocyte/macrophage lineage, and the precursor cells express various cytokine receptors. Inflammatory cytokines that are mainly produced by macrophages such as IL-1, TNF-α, and IL-6 promote osteoclastogenesis and are also called osteolytic cytokines on the basis of their bone-resorptive effect *in vivo* (Kwan Tat et al., 2004; Lee et al., 2008). IL-1, TNF-α, and IL-6 indirectly facilitate osteoclastogenesis by acting on the osteoblasts through induction of RANKL (Suda et al., 1999; Palmqvist et al., 2002; Sato et al., 2004). IL-1 also stimulates TRAF6 (and therefore activates NF-κB and MAPKs) and synergizes with RANKL to promote the bone-resorbing activity of mature osteoclasts, but interestingly IL-1 alone cannot induce differentiation, indicating that TRAF6 activation is not sufficient. TNF-α stimulates the activation of NF-κB mainly through TRAF2. Although TNF-α alone cannot induce osteoclastogenesis *in vivo*, nor can TNF-α overexpression rescue the deficiency of RANKL (Lam et al., 2000; Li et al., 2004), TNF-α plus transforming growth factor-β (TGF-β) was reported to induce *in vitro* osteoclastogenesis even in the absence of RANK or TRAF6 (Kim et al., 2005). In addition, TNF-α enhances the osteoclastogenic potential of osteoclast precursor cells through inducing PIR-A (Ochi et al., 2007).

Type I interferons (IFN-α and IFN-β) are essential for host defense against pathogens such as viruses. RANKL induces the *IFN-β* gene in osteoclast precursor cells, and IFN-β functions as a negative-feedback regulator that inhibits the differentiation of osteoclasts by interfering with the RANKL-induced expression of c-Fos. The importance of type I IFNs in bone homeostasis was underscored by the observation that mice deficient in the type I IFN-receptor component IFNAR1 spontaneously develop marked osteopenia, accompanied by enhanced osteoclastogenesis (Takayanagi et al., 2002b).

MECHANISM OF BONE DESTRUCTION IN RA

THE ESSENTIAL ROLE OF OSTEOCLASTS IN BONE DESTRUCTION IN RA

As described earlier, efficient osteoclast formation was observed in synovial cell cultures obtained from patients with RA (Takayanagi et al., 1997). Moreover, the expression of RANKL was detected specifically in the synovium of patients with RA but not in the synovium of patients with other bone diseases (Gravallese et al., 2000; Takayanagi et al., 2000a). Recent studies have provided further direct genetic evidence: RANKL-deficient mice, which lack osteoclasts, were protected from bone destruction in an arthritis model induced by serum transfer (Pettit et al., 2001). Bone erosion was not observed in osteopetrotic $Fos^{-/-}$ mice, even when they were crossed with TNF-α transgenic mice that develop erosive arthritis spontaneously (Redlich et al., 2002). In both cases, a similar level of inflammation was observed, indicating that RANKL and osteoclasts are indispensable for the bone loss but not for the inflammation. Consistent with this, anti-RANKL and antiosteoclast therapies was shown to be beneficial in the treatment of bone damage in animal models of arthritis (Kong et al., 1999a; Takayanagi et al., 1999). Inflammatory cytokines such as TNF-α, IL-1, and IL-6 are important accelerators of the bone destruction in RA. Especially, TNF-α is considered important because anti-TNF therapy reduces bone erosion as well as inflammation (Lipsky et al., 2000; Redlich et al., 2003; Catrina et al., 2005; Lange et al., 2005; Takayanagi, 2009).

EFFECT OF T CELLS ON OSTEOCLASTOGENESIS

As infiltration of T cells into the synovium is a hallmark pathological finding of RA, it is vital to address how T-cell immunity is linked to the enhanced expression of RANKL and osteoclastic bone resorption. More specifically, as RANKL is known to be expressed in activated T cells, it is important to determine whether this source of RANKL can directly induce osteoclast differentiation. In 1999, Kong et al. showed that RANKL expressed on activated T cells directly acts on osteoclast precursor cells and induces osteoclastogenesis *in vitro* (Kong et al., 1999a). Horwood et al. (1999) also reported that osteoclastogenesis could be induced *in vitro* by activated T cells. However, it is important to note that T cells produce various cytokines, including IFN-γ, IL-4, and IL-10, which exert potent inhibitory effects on osteoclast differentiation (Takayanagi, 2007). In the former study, the T cells were fixed by formaldehyde and could not release any humoral factors (Kong et al., 1999a). In the latter study, the T cells and the osteoclast precursor cells were derived from different species, suggesting that the effect of cytokines would be much lower than that on cells of the same species (Horwood et al., 1999). The question then arises as to how T-cell cytokines other than RANKL affect osteoclast differentiation.

Upon activation, naive CD4$^+$ T cells differentiate into different lineages of Th cells, depending on the cytokine milieu (Zhou et al., 2009). Th1 and Th2 cells are traditionally thought to be the major subsets generated on antigenic stimulation. Th1 cells, which are induced by IL-12, produce mainly IFN-γ and are involved in cellular immunity; Th2 cells mainly produce IL-4, IL-5, and IL-10 and contribute to humoral immunity. RA was considered to be a disease in which the Th1–Th2 balance is skewed toward Th1. However, IFN-γ are not highly expressed in the joints of RA patients (Firestein and Zvaifler, 1990). Notably, IFN-γ strongly inhibits osteoclastogenesis even at minute concentrations through ubiquitin-proteasome-mediated degradation of TRAF6 (Takayanagi et al., 2000b). Moreover, the severity of collagen-induced arthritis was reported to be exaggerated in the absence of IFN-γ signaling (Manoury-Schwartz et al., 1997; Vermeire et al., 1997), suggesting that Th1 cells are not linked to bone damage in arthritis.

TH17 CELLS FUNCTION AS THE OSTEOCLASTOGENIC TH CELLS

It is worthwhile to define what we believe to be a very rare but pathologically important Th cell subset responsible for abnormal bone resorption as osteoclastogenic Th cells. Previous investigations in our laboratory and other studies on synovial T cells in RA clarified the characteristics of osteoclastogenic Th cells in autoimmune arthritis (Sato and Takayanagi, 2006; Takayanagi, 2005). First, osteoclastogenic Th cells do not produce a large amount of IFN-γ. Second, they trigger local inflammation and the production of inflammatory cytokines that induce RANKL expression on synovial fibroblasts. Third, osteoclastogenic Th cells express RANKL and might directly participate in accelerated osteoclastogenesis. Because these Th cells have such osteoclastogenic characteristics, they can tip the balance in favor of osteoclastogenesis in various aspects.

IL-17-producing helper T (Th17) cells have recently been identified as a new subset of effector Th cells, which is characterized by the production of proinflammatory cytokines including IL-17, IL-17F, IL-21, and IL-22. Th17 cell differentiation is induced by the combination of IL-6 and TGF-β. IL-23 is dispensable for lineage commitment of Th17 cells but required for the growth, survival, and effector functions of Th17 cells (Kastelein et al., 2007; Korn et al., 2009). Importantly, this unique subset plays a critical role in host defense against certain extracellular pathogens and also contributes to the pathogenesis of various autoimmune diseases (Korn et al., 2009; Dong, 2008). Recent data from our laboratory indicate that Th17 cells represent the long sought-after osteoclastogenic Th cell subset, fulfilling all the criteria mentioned earlier (Sato et al., 2006b). IL-17 induces RANKL on osteoclastogenesis-supporting mesenchymal cells such as osteoblasts and synovial fibroblasts (Kotake et al., 1999). IL-17 also enhances local inflammation and increases the production of inflammatory cytokines, which further promote RANKL expression and activity. Therefore, the infiltration of Th17 cells into the inflammatory lesion links the abnormal T-cell response to bone damage (Figure 5.2).

NOVEL INSIGHTS INTO THE MECHANISMS OF TH17 INDUCTION IN AUTOIMMUNITY

Th17 cell subset has emerged as attractive therapeutic targets for both inflammation and bone destruction. It is therefore important to understand the molecular mechanism underlying Th17 development to develop novel therapeutic strategies.

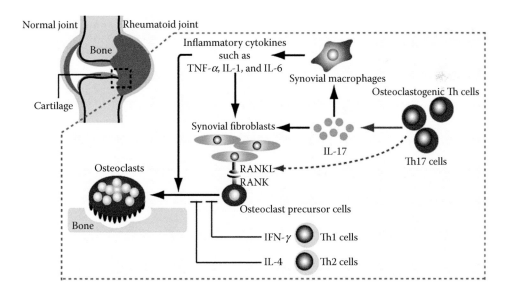

FIGURE 5.2 (See color insert.) Regulation of osteoclast differentiation by T cells in RA, Th17 cells have stimulatory effects on osteoclastogenesis and play an important role in the pathogenesis of RA through IL-17, whereas Th1 and Th2 cells have inhibitory effects on osteoclastogenesis through IFN-γ and IL-4, respectively. IL-17 not only induces RANKL on synovial fibroblasts of mesenchymal origin but also activates local inflammation, leading to the upregulation of proinflammatory cytokines, such as TNF-α, IL-1, and IL-6. These cytokines activate osteoclastogenesis by either directly acting on osteoclast precursor cells or inducing RANKL on synovial fibroblasts. Th17 cells also express RANKL on their membrane, which partly contributes to the enhanced osteoclastogenesis.

A Novel Role of Cathepsin K in Autoimmunity

Cathepsin K is a lysosomal cysteine protease that plays a pivotal role in osteoclast-mediated degradation of the bone matrices (Gelb et al., 1996; Brix et al., 2008). Thus, cathepsin K has been considered as a potential therapeutic target for the treatment of bone diseases such as osteoporosis. We developed a new orally active cathepsin K inhibitor, NC-2300, and examined the effect of the inhibitor in osteoporosis as well as arthritis models (Asagiri et al., 2008). We observed unexpected results that cathepsin K suppression leads to the reduction of inflammation in the latter model. Cathepsin K, despite a low expression level in dendritic cells, plays an important role in the activation of TLR-9 signaling. CpG (cytosine followed by guanine) DNA (a TLR-9 ligand)-induced production of cytokines such as IL-6 and IL-23 was found to be impaired in cathepsin K inhibitor–treated or cathepsin K–deficient dendritic cells. The immune function of cathepsin K was further analyzed in experimental autoimmune encephalomyelitis (EAE), a mouse model of multiple sclerosis, and the severity of the disease was markedly suppressed in cathepsin K–deficient mice. The suppression of inflammation was associated with the reduced induction of Th17 cells, indicating that cathepsin K contributes to autoimmune inflammation by inducing Th17 cells, possibly through cytokines such as IL-6 and IL-23 in dendritic cells.

The detailed mechanism by which cathepsin K regulates TLR-9 signaling remains elusive, but it has been reported that functional maturation of TLR-9 requires its proteolytic cleavage (Ewald et al., 2008; Park et al., 2008), to which cathepsin K might contribute. As cathepsin K is now known to be expressed by other cell types including synovial cells (Hummel et al., 1998; Hou et al., 2001), we cannot exclude the possibility that NC-2300 exerted an antiarthritic effect through other cells. However, cathepsin K is an interesting example of a molecule that was originally found in bone and subsequently shown to regulate the immune system. Our study identified cathepsin K as a novel dendritic cell-specific regulator of TLR-9 signaling and as a potential target of therapeutic intervention into inflammation-associated bone loss (Figure 5.3).

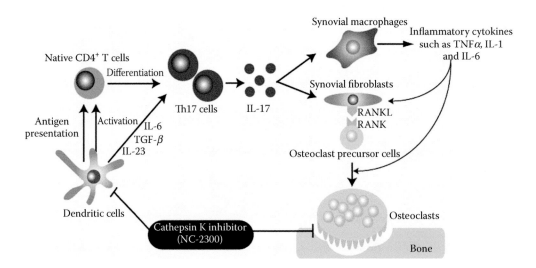

FIGURE 5.3   (See color insert.) A cathepsin K inhibitor inhibits both Th17 development and osteoclastogenesis. Cathepsin K is involved in the TLR-9-mediated activation of dendritic cells as well as osteoclastic bone resorption. Cathepsin K inhibition results in the reduced expression of inflammatory cytokines such as IL-6 and IL-23, which are important for the induction of Th17 cells. Therefore, a cathepsin K inhibitor (NC-2300) has dual benefits in the treatment of autoimmune arthritis.

The Essential Role of IκBζ in Th17 Development

Coordinated cytokine signaling induces the activation of specific transcription factors to promote lineage-specific cytokine production in Th cells (Zhou et al., 2009). For example, T-box-containing protein expressed in T cells, activated by IL-12 and IFN-γ, is required for Th1 cell differentiation. Th2 cell differentiation requires the function of GATA binding protein 3 induced by IL-4-activated signal transducer and activator of transcription (Stat) 6.

Soon after the discovery of Th17 cells, Dr. Littman et al. reported that retinoid-related orphan receptor γt (RORγt) is selectively expressed in Th17 cells and required for Th17 cell differentiation (Ivanov et al., 2006). RORγt expression is induced by the combination of IL-6 and TGF-β through Stat3. Furthermore, RORγt deficiency led to an impairment of Th17 cell differentiation *in vitro* and *in vivo*. Subsequent studies by Dr. Dong et al. showed that another ROR family member, RORα, is also highly induced during Th17 cell differentiation in a Stat3-dependent manner (Yang et al. 2008). Although RORα deletion in mice had minimal effect on IL-17 production, deficiency of both RORα and RORγt completely abolished IL-17 production and protected mice from EAE. Thus, RORγt and RORα have redundant functions, but RORγt seems to be a major player in Th17 cell differentiation. However, the mechanisms by which the ROR nuclear receptor drives Th17 development have not yet been fully elucidated. Notably, several groups reported that the ectopic expression of RORγt or RORα leads to only a modest IL-17 production in the absence of IL-6 and TGF-β (Yang et al. 2008; Brustle et al., 2007).

Our group found that the expression of a nuclear IκB family member, IκBζ, was most highly expressed in Th17 cells among Th cell subsets (Okamoto et al., 2010). IκBζ is a nuclear protein highly homologous to Bcl-3, which interacts with the NF-κB subunit via the ankyrin repeat domain (Muta, 2006). Its expression is rapidly induced by TLR ligands or IL-1 stimulation in peritoneal macrophages. Yamamoto et al. demonstrated using IκBζ-deficient mice that IκBζ is essential for the induction of a subset of secondary response genes, including IL-6 and IL-12 p40 subunit in macrophages (Yamamoto et al., 2004). However, no attempt was made to determine the function of IκBζ in T cells in their study.

IκBζ expression was upregulated by the combination of IL-6 and TGF-β. IκBζ induction was mediated by Stat3, but not by RORγt, in Th17 cells. Importantly, not only IκBζ-deficient mice but also Rag2-deficient mice transferred with IκBζ-deficient CD4+ T cells were highly resistant to EAE. When naive CD4+ T cells were activated *in vitro* under Th1- and Th2-polarizing conditions, IκBζ-deficient naive CD4+ T cells normally produced IFN-γ and IL-4, respectively. On the other hand, when activated under Th17-polarizing conditions, IL-17 production in IκBζ-deficient T cells was markedly reduced compared with wild-type T cells. Since the expression of RORγt and RORα was normal in IκBζ-deficient T cells, it is unlikely that ROR nuclear receptors function downstream of IκBζ or vice versa.

In the absence of IL-6 and TGF-β, the ectopic expression of IκBζ in naive CD4+ T cells did not induce IL-17 production. Interestingly, even in the absence of IL-6 and TGF-β, the ectopic expression of IκBζ together with RORγt or RORα potently induced IL-17 production. The reporter assay showed that IκBζ moderately activated the promoter of the mouse *Il17* gene as well as RORγt and RORα. When ROR nuclear receptor was expressed, IκBζ highly activated the *Il17* promoter. Previous studies showed that an evolutionarily conserved noncoding sequences 2 (CNS2) region in the *Il17* locus is associated with histone H3 acetylation in a Th17 lineage-specific manner and that ROR nuclear receptor is recruited to the CNS2 region during Th17 development (Akimzhanov et al., 2007; Yang et al., 2008; Zhang et al., 2008). In combination with RORγt and RORα, IκBζ strongly induced the CNS2 enhancer activity. IκBζ was recruited to the CNS2 region in Th17 cells, and recruitment of IκBζ to the CNS2 region was dependent on RORγt function (Figure 5.4). Moreover, the expression of IL-17F, IL-21, and IL-23 receptor was decreased in IκBζ-deficient T cells. IκBζ also bound to the promoter or the enhancer region of these genes in Th17 cells. Collectively, these findings indicated that IκBζ is critical for the transcriptional program in Th17 cell lineage commitment (Okamoto et al. 2010).

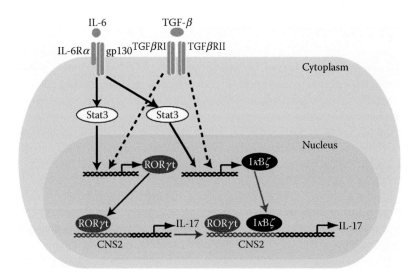

FIGURE 5.4 **(See color insert.)** IκBζ and ROR nuclear receptors synergistically promote Th17 development. IL-6 and TGF-β induce Th17 cell differentiation, in which ROR nuclear receptors, RORγt and RORα, have an indispensable role. The expression of IκBζ is induced by the combination of IL-6 and TGF-β. IκBζ induction is mediated by Stat3, but not RORγt. IκBζ and ROR nuclear receptor bind directly to the CNS2 region of the *Il17* promoter and cooperatively activate the *Il17* promoter. Notably, recruitment of IκBζ to the CNS2 region was dependent on RORγt, suggesting that the binding of both IκBζ and ROR nuclear receptors to the *Il17* promoter leads to an efficient recruitment of transcriptional coactivators with histone acetylase activity.

CONCLUSIONS

The emerging field of osteoimmunology originates from studies on bone destruction in RA. Increasing evidence suggests that the skeletal and immune systems are connected in complex ways, and it would be difficult to understand either system adequately without the insights afforded by studying their interaction in an osteoimmunologic context. The findings in RA might be applicable to numerous inflammatory or neoplastic diseases, such as periodontitis, infectious diseases, and primary or metastatic bone tumors; however, the role of the immune system in osteoporosis and/or osteoarthritis still remains largely unclear.

Clearly, Th17 cell subset is an auspicious target for future therapeutic investigation, and cytokines related to Th17 cell differentiation and function will be of great clinical importance. Antibodies against IL-17 or IL-23 could be expected to exert beneficial effects in autoimmune diseases, and antibodies targeting the IL-6 receptor might also inhibit Th17 development in RA, in addition to direct inhibition of local inflammation and osteoclastogenesis (Takatori et al., 2008; Mihara et al., 2009). The mechanism of Th17 development is currently one of the most important subjects in immunology. In recent years, several transcriptional regulators of Th17 development have been reported including IFN regulatory factor 4, B-cell-activating transcription factor, aryl hydrocarbon receptor, and runt-related transcription factor 1 (Brustle et al., 2007; Quintana et al., 2008; Veldhoen et al., 2008; Zhang et al., 2008; Schraml et al., 2009). Although further studies will be required to determine whether or how IκBζ synergizes with other transcriptional regulators of Th17 cells, our results raise the possibility that targeting of IκBζ may prove effective for the treatment of autoimmune diseases.

Importantly, Th17 cells are also implicated in host defense against a number of microorganisms. Inhibition of Th17 cells might have the risk of increasing susceptibility to infection. Therefore, careful efforts will be necessary to prevent autoimmune diseases without compromising the host defense system. Understanding of the precise role of Th17 cells in human autoimmune disorders will be required for the development of effective therapeutic interventions.

ACKNOWLEDGMENTS

This work was supported in part by Grants-in-Aid for GCOE Program from the Ministry of Education, Culture, Sports, Science and Technology of Japan (MEXT) and the ERATO, Takayanagi Osteonetwork Project, from JST. It was also supported by grants from Takeda Life Science Foundation and Yokoyama Foundation for Clinical Pharmacology and the Ichiro Kanehara Foundation.

REFERENCES

Akimzhanov AM, Yang XO, Dong C. Chromatin remodeling of interleukin-17 (IL-17)-IL-17F cytokine gene locus during inflammatory helper T cell differentiation. J Biol Chem 2007;282(9):5969–5972.

Aliprantis AO, Ueki Y, Sulyanto R, Park A, Sigrist KS, Sharma SM, Ostrowski MC, Olsen BR, Glimcher LH. NFATc1 in mice represses osteoprotegerin during osteoclastogenesis and dissociates systemic osteopenia from inflammation in cherubism. J Clin Invest 2008;118(11):3775–3789.

Anderson DM, Maraskovsky E, Billingsley WL, Dougall WC, Tometsko ME, Roux ER, Teepe MC, DuBose RF, Cosman D, Galibert L. A homologue of the TNF receptor and its ligand enhance T-cell growth and dendritic-cell function. Nature 1997;390(6656):175–179.

Asagiri M, Hirai T, Kunigami T, Kamano S, Gober HJ, Okamoto K, Nishikawa K, et al. Cathepsin K–dependent toll-like receptor 9 signaling revealed in experimental arthritis. Science 2008;319(5863):624–627.

Asagiri M, Sato K, Usami T, Ochi S, Nishina H, Yoshida H, Morita I, et al. Autoamplification of NFATc1 expression determines its essential role in bone homeostasis. J Exp Med 2005;202(9):1261–1269.

Bai S, Kitaura H, Zhao H, Chen J, Muller JM, Schule R, Darnay B, Novack DV, Ross FP, Teitelbaum SL. FHL2 inhibits the activated osteoclast in a TRAF6-dependent manner. J Clin Invest 2005; 115(10): 2742–2751.

Bohm C, Hayer S, Kilian A, Zaiss MM, Finger S, Hess A, Engelke K, et al. The α-isoform of p38 MAPK specifically regulates arthritic bone loss. J Immunol 2009;183(9):5938–5947.

Brix K, Dunkhorst A, Mayer K, Jordans S. Cysteine cathepsins: cellular roadmap to different functions. Biochimie 2008;90(2):194–207.

Bromley M, Woolley DE. Chondroclasts and osteoclasts at subchondral sites of erosion in the rheumatoid joint. Arthritis Rheum 1984;27(9):968–975.

Brustle A, Heink S, Huber M, Rosenplanter C, Stadelmann C, Yu P, Arpaia E, Mak TW, Kamradt T, Lohoff M. The development of inflammatory T$_H$-17 cells requires interferon-regulatory factor 4. Nat Immunol 2007;8(9):958–966.

Bucay N, Sarosi I, Dunstan CR, Morony S, Tarpley J, Capparelli C, Scully S, Tan HL, et al. *Osteoprotegerin-* deficient mice develop early onset osteoporosis and arterial calcification. Genes Dev 1998;12(9): 1260–1268.

Catrina AI, Trollmo C, af Klint E, Engstrom M, Lampa J, Hermansson Y, Klareskog L, Ulfgren AK. Evidence that anti-tumor necrosis factor therapy with both etanercept and infliximab induces apoptosis in macrophages, but not lymphocytes, in rheumatoid arthritis joints: extended report. Arthritis Rheum 2005;52(1):61–72.

Dong C. T$_H$17 cells in development: an updated view of their molecular identity and genetic programming. Nature Rev. Immunol 2008;8(5):337–348.

Dougall WC, Glaccum M, Charrier K, Rohrbach K, Brasel K, De Smedt T, Daro E, et al. RANK is essential for osteoclast and lymph node development. Genes Dev 1999;13(18):2412–2424.

Ewald SE, Lee BL, Lau L, Wickliffe KE, Shi GP, Chapman HA, Barton GM. The ectodomain of Toll-like receptor 9 is cleaved to generate a functional receptor. Nature 2008;456(7222):658–662.

Firestein GS, Zvaifler NJ. How important are T cells in chronic rheumatoid synovitis? Arthritis Rheum 1990;33(6):768–773.

Franzoso G, Carlson L, Xing L, Poljak L, Shores EW, Brown KD, Leonardi A, Tran T, Boyce BF, Siebenlist U. Requirement for NF-κB in osteoclast and B-cell development. Genes Dev 1997; 11(24): 3482–3496.

Gelb BD, Shi GP, Chapman HA, Desnick RJ. Pycnodysostosis, a lysosomal disease caused by cathepsin K deficiency. Science 1996;273(5279):1236–1238.

Gohda J, Akiyama T, Koga T, Takayanagi H, Tanaka S, Inoue J. RANK-mediated amplification of TRAF6 signaling leads to NFATc1 induction during osteoclastogenesis. EMBO J 2005;24(4):790–799.

Gravallese EM, Harada Y, Wang JT, Gorn AH, Thornhill TS, Goldring SR. Identification of cell types responsible for bone resorption in rheumatoid arthritis and juvenile rheumatoid arthritis. Am J Pathol 1998;152(4):943–951.

Gravallese EM, Manning C, Tsay A, Naito A, Pan C, Amento E, Goldring SR. Synovial tissue in rheumatoid arthritis is a source of osteoclast differentiation factor. Arthritis Rheum 2000;43(2):250–258.

Guerrini MM, Sobacchi C, Cassani B, Abinun M, Kilic SS, Pangrazio A, Moratto D, et al. Human osteoclast-poor osteopetrosis with hypogammaglobulinemia due to *TNFRSF11A(RANK)* mutations. Am J Hum Genet 2008;83(1):64–76.

Horwood NJ, Kartsogiannis V, Quinn JM, Romas E, Martin TJ, Gillespie MT. Activated T lymphocytes support osteoclast formation *in vitro*. Biochem Biophys Res Commun 1999;265(1):144–150.

Hou WS, Li Z, Gordon RE, Chan K, Klein MJ, Levy R, Keysser M, Keyszer G, Bromme D. Cathepsin K is a critical protease in synovial fibroblast-mediated collagen degradation. Am J Pathol 2001;159(6):2167–2177.

Hughes AE, Ralston SH, Marken J, Bell C, MacPherson H, Wallace RG, van Hul W, et al. Mutations in *TNFRSF11A*, affecting the signal peptide of RANK, cause familial expansile osteolysis. Nat Genet 2000;24(1):45–48.

Hummel KM, Petrow PK, Franz JK, Muller-Ladner U, Aicher WK, Gay RE, Bromme D, Gay S. Cysteine pro-teinase cathepsin K mRNA is expressed in synovium of patients with rheumatoid arthritis and is detected at sites of synovial bone destruction. J Rheumatol 1998;25(10):1887–1894.

Iotsova V, Caamano J, Loy J, Yang Y, Lewin A, Bravo R. Osteopetrosis in mice lacking NF-κB1 and NF-κB2. Nat Med 1997;3(11):1285–1289.

Ivanov II, McKenzie BS, Zhou L, Tadokoro CE, Lepelley A, Lafaille JJ, Cua DJ, Littman DR. The orphan nuclear receptor RORγt directs the differentiation program of proinflammatory IL-17+ T helper cells. Cell 2006;126(6):1121–1133.

Kastelein RA, Hunter CA, Cua DJ. Discovery and biology of IL-23 and IL-27: related but functionally distinct regulators of inflammation. Annu Rev Immunol 2007;25:221–242.

Kim N, Kadono Y, Takami M, Lee J, Lee SH, Okada F, Kim JH, et al. Osteoclast differentiation independent of the TRANCE–RANK–TRAF6 axis. J Exp Med 2005;202(5):589–595.

Kobayashi N, Kadono Y, Naito A, Matsumoto K, Yamamoto T, Tanaka S, Inoue J. Segregation of TRAF6-mediated signaling pathways clarifies its role in osteoclastogenesis. EMBO J 2001; 20(6):1271–1280.

Koga T, Inui M, Inoue K, Kim S, Suematsu A, Kobayashi E, Iwata T, et al. Costimulatory signals mediated by the ITAM motif cooperate with RANKL for bone homeostasis. Nature 2004;428(6984):758–763.

Kong YY, Feige U, Sarosi I, Bolon B, Tafuri A, Morony S, Capparelli C, et al. Activated T cells regu-late bone loss and joint destruction in adjuvant arthritis through osteoprotegerin ligand. Nature 1999a;402(6759):304–309.

Kong YY, Yoshida H, Sarosi I, Tan HL, Timms E, Capparelli C, Morony S, et al. OPGL is a key reg-ulator of osteoclastogenesis, lymphocyte development and lymph-node organogenesis. Nature 1999b;397(6717):315–323.

Korn T, Bettelli E, Oukka M, Kuchroo VK. IL-17 and Th17 cells. Annu Rev Immunol 2009;27:485–517.

Kotake S, Udagawa N, Takahashi N, Matsuzaki K, Itoh K, Ishiyama S, Saito S, et al. IL-17 in synovial flu-ids from patients with rheumatoid arthritis is a potent stimulator of osteoclastogenesis. J Clin Invest 1999;103(9):1345–1352.

Kwan Tat S, Padrines M, Theoleyre S, Heymann D, Fortun Y. IL-6, RANKL, TNF-α/IL-1: interrelations in bone resorption pathophysiology. Cytokine Growth Factor Rev 2004;15(1):49–60.

Lacey DL, Timms E, Tan HL, Kelley MJ, Dunstan CR, Burgess T, Elliott R, et al. Osteoprotegerin ligand is a cytokine that regulates osteoclast differentiation and activation. Cell 1998;93(2):165–176.

Lagasse E, Weissman IL. Enforced expression of Bcl-2 in monocytes rescues macrophages and partially reverses osteopetrosis in *op/op* mice. Cell 1997;89(7):1021–1031.

Lam J, Takeshita S, Barker JE, Kanagawa O, Ross FP, Teitelbaum SL. TNF-α induces osteoclastogenesis by direct stimulation of macrophages exposed to permissive levels of RANK ligand. J Clin Invest 2000;106(12):1481–1488.

Lange U, Teichmann J, Muller-Ladner U, Strunk J. Increase in bone mineral density of patients with rheu-matoid arthritis treated with anti-TNF-α antibody: a prospective open-label pilot study. Rheumatology (Oxford) 2005;44(12):1546–1548.

Lee SH, Kim TS, Choi Y, Lorenzo J. Osteoimmunology: cytokines and the skeletal system. BMB Rep 2008;41(7):495–510.

Li J, Sarosi I, Yan XQ, Morony S, Capparelli C, Tan HL, McCabe S, et al. RANK is the intrinsic hematopoietic cell surface receptor that controls osteoclastogenesis and regulation of bone mass and calcium metabo-lism. Proc Natl Acad Sci U S A 2000;97(4):1566–1571.

Li P, Schwarz EM, O'Keefe RJ, Ma L, Boyce BF, Xing L. RANK signaling is not required for TNFα-mediated increase in CD11[hi] osteoclast precursors but is essential for mature osteoclast formation in TNFα-mediated inflammatory arthritis. J Bone Miner Res 2004;19(2):207–213.

Lipsky PE, van der Heijde DM, St Clair EW, Furst DE, Breedveld FC, Kalden JR, Smolen JS, et al. Infliximab and methotrexate in the treatment of rheumatoid arthritis. Anti-Tumor Necrosis Factor Trial in Rheumatoid Arthritis with Concomitant Therapy Study Group. N Engl J Med 2000;343(22):1594–1602.

Lomaga MA, Yeh WC, Sarosi I, Duncan GS, Furlonger C, Ho A, Morony S, et al. TRAF6 deficiency results in osteopetrosis and defective interleukin-1, CD40, and LPS signaling. Genes Dev 1999;13(8):1015–1024.

Manoury-Schwartz B, Chiocchia G, Bessis N, Abehsira-Amar O, Batteux F, Muller S, Huang S, Boissier MC, Fournier C. High susceptibility to collagen-induced arthritis in mice lacking IFN-γ receptors. J Immunol 1997;158(11):5501–5506.

Mihara M, Ohsugi Y, Kishimoto T. Evidence for the role of Th17 cell inhibition in the prevention of autoimmune diseases by anti-interluekin-6 receptor antibody. Biofactors 2009;35(1):47–51.

Mizuno A, Amizuka N, Irie K, Murakami A, Fujise N, Kanno T, Sato Y, et al. Severe osteoporosis in mice lacking osteoclastogenesis inhibitory factor/osteoprotegerin. Biochem Biophys Res Commun 1998;247(3):610–615.

Mocsai A, Humphrey MB, Van Ziffle JA, Hu Y, Burghardt A, Spusta SC, Majumdar S, Lanier LL, Lowell CA, Nakamura MC. The immunomodulatory adapter proteins DAP12 and Fc receptor γ-chain (FcRγ) regulate development of functional osteoclasts through the Syk tyrosine kinase. Proc Natl Acad Sci U S A 2004;101(16):6158–6163.

Muta T. IκB-ζ: an inducible regulator of nuclear factor-κB. Vitam Horm 2006;74:301–316.

Naito A, Azuma S, Tanaka S, Miyazaki T, Takaki S, Takatsu K, Nakao K, et al. Severe osteopetrosis, defective interleukin-1 signalling and lymph node organogenesis in *TRAF6*-deficient mice. Genes Cells 1999;4(6):353–362.

Negishi-Koga T, Takayanagi H. Ca^{2+}-NFATc1 signaling is an essential axis of osteoclast differentiation. Immunol Rev 2009;231(1):241–256.

Ochi S, Shinohara M, Sato K, Gober HJ, Koga T, Kodama T, Takai T, Miyasaka N, Takayanagi H. Pathological role of osteoclast costimulation in arthritis-induced bone loss. Proc Natl Acad Sci U S A 2007;104(27):11394–11399.

Okada Y, Nagase H, Harris ED Jr. Matrix metalloproteinases 1, 2, and 3 from rheumatoid synovial cells are sufficient to destroy joints. J Rheumatol 1987;14 Spec No:41–42.

Okamoto K, Iwai Y, Oh-hora M, Yamamoto M, Morio T, Aoki K, Ohya K, et al. IκBζ regulates T$_H$17 development by cooperating with ROR nuclear receptors. Nature 2010;464(7293):1381–1385.

Palmqvist P, Persson E, Conaway HH, Lerner UH. IL-6, leukemia inhibitory factor, and oncostatin M stimulate bone resorption and regulate the expression of receptor activator of NF-κB ligand, osteoprotegerin, and receptor activator of NF-κB in mouse calvariae. J Immunol 2002;169(6):3353–3362.

Park B, Brinkmann MM, Spooner E, Lee CC, Kim YM, Ploegh HL. Proteolytic cleavage in an endolysosomal compartment is required for activation of Toll-like receptor 9. Nat Immunol 2008;9(12):1407–1414.

Pettit AR, Ji H, von Stechow D, Muller R, Goldring SR, Choi Y, Benoist C, Gravallese EM. TRANCE/RANKL knockout mice are protected from bone erosion in a serum transfer model of arthritis. Am J Pathol 2001;159(5):1689–1699.

Quintana FJ, Basso AS, Iglesias AH, Korn T, Farez MF, Bettelli E, Caccamo M, Oukka M, Weiner HL. Control of T$_{reg}$ and T$_H$17 cell differentiation by the aryl hydrocarbon receptor. Nature 2008;453(7191):65–71.

Redlich K, Hayer S, Ricci R, David JP, Tohidast-Akrad M, Kollias G, Steiner G, Smolen JS, Wagner EF, Schett G. Osteoclasts are essential for TNF-α-mediated joint destruction. J Clin Invest 2002; 110(10): 1419–1427.

Redlich K, Schett G, Steiner G, Hayer S, Wagner EF, Smolen JS. Rheumatoid arthritis therapy after tumor necrosis factor and interleukin-1 blockade. Arthritis Rheum 2003;48(12):3308–3319.

Sato K, Suematsu A, Nakashima T, Takemoto-Kimura S, Aoki K, Morishita Y, Asahara H, et al. Regulation of osteoclast differentiation and function by the CaMK–CREB pathway. Nat Med 2006a;12(12):1410–1416.

Sato K, Suematsu A, Okamoto K, Yamaguchi A, Morishita Y, Kadono Y, Tanaka S, et al. Th17 functions as an osteoclastogenic helper T cell subset that links T cell activation and bone destruction. J Exp Med 2006b;203(12):2673–2682.

Sato K, Takayanagi H. Osteoclasts, rheumatoid arthritis, and osteoimmunology. Curr Opin Rheumatol 2006;18(4):419–426.

Sato N, Takahashi N, Suda K, Nakamura M, Yamaki M, Ninomiya T, Kobayashi Y, et al. MyD88 but not TRIF is essential for osteoclastogenesis induced by lipopolysaccharide, diacyl lipopeptide, and IL-1α. J Exp Med 2004;200(5):601–611.

Schraml BU, Hildner K, Ise W, Lee WL, Smith WA, Solomon B, Sahota G, et al. The AP-1 transcription factor Batf controls T_H17 differentiation. Nature 2009;460(7253):405–409.

Seeman E, Delmas PD. Bone quality—the material and structural basis of bone strength and fragility. N Engl J Med 2006;354(21):2250–2261.

Shinohara M, Koga T, Okamoto K, Sakaguchi S, Arai K, Yasuda H, Takai T, et al. Tyrosine kinases Btk and Tec regulate osteoclast differentiation by linking RANK and ITAM signals. Cell 2008; 132(5):794–806.

Simonet WS, Lacey DL, Dunstan CR, Kelley M, Chang MS, Luthy R, Nguyen HQ, et al. Osteoprotegerin: a novel secreted protein involved in the regulation of bone density. Cell 1997;89(2):309–319.

Sobacchi C, Frattini A, Guerrini MM, Abinun M, Pangrazio A, Susani L, Bredius R, et al. Osteoclast-poor human osteopetrosis due to mutations in the gene encoding RANKL. Nat Genet 2007;39(8):960–962.

Suda T, Takahashi N, Udagawa N, Jimi E, Gillespie MT, Martin TJ. Modulation of osteoclast differentiation and function by the new members of the tumor necrosis factor receptor and ligand families. Endocr Rev 1999;20(3):345–357.

Takahashi N, Akatsu T, Udagawa N, Sasaki T, Yamaguchi A, Moseley JM, Martin TJ, Suda T. Osteoblastic cells are involved in osteoclast formation. Endocrinology 1988a;123(5):2600–2602.

Takahashi N, Yamana H, Yoshiki S, Roodman GD, Mundy GR, Jones SJ, Boyde A, Suda T. Osteoclast-like cell formation and its regulation by osteotropic hormones in mouse bone marrow cultures. Endocrinology 1988b;122(4):1373–1382.

Takatori H, Kanno Y, Chen Z, O'Shea JJ. New complexities in helper T cell fate determination and the implications for autoimmune diseases. Mod Rheumatol 2008;18(6):533–541.

Takayanagi H. Inflammatory bone destruction and osteoimmunology. J Periodontal Res 2005;40(4):287–293.

Takayanagi H. Osteoimmunology: shared mechanisms and crosstalk between the immune and bone systems. Nat Rev Immunol 2007;7(4):292–304.

Takayanagi H. Osteoimmunology and the effects of the immune system on bone. Nat Rev Rheumatol 2009;5(12):667–676.

Takayanagi H, Iizuka H, Juji T, Nakagawa T, Yamamoto A, Miyazaki T, Koshihara Y, Oda H, Nakamura K, Tanaka S. Involvement of receptor activator of nuclear factor κB ligand/osteoclast differentiation factor in osteoclastogenesis from synoviocytes in rheumatoid arthritis. Arthritis Rheum 2000a;43(2):259–269.

Takayanagi H, Juji T, Miyazaki T, Iizuka H, Takahashi T, Isshiki M, Okada M, et al. Suppression of arthritic bone destruction by adenovirus-mediated *csk* gene transfer to synoviocytes and osteoclasts. J Clin Invest 1999;104(2):137–146.

Takayanagi H, Kim S, Koga T, Nishina H, Isshiki M, Yoshida H, Saiura A, et al. Induction and activation of the transcription factor NFATc1(NFAT2) integrate RANKL signaling in terminal differentiation of osteoclasts. Dev Cell 2002a;3(6):889–901.

Takayanagi H, Kim S, Matsuo K, Suzuki H, Suzuki T, Sato K, Yokochi T, et al. RANKL maintains bone homeostasis through c-Fos-dependent induction of interferon-β. Nature 2002b;416(6882):744–749.

Takayanagi H, Oda H, Yamamoto S, Kawaguchi H, Tanaka S, Nishikawa T, Koshihara Y. A new mechanism of bone destruction in rheumatoid arthritis: synovial fibroblasts induce osteoclastogenesis. Biochem Biophys Res Commun 1997;240(2):279–286.

Takayanagi H, Ogasawara K, Hida K, Chiba T, Murata S, Sato K, Takaoka A, et al. T-cell-mediated regulation of osteoclastogenesis by signalling cross-talk between RANKL and IFN-γ. Nature 2000b;408(6812):600–605.

Theill LE, Boyle WJ, Penninger JM. RANK-L and RANK: T cells, bone loss, and mammalian evolution. Annu Rev Immunol 2002;20:795–823.

Tsuda E, Goto M, Mochizuki S, Yano K, Kobayashi F, Morinaga T, Higashio K. Isolation of a novel cytokine from human fibroblasts that specifically inhibits osteoclastogenesis. Biochem Biophys Res Commun 1997;234(1):137–142.

Veldhoen M, Hirota K, Westendorf AM, Buer J, Dumoutier L, Renauld JC, Stockinger B. The aryl hydrocarbon receptor links T_H17-cell-mediated autoimmunity to environmental toxins. Nature 2008;453(7191): 106–109.

Vermeire K, Heremans H, Vandeputte M, Huang S, Billiau A, Matthys P. Accelerated collagen-induced arthritis in IFN-γ receptor-deficient mice. J Immunol 1997;158(11):5507–5513.

Wada T, Nakashima T, Oliveira-dos-Santos AJ, Gasser J, Hara H, Schett G, Penninger JM. The molecular scaffold Gab2 is a crucial component of RANK signaling and osteoclastogenesis. Nat Med 2005; 11(4):394–399.

Wagner EF, Eferl R. Fos/AP-1 proteins in bone and the immune system. Immunol Rev 2005;208:126–140.

Whyte MP, Obrecht SE, Finnegan PM, Jones JL, Podgornik MN, McAlister WH, Mumm S. Osteoprotegerin deficiency and juvenile Paget's disease. N Engl J Med 2002;347(3):175–184.

Winslow MM, Pan M, Starbuck M, Gallo EM, Deng L, Karsenty G, Crabtree GR. Calcineurin/NFAT signaling in osteoblasts regulates bone mass. Dev Cell 2006;10(6):771–782.

Wong BR, Rho J, Arron J, Robinson E, Orlinick J, Chao M, Kalachikov S, et al. TRANCE is a novel ligand of the tumor necrosis factor receptor family that activates c-Jun N-terminal kinase in T cells. J Biol Chem 1997;272(40):25190–25194.

Yamamoto M, Yamazaki S, Uematsu S, Sato S, Hemmi H, Hoshino K, Kaisho T, et al. Regulation of Toll/IL-1-receptor-mediated gene expression by the inducible nuclear protein IκBζ. Nature 2004;430(6996): 218–222.

Yamashita T, Yao Z, Li F, Zhang Q, Badell IR, Schwarz EM, Takeshita S, et al. NF-κB p50 and p52 regulate receptor activator of NF-κB ligand(RANKL) and tumor necrosis factor-induced osteoclast precursor differentiation by activating c-Fos and NFATc1. J Biol Chem 2007;282(25):18245–18253.

Yang XO, Pappu BP, Nurieva R, Akimzhanov A, Kang HS, Chung Y, Ma L, et al. T helper 17 lineage differentiation is programmed by orphan nuclear receptors RORα and RORγ. Immunity 2008;28(1):29–39.

Yasuda H, Shima N, Nakagawa N, Yamaguchi K, Kinosaki M, Mochizuki S, Tomoyasu A, et al. Osteoclast differentiation factor is a ligand for osteoprotegerin/osteoclastogenesis-inhibitory factor and is identical to TRANCE/RANKL. Proc Natl Acad Sci U S A 1998;95(7):3597–3602.

Yoshida H, Hayashi S, Kunisada S, Ogawa M, Nishikawa S, Okamura H, Sudo T, Shultz LD. The murine mutation osteopetrosis is in the coding region of the macrophage colony stimulating factor gene. Nature 1990;345(6274):442–444.

Zhang F, Meng G, Strober W. Interactions among the transcription factors Runx1, RORγt and Foxp3 regulate the differentiation of interleukin 17-producing T cells. Nature Immunol 2008;9(11):1297–1306.

Zhou L, Chong MM, Littman DR. Plasticity of CD4+ T cell lineage differentiation. Immunity 2009;30(5): 646–655.

6 WNT/β-Catenin Signaling Modulating Osteoarthritis

Maripat Corr

CONTENTS

Osteoarthritis (OA) is a chronic disease that is variable in its progression (Felson et al., 2000). In this disease, there is active bone remodeling, seen with osteophyte formation, and compromise to the overlying cartilage (Felson et al., 2000). Although it remains to be determined whether OA is primarily a disease of bone or cartilage, the current data suggest that this disease is not a passive process of degeneration but an active result of multiple molecular signaling pathways. The enhanced turnover of cartilage and bone matrix components suggests that mechanisms of self-renewal and homeostasis are not operating effectively in this disease. A growing body of evidence indicates that the WNT/β-catenin pathway is one of the key pathways involved in the pathogenesis of OA.

WNT SIGNALING PATHWAYS

Wnt/frizzled pathways have been previously implicated in embryogenesis, wound healing, tumorigenesis, and metabolic syndrome (McMahon and Moon, 1989; Logan and Nusse, 2004; Clevers, 2006; Katz et al., 2010). The names of the key proteins in this pathway largely stem from research done in *Drosophila*. The gene identified in wingless (*Wg*) flies was linked to the vertebrate oncogene *int-1*, and a fusion of nomenclature resulted for the WNT family of glycoproteins (Rijsewijk et al., 1987). To date, there have been 19 human WNT isoforms and at least 10 frizzled (fzd) receptors reported. The diversity in signaling is not merely a result of the mathematical combinations of ligand and receptor pairing. There are multiple signaling pathways that use these proteins, which are generally categorized as canonical and noncanonical pathways as depicted in Figure 6.1.

The canonical pathway involves the translocation of β-catenin to the nucleus and has been investigated in detail. However, other WNT signaling pathways exist and are referred to as β-catenin-independent pathways because some of these activate Ca^{2+} and c-Jun N-terminal kinase (JNK) pathways (Veeman et al., 2003). Each WNT ligand is not necessarily relegated to a specific pathway, and signaling is often context dependent. For example, WNT-5a can activate migration through

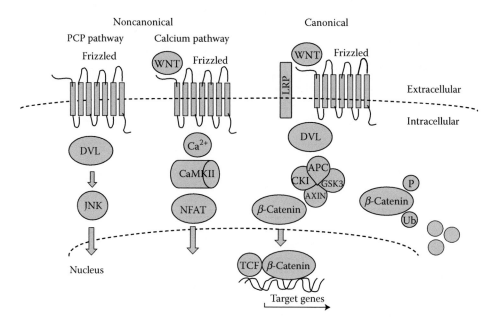

FIGURE 6.1   Simplified schematic of WNT pathways. The noncanonical pathways are β-catenin-independent pathways. The planar cell polarity pathway is not well defined and can activate the cytosolic protein Disheveled (DVL). The JNK pathways can in turn be activated. Alternatively, WNT can signal through the seven trans-membrane frizzled receptors and activate the calcium pathway through CaM kinase (CaMKII) and transmit nuclear signals through NFAT. In the canonical pathway, WNT ligands bind to the frizzled receptor and the LRP coreceptor. Disheveled (DVL) is recruited to the membrane complex and then AXIN. β-Catenin is released from the destruction complex and translocates to the nucleus. In the nucleus, it complexes with other transcription factors including TCF and initiates transcription of target genes. The destruction complex with GSK3β, AXIN, adenomatous polyposis coli, and CKIα phosphorylates β-catenin and targets it for ubiquitination (Ub) and proteosomal destruction.

JNK-dependent signals but can also signal through the canonical pathway (Mikels and Nusse, 2006). In some instances, WNT proteins interact with alternative receptors including ROR and Ryk (Harris and Beckendorf, 2007; Hendrickx and Leyns, 2008). Alternatively, the frizzled receptors can be activated after binding to non-WNT ligands such as Norrin and R-spondin (Xu et al., 2004; Nam et al., 2006; Hendrickx and Leyns, 2008). The planar cell polarity pathway is descriptively named for the process of cells orienting themselves relative to the plane of tissue (Veeman et al., 2003). Although this pathway involves the proteins encoded by frizzled and disheveled genes, which are named for altered polarity phenotypes, the involvement of WNT ligands in this pathway has yet to be definitively established. Collectively, these pathways contribute to the complex functions of WNT/frizzled signaling, which include cell fate determination, tissue polarity, and cell migration (Wada and Okamoto, 2009).

Canonical WNT signaling is regulated intracellularly by phosphorylation, poly(ADP-ribosyl) ation, and ubiquitination (McMahon and Moon, 1989; Yost et al., 1996; Huang et al., 2009). In the absence of canonical WNT signaling, β-catenin is complexed with the adenomatous polyposis coli (APC) tumor suppressor protein, AXIN, and glycogen synthetase 3 beta (GSK3β), which is often referred to as the "destruction complex" (Rubinfeld et al., 1996). Casein kinase (CKIα) and GSK3β negatively regulate β-catenin by facilitating phosphorylation near the amino terminus, thereby accelerating its ubiquitination and proteolytic degradation (Yost et al., 1996). Canonical signaling is initiated by lipid modified WNT glycoproteins binding to seven transmembrane domain G-protein-coupled frizzled receptors (Bhanot et al., 1996; Yang-Snyder et al., 1996). After WNT binds to frizzled, disheveled (DVL) is phosphorylated by CKIα and then binds to the frizzled receptor (Cong et al., 2004). Signal transmission is further facilitated by frizzled complexing with its coreceptor, LDL-related protein (LRP) 5/6, which is then phosphorylated by GSK3β (Cong et al., 2004). AXIN is recruited to the membrane and binds to phosphorylated LRP (Cong et al., 2004). β-Catenin is then released from the destruction complex, accumulates in the cytoplasm, and translocates into the nucleus. In the nucleus, β-catenin complexes with other transcription factors, including the lymphoid-enhancing factor or T-cell factor (TCF) (Behrens et al., 1996), and initiates transcription of targets genes such as *c-myc*, *cyclin D1*, matrix metalloproteinase 3 (*MMP-3*), and *CD44* (He et al., 1998; Li et al., 1999; Shtutman et al., 1999; Wielenga et al., 1999).

There are other intracellular checkpoints that regulate canonical signaling. For example, tankyrase activity modulates the amount of cytoplasmic axin by negative regulation through poly(ADP-ribosyl)ation and subsequent degradation (Huang et al., 2009). The level of cytoplasmic β-catenin is also regulated by interacting with multiple other proteins such as cadherin. The cadherins bind to β-catenin at the cell surface, linking it to the cytoskeleton (Aberle et al., 1994; Hoschuetzky et al., 1994). Loss of cadherin at the cell surface can lead to a redistribution of β-catenin to the cytoplasm and subsequent nuclear translocation and transcriptional activation of target genes (Nelson and Nusse, 2004). In addition, the disheveled proteins can regulate both canonical and JNK signaling in mammalian cells (Boutros et al., 1998; Li et al., 1999).

Extracellular proteins as well as intracellular proteins regulate the WNT pathway. These include secreted frizzled receptor protein (SFRP) family members (Baranski et al., 2000), Dickkopf (DKK) proteins (Glinka et al., 1998), WNT inhibitory factor (Hsieh et al., 1999), sclerostin (SOST) (Brunkow et al., 2001), WNT-1-induced secreted protein (Itasaki et al., 2003), and Cerbrus (Piccolo et al., 1999). There are five SFRP family members and four DKK family members. DKK and SOST bind to the LRP coreceptor and primarily inhibit the canonical signaling pathway (Semenov et al., 2001). The other inhibitors function as soluble competitors for frizzled receptor engagement by binding directly to WNT proteins. For example, the SFRP family has an amino terminal domain, which is homologous to the cysteine-rich WNT binding domain in FZD receptors and binds to WNT proteins (Lin et al., 1997). The inhibitors influence different aspects of the various WNT signaling pathways and thus perform distinct functions in different tissues.

GENETIC EVIDENCE FOR THE ROLE OF WNT SIGNALING IN OA

Both the canonical and the noncanonical pathways are critical for the development of the skeletal structure as evidenced by human congenital defects and animal models (Hartmann and Tabin, 2000, 2001; Hartmann, 2007). For example, noncanonical WNT-5a signaling is involved in pattern formation along the proximal-distal axis by regulating chondrogenic differentiation (Kawakami et al., 1999). The canonical pathway is also critical for chondrocyte maturation, long bone formation, and interzone of the joint cavity formation (Hartmann and Tabin, 2000, 2001; Hartmann, 2002, 2007). Human genetic syndromes of van Buchem's disease (variants of SOST) (Wergedal et al., 2003) and Robinow syndrome (variants of WNT-5a and ROR) (van Bokhoven et al., 2000; Person et al., 2010) suggest that polymorphisms rather than genetic ablation are not neonatally lethal and indicate that both canonical and noncanonical signaling are necessary for development and homeostasis of the musculoskeletal system. Mutations in the CCN gene family member WNT-induced signaling protein 3 result in progressive pseudorheumatoid dysplasia (Hurvitz et al., 1999). In pseudorheumatoid dysplasia, cartilage is affected after birth and patients experience advanced cartilage loss and destructive bone changes, often requiring joint replacement surgery by the third decade of life (Hurvitz et al., 1999). Small perturbations in development could lead to subtle anatomic changes such as hip shape, which would lead to impaired responses to mechanical loading and OA later in life.

Further supporting evidence that WNT signaling might contribute to the development or progression of OA stemmed from genome-wide association studies (Loughlin et al., 1999; Slagboom et al., 2000; Demissie et al., 2002; Stefansson et al., 2003). These studies identified several regions that contained the genes for *FZD5, FZD7, LRP,* and *FRZB. LRP5* is in close proximity to the OA susceptibility locus on chromosome 11q (Chapman et al., 1999; Demissie et al., 2002) and is the fzd coreceptor that enables FZD to preferentially signal through the canonical pathway. Increased bone density has been described as a risk factor for developing OA, and *LRP5* variants result in altered bone accrual in adults (Boyden et al., 2002; Li et al., 2002; Gong et al., 2001). Individuals with two copies of variant *LRP5* alleles, which completely abrogate the function of the protein, are born with osteoporosis-pseudoglioma syndrome (Gong et al., 2001). Carriers of single *LRP5* polymorphisms have reduced bone density compared with control subjects (Boyden et al., 2002; Van Wesenbeeck et al., 2003). Alternatively, gain-of-function mutations in *LRP5*-related signaling pathway or variants that disrupt *LRP5* interaction with DKK increase bone accrual in adults (Boyden et al., 2002; Little et al., 2002). A single polymorphism (Q89R) in *LRP5* was associated with an increase risk of spinal OA (Urano et al., 2007). However, more complex haplotypes in this gene were associated with susceptibility to knee OA (Smith et al., 2005). It remains to be determined if the effects of these polymorphisms are directly attributable to changes in bone density or if another mechanism is associated with the increased susceptibility to OA.

In addition to the region on 11q, genome-wide scans detected an OA susceptibility locus on chromosome 2q (Loughlin et al., 1999; Slagboom et al., 2000). Finer mapping revealed that single nucleotide polymorphisms in the *FRZB* gene were associated with primary hip OA in Caucasian women (Loughlin et al., 2004). *FRZB*, which is abbreviated for frizzled motif associated with bone development, encodes SFRP-3. The haplotype with substitutions at two highly conserved arginine residues in *FRZB* at positions 200 and 324 (R200W and R324G) was the strongest risk factor for primary hip OA, with an odds ratio of 4.1 (Loughlin et al., 2004). A second larger study of elderly Caucasian women with radiographically defined hip OA (RHOA) confirmed that the R200W/R324G haplotype showed the greatest proportionate increase in risk (Lane et al., 2006).

Functional studies suggested that the R324G but not the R200W substitution reduced the ability of SFRP-3 to antagonize WNT signaling and translocation of β-catenin to the nucleus (Loughlin et al., 2004). These findings suggest that abnormal functioning of SFRP-3 might influence development and progression of OA by at least two different mechanisms. Further genetic studies indicated that bone and cartilage processes might be affected by separate functions of SFRP. Women homozygous for the minor allele of the R200W substitution in *FRZB* had over a threefold higher risk of developing RHOA characterized by femoral osteophytes (Lane et al., 2006), although inheritance of a variant coding for the R324G substitution was a susceptibility factor for developing RHOA characterized by moderate to severe joint space narrowing suggesting cartilage loss (Lane et al., 2006). This polymorphism was also noted to be transmitted in a multigenerational family study with a cartilage debonding syndrome (Holderbaum et al., 2005).

In Caucasian populations, the *FRZB* haplotype encoding both R200W and R324G was associated with the susceptibility of developing hip and knee OA in women (Loughlin et al., 2004; Valdes et al., 2007). This sex-related difference suggested that either subtle anatomic difference in skeletal morphology, like hip shape, in women might be a congenital effect of these polymorphisms. In a European population, the R324G polymorphism was associated with an increased risk of generalized OA, suggesting a more global influence rather than a site-specific anatomic variation (Min et al., 2005). Further evidence for a systemic effect of altered SFRP function was the differential association of the *FRZB* R200W single-nucleotide polymorphism with hip OA and bone loss (osteoporosis) (Min et al., 2005). Increases in β-catenin transcriptional activity were associated with relative bone formation, whereas higher levels of β-catenin were seen in areas of compromised cartilage. In general, the genetic profiles for OA susceptibility suggested that diminished suppression of WNT signaling might lead to an increased risk of developing OA. However, joint-specific and sex-related differences need to be further studied.

WNT-ASSOCIATED GENE EXPRESSION PROFILING IN OA TISSUES

An increase in the expression of WNT pathway–associated genes was reported in both the cartilage and the bone in OA specimens (Hopwood et al., 2007; Weng et al., 2009). Overexpression of WNT target genes in OA bone specimens has been reported (Hopwood et al., 2007). Microarray gene expression profiling of bone from patients undergoing joint replacement surgery for degenerative hip OA compared with bone harvested postmortem from deceased individuals with no evidence of joint disease also demonstrated sex-related differences in gene expression (Hopwood et al., 2007). In another study, the expression of WNT-related genes was analyzed in bone samples and osteoblast primary cultures from patients with hip fractures and hip or knee OA. Seven genes were consistently upregulated both in tissue samples and in cell cultures from patients with knee OA: *BCL9*, *FZD5*, *DVL2*, *EP300*, *FRZB*, *LRP5*, and *TCF7L1* (Velasco et al., 2010). The upregulation of expression of genes in the WNT pathway in OA bone specimens suggested their involvement not only in cartilage pathology but also in subchondral bone changes (Velasco et al., 2010).

Differential gene expression profiles of damaged versus intact cartilage areas within the same joint of patients with knee OA were examined using whole-genome oligonucleotide arrays (Geyer et al., 2009). WNT-induced signaling protein 1 was one of six genes that were found to be upregulated in the affected cartilage of all patients (Geyer et al., 2009). In a separate study, *LRP5* mRNA was reported to be overexpressed in OA cartilage and correlated with an increase in β-catenin (Papathanasiou et al., 2010). In addition, WNT-16 is increased (Dell'Accio et al., 2008) and SFRP-3 mRNA expression is reduced in response to *in vitro* mechanical cartilage injury (Loughlin et al., 2004; Dell'Accio et al., 2006).

Interestingly DKK-1, a soluble WNT inhibitor, mRNA expression was increased in articular cartilage specimens harvested from nine patients with knee OA compared with controls with femoral neck fractures (Weng et al., 2009). Interleukin-1β (IL-1β) is a major catabolic cytokine, which plays a pivotal role in cartilage destruction. The expression of DKK-1 correlated with IL-1β and tumor necrosis factor expression and apoptotic areas in OA cartilage tissues (Weng et al., 2009). Functional studies suggested that IL-1β-induced chondrocyte death could be modulated by DKK-1 (Weng et al., 2009). Hence, WNT-associated proteins in cartilage might be actively involved in the catabolic process.

WNT IN CARTILAGE AND BONE BIOLOGY

In articular cartilage, the homeostasis of the extracellular matrix is maintained through a balance of anabolic and catabolic processes. In addition to the differential expression patterns of WNT proteins and inhibitors seen in OA and RA synovium (Sen et al., 2000; Ijiri et al., 2002; Imai et al., 2006), the biochemical effects of excessive WNT signaling have been shown to contribute to cartilage degradation. Increased levels of β-catenin have been reported in chondrocytes within areas of degenerative cartilage (Kim et al., 2002; Hwang et al., 2005). Consistent with a catabolic role for β-catenin in cartilage, β-catenin overexpression in chondrocytes strongly stimulated expression of matrix degradation enzymes (Tamamura et al., 2005). Biochemical alterations in either glycosaminoglycan sulfation or matrix content affected the response of human articular chondrocytes to a canonical WNT stimulus (Shortkroff and Yates, 2007). Thus, WNT/β-catenin signals may activate cartilage matrix catabolism and have a role in cartilage destruction under pathological conditions.

Activation of β-catenin in mature cartilage cells stimulates hypertrophy, matrix mineralization, expression of MMP-13, and vascular endothelial growth factor (Day et al., 2005; Tamamura et al., 2005). Similarly, β-catenin overexpression in chondrocytes strongly stimulated expression of matrix degradation enzymes (Tamamura et al., 2005). Also, reducing LRP5 expression with siRNA resulted in a significant decrease in MMP-13 expression (Papathanasiou et al., 2010). These findings further implicated a catabolic role for the WNT/β-catenin pathway in human OA.

The catabolic effects of WNT signaling may not be exclusively mediated by the canonical pathway. Treatment of chondrocytes with IL-1β upregulated WNT-5a and downregulated WNT-11 expression (Ryu and Chun, 2006). WNT-5a and WNT-11, signaling through distinct noncanonical WNT pathways, had opposing effects on type II collagen expression by chondrocytes (Ryu and Chun, 2006). In addition, stimulation of WNT-5a resulted in MMP production through the JNK pathway (Ge et al., 2009). Thus, β-catenin-independent signals may also impact cartilage destruction under pathological conditions.

Canonical β-catenin signaling does have a role in normal cartilage homeostasis. The adhesion molecule, E-cadherin, is stabilized by β-catenin at the cell membrane, and β-catenin is involved in transcriptional regulation of the hyaluronan receptor (CD44) expression (Wielenga et al., 1999). Articular chondrocytes express CD44 and integrins, which interact with surrounding extracellular matrix to preserve cartilage integrity (Knudson and Loeser, 2002). Cartilage slices treated with antisense oligonucleotides have been shown to inhibit CD44 protein expression, which exhibited a chondrolysis with near-total loss of detectable proteoglycan-rich matrix (Chow et al., 1998). Maintenance of cell surface adhesion molecules is just one potential role for WNT signaling in maintaining cartilage health.

The impact of the WNT pathway on the development and susceptibility to OA is not limited to the effects on chondrocytes. The WNT pathway directly impacts global bone density, and local changes in the subchondral bone could also be regulated by this pathway. The activity of LRP5 has been clearly demonstrated to affect bone density (Gong et al., 2001; Boyden et al., 2002; Li et al., 2002). The WNT signaling antagonists might also influence local changes. SFRP-1 binds to RANKL (Hausler et al., 2004), and DKK-1 stimulates osteoprotegerin secretion (Diarra et al., 2007). Osteoprotegerin and RANKL regulate osteoclast and osteoblast development. By reducing the availability of RANKL, SFRP-1 would decrease effective osteoclast differentiation. This could be counterbalanced by the effects of soluble WNT antagonists DKK-1 and SFRP-2, which inhibit osteoblast differentiation (Tian et al., 2003; Oshima et al., 2005).

WNT IN GENETIC MOUSE MODELS OF OA

Several mutant mouse models of OA have been developed. Although these models provide evidence that weakened matrix or abnormal mechanical stresses from loading result in changes in chondrocytes leading to the development of OA, none of them fully recapitulate human disease. Recently, several models have been reported that directly address the effects of WNT-associated proteins on the development of OA in mice. *frzb*-deficient mice appear normal at birth; however, they have accelerated cartilage loss with age (Lories et al., 2007). They also developed advanced histological cartilage damage and sulfated proteoglycan loss after the induction of arthritis (Lories et al., 2007). The cartilage loss was associated with a trend in increased β-catenin levels in the damaged cartilage. These data imply that SFRP-3 might protect against the development or progression of cartilage loss.

In *frzb*-deficient mice, cartilage damage was also associated with an increase in MMP-3 expression and activity (Lories et al., 2007). This increase in MMP-3 may not have been solely due to increased gene expression, as SFRP-3 inhibited the activities of MMP-2 and MMP-3 *in vitro* (Lories et al., 2007). SFRP proteins have two domains. The amino terminal domain is homologous to the cysteine rich of *FZD* receptors and binds to WNT (Lin et al., 1997). The mid region has a netrin-like domain, similar to the N-terminal domain of tissue inhibitors of metalloproteinases, and binds to other proteins. Direct protein binding the MMPs has not been formally demonstrated; however, the diminished MMP activity may have been mediated through the netrin domain in SFRP-3.

There may be an additional influence of the WNT pathway in the development of OA in mechanosensing by bone. The effect of bone loading and the response of WNT signaling were assessed in mice transgenic for LRP5 with a gain-of-function mutation. These mice had high levels of WNT signaling and an increase in trabecular bone mass, trabecular number, strength, and density (Akhter et al., 2004). In a four-point tibia bending model, they had increased bone formation and required a lower level of strain to initiate a bone-forming response compared with control mice (Robinson et al., 2006). Additional supporting data come from $frzb^{-/-}$ mice, which have stiffer bones as demonstrated by their stress–strain relationship and an increased periosteal anabolic response to mechanical loading than wild-type mice (Lories et al., 2007).

Additional mouse model evidence used a sophisticated conditional tamoxifen-inducible Cre recombinase and the *Col2a1* promoter (Zhu et al., 2009). This promoter was chondrocyte specific and activated when mice were treated with the estrogen antagonist tamoxifen or an active metabolite 4-OH-tamoxifen. Tamoxifen was used to stimulate the deletion of exon 3 in the β-catenin gene in type II collagen–expressing cells, namely, cartilage (Zhu et al., 2009). GSK3β phosphorylation of residues encoded by exon 3 of β-catenin targets it for degradation. Hence, deletion of exon 3 of the β-catenin gene resulted in the production of higher levels of stable transcriptionally active protein. The articular cartilage phenotype of these mice was analyzed by histological study, showing loss of the articular cartilage, particularly in the weight-bearing areas in 5- and 8-month-old mice (Zhu et al., 2009). At 8 months of age, there was progression to severe destruction of articular cartilage with surface fibrillation and vertical clefts (Zhu et al., 2009). Furthermore, MMP-13 mRNA and protein expression were significantly increased (Zhu et al., 2009). Overall, when β-catenin was stabilized in chondrocytes these phenotypic changes grossly resembled the clinical features in OA.

CONCLUSION

The pathogenesis of OA is complex, involving genetic, developmental, and environmental factors (Felson et al., 2000). Clearly, the WNT signaling pathways influence the progression if not the susceptibility to OA. The oncogenic potential of this pathway, however, may limit intervention in this chronic disease. Given the specificity of some of the known protein inhibitors, these molecules warrant investigation for their potential as biologic disease modifiers.

REFERENCES

Aberle H, Butz S, Stappert J, Weissig H, Kemler R, Hoschuetzky H. Assembly of the cadherin-catenin complex in vitro with recombinant proteins. J Cell Sci 1994;107(Pt 12):3655–3663.

Akhter MP, Wells DJ, Short SJ, Cullen DM, Johnson ML, Haynatzki GR, Babij P, et al. Bone biomechanical properties in LRP5 mutant mice. Bone 2004;35(1):162–169.

Baranski M, Berdougo E, Sandler JS, Darnell DK, Burrus LW. The dynamic expression pattern of frzb-1 suggests multiple roles in chick development. Dev Biol 2000;217(1):25–41.

Behrens J, von Kries JP, Kuhl M, Bruhn L, Wedlich D, Grosschedl R, Birchmeier W. Functional interaction of beta-catenin with the transcription factor LEF-1. Nature 1996;382(6592):638–642.

Bhanot P, Brink M, Samos CH, Hsieh JC, Wang Y, Macke JP, Andrew D, Nathans J, Nusse R. A new member of the frizzled family from Drosophila functions as a Wingless receptor. Nature 1996;382(6588):225–230.

Boutros M, Paricio N, Strutt DI, Mlodzik M. Dishevelled activates JNK and discriminates between JNK pathways in planar polarity and wingless signaling. Cell 1998;94(1):109–118.

Boyden LM, Mao J, Belsky J, Mitzner L, Farhi A, Mitnick MA, Wu D, Insogna K, Lifton RP. High bone density due to a mutation in LDL-receptor-related protein 5. N Engl J Med 2002;346(20):1513–1521.

Brunkow ME, Gardner JC, Van Ness J, Paeper BW, Kovacevich BR, Proll S, Skonier JE, et al. Bone dysplasia sclerosteosis results from loss of the SOST gene product, a novel cystine knot-containing protein. Am J Hum Genet 2001;68(3):577–589.

Chapman K, Mustafa Z, Irven C, Carr AJ, Clipsham K, Smith A, Chitnavis J, et al. Osteoarthritis-susceptibility locus on chromosome 11q, detected by linkage. Am J Hum Genet 1999;65(1):167–174.

Chow G, Nietfeld JJ, Knudson CB, Knudson W. Antisense inhibition of chondrocyte CD44 expression leading to cartilage chondrolysis. Arthritis Rheum 1998;41(8):1411–1419.

Clevers H. Wnt/beta-catenin signaling in development and disease. Cell 2006;127(3):469–480.

Cong F, Schweizer L, Varmus H. Wnt signals across the plasma membrane to activate the beta-catenin pathway by forming oligomers containing its receptors, Frizzled and LRP. Development 2004;131(20):5103–5115.

Day TF, Guo X, Garrett-Beal L, Yang Y. Wnt/beta-catenin signaling in mesenchymal progenitors controls osteoblast and chondrocyte differentiation during vertebrate skeletogenesis. Dev Cell 2005;8(5):739–750.

Dell'Accio F, De Bari C, El Tawil NM, Barone F, Mitsiadis TA, O'Dowd J, Pitzalis C. Activation of WNT and BMP signaling in adult human articular cartilage following mechanical injury. Arthritis Res Ther 2006;8(5):R139.

Dell'Accio F, De Bari C, Eltawil NM, Vanhummelen P, Pitzalis C. Identification of the molecular response of articular cartilage to injury, by microarray screening: Wnt-16 expression and signaling after injury and in osteoarthritis. Arthritis Rheum 2008;58(5):1410–1421.

Demissie S, Cupples LA, Myers R, Aliabadi P, Levy D, Felson DT. Genome scan for quantity of hand osteoarthritis: the Framingham Study. Arthritis Rheum 2002;46(4):946–952.

Diarra D, Stolina M, Polzer K, Zwerina J, Ominsky MS, Dwyer D, Korb A, et al. Dickkopf-1 is a master regulator of joint remodeling. Nat Med 2007;13(2):156–163.

Felson DT, Lawrence RC, Dieppe PA, Hirsch R, Helmick CG, Jordan JM, Kington RS, Lane NE, Nevitt MC, Zhang Y. Osteoarthritis: new insights. Part 1: the disease and its risk factors. Ann Intern Med 2000;133(8):635–646.

Ge X, Ma X, Meng J, Zhang C, Ma K, Zhou C. Role of Wnt-5A in interleukin-1beta-induced matrix metalloproteinase expression in rabbit temporomandibular joint condylar chondrocytes. Arthritis Rheum 2009;60(9):2714–2722.

Geyer M, Grassel S, Straub RH, Schett G, Dinser R, Grifka J, Gay S, Neumann E, Muller-Ladner U. Differential transcriptome analysis of intraarticular lesional vs intact cartilage reveals new candidate genes in osteoarthritis pathophysiology. Osteoarthritis Cartilage 2009;17(3):328–335.

Glinka A, Wu W, Delius H, Monaghan AP, Blumenstock C, Niehrs C. Dickkopf-1 is a member of a new family of secreted proteins and functions in head induction. Nature 1998;391(6665):357–362.

Gong Y, Slee RB, Fukai N, Rawadi G, Roman-Roman S, Reginato AM, Wang H, et al. LDL receptor-related protein 5 (LRP5) affects bone accrual and eye development. Cell 2001;107(4):513–523.

Harris KE, Beckendorf SK. Different Wnt signals act through the Frizzled and RYK receptors during Drosophila salivary gland migration. Development 2007;134(11):2017–2025.

Hartmann C. Wnt-signaling and skeletogenesis. J Musculoskelet Neuronal Interact 2002;2(3):274–276.

Hartmann C. Skeletal development—Wnts are in control. Mol Cells 2007;24(2):177–184.

Hartmann C, Tabin CJ. Dual roles of Wnt signaling during chondrogenesis in the chicken limb. Development 2000;127(14):3141–3159.

Hartmann C, Tabin CJ. Wnt-14 plays a pivotal role in inducing synovial joint formation in the developing appendicular skeleton. Cell 2001;104(3):341–351.

Hausler KD, Horwood NJ, Chuman Y, Fisher JL, Ellis J, Martin TJ, Rubin JS, Gillespie MT. Secreted frizzled-related protein-1 inhibits RANKL-dependent osteoclast formation. J Bone Miner Res 2004;19(11):1873–1881.

He TC, Sparks AB, Rago C, Hermeking H, Zawel L, da Costa LT, Morin PJ, Vogelstein B, Kinzler KW. Identification of c-MYC as a target of the APC pathway. Science 1998;281(5382):1509–1512.

Hendrickx M, Leyns L. Non-conventional Frizzled ligands and Wnt receptors. Dev Growth Differ 2008;50(4):229–243.

Holderbaum D, Malvitz T, Ciesielski CJ, Carson D, Corr MP, Moskowitz RW. A newly described hereditary cartilage debonding syndrome. Arthritis Rheum 2005;52(10):3300–3304.

Hopwood B, Tsykin A, Findlay DM, Fazzalari NL. Microarray gene expression profiling of osteoarthritic bone suggests altered bone remodelling, WNT and transforming growth factor-beta/bone morphogenic protein signalling. Arthritis Res Ther 2007;9(5):R100.

Hoschuetzky H, Aberle H, Kemler R. Beta-catenin mediates the interaction of the cadherin–catenin complex with epidermal growth factor receptor. J Cell Biol 1994;127(5):1375–1380.

Hsieh JC, Kodjabachian L, Rebbert ML, Rattner A, Smallwood PM, Samos CH, Nusse R, Dawid IB, Nathans J. A new secreted protein that binds to Wnt proteins and inhibits their activities. Nature 1999;398(6726):431–436.

Huang SM, Mishina YM, Liu S, Cheung A, Stegmeier F, Michaud GA, Charlat O, et al. Tankyrase inhibition stabilizes axin and antagonizes Wnt signalling. Nature 2009;461(7264):614–620.

Hurvitz JR, Suwairi WM, Van Hul W, El-Shanti H, Superti-Furga A, Roudier J, Holderbaum D, et al. Mutations in the CCN gene family member WISP3 cause progressive pseudorheumatoid dysplasia. Nat Genet 1999;23(1):94–98.

Hwang SG, Yu SS, Ryu JH, Jeon HB, Yoo YJ, Eom SH, Chun JS. Regulation of beta-catenin signaling and maintenance of chondrocyte differentiation by ubiquitin-independent proteasomal degradation of alpha-catenin. J Biol Chem 2005;280(13):12758–12765.

Ijiri K, Nagayoshi R, Matsushita N, Tsuruga H, Taniguchi N, Gushi A, Sakakima H, Komiya S, Matsuyama T. Differential expression patterns of secreted frizzled related protein genes in synovial cells from patients with arthritis. J Rheumatol 2002;29(11):2266–2270.

Imai K, Morikawa M, D'Armiento J, Matsumoto H, Komiya K, Okada Y. Differential expression of WNTs and FRPs in the synovium of rheumatoid arthritis and osteoarthritis. Biochem Biophys Res Commun 2006;345(4):1615–1620.

Itasaki N, Jones CM, Mercurio S, Rowe A, Domingos PM, Smith JC, Krumlauf R. Wise, a context-dependent activator and inhibitor of Wnt signalling. Development 2003;130(18):4295–4305.

Katz JD, Agrawal S, Velasquez M. Getting to the heart of the matter: osteoarthritis takes its place as part of the metabolic syndrome. Curr Opin Rheumatol 2010;22(5):512–519.

Kawakami Y, Wada N, Nishimatsu SI, Ishikawa T, Noji S, Nohno T. Involvement of Wnt-5a in chondrogenic pattern formation in the chick limb bud. Dev Growth Differ 1999;41(1):29–40.

Kim SJ, Im DS, Kim SH, Ryu JH, Hwang SG, Seong JK, Chun CH, Chun JS. Beta-catenin regulates expression of cyclooxygenase-2 in articular chondrocytes. Biochem Biophys Res Commun 2002;296(1):221–226.

Knudson W, Loeser RF. CD44 and integrin matrix receptors participate in cartilage homeostasis. Cell Mol Life Sci 2002;59(1):36–44.

Lane NE, Lian K, Nevitt MC, Zmuda JM, Lui L, Li J, Wang J, et al. Frizzled-related protein variants are risk factors for hip osteoarthritis. Arthritis Rheum 2006;54(4):1246–1254.

Li L, Mao J, Sun L, Liu W, Wu D. Second cysteine-rich domain of Dickkopf-2 activates canonical Wnt signaling pathway via LRP-6 independently of dishevelled. J Biol Chem 2002;277(8):5977–5981.

Li L, Yuan H, Xie W, Mao J, Caruso AM, McMahon A, Sussman DJ, Wu D. Dishevelled proteins lead to two signaling pathways. Regulation of LEF-1 and c-Jun N-terminal kinase in mammalian cells. J Biol Chem 1999;274(1):129–134.

Lin K, Wang S, Julius MA, Kitajewski J, Moos M Jr., Luyten FP. The cysteine-rich frizzled domain of Frzb-1 is required and sufficient for modulation of Wnt signaling. Proc Natl Acad Sci U S A 1997;94(21):11196–11200.

Little RD, Carulli JP, Del Mastro RG, Dupuis J, Osborne M, Folz C, Manning SP, et al. A mutation in the LDL receptor-related protein 5 gene results in the autosomal dominant high-bone-mass trait. Am J Hum Genet 2002;70(1):11–19.

Logan CY, Nusse R. The Wnt signaling pathway in development and disease. Annu Rev Cell Dev Biol 2004;20:781–810.

Lories RJ, Peeters J, Bakker A, Tylzanowski P, Derese I, Schrooten J, Thomas JT, Luyten FP. Articular cartilage and biomechanical properties of the long bones in Frzb-knockout mice. Arthritis Rheum 2007;56(12):4095–4103.

Loughlin J, Dowling B, Chapman K, Marcelline L, Mustafa Z, Southam L, Ferreira A, Ciesielski C, Carson DA, Corr M. Functional variants within the secreted frizzled-related protein 3 gene are associated with hip osteoarthritis in females. Proc Natl Acad Sci U S A 2004;101(26):9757–9762.

Loughlin J, Mustafa Z, Irven C, Smith A, Carr AJ, Sykes B, Chapman K. Stratification analysis of an osteoarthritis genome screen-suggestive linkage to chromosomes 4, 6, and 16. Am J Hum Genet 1999;65(6):1795–1798.

McMahon AP, Moon RT. Ectopic expression of the proto-oncogene int-1 in Xenopus embryos leads to duplication of the embryonic axis. Cell 1989;58(6):1075–1084.

Mikels AJ, Nusse R. Purified Wnt5a protein activates or inhibits beta-catenin-TCF signaling depending on receptor context. PLoS Biol 2006;4(4):e115.

Min JL, Meulenbelt I, Riyazi N, Kloppenburg M, Houwing-Duistermaat JJ, Seymour AB, Pols HA, van Duijn CM, Slagboom PE. Association of the Frizzled-related protein gene with symptomatic osteoarthritis at multiple sites. Arthritis Rheum 2005;52(4):1077–1080.

Nam JS, Turcotte TJ, Smith PF, Choi S, Yoon JK. Mouse cristin/R-spondin family proteins are novel ligands for the Frizzled 8 and LRP6 receptors and activate beta-catenin-dependent gene expression. J Biol Chem 2006;281(19):13247–13257.

Nelson WJ, Nusse R. Convergence of Wnt, beta-catenin, and cadherin pathways. Science 2004;303(5663):1483–1487.

Oshima T, Abe M, Asano J, Hara T, Kitazoe K, Sekimoto E, Tanaka Y, et al. Myeloma cells suppress bone formation by secreting a soluble Wnt inhibitor, sFRP-2. Blood 2005;106(9):3160–3165.

Papathanasiou I, Malizos KN, Tsezou A. Low-density lipoprotein receptor-related protein 5 (LRP5) expression in human osteoarthritic chondrocytes. J Orthop Res 2010;28(3):348–353.

Person AD, Beiraghi S, Sieben CM, Hermanson S, Neumann AN, Robu ME. Schleiffarth JR, et al. WNT5A mutations in patients with autosomal dominant Robinow syndrome. Dev Dyn 2010;239(1):327–337.

Piccolo S, Agius E, Leyns L, Bhattacharyya S, Grunz H, Bouwmeester T, De Robertis EM. The head inducer cerberus is a multifunctional antagonist of nodal, BMP and Wnt signals. Nature 1999;397(6721):707–710.

Rijsewijk F, Schuermann M, Wagenaar E, Parren P, Weigel D, Nusse R. The Drosophila homolog of the mouse mammary oncogene int-1 is identical to the segment polarity gene wingless. Cell 1987;50(4):649–657.

Robinson JA, Chatterjee-Kishore M, Yaworsky PJ, Cullen DM, Zhao W, Li C, Kharode Y, et al. Wnt/beta-catenin signaling is a normal physiological response to mechanical loading in bone. J Biol Chem 2006;281(42):31720–31728.

Rubinfeld B, Albert I, Porfiri E, Fiol C, Munemitsu S, Polakis P. Binding of GSK3beta to the APC-beta-catenin complex and regulation of complex assembly. Science 1996;272(5264):1023–1026.

Ryu JH, Chun JS. Opposing roles of WNT-5A and WNT-11 in interleukin-1beta regulation of type II collagen expression in articular chondrocytes. J Biol Chem 2006;281(31):22039–22047.

Semenov MV, Tamai K, Brott BK, Kuhl M, Sokol S, He X. Head inducer Dickkopf-1 is a ligand for Wnt coreceptor LRP6. Curr Biol 2001;11(12):951–961.

Sen M, Lauterbach K, El-Gabalawy H, Firestein GS, Corr M, Carson DA. Expression and function of wingless and frizzled homologs in rheumatoid arthritis. Proc Natl Acad Sci U S A 2000;97(6):2791–2796.

Shortkroff S, Yates KE. Alteration of matrix glycosaminoglycans diminishes articular chondrocytes' response to a canonical Wnt signal. Osteoarthritis Cartilage 2007;15(2):147–154.

Shtutman M, Zhurinsky J, Simcha I, Albanese C, D'Amico M, Pestell R, Ben-Ze'ev A. The cyclin D1 gene is a target of the beta-catenin/LEF-1 pathway. Proc Natl Acad Sci U S A 1999;96(10):5522–5527.

Slagboom PE, Heijmans BT, Beekman M, Westendorp RG, Meulenbelt I. Genetics of human aging. The search for genes contributing to human longevity and diseases of the old. Ann N Y Acad Sci 2000;908:50–63.

Smith AJ, Gidley J, Sandy JR, Perry MJ, Elson CJ, Kirwan JR, Spector TD, Doherty M, Bidwell JL, Mansell JP. Haplotypes of the low-density lipoprotein receptor-related protein 5 (LRP5) gene: are they a risk factor in osteoarthritis? Osteoarthritis Cartilage 2005;13(7):608–613.

Stefansson SE, Jonsson H, Ingvarsson T, Manolescu I, Jonsson HH, Olafsdottir G, Palsdottir E, et al. Genomewide scan for hand osteoarthritis: a novel mutation in matrilin-3. Am J Hum Genet 2003;72(6):1448–1459.

Tamamura Y, Otani T, Kanatani N, Koyama E, Kitagaki J, Komori T, Yamada Y. Developmental regulation of Wnt/beta-catenin signals is required for growth plate assembly, cartilage integrity, and endochondral ossification. J Biol Chem 2005;280(19):19185–19195.

Tian E, Zhan F, Walker R, Rasmussen E, Ma Y, Barlogie B, Shaughnessy JD Jr. The role of the Wnt-signaling antagonist DKK1 in the development of osteolytic lesions in multiple myeloma. N Engl J Med 2003;349(26):2483–2494.

Urano T, Shiraki M, Narusawa K, Usui T, Sasaki N, Hosoi T, Ouchi Y, Nakamura T, Inoue S. Q89R polymorphism in the LDL receptor-related protein 5 gene is associated with spinal osteoarthritis in postmenopausal Japanese women. Spine 2007;32(1):25–29.

Valdes AM, Loughlin J, Oene MV, Chapman K, Surdulescu GL, Doherty M, Spector TD. Sex and ethnic differences in the association of ASPN, CALM1, COL2A1, COMP, and FRZB with genetic susceptibility to osteoarthritis of the knee. Arthritis Rheum 2007;56(1):137–146.

van Bokhoven H, Celli J, Kayserili H, van Beusekom E, Balci S, Brussel W, Skovby F, et al. Mutation of the gene encoding the ROR2 tyrosine kinase causes autosomal recessive Robinow syndrome. Nat Genet 2000;25(4):423–426.

Van Wesenbeeck L, Cleiren E, Gram J, Beals RK, Benichou O, Scopelliti D, Key L, et al. Six novel missense mutations in the LDL receptor-related protein 5 (LRP5) gene in different conditions with an increased bone density. Am J Hum Genet 2003;72(3):763–771.

Veeman MT, Axelrod JD, Moon RT. A second canon. Functions and mechanisms of beta-catenin-independent Wnt signaling. Dev Cell 2003;5(3):367–377.

Velasco J, Zarrabeitia MT, Prieto JR, Perez-Castrillon JL, Perez-Aguilar MD, Perez-Nunez MI, Sanudo C, et al. Wnt pathway genes in osteoporosis and osteoarthritis: differential expression and genetic association study. Osteoporos Int 2010;21(1):109–118.

Wada H, Okamoto H. Roles of planar cell polarity pathway genes for neural migration and differentiation. Dev Growth Differ 2009;51(3):233–240.

Weng LH, Wang CJ, Ko JY, Sun YC, Su YS, Wang FS. Inflammation induction of Dickkopf-1 mediates chondrocyte apoptosis in osteoarthritic joint. Osteoarthritis Cartilage 2009;17(7):933–943.

Wergedal JE, Veskovic K, Hellan M, Nyght C, Balemans W, Libanati C, Vanhoenacker FM, Tan J, Baylink DJ, Van Hul W. Patients with Van Buchem disease, an osteosclerotic genetic disease, have elevated bone formation markers, higher bone density, and greater derived polar moment of inertia than normal. J Clin Endocrinol Metab 2003;88(12):5778–5783.

Wielenga VJ, Smits R, Korinek V, Smit L, Kielman M, Fodde R, Clevers H, Pals ST. Expression of CD44 in Apc and Tcf mutant mice implies regulation by the WNT pathway. Am J Pathol 1999;154(2):515–523.

Xu Q, Wang Y, Dabdoub A, Smallwood PM, Williams J, Woods C, Kelley MW, et al. Vascular development in the retina and inner ear: control by Norrin and Frizzled-4, a high-affinity ligand-receptor pair. Cell 2004;116(6):883–895.

Yang-Snyder J, Miller JR, Brown JD, Lai CJ, Moon RT. A frizzled homolog functions in a vertebrate Wnt signaling pathway. Curr Biol 1996;6(10):1302–1306.

Yost C, Torres M, Miller JR, Huang E, Kimelman D, Moon RT. The axis-inducing activity, stability, and subcellular distribution of beta-catenin is regulated in Xenopus embryos by glycogen synthase kinase 3. Genes Dev 1996;10(12):1443–1454.

Zhu M, Tang D, Wu Q, Hao S, Chen M, Xie C, Rosier RN, O'Keefe RJ, Zuscik M, Chen D. Activation of beta-catenin signaling in articular chondrocytes leads to osteoarthritis-like phenotype in adult beta-catenin conditional activation mice. J Bone Miner Res 2009;24(1):12–21.

7 Psoriatic Arthritis
Epidemiology, Risk Factors, and Quality of Life

Arathi R. Setty

CONTENTS

INTRODUCTION

Psoriatic arthritis (PsA) is a chronic, seronegative inflammatory arthritis that is often associated with psoriasis. It is a heterogeneous disease with varied presentation. On the basis of clinical and immunohistopathological characteristics and HLA associations, PsA is classified as a spondyloarthropathy [1–3]. Clinical manifestations are diverse and range from dactylitis, enthesitis, monoarthritis, oligoarthritis, symmetric polyarthritis, distal interphalangeal (DIP) predominant arthritis, sacroiliitis, spondylitis, and arthritis mutilans. The clinical manifestations can occur in combination. Early in PsA, the disease is usually oligoarticular and mild; over time, it can evolve into a polyarticular disease with increased severity [1].

Recent studies have added to our knowledge of the epidemiology of PsA across various populations. However, absence of a standard case definition of PsA for population studies and its relative rarity has contributed to the general paucity of available data. Although there are a number of classification criteria available, epidemiologic studies often use the presence of arthritis in patients with psoriasis or the European Spondyloarthropathy Study Group (ESSG) criteria for classifying patients as having PsA. Issues with these methods include the poor sensitivity of ESSG criteria at 74% [4] and the fact that that even if a patient with psoriasis has an inflammatory arthritis it may not be PsA.

Sensitivity for the Vasey and Espinoza method was 97%, for the McGonagle method 98%, and for the Moll and Wright method 91% [4]. Although the sensitivities of the first two methods are higher than the ESSG criteria, they have not been used in studies of PsA prevalence and incidence.

The oldest of the classification schemes is the Moll and Wright criteria, and although this is a diagnostic criteria, studies have used it as classification criteria [5]. The Classification of Psoriatic Arthritis (CASPAR) study group criteria were developed on the basis of an extensive analysis of more than 500 patients with PsA and 500 patients with another type of inflammatory arthritis serving as controls [4]. In patients with long-standing PsA, the sensitivity was 91.4% and specificity 98.7%. The CASPAR criteria allow for the classification of patients as having PsA in the absence of current, past, or family history of psoriasis. In this study, only 20 patients (3.4%) had PsA without psoriasis, and of those 10 had a family history of psoriasis, 8 had dactylitis, 4 had dystrophic nails, 0 had positive anti-CCPs, and only 1 had a positive rheumatoid factor [4]. The CASPAR criteria have excellent sensitivity and specificity in early PsA [6].

ASSOCIATION BETWEEN PSORIASIS AND INFLAMMATORY ARTHRITIS

Investigators have recognized an increase in the prevalence of inflammatory polyarthritis in patients with psoriasis. A Swedish study investigated the prevalence of inflammatory joint manifestations in patients with psoriasis, identifying them from a community and a hospital-based registry [7]. Forty-eight percent of psoriatics identified themselves as having or having had an inflammatory manifestation, and 33% had peripheral arthritis and/or axial disease, as diagnosed by a rheumatologist [7]. Of these patients, 45% had not been previously diagnosed, and of the patients with peripheral arthritis, nearly half had evidence of radiographic changes and/or deforming disease.

As a corollary, it appears that psoriasis occurs more commonly in patients with inflammatory arthritis. More than 5% of patients with early inflammatory polyarthritis had psoriasis on examination [8]. Although this prevalence is thought to be higher than the general prevalence of psoriasis among Caucasians, the study did not have an internal control group to allow for a direct comparison.

PREVALENCE

Published data on the prevalence of PsA are summarized in Table 7.1 [9–17]. The prevalence of PsA in studies published before 2000 ranged from 0.02% to 0.05%. These estimates appear to be lower than those from more recent studies (ranging from 0.06% to 0.25%) and are discussed in detail below. The observed variations may be due to secular trends, increased detection of PsA, differences in the case definitions, dissimilar study populations, environmental exposures, and other methodological aspects.

The Rochester Epidemiology Project screened the medical records of Olmsted County, Minnesota, residents for a diagnosis consistent with psoriasis [12]. They identified 66 cases of PsA from 1056 cases of dermatologist-confirmed psoriasis between 1982 and 1991. PsA was defined as an inflammatory arthritis (i.e., inflammatory back pain for 3 months or more with radiographic evidence of sacroiliitis) associated with psoriasis. Other causes of inflammatory arthropathy were excluded. The age- and the sex-adjusted prevalence of PsA was estimated at 0.1% (95% confidence interval [CI] = 0.08–0.12) [12]. The average age at diagnosis was 40.7 years, with 91%, 6%, and 3% of the patients with oligoarthritis, spondylitis, and polyarthritis, respectively.

A study in northwest Greece of a homogenous Caucasian population of 500,000 found the age-adjusted prevalence of PsA at 0.06% [13]. Cases were identified in the context of a systematic recording system for autoimmune rheumatic diseases that had been developed for this area of Greece. The system recorded cases from in- and outpatients referred to two area hospitals and eight private rheumatology clinics. The authors felt that these sources represented all points where patients diagnosed with PsA could have been referred to in the study area. They identified 221 new

TABLE 7.1
Prevalence of PsA

Author	Country	Year	Prevalence (%)	Case Definition
Lomholt [9]	Faroe Islands	1963	0.04	Psoriasis with arthritis of the DIP joints
Hellgren [10]	Sweden	1969	0.02	ARA criteria for RA and typical feature of PsA and psoriasis
van Romunde et al. [11]	Netherlands	1984	0.05	As defined after examination by a rheumatologist
Shbeeb et al. [12]	United States (Olmsted County)	2000	0.1	Inflammatory arthritis amongst those with dermatologist-confirmed psoriasis
Alamanos et al. [13]	Greece	2003	0.06	ESSG criteria
Trontzas et al. [14]	Greece	2005	0.17	Interview and physical examination by a rheumatologist
Madland et al. [15]	Norway	2005	0.20	As defined after examination by a rheumatologist
Gelfand et al. [16]	United States	2005	0.25	Patient report of physician diagnosed psoriasis and PsA
Wilson et al. [17]	United States (Olmsted County)	2009	0.16	CASPAR

cases of PsA between 1982 and 2001 using the ESSG criteria. It is conceivable that mild cases may have not have been presented to a rheumatologist and may have remained undiagnosed or were treated by a general practitioner.

A cross-sectional Greek study from 2005 screened patients using a standardized questionnaire, followed by an evaluation by a rheumatologist to ascertain the ESSG criteria and the presence of typical psoriatic skin or nail lesion [14]. The subjects in this study, a target Greek population of 14,233 adults, were ethnically homogeneous in that 98.3% were Caucasian Greeks. The participation rate was 81.2%, and the prevalence of PsA was estimated at 0.17%. The average age of onset of PsA in this study was 45.24 years, similar to what was found in Olmsted County [12, 14]. The study also reported that rheumatologists had correctly diagnosed 87.5% of the cases, whereas nonrheumatologists were able to diagnose only 7.7% of the cases. This finding highlights the difficulty of having a nonrheumatologist diagnose PsA.

Review of medical records from rheumatology centers that served a population of 442,000 in Norway from 1999 to 2002 found 634 prevalent cases of PsA [15]. Cases with psoriasis and peripheral arthritis and/or radiographic evidence of spondylarthritis were considered to have PsA, whereas those with other arthritides were excluded. The prevalence was estimated to be 0.20% (95% CI = 0.18–0.21). The prevalence was highest between the ages of 40 and 59 years, and there were no significant differences between men and women.

On the basis of a national telephone survey of 27,220 adults, the prevalence of PsA in the United States was estimated at 0.25% (95% CI = 0.18–0.31), with a projected total of 520,000 PsA cases [16]. PsA cases were based on participants' self-report of a physician diagnosis of psoriasis and PsA. Given the case ascertainment methods, there may have been overestimation because of misclassification of cases and potential responder bias (i.e., increased response rate among those with PsA). Nonetheless, the study provides a nationally representative estimate of the prevalence of PsA.

The prevalence of PsA in Asian countries is less than what has been reported in Europe and in the United States and ranges from 1% to 9%. PsA was observed in 9% of patients with psoriasis in Iran, Korea, and India, 5% in China, 2% in Turkey, and 1% in Japan [18]. Divergent distribution of

HLA and its subtypes may account for some of this discrepancy. HLA-B16, HLA-B17, HLA-B27, and HLA-Cw6 are associated with PsA in Caucasians, whereas HLA-A2, HLA-B46, HLA-DR8, and HLA-B27 were associated with PsA in the Japanese [18]. In Taiwan HLA-Cw12 was associated with risk of PsA, whereas HLA-B58 and HLA-DR17 were protective. HLA-B27 was not associated in PsA in Israeli or Korean patients [18]. The lowest prevalence rate of PsA was in Japan at 0.1 to 1 per 100,000 [19]. This is likely related to the low prevalence of 0.5% or less of HLA-B27 in the Japanese population. To date, Asian studies of prevalence or incidence estimates have been limited by small cross-sectional studies, limited time of follow-up, and use of PsA criteria lacking diagnostic sensitivity [18].

Some of the prevalence estimates may have been underestimated because of several factors. First, it is difficult to account for patients with mild or no psoriasis at the time of the study. Second, PsA is variable in its clinical course and may enter a period of remission. Third, arthritis that precedes psoriatic skin lesions would not be recognized as PsA, and arthritis that is confined to the spine or sacroiliac joints could remain unrecognized, unless patients were radiographically accessed [20].

INCIDENCE RATE

Studies of the incidence rate of PsA are methodologically more challenging. To achieve a reasonable precision in an incidence estimate, a large population needs to be followed for sufficient duration. Recent studies that addressed the incidence of PsA are summarized in Table 7.2 [8, 12, 13, 17, 21].

A study using drug reimbursement data for PsA in a Finnish population of approximately 1 million adults in 1990 identified 65 incident PsA cases, resulting in an incidence rate of 6 per 100,000 [21]. The authors used the nationwide sickness insurance scheme to identify patients who were

TABLE 7.2
Incidence Rate of PsA

Author	Country of Study	Year	Incidence Rate per 100,000	Age at Diagnosis (year)[a]	Male-to-Female Ratio	Case Definition
Kaipiainen-Seppanen [21]	Finland	1996	6.1	46.8	1.3:1	Psoriatic skin and/or nail involvement and arthritis and/or spinal involvement
Harrison et al. [8]	United Kingdom	1997	3.6 for men 3.4 for women	52 (median age at onset)	1:1.04	Polyarthritis of at least 2 joint areas for 4 weeks with psoriasis at time of exam
Shbeeb et al. [12]	United States (Olmsted County)	2000	6.59	40.7	1:1.06	Inflammatory arthritis amongst those with dermatologist-confirmed psoriasis
Alamanos et al. [13]	Greece	2003	3.02 (2.87 for men and 3.14 for women)	47.7	1:1.05	ESSG criteria
Wilson et al. [17]	United States (Olmsted County)	2009	7.2 (9.1 for men and 5.4 for women)	42.7	1:0.63	CASPAR

[a] Mean unless otherwise noted.

receiving reimbursement for drugs used to treat PsA. Cases were defined on the basis of psoriatic involvement of the skin or nails and arthritis with or without spinal involvement. Hospital records were used when information contained in the reimbursement certificates was insufficient.

Investigators determined the incidence rate of PsA in the Norfolk Arthritis Register (NOAR) at 3.4 per 100,000 for women and 3.6 per 100,000 for men [8]. NOAR consists of a cohort of incident cases of inflammatory polyarthritis (i.e., swelling of two or more joint areas for 4 weeks) presenting to primary care within the Norwich Health Authority in the United Kingdom. Of the 966 patients that fit the inclusion criteria, 71 patients (7.3%) had a self-reported history of psoriasis and 51 cases (5.3%) were found to have psoriasis on examination by a research nurse. Of note, by the inclusion criteria, NOAR did not include patients with monoarthritis or spondyloarthropathy.

In Olmsted County, the age- and the sex-adjusted incidence of PsA between 1982 and 1991 was estimated at 6.59 per 100,000 [12], whereas the age-adjusted incidence of PsA in northwest Greece was 3.02 cases per 100,000 [13]. The lower incidence in the Greek population could be due to the fact that the Greek study used the ESSG criteria [13].

Using the CASPAR criteria, an Olmsted County study from January 1, 1970, to December 31, 1999, found that the age- and sex-adjusted incidence of PsA has been increasing over the past 30 years [17]. It increased from 3.6 per 100,000 for 1970–1979 to 9.8 per 100,000 for 1990–2000. This may be due to a true change in incidence, greater physician awareness, or better diagnostic techniques. The authors extrapolated that between 162,000 and 589,000 adults 18 years or older were affected with PsA in the United States in 2000, with 8000 to 27,000 new cases occurring each year.

It is important to note that the methods and sources of information retrieval differed among the studies reporting incidence of PsA. The first study from Olmsted County study was based on medical records of patients with psoriasis who had arthritis, whereas the study from Finland identified patients with an inflammatory arthritis by using a certified drug treatment for arthritis and then identified patients with psoriasis [12, 21]. The Finnish study excluded patients with onset of psoriasis after the development of arthritis, whereas the Olmsted County and Greek studies included these patients [12, 13, 21]. In addition, the differences in the incidence rate could also be due to variation in their genetic and ethnic composition and environmental factors.

POTENTIAL RISK FACTORS FOR PsA

DEMOGRAPHIC FACTORS

The mean age at the time of diagnosis is similar across the studies. Studies from the United States, Europe, and Asia have found that many of the cases occur when patients are in their early to mid forties, with the majority occurring in the 45- to 64-year age category [8, 12, 13, 17, 21].

SEX

The prevailing belief is that PsA occurs equally in both sexes [20]. A recent study found that the incidence of PsA in women is less than the incidence of men until the sixth decade of life [17]. Similar patterns have been observed for the incidence of psoriasis in Olmsted County and in the United Kingdom [17]. PsA affects both sexes almost equally in Chinese, Japanese, and Iranians, with an increased prevalence in men in Indians, Malay, Thai, and Koreans [18].

INFECTION

The role of infection as an etiological agent has long been speculated for both psoriasis and PsA. The link is more evident for certain subtypes of psoriasis than others. Acute episodes of guttate psoriasis, for example, have been associated with streptococcal infection [22]. There is an increased association of psoriasis and PsA in patients with HIV [23]. The prevalence of PsA in those with HIV in North American populations varies from 5.7% in Toronto, Canada, to less than 1% in Cincinnati,

Ohio [24]. However, among certain African populations with PsA, there is an almost universal finding of HIV infection. In a cohort of black Zambians attending an arthritis clinic, the prevalence of HIV seropositivity was 94% in those with PsA [25]. This high prevalence of HIV seropositivity is in contrast to the 30% and 50% seropositivity in the adult urban and hospital outpatient population in that area, respectively [25]. In the black Zambian population, PsA is almost universally associated with HIV, with clinical features similar to what has been described in Caucasians with HIV-associated PsA [26]. Previous to the HIV epidemic in sub-Saharan countries, seronegative spondyloarthropathies were felt to be uncommon in Africans because of the low prevalence of HLA-B27 [27]. A study in Zambian patients with HIV found that HLA-B*5703 appears to be protective against the progression of HIV infection, and that could account for the increase in the incidence of spondyloarthropathies seen in this population [28]. In this case, the gene–environment interaction appears to require an environmentally triggered expression of HIV for the development of a spondyloarthropathy [28].

FEATURES OF PSORIASIS

Approximately two-thirds of patients develop the skin disease before the joint disease, and the type of psoriasis itself may have a role in determining the onset of PsA [29]. A study comparing the onset of PsA in the two types of psoriasis found that those with type I psoriasis (i.e., early onset, heritable form) develop skin disease 9 years before developing the joint disease, whereas those with type II psoriasis (i.e., late onset, more sporadic form) develop the skin and joint manifestation within a year of each other [30]. Although this may be due to differing environmental and genetic influences, it may also simply imply that an inflammatory arthritis is more common with advancing age, and thus if psoriasis develops later in life, the chance of the arthritis occurring closer to the onset of the skin disease is more likely.

Several studies have also investigated the potential link between certain features of psoriasis and the presence of PsA. Nail changes were present in 63% of the PsA patients and in 37% of psoriatics without arthritis [29]. In 88% of patients in whom the joint disease preceded the skin disease, nail changes appeared before the appearance of the skin lesions [29]. Evidence of nail disease was more common in patients with involvement of the DIP joints and was significantly associated with disease in the adjacent DIP joint [31]. Scalp lesions have been associated with almost a fourfold increased risk of PsA, whereas dystrophic nails and intergluteal/perianal lesions were associated with a threefold and over a twofold risk of PsA, respectively [32]. In Asian patients, almost all (51.2%–97.5%) developed arthritis after the onset of psoriasis, and psoriasis vulgaris was the most common form [18].

The prevalence of PsA is significantly increased in psoriatic patients who had increased involvement of their skin, as measured by the percentage of body surface area [16]. This was confirmed by a more recent study that found that the risk of PsA was heightened in patients with at least three areas of skin involvement by psoriasis, suggesting that the risk of PsA is higher in psoriasis patients with more extensive disease [32].

FEATURES OF PsA

Of the five clinical patterns of PsA described by Moll and Wright [5], polyarthritis developing on the fourth decade was the most common pattern of arthritis in Chinese from Hong Kong, Singaporeans, Indians, Iranians, and Kuwaiti Arabs, whereas oligoarthritis was the predominant pattern in patients from Israel, Japan, and Rural India [18]. Clinically apparent lumbar spondylitis was more common in Indians than that in Chinese from Singapore [18]. When spondylitis was present in Chinese patients, 45% were asymptomatic, and it was detected on radiological exam. Arthritis mutilans was rare in all studies from the Asian region, and eye involvement was rarely reported in Asian countries [18].

In a study of incident cases of PsA in Olmsted County, more subjects had asymmetrical joint involvement (78%) than symmetric (22%), 32% had erosive disease, 10.7% had evidence of inflammatory spinal disease, and 24% had active dactylitis [17]. In this study, 94% had psoriasis at PsA incidence and 21% had family history of psoriasis. The actual incidence of family history of psoriasis might have been higher as 60% of the medical records lacked family history. Oligoarticular arthritis with enthesitis was the predominant pattern in this study [17], and this is in contrast with studies of prevalent cases of PsA where the predominant pattern was polyarticular. This may be because at its onset, PsA is oligoarticular and with time there is more joint involvement and it evolves into polyarticular disease.

OTHER RISK FACTORS

Corticosteroid use in the 2 years before the onset of psoriasis through the inception of PsA increased the risk of developing PsA by greater than fourfold [33]. However, pregnancy during the same period of time was protective and decreased the risk of developing PsA with an odds ratio of 0.19 (95% CI = 0.04–0.95) [33]. In this nested case–control study, ethnicity, trauma, infection, comorbidities, extent of psoriasis, type of psoriasis, and therapy for psoriasis were not significantly associated with an increase in the risk of developing PsA [33]. Limitations of the study include a relatively small sample size, a retrospective ascertainment of exposure, and a low response rate of 54%. Nonetheless, the study highlights the difficulties involved in studying incident cases of PsA and provides useful data and a basis for further investigation. The pregnancy associations have been confirmed by another study where they found that pregnancy was associated with reduced likelihood of PsA and that PsA improved during pregnancy but flares were common in the postpartum period [17]. These studies suggest a possible hormonal influence in the onset of PsA.

QUALITY OF LIFE

A quality of life (QOL) study in the Nordic Psoriasis Association found that, compared with those with only psoriasis, patients who also had arthritis had a greater impairment of their QOL. In another recent study of self-reported QOL using a single global question on the basis of a 10-point scale, 39% of the patients found PsA to be a large problem in their lives, whereas 12% of patients with only psoriasis felt the same [34]. Female patients tended to report greater impairment in their QOL than did male patients, and age tended to be unrelated to alterations in the QOL [35]. Not surprisingly, the extent of skin involvement was associated with increased impairment in the QOL [35].

Two recent studies suggest that QOL in PsA is similar to that in RA. The first study compared QOL between PsA and RA and found that the psychosocial reflection of QOL and life satisfaction were the same in both groups [36]. This was despite increased peripheral joint damage, inflammation, and physical disability in those with RA. Similarly, another study compared the QOL between RA and PsA patients after matching for disease duration and found no difference in the Health Assessment Questionnaire or the EuroQol-5D scores between the two groups [37]. The impairment in the QOL measures may be due to the additional impact of the skin disease in those with PsA.

MORBIDITY AND MORTALITY

The association between inflammatory joint disease, psoriasis, medications used to treat these diseases, and malignancy has been challenging to characterize. Inflammatory joint diseases such as rheumatoid arthritis (RA) have been linked to an increased risk of malignancy [38]. A cohort analysis of 665 patients with PsA who were prospectively followed from 1978 to 2004 at the University of Toronto found that 10% developed malignancies, the most frequent being breast, lung, and prostate [38]. The incidence of malignancy in this cohort did not differ from that of the general population both overall and by sex. These findings differ from those in RA but are consistent with known data regarding other seronegative disorders such as ankylosing spondylitis. Age at the onset of psoriasis and PsA, joint activity as measured by the number of joints with active disease, and the number of joints with effusions were not found to be associated with increased risk of malignancy. There was no evidence that treatments for PsA such as nonsteroidal anti-inflammatory drugs (NSAIDs), immunosuppressive agents, disease-modifying anti-rheumatic drugs (DMARDs), methotrexate (MTX) or biologics were associated with increased risk of malignancy. However, elevated erythrocyte sedimentation rate was predictive of the development of malignancy in patients with PsA [38].

The Olmsted County and the Greek population studies found the mortality rate in PsA patients similar to that of the general population [12, 13]. This is in contrast to results from the University of Toronto Psoriatic Arthritis Clinic, where the combined standardized mortality rate for men and women was increased [39]. This disparity in the mortality data between the studies is likely due to the difference in the study populations. Patients at the University of Toronto Psoriatic Arthritis Clinic were more likely to be referred to the center and likely represent a cohort of patients whose disease is more severe. In the Olmsted County study, there were some cases that had never been seen by a rheumatologist and may represent a subset of patients with milder disease. The most frequent cause of mortality was due to circulatory and respiratory system disorders, followed by malignancies and injury/poisoning [39]. Deaths due to injury/poisoning exceeded the rate for the general population in men only. The cause for the increase in cardiovascular mortality seen in some centers has been addressed by a recent study that found that even low-risk patients with PsA have a marked increase in carotid atherosclerosis independent of traditional risk factors [40]. Limitations of this study include its cross-sectional nature, limiting inferences of causality, and exclusion of controls who smoked or had known cardiovascular risk factors and that it is based on a Chinese population [40]. Further studies on this subject need to be prospective and include heterogeneous populations.

A multivariate analysis revealed that an erythrocyte sedimentation rate greater than 15 mm/h, medications used before initial clinic visit, radiological damage, and absence of nail lesions were associated with an increased overall mortality rate [41]. The presence of nail disease in this study appeared to be a protective factor and had the most clinical importance in the setting of previously active and severe disease [41].

CONCLUSIONS

Recent studies have added to our knowledge of the epidemiology of PsA across various populations. However, absence of a standard case definition of PsA for population studies and its relative rarity has likely contributed to the general paucity of available data. Reported prevalence estimates appear to vary more than incidence estimates, which generally appear to converge. Some of the heterogeneity among the prevalence estimates may be due to differences in genetic factors, exposure to environmental factors, and study methods. Overall, the available data suggest that QOL in PsA patient's is substantially reduced and is similar to that in patients with rheumatoid arthritis. The paucity of relevant data about important outcomes of PsA, including mortality and cardiovascular complications, calls for further investigation.

REFERENCES

1. Gladman DD, Antoni C, Mease P, Clegg DO, Nash P. Psoriatic arthritis: epidemiology, clinical features, course, and outcome. Ann Rheum Dis 2005;64 Suppl 2:ii14-ii17.
2. Kruithof E, Baeten D, De Rycke L, Vandooren B, Foell D, Roth J, et al. Synovial histopathology of psoriatic arthritis, both oligo- and polyarticular, resembles spondyloarthropathy more than it does rheumatoid arthritis. Arthritis Res Ther 2005;7:R569–580.
3. Mease P. Psoriatic arthritis update. Bull NYU Hosp Jt Dis 2006;64:25–31.
4. Taylor W, Gladman D, Helliwell P, Marchesoni A, Mease P, Mielants H. Classification criteria for psoriatic arthritis: development of new criteria from a large international study. Arthritis Rheum 2006;54:2665–2673.
5. Moll JM, Wright V. Psoriatic arthritis. Semin Arthritis Rheum 1973;3:55–78.

6. Chandran V, Schentag CT, Gladman DD. Sensitivity of the classification of psoriatic arthritis criteria in early psoriatic arthritis. Arthritis Rheum 2007;57:1560–1563.
7. Alenius GM, Stenberg B, Stenlund H, Lundblad M, Dahlqvist SR. Inflammatory joint manifestations are prevalent in psoriasis: prevalence study of joint and axial involvement in psoriatic patients, and evaluation of a psoriatic and arthritic questionnaire. J Rheumatol 2002;29:2577–2582.
8. Harrison BJ, Silman AJ, Barrett EM, Scott DG, Symmons DP. Presence of psoriasis does not influence the presentation or short-term outcome of patients with early inflammatory polyarthritis. J Rheumatol 1997;24:1744–1749.
9. Lomholt G. Psoriasis: Prevalence, Spontaneous Course and Genetics: A Census Study on the Prevalence of Skin Diseases on the Faroe Islands. Copenhagen: GEC CAD; 1963.
10. Hellgren L. Association between rheumatoid arthritis and psoriasis in total populations. Acta Rheumatol Scand 1969;15:316–326.
11. van Romunde LK, Valkenburg HA, Swart-Bruinsma W, Cats A, Hermans J. Psoriasis and arthritis. I. A population study. Rheumatol Int 1984;4:55–60.
12. Shbeeb M, Uramoto KM, Gibson LE, O'Fallon WM, Gabriel SE. The epidemiology of psoriatic arthritis in Olmsted County, Minnesota, USA, 1982–1991. J Rheumatol 2000;27:1247–1250.
13. Alamanos Y, Papadopoulos NG, Voulgari PV, Siozos C, Psychos DN, Tympanidou M, Drosos AA. Epidemiology of psoriatic arthritis in northwest Greece, 1982–2001. J Rheumatol 2003;30:2641–2644.
14. Trontzas P, Andrianakos A, Miyakis S, Pantelidou K, Vafiadou E, Garantziotou V, Voudouris C, ESORDIG study group. Seronegative spondyloarthropathies in Greece: a population-based study of prevalence, clinical pattern, and management. The ESORDIG study. Clin Rheumatol 2005;24:583–589.
15. Madland TM, Apalset EM, Johannessen AE, Rossebo B, Brun JG. Prevalence, disease manifestations, and treatment of psoriatic arthritis in Western Norway. J Rheumatol 2005;32:1918–1922.
16. Gelfand JM, Gladman DD, Mease PJ, Smith N, Margolis DJ, Nijsten T, Stern RS, Feldman SR, Rolstad T. Epidemiology of psoriatic arthritis in the population of the United States. J Am Acad Dermatol 2005;53:573.
17. Wilson FC, Icen M, Crowson CS, McEvoy MT, Gabriel SE, Kremers HM. Time trends in epidemiology and characteristics of psoriatic arthritis over 3 decades: a population-based study. J Rheumatol 2009;36:361–367.
18. Tam LS, Leung YY, Li EK. Psoriatic arthritis in Asia. Rheumatology (Oxford, England) 2009;48: 1473–1477.
19. Hukuda S, Minami M, Saito T, Mitsui H, Matsui N, Komatsubara Y, Makino H, et al. Spondyloarthropathies in Japan: nationwide questionnaire survey performed by the Japan Ankylosing Spondylitis Society. J Rheumatol 2001;28:554–559.
20. Setty AR, Choi HK. Psoriatic arthritis epidemiology. Curr Rheumatol Rep 2007;9:449–454.
21. Kaipiainen-Seppanen O. Incidence of psoriatic arthritis in Finland. Br J Rheumatol 1996;35:1289–1291.
22. Mallbris L, Larsson P, Bergqvist S, Vingard E, Granath F, Stahle M. Psoriasis phenotype at disease onset: clinical characterization of 400 adult cases. J Invest Dermatol 2005;124:499–504.
23. Solinger AM, Hess EV. Rheumatic diseases and AIDS—is the association real? J Rheumatol 1993;20:678–683.
24. Espinoza LR, Jara LJ, Espinoza CG, Silveira LH, Martinez-Osuna P, Seleznick M. There is an association between human immunodeficiency virus infection and spondyloarthropathies. Rheum Dis Clin North Am 1992;18:257–266.
25. Njobvu P, McGill P, Kerr H, Jellis J, Pobee J. Spondyloarthropathy and human immunodeficiency virus infection in Zambia. J Rheumatol 1998;25:1553–1559.
26. Njobvu P, McGill P. Psoriatic arthritis and human immunodeficiency virus infection in Zambia. J Rheumatol 2000;27:1699–1702.
27. Mijiyawa M, Oniankitan O, Khan MA. Spondyloarthropathies in sub-Saharan Africa. Curr Opin Rheumatol 2000;12:281–286.
28. Lopez-Larrea C, Njobvu PD, Gonzalez S, Blanco-Gelaz MA, Martinez-Borra J, Lopez-Vazquez A. The HLA-B*5703 allele confers susceptibility to the development of spondylarthropathies in Zambian human immunodeficiency virus-infected patients with slow progression to acquired immunodeficiency syndrome. Arthritis Rheum 2005;52:275–279.
29. Scarpa R, Oriente P, Pucino A, Torella M, Vignone L, Riccio A, Biondi Oriente C. Psoriatic arthritis in psoriatic patients. Br J Rheumatol 1984;23:246–250.
30. Rahman P, Schentag CT, Gladman DD. Immunogenetic profile of patients with psoriatic arthritis varies according to the age at onset of psoriasis. Arthritis Rheum 1999;42:822–823.

31. Jones SM, Armas JB, Cohen MG, Lovell CR, Evison G, McHugh NJ. Psoriatic arthritis: outcome of disease subsets and relationship of joint disease to nail and skin disease. Br J Rheumatol 1994;33:834–839.
32. Wilson FC, Icen M, Crowson CS, McEvoy MT, Gabriel SE, Kremers HM. Incidence and clinical predictors of psoriatic arthritis in patients with psoriasis: a population-based study. Arthritis Rheum 2009;61:233–239.
33. Thumboo J, Uramoto K, Shbeeb MI, O'Fallon WM, Crowson CS, Gibson LE, Michet CJ Jr, Gabriel SE. Risk factors for the development of psoriatic arthritis: a population based nested case control study. J Rheumatol 2002;29:757–762.
34. Zachariae H, Zachariae R, Blomqvist K, Davidsson S, Molin L, Mork C, Sigurgeirsson B. Quality of life and prevalence of arthritis reported by 5,795 members of the Nordic Psoriasis Associations. Data from the Nordic Quality of Life Study. Acta Derm Venereol 2002;82:108–113.
35. Borman P, Toy GG, Babaoglu S, Bodur H, Ciliz D, Alli N. A comparative evaluation of quality of life and life satisfaction in patients with psoriatic and rheumatoid arthritis. Clin Rheumatol 2007;26:330–334.
36. Gelfand JM, Feldman SR, Stern RS, Thomas J, Rolstad T, Margolis DJ. Determinants of quality of life in patients with psoriasis: a study from the US population. J Am Acad Dermatol 2004;51:704–708.
37. Sokoll KB, Helliwell PS. Comparison of disability and quality of life in rheumatoid and psoriatic arthritis. J Rheumatol 2001;28:1842–1846.
38. Rohekar S, Tom BD, Hassa A, Schentag CT, Farewell VT, Gladman DD. Prevalence of malignancy in psoriatic arthritis. Arthritis Rheum 2008;58:82–87.
39. Wong K, Gladman DD, Husted J, Long JA, Farewell VT. Mortality studies in psoriatic arthritis: results from a single outpatient clinic. I. Causes and risk of death. Arthritis Rheum 1997;40:1868–1872.
40. Tam LS, Shang Q, Li EK, Tomlinson B, Chu TT, Li M, Leung YY, et al. Subclinical carotid atherosclerosis in patients with psoriatic arthritis. Arthritis Rheum 2008;59:1322–1331.
41. Gladman DD, Farewell VT, Wong K, Husted J. Mortality studies in psoriatic arthritis: results from a single outpatient center. II. Prognostic indicators for death. Arthritis Rheum 1998;41:1103–1110.

Section II

Consequences

8 Arthritis, Obesity, Increased Cardiovascular Risk, and Disability

Shampa Chatterjee

CONTENTS

INTRODUCTION

Arthritis (either rheumatoid arthritis (RA) or osteoarthritis) is a chronic inflammatory disease, characterized by inflammation of the synovial tissues lining the joints [1–4]. Inflammation starts with the infiltration of inflammatory cells, including monocytes and activated leukocytes, into the joints [5–10]. These cells release enzymes and proinflammatory and other factors that degrade and destroy synovial tissue [8–10]. Inflammation eventually leads to coagulation and fibrin deposits on the synovial membrane and in the intracellular matrix of the joints. This fibrin develops into granulation tissue called pannus, which is considered as a scar tissue in the healing process. Pannus tissue around the joint eventually immobilizes the joint. In addition to this process, synovial membrane cells abnormally proliferate and enlarge and eventually occlude small blood causing reduced blood flow or ischemia. This causes hypoxia and metabolic acidosis. Acidosis stimulates the release of hydrolytic enzymes from synovial cells into the surrounding tissue, initiating erosion of the cartilage and bone and finally joint deformity and functional disability [11–14].

Arthritis has been related to several other diseases such as obesity and cardiovascular disease. For many years, the association of obesity and arthritis had been attributed to the effects of overload on weight-bearing joints [15, 16]. This was also supported by epidemiological studies where a correlation between increased body mass index and the severity of arthritis, specifically arthritic pain of the knee or hip, was observed [17, 18]. However, a growing body of evidence now supports that obesity is a complex syndrome in which an abnormal activation of proinflammatory pathways leads to an altered control of food intake, fat expansion, and metabolic changes. Activated white adipose tissue increases the synthesis of proinflammatory cytokines, interleukins (ILs) such as IL-6, IL-1, IL-8, tumor necrosis factor α (TNF-α), and IL-18, whereas regulatory cytokines, such as IL-10, are decreased [19–21]. Adipocytes also produce cytokines and adipokines that exert multiple effects, and promote synovial inflammation, cartilage degrading enzymes, and bone matrix remodeling [21–25].

Cardiovascular risk, which has been linked to obesity, is also being seen as a low-grade inflammation disorder. It is now beyond dispute that inflammation is a key player in the development of atherosclerosis. In individuals with an excess of visceral/ectopic fat, it plays an important role in several cardiovascular disorders. In addition to atherosclerosis, in which the involvement of inflammation is well known, other cardiovascular disorders, such as calcific aortic stenosis and aortic aneurysms, are strongly influenced by the inflammatory components of visceral obesity. In terms of its proinflammatory and metabolic features (which have intricate and reciprocal relationships), visceral obesity is an emergent powerful but modifiable risk factor for cardiovascular disease.

Thus, inflammation in arthritis clusters with metabolic syndrome of obesity and an increased risk of cardiovascular disease. In exploring the link between arthritis, obesity, and cardiovascular disorder, this chapter summarizes the role of inflammation as a key link between these diseases.

OBESITY AND ARTHRITIS

Obesity is a global problem leading to excess morbidity and mortality. According to the latest World Health Organization projections, more than 1.6 billion adults are overweight and at least 400 million are obese worldwide [26, 27]. Although obesity is a known risk factor for arthritis, it is now well accepted that proinflammatory pathways triggered by it may be the key in promoting arthritis [20–23, 28–32].

Activated white adipose tissue increases the synthesis of proinflammatory cytokines such as IL-6, IL-1, IL-8, TNF-α, and IL-18 and decreases regulatory cytokines such as IL-10 [19–21]. As mentioned earlier, adipocytes trigger production of cytokines that cause increased inflammation and bone matrix remodeling [21–25]. Furthermore, proinflammatory cytokines stimulate adipocytes to synthesize neuropeptides such as substance P and nerve growth factor that have been shown to be critical in regulating both appetite and cartilage homeostasis [21, 33–35]. Thus, the influence of obesity on arthritis seems to stem from a complex interaction of inflammatory and metabolic factors.

IL-6 stimulates the hepatic production of C-reactive protein (CRP). A positive correlation has been found between CRP levels and abdominal obesity. It has, therefore, been suggested that obesity may be a risk factor for inflammatory arthritis. The discovery of the leptin system has led to examining its role in the pathogenesis of inflammatory arthritis [36]. Leptin belongs to the type I cytokine family, and its expression is regulated by proinflammatory mediators. Murine models of autoimmune diseases such as antigen-induced arthritis and leptin-deficient mouse (ob/ob) showed reduced susceptibility to arthritis [36]. Leptin levels have been shown to be higher in patients with arthritis as compared with healthy controls [37], and exogenous leptin administration decreased the severity of septic arthritis [38]. However, other studies have found no differences between leptin levels of patients with arthritis and healthy controls [39–41]. Thus, the precise role of leptin in arthritis (specifically RA) remains unclear.

In a study on patients with RA, Chung et al. [42] showed that insulin resistance was associated with several markers of inflammation, including TNF-α, IL-6, and CRP, and in patients with RA, insulin resistance was associated with coronary calcification. These results highlight the link between obesity, metabolic syndrome, and inflammation in the pathogenesis of coronary atherosclerosis in arthritis.

OBESITY AND CARDIOVASCULAR DYSFUNCTION

It is now beyond dispute that inflammation is one of the important causes of cardiovascular disease and a key player in the development of atherothrombosis. Inflammation is also considered to be at the center stage of metabolic dysfunction. Insulin resistance is strongly influenced by several proinflammatory signals. Both insulin resistance and the presence of a proinflammatory status may account for the development of endothelial dysfunction, an early step in the atherogenesis process observed in patients with RA [43–45].

In the past decade or so, data from studies by various investigators have shown that chronic low-grade inflammation is encountered in individuals with an excess of visceral/ectopic fat, which plays an important role in several cardiovascular disorders. Thus, in terms of its proinflammatory and metabolic features, obesity is an emergent risk factor for cardiovascular disease [46–49].

Under normal conditions, the endothelial cells of the arterial wall resist adhesion and aggregation of leukocytes and promote fibrinolysis. When activated by stimuli such as obesity, insulin resistance, or inflammation, the endothelial cells express a series of adhesion molecules that selectively recruit various classes of leukocytes. Inflammatory cells such as blood monocytes now adhere to the "adherent" endothelial surface by binding to leukocyte adhesion molecules. After adhesion of monocytes, proinflammatory proteins also called chemokines are produced, and these provide a chemotactic stimulus that induces them to enter the intima. Within the intima, the monocytes mature into macrophages, which express scavenger receptors. These receptors allow macrophages to engulf oxidized or modified lipoprotein particles. The macrophages also proliferate within the intima and after being filled with lipid particles get a frothy appearance of the foam cells found in atherosclerotic lesions [50–53]. These cells also release several growth factors and cytokines, including enzymes such as matrix metalloproteinases and the procoagulant tissue factor that can destroy the vessel wall matrix.

SYSTEMIC INFLAMMATORY CONDITIONS

Inflammatory mediators are the critical factors that link obesity and cardiovascular disease with arthritis. In all these cases, inflammation, which causes vascular dysfunction, also inflames synovial tissue in joints. Blood monocytes, activated macrophages, and synovial fibroblasts accumulate in the region of the joint and produce proinflammatory cytokines, including TNF-α, IL-1, IL-6, and IL-17, and growth factors, such as M-CSF, in and around the vicinity of synovial tissue. Eventually, cells of monocyte–macrophage lineage form osteoclasts, which secrete proteases and create an acidic environment that causes bone destruction [54–56]. Normally, bone destruction is compensated by osteoblasts or cells that arise from mesenchymal stem cells and undergo maturation and differentiation to form bone matrix. However, joint inflammation is reported to suppress osteoblast growth.

In RA, anti-TNF-α agents are now being used for therapy. This is because TNF-α is a dominant proinflammatory cytokine in the pathophysiology of RA. Both of the newer TNF-α antagonists, certolizumab pegol and golimumab [57–60] when administered either alone or in combination with methotrexate, have also significantly reduced clinical evidence of disease activity and affected clinical remission in some patients. Recombinant human IL-1Rα (anakinra) reduces the rate of radiographic progression of RA compared with treatment with placebo [61]. In the same way, anti-IL-6 receptor monoclonal antibody binds to the membrane-bound and soluble forms of the IL-6 receptor and blocks binding of IL-6 to its receptor, thereby preventing signaling [62].

ATHEROSCLEROTIC CARDIOVASCULAR DISEASE IN RA

As has been mentioned in the previous sections, arthritis involves increased generation of IL-1 or TNF-α and other inflammatory cytokines produced in the joints. These eventually spill into the circulation, where they can cause increased production of adhesion molecules and other proinflammatory molecules such as chemokines and chemotaxic substances. This leads to monocyte and leukocyte adhesion to the endothelial cells of the vessel wall followed by chemotaxis of these into vessel walls, which ultimately leads to atherosclerosis [52, 53].

In addition, CRP also increases with arthritis-associated inflammation. CRP stimulates macrophages to produce tissue factor, an important procoagulant found in atherosclerotic plaques. Thus, inflammatory and immune responses link joint damage and atherosclerosis. Studies on patients with unstable angina showed that they have an increase of CD4-positive T cells. These cells have been reported earlier to increase in patients with severe RA [63]. In addition, studies have documented an increased incidence and prevalence of cardiovascular conditions in patients with RA compared with individuals without RA. Also, a number of studies using noninvasive means to detect atherosclerosis have shown that patients with RA may be prone to atherosclerosis. Moreover, vascular dysfunction has been well documented in patients with RA by means of flow-mediated dilation of brachial artery and increased arterial stiffness in cardiovascular disease–free patients [64, 65].

Also, there is remarkable resemblance between conditions that drive both atherosclerosis and arthritis. Unstable coronary lesions often follow inflammatory synovitis in RA with abundant presence of cytokines, activated macrophages, T cells, expression of adhesion molecules (intercellular adhesion molecule 1, vascular cell adhesion molecule 1, E-selectin), and release of proteolytic enzymes (matrix metalloproteinases). All play an important role in the process in arterial wall injury and destruction. Other changes that are also shared between the two conditions are increased reactivity against bacterial and human heat shock protein 60/65 and proliferation of the T-lymphocyte subtype characterized by proinflammatory and aggressive tissue-damaging properties [63, 66–70].

ADIPOCYTOKINES AND INSULIN RESISTANCE IN RA

Adipokine is used to denote biologically active substances found in the adipocytes of white adipose tissue. Adipokines are specific adipose tissue–derived peptides. Adipokines include a variety of proinflammatory peptides including TNF-α. As mentioned in the course of this review, these proinflammatory adipokines appear to contribute to the "low-grade inflammatory state" of obese subjects, setting up a cluster of metabolic aberrations including cardiovascular complications and autoimmune inflammatory diseases such as arthritis [71–75].

Some adipokines such as leptin have neuroendocrine functions. Leptin receptors are expressed on monocytes/macrophages, T cells, and natural killer cells. In isolated monocytes/macrophages, leptin induces the production of TNF-α and IL-6. Leptin-deficient mice are less prone than nonleptin-deficient mice to develop inflammatory diseases [76, 77].

However, the role of leptin in atherogenesis is not very clear. Leptin-deficient ob/ob mice exhibit early onset obesity yet are resistant to diet-induced atherosclerosis [78, 79]. Exogenous administration of leptin reduces adiposity in leptin-deficient children, whereas it has been shown to induce vascular neointimal proliferation in rodents [33, 80].

In patients with RA, circulating leptin levels have been described as either higher or unmodified in comparison with healthy controls. However, a fasting-induced reduction in circulating leptin is associated with decreased CD4+ lymphocyte reactivity. *In vivo*, an experimental antigen-induced arthritis is less severe in leptin-deficient *ob/ob* mice than that in wild-type mice. In osteoarthritis, leptin production is much higher in osteoarthritic human cartilage than that in normal cartilage. The finding that administration of exogenous leptin increases transforming growth factor β1 production by rat knee-joint cartilage has suggested that high circulating leptin levels in obese individuals might protect cartilage from osteoarthritic degeneration. Other novel adipokines that supposedly exert action in inflammation and immunity are apelin, omentin, hepcidin, and vaspin [77].

It is now clear that adipokines have multiple important roles in the body and that there is a complex adipokine-mediated interplay between obesity, metabolic disorders, inflammatory diseases, and autoimmune disorders like arthritis.

REFERENCES

1. Myasoedova E, Davis JM 3rd, Crowson CS, Gabriel SE. Epidemiology of rheumatoid arthritis: rheumatoid arthritis and mortality. Curr Rheumatol Rep 2010;12(5):379–385.
2. Damasio MB, Malattia C, Martini A, Toma P. Synovial and inflammatory diseases in childhood: role of new imaging modalities in the assessment of patients with juvenile idiopathic arthritis. Pediatr Radiol 2010;40:985–998.
3. Goronzy JJ, Weyand CM. Developments in the scientific understanding of rheumatoid arthritis. Arthritis Res Ther 2009;11:249.

4. Szekanecz Z, Besenyei T, Paragh G, Koch AE. New insights in synovial angiogenesis. Joint Bone Spine 2009;77:13–19.
5. Manicourt DH, Triki R, Fukuda K, Devogelaer JP, Nagant de Deuxchaisnes C, Thonar EJ. Levels of circulating tumor necrosis factor alpha and interleukin-6 in patients with rheumatoid arthritis. Relationship to serum levels of hyaluran and antigenic keratan sulfate. Arthritis Rheum 1993;36:490–499.
6. Tetta C, Camussi G, Modena V, Di Vittorio C, Baglioni C. Tumor necrosis factor in serum and synovial fluid of patients with active and severe rheumatoid arthritis. Ann Rheum Dis 1990;49:665–667.
7. Wolfe F. Comparative usefulness of C-reactive protein and erythrocyte sedimentation rate in patients with rheumatoid arthritis. J Rheumatol 1997;24:1477–1485.
8. Van Leuven SI, Franssen R, Kastelein JJ, Levi M, Stroes ES, Tak PP. Systemic inflammation as a risk factor for atherothrombosis. Rheumatology 2008;47:3–7.
9. Gonzalez-Gay MA, Gonzalez-Juanatey C, Pineiro A, Garcia-Porrua C, Testa A, Llorca J. High-grade C-reactive protein elevation correlates with accelerated atherogenesis in patients with rheumatoid arthritis. J Rheumatol 2005;32:1219–1223.
10. Gonzalez-Gay MA, Gonzalez-Juanatey C, Martin J. Rheumatoid arthritis: a disease associated with accelerated atherogenesis. Semin Arthritis Rheum 2005;35:8–17.
11. Paleolog EM. Angiogenesis in rheumatoid arthritis. Arthritis Res 2002;4:S81–S90.
12. Wick G, Knoflach M, Xu Q. Autoimmune and inflammatory mechanisms in atherosclerosis. Annu Rev Immunol 2004;22:361–403.
13. Rothschild BM, Masi AT. Pathogenesis of rheumatoid arthritis: a vascular hypothesis. Semin Arthritis Rheum 1982;12:11–31.
14. Paleolog EM. Angiogenesis in rheumatoid arthritis. Arthritis Res 2002;4:S81–S90.
15. Felson DT, Anderson JJ, Naimark A, Walker AM, Meenan RF. Obesity and knee osteoarthritis. The Framingham Study. Ann Intern Med 1988;109:18–24
16. Hart DJ, Doyle DV, Spector TD. Incidence and risk factors for radiographic knee osteoarthritis in middle-aged women: the Chingford Study. Arthritis Rheum 1999;42:17–24.
17. Felson DT, Zhang Y, Hannan MT, Naimark A, Weissman B, Aliabadi P, Levy D. Risk factors for incident radiographic knee osteoarthritis in the elderly: the Framingham Study. Arthritis Rheum 1997;40:728–33.
18. Reijman M, Pols HA, Bergink AP, Hazes JM, Belo JN, Lievense AM, Bierma-Zeinstra SM. Body mass index associated with onset and progression of osteoarthritis of the knee but not of the hip: the Rotterdam Study. Ann Rheum Dis 2007;66:158–162.
19. Wellen KE, Hotamisligil GS. Inflammation, stress, and diabetes. J Clin Invest 2005;115:1111–1119.
20. Coppack SW. Pro-inflammatory cytokines and adipose tissue. Proc Nutr Soc 2001;60:349–356.
21. Iannone F, Lapadula G. Obesity and inflammation—targets for OA therapy. Curr Drug Targets 2001;11:586–598.
22. Dayer JM, Chicheportiche R, Juge-Aubry C, Meier C. Adipose tissue has anti-inflammatory properties: focus on IL-1 receptor antagonist (IL-1Ra). Ann N Y Acad Sci 2006;1069:444–453.
23. Otero M, Lago R, Gomez R, Dieguez C, Lago F, Gomez-Reino J, Gualillo O. Towards a pro-inflammatory and immunomodulatory emerging role of leptin. Rheumatology (Oxford) 2006;45:944–950.
24. Edwards JCW. Fibroblast biology. Development and differentiation of synovial fibroblasts in arthritis. Arthritis Res 2000;2:344–347.
25. Magliano M. Obesity and arthritis. Menopause Int 2008;14:149–154.
26. Obesity and Overweight. World Health Organization. http://www.whoint/mediacentre/factsheets/fs311/en/indexhtml. Accessed 2006.
27. Nguyen DM, El-Serag HB. The epidemiology of obesity. Gastroenterol Clin North Am. 2010;39:1–7.
28. Voigt LF, Koepsell TD, Nelson JL, Dugowson CE, Daling JR. Smoking, obesity, alcohol consumption, and the risk of rheumatoid arthritis. Epidemiology 1994;5:525–532.
29. Symmons DP, Bankhead CR, Harrison BJ, Brennan P, Barrett EM, Scott DG, Silman AJ. Blood transfusion, smoking, and obesity as risk factors for the development of rheumatoid arthritis: results from a primary care-based incident case-control study in Norfolk, England. Arthritis Rheum 1997;40:1955–1961.
30. Despres JP. Inflammation and cardiovascular disease: is abdominal obesity the missing link? Int J Obes Relat Metab Disord 2003;27:S22–S24.
31. Cartier A, Lemieux I, Almeras N, Tremblay A, Bergeron J, Despres JP. Visceral obesity and plasma glucose-insulin homeostasis: contributions of interleukin-6 and tumor necrosis factor-alpha in men. J Clin Endocrinol Metab 2008;93:1931–1938.

32. Blackburn P, Després JP, Lamarche B, Tremblay A, Bergeron J, Lemieux I, Couillard C. Postprandial variations of plasma inflammatory markers in abdominally obese men. Obesity 2006;14:1747–1754.
33. Mathieu P, Lemieux I, Després JP. Obesity, inflammation, and cardiovascular risk. Clin Pharmacol Ther 2010;87:407–416.
34. Matsuzawa, Y. The metabolic syndrome and adipocytokines. FEBS Lett 2006;580:2917–2921.
35. Cote M, Mauriège P, Bergeron J, Alméras N, Tremblay A, Lemieux I, Després JP. Adiponectinemia in visceral obesity: impact on glucose tolerance and plasma lipoprotein and lipid levels in men. J Clin Endocrinol Metab 2005;90:1434–1439.
36. Otero M, Lago R, Gomez R, Dieguez C, Lago F, Gómez-Reino J, Gualillo O. Towards a proinflammatory and immunomodulatory emerging role of leptin. Rheumatology (Oxford) 2006;45:944–950.
37. Popa C, Netea MG, Radstake TR, van Riel PL, Barrera P, van der Meer JW. Markers of inflammation are negatively correlated with serum leptin in rheumatoid arthritis. Ann Rheum Dis 2005;64:1195–1198.
38. Hultgren OH, Tarkowski A. Leptin in septic arthritis: decreased levels during infection and amelioration of disease activity upon its administration. Arthritis Res 2001;3:389–394.
39. Hizmetli S, Kisa M, Gokalp N, Bakici MZ. Are plasma and synovial fluid leptin levels correlated with disease activity in rheumatoid arthritis? Rheumatol Int 2007;27:335–338.
40. Harle P, Sarzi-Puttini P, Cutolo M, Straub RH. No change of serum levels of leptin and adiponectin during anti-tumour necrosis factor antibody treatment with adalimumab in patients with rheumatoid arthritis. Ann Rheum Dis 2006;65:970–971.
41. Wisłowska M, Rok M, Jaszczyk B, Stepień K, Cicha M. Serum leptin in rheumatoid arthritis. Rheumatol Int 2007;27:947–954.
42. Chung CP, Oeser A, Solus JF, Gebretsadik T, Shintani A, Avalos I, Sokka T, Raggi P, Pincus T, Stein CM. Inflammation-associated insulin resistance: differential effects in rheumatoid arthritis and systemic lupus erythematosus define potential mechanisms. Arthritis Rheum 2008;58:2105–2112.
43. Xu H, Barnes GT, Yang Q, Tan G, Yang D, Chou CJ, Sole J, et al. Chronic inflammation in fat plays a crucial role in the development of obesity-related insulin resistance. J Clin Invest 2003;112:1821–1830.
44. Poirier P, Lemieux I, Mauriège P, Dewailly E, Blanchet C, Bergeron J, Després JP. Impact of waist circumference on the relationship between blood pressure and insulin: the Quebec Health Survey. Hypertension 2005;45:363–367.
45. Engeli S, Böhnke J, Gorzelniak K, Janke J, Schling P, Bader M, Luft FC, Sharma AM. Weight loss and the renin–angiotensin–aldosterone system. Hypertension 2005;45:356–362.
46. Gade W, Schmit J, Collins M, Gade J. Beyond obesity: the diagnosis and pathophysiology of metabolic syndrome. Clin Lab Sci 2010;23:51–61.
47. Kirk EP, Klein S. Pathogenesis and pathophysiology of the cardiometabolic syndrome. J Clin Hypertens (Greenwich) 2010;11:761–765.
48. Mathieu P, Pibarot P, Larose E, Poirier P, Marette A, Despres JP. Visceral obesity and the heart. Int J Biochem Cell Biol 2008;40:821–836.
49. Andersson CX, Gustafson B, Hammarstedt A, Hedjazifar S, Smith U. Inflamed adipose tissue, insulin resistance and vascular injury. Diabetes Metab Res Rev 2008;24:595–603.
50. Manicourt DH, Triki R, Fukuda K, Devogelaer JP, Nagant de Deuxchaisnes C, Thonar EJ. Levels of circulating tumor necrosis factor alpha and interleukin-6 in patients with rheumatoid arthritis. Relationship to serum levels of hyaluran and antigenic keratan sulfate. Arthritis Rheum 1993;36:490–499.
51. Tetta C, Camussi G, Modena V, Di Vittorio C, Baglioni C. Tumor necrosis factor in serum and synovial fluid of patients with active and severe rheumatoid arthritis. Ann Rheum Dis 1990;49:665–667.
52. Libby P. Molecular and cellular mechanisms of the thrombotic complications of atherosclerosis. J Lipid Res 2009;50:S352–S357.
53. Zaman AG, Helft G, Worthley SG, Badimon JJ. The role of plaque rupture and thrombosis in coronary artery disease. Atherosclerosis 2000;149:251–266.
54. Kinne RW, Bräuer R, Stuhlmüller B, Palombo-Kinne E, Burmester GR. Macrophages in rheumatoid arthritis. Arthritis Res 2000;2:189–202.
55. Suzuki Y, Tsutsumi Y, Nakagawa M, Suzuki H, Matsushita K, Beppu M, Aoki H, Ichikawa Y, Mizushima Y. Osteoclast-like cells in an in vitro model of bone destruction by rheumatoid synovium. Rheumatology (Oxford) 2001;40:673–682.
56. Karmakar S, Kay J, Gravallese EM. Bone damage in rheumatoid arthritis: mechanistic insights and approaches to prevention. Rheum Dis Clin North Am 2010;36:385–404.
57. Fleischmann R, Vencovsky J, van Vollenhoven RF, Borenstein D, Box J, Coteur G, Goel N, Brezinschek HP, Innes A, Strand V. Efficacy and safety of certolizumab pegol monotherapy every 4

weeks in patients with rheumatoid arthritis failing previous disease-modifying antirheumatic therapy: the FAST4- WARD study. Ann Rheum Dis 2009;68:805–811.

58. Smolen J, Landewe RB, Mease P, Brzezicki J, Mason D, Luijtens K, van Vollenhoven RF, et al. Efficacy and safety of certolizumab pegol plus methotrexate in active rheumatoid arthritis: the RAPID 2 study. A randomised controlled trial. Ann Rheum Dis 2009;68:797–804.

59. Kay J, Matteson EL, Dasgupta B, Nash P, Durez P, Hall S, Hsia EC, et al. Golimumab in patients with active rheumatoid arthritis despite treatment with methotrexate: a randomized, doubleblind, placebo-controlled, dose-ranging study. Arthritis Rheum 2008;58:964–975.

60. Emery P, Fleischmann RM, Moreland LW, Hsia EC, Strusberg I, Durez P, Nash P, et al. Golimumab, a human anti-tumor necrosis factor alpha monoclonal antibody, injected subcutaneously every four weeks in methotrexate-naive patients with active rheumatoid arthritis: twenty-four-week results of a phase III, multicenter, randomized, double-blind, placebo-controlled study of golimumab before methotrexate as first-line therapy for early-onset rheumatoid arthritis. Arthritis Rheum 2009;60:2272–2283.

61. Jiang Y, Genant HK, Watt I, Cobby M, Bresnihan B, Aitchison R, McCabe D. A multicenter, double-blind, dose-ranging, randomized, placebo-controlled study of recombinant human interleukin-1 receptor antagonist in patients with rheumatoid arthritis: radiologic progression and correlation of Genant and Larsen scores. 2000 Arthritis Rheum 2000;43:1001–1009.

62. Genovese MC, McKay JD, Nasonov EL, Mysler EF, da Silva NA, Alecock E, Woodworth T, Gomez-Reino JJ. Interleukin-6 receptor inhibition with tocilizumab reduces disease activity in rheumatoid arthritis with inadequate response to disease-modifying antirheumatic drugs: the tocilizumab in combination with traditional disease-modifying antirheumatic drug therapy study. Arthritis Rheum 2008;58:2968–2980.

63. Liuzzo G, Kopecky SL, Frye RL, O'Fallon WM, Maseri A, Goronzy JJ, Weyand CM. Perturbation of the T-cell repertoire in patients with unstable angina. Circulation 1999;100:2135–2139.

64. Soltész P, Dér H, Kerekes G, Szodoray P, Szücs G, Dankó K, Shoenfeld Y, Szegedi G, Szekanecz Z. A comparative study of arterial stiffness, flow-mediated vasodilation of the brachial artery, and the thickness of the carotid artery intima-media in patients with systemic autoimmune diseases. Clin Rheumatol 2009;28:655–662.

65. Vaudo G, Marchesi S, Gerli R, Allegrucci R, Giordano A, Siepi D, Pirro M, Shoenfeld Y, Schillaci G, Mannarino E. Endothelial dysfunction in young patients with rheumatoid arthritis and low disease activity. Ann Rheum Dis 2004;63:31–35.

66. Pasceri V, Yeh ET. A tale of two diseases: atherosclerosis and rheumatoid arthritis. Circulation 1999;100:2124–2126.

67. Stevens RJ, Douglas KM, Saratzis AN, Kitas GD. Inflammation and atherosclerosis in rheumatoid arthritis. Expert Rev Mol Med 2005;7:1–24.

68. Rajaiah R, Moudgil KD. Heat-shock proteins can promote as well as regulate autoimmunity. Autoimmun Rev 2009;8:388–393.

69. Mayr M, Kiechl S, Willeit J, Wick G, Xu Q. Infections, immunity, and atherosclerosis: associations of antibodies to *Chlamydia pneumoniae, Helicobacter pylori,* and cytomegalovirus with immune reactions to heat shock protein 60 and carotid or femoral atherosclerosis. Circulation 2000;102:833–839.

70. Ward JR, Wilson HL, Francis SE, Crossman DC, Sabroe I. Translational mini-review series on immunology of vascular disease: inflammation, infections and Toll-like receptors in cardiovascular disease. Clin Exp Immunol 2009;156:386–394.

71. Trayhurn P, Wood IS. Adipokines: inflammation and the pleiotropic role of white adipose tissue. Br J Nutr 2004;92:347–355.

72. Cousin B, Munoz O, Andre M, Fontanilles AM, Dani C, Cousin JL, Laharrague P, Casteilla L, Pénicaud L. A role for preadipocytes as macrophage-like cells. FASEB J 1999;13:305–312.

73. Villena JA, Cousin B, Pénicaud L, Casteilla L. Adipose tissues display differential phagocytic and microbicidal activities depending on their localization. Int J Obes Relat Metab Disord 2001;25:1275–1280.

74. Trayhurn P, Wood IS. Signalling role of adipose tissue: adipokines and inflammation in obesity. Biochem Soc Trans 2005;33:1078–1081.

75. Xu H, Barnes GT, Yang Q, Tan G, Yang D, Chou CJ, Sole J, et al. Chronic inflammation in fat plays a crucial role in the development of obesity-related insulin resistance. J Clin Invest 2003;112:1821–1830.

76. Otero M, Lago R, Lago F, Casanueva FF, Dieguez C, Gómez-Reino JJ, Gualillo O. Leptin, from fat to inflammation: old questions and new insights. FEBS Lett 2005;579:295–301.

77. Gualillo O, González-Juanatey JR, Lago F. The emerging role of adipokines as mediators of cardiovascular function: physiologic and clinical perspectives. Trends Cardiovasc Med 2007;17:275–283.

78. Nishina PM, Naggert JK, Verstuyft J, Paigen B. Atherosclerosis in genetically obese mice: the mutants obese, diabetes, fat, tubby, and lethal yellow. Metabolism 1994;43:554–558.
79. Silver DL, Jiang XC, Tall AR. Increased high density lipoprotein (HDL), defective hepatic catabolism of apoA-I and apoA-II, and decreased apoA-I mRNA in ob/ob mice. J Biol Chem 1999;274:4140–4146.
80. Wallace, AM. McMahon AD, Packard CJ, Kelly A, Shepherd J, Gaw A, Sattar N. Plasma leptin and the risk of cardiovascular disease in the west of Scotland coronary prevention study (WOSCOPS). Circulation 2001;104:3052–3056.

Section III

Antiarthritic Drugs

9 An Overview
Use of Traditional Antiarthritic Drugs and Update on Drug Development

Gabriela Schmajuk and Michael G. Lyon

CONTENTS

INTRODUCTION

Arthritic symptoms are among the most common reasons for visits to physicians. Arthritic disorders may cause a variety of symptoms, but among the most common of these are pain and impairment of function. Functional impairment may be caused by pain, structural joint damage, or both. Relief of pain and prevention of joint damage should therefore be the primary goals of arthritis therapies. The extent to which these goals are attainable with traditional drug therapies will differ according to the particular type of arthritis being treated.

In the inflammatory arthritides, of which rheumatoid arthritis (RA) is the prototype, pain and structural joint damage are caused by autoimmune mediated inflammation. Nonsteroidal anti-inflammatory drugs (NSAIDs) suppress inflammation and also exert analgesic effects. The disease-modifying antirheumatic drugs (DMARDs) may downregulate the abnormal immune response in RA, thereby preventing or suppressing structural damage to the joint.

In the case of osteoarthritis (OA), joint damage and pain are ultimately the result of cartilage breakdown and the abnormal joint mechanics that result from this process. Inflammation, although present in the OA joint, is much less important pathophysiologically than it is in RA. Therefore, although NSAIDs can have a role in pain therapy of OA, acetaminophen and other pure analgesics are often safer and more effective. To date, there are no pharmacologic agents that are remission inducing in OA; hence, preservation of joint function is best attempted through physical therapy and other nondrug modalities.

PAIN CONTROL IN ARTHRITIS

The pharmacotherapy of pain in arthritis includes many components. These components will be more or less appropriate according to the particular type of arthritis being treated.

Nonsteroidal Anti-inflammatory Drugs

NSAIDs are the most commonly prescribed class of medication for pain relief in the arthritic diseases. Some NSAIDs are available over the counter in many countries. They are also prescribed for nonarthritic conditions, such as headache and dysmenorrhea, and for certain nonpainful conditions like hereditary polyposis coli and Alzheimer's disease. There are now more than 20 different NSAID preparations (Table 9.1), and there are important differences in the chemical structure, dosing, adverse effects, and pharmacokinetics between the various agents. All NSAIDs have anti-pyretic, analgesic, and anti-inflammatory properties.

Mechanism of Action

Inhibition of prostaglandin synthesis is the primary therapeutic mechanism of action of all currently available NSAIDs. E-series prostanoic acids are proinflammatory, increase sensitivity to the release

TABLE 9.1
Commonly Available NSAIDs

Chemical Class	Generic Name	Usual Dose
Carboxylic acids		
Salicylic acid and esters	Aspirin	2–6 g/24 h in divided doses
	Diflunisal	250–750 mg bid
Phenyl acetic acids	Diclofenac sodium	25–75 mg bid
Carbo- and heterocyclic acids	Et odolac	200, 300, or 400 mg bid–qid (maximum 1200 mg/24 h)
	Indomethacin	25–50 mg tid
	Ketorolac	po, iv, or im 60–120 mg total/24 h for 5 days maximum
	Sulindac	150–200 mg bid
	Tolmetin sodium	400–800 mg tid–qid (maximum 2400 mg/24 h)
Propionic acids	Flurbiprofen	100 mg bid–tid
	Ketoprofen	50–75 mg tid
	Oxaprozin	600–1200 g once daily
	Naproxen	250–500 mg bid (maximum 1 g/24 h)
	Ibuprofen	250–500 mg bid (maximum 1 g/24 h)
Fenamic acids	Meclofenamate sodium	50–100 mg tid–qid
Enolic acids	Pioxicam	10 or 20 mg once daily
	Meloxicam	7.5 or 15 mg once daily
Napthylkanones	Nabumetone	500–750 mg bid
Nonacetylated salicylates	Salaslate	500–1500 mg bid
	Choline magnesium trisalicylate	500–1500 mg bid
COX-2 selective	Celecoxib	100–200 mg once daily

Abbreviation: COX, Cyclooxygenase.

of bradykinins, and increase vascular permeability. The reduced levels of prostaglandin E result in anti-inflammatory and analgesic effects. NSAIDs also inhibit the formation of prostacyclin and thromboxane, with corresponding complex effects on vascular permeability and platelet aggregation. NSAIDs ultimately reduce prostaglandin levels via the inhibition of cyclooxygenase (COX), the critical enzyme in the conversion of arachidonic acid to prostaglandin. Except in the case of aspirin, the inhibition of COX by NSAIDs is reversible.

There are two isoforms of COX, which are designated as COX-1 and COX-2. COX-1, the constitutive form, is normally expressed in most tissues and is responsible for maintaining normal gastric mucosal function. COX-2 is an inducible enzyme, levels of which are not normally detectable in many body tissues, but which increase in response to inflammation. All currently available NSAIDs that inhibit COX-1 also inhibit COX-2, with the exception of low-dose aspirin, which is COX-1 specific.

Administration

Most NSAIDs are given orally as a tablet or capsule. Ibuprofen, meloxicam, and some others are available in liquid form as well. Ketorolac is also available for intramuscular or intravenous injection for the short-term treatment of acute pain.

Adverse Effects

Most NSAID toxicity is related to the inhibition of the normal functions of prostaglandins. The toxicity potential of NSAIDs differs in some organ systems, depending on the degree of COX-2 selectivity

(Table 9.2). Upper gastrointestinal (GI) injury is the most important toxicity associated with NSAIDs. The risk of serious GI complications is 0.5% per year. Age, use of glucocorticoids or anticoagulants, prior history of ulcer disease, and RA all further increase the risk of serious GI toxicity (Singh et al., 1996). The GI risk can be reduced through the use of concomitant proton pump inhibitor medicines or misoprostol or by using NSAIDs with greater COX-2 selectivity (Rostom et al., 2002).

Renal toxicity is increasingly recognized as an important problem in patients on NSAIDs. It is clear that COX-2 specific NSAIDs have similar deleterious effects on renal function to the nonselective NSAIDs. There are known risk factors for renal toxicity with NSAIDs, the most important of which include volume depletion, congestive heart failure, cirrhosis, and comorbid renal disease.

Monitoring and Patient Education

The American College of Rheumatology recommends baseline and yearly complete blood count (CBC), creatinine, aspartate aminotransferase, and alanine aminotransferase for patients starting long-term NSAID therapy. In addition, periodic screening for dyspepsia, nausea/vomiting, abdominal pain, edema, shortness of breath, and bloody or tarry stool is appropriate. The concomitant administration of misoprostol, proton pump inhibitors, or double-dose H2 receptor antagonists has been shown effective in the prevention of NSAID-related gastric and duodenal ulcers.

TABLE 9.2
Adverse Effects of Nonspecific and COX-2-Specific Nonsteroidal Anti-inflammatories

Organ System	Nonspecific NSAIDs	Differences with COX-2-Specific NSAIDs
GI	Dyspepsia	Decreased UGI ulceration
	Gastroduodenal ulceration	Decreased bleeding
	Bleeding (all levels)	
	Colitis	
Renal	Hypertension	
	Edema	
	Acute renal failure	
	Interstitial nephritis	
	Papillary necrosis	
Hepatic	Elevated transaminases	
	Rare severe hepatic reactions	
Asthma	Exacerbation of AERD	No cross-reactivity in AERD
Allergic reactions	Hypersensitivity reactions	Celecoxib contraindicated in patients with sulfonamide allergies
Cardiovascular	Platelet dysfunction	Arterial thrombosis in high-risk patients with high-dose, long-acting, highly specific inhibitors (rofecoxib)
Central nervous system	Dizziness	
	Somnolence	
	Cognitive dysfunction	
	Aseptic meningitis	

Source: From Klippel, J.H., ed., *Primer on the Rheumatic Diseases*, 13th ed., Table 41-2. Springer, New York, 2008. With permission.

Abbreviations: AERD, aspirin-exacerbated respiratory disease; NSAIDs, nonsteroidal anti-inflammatory drugs; UGI, upper gastrointestinal tract.

ACETAMINOPHEN

Acetaminophen is often an effective analgesic in arthritis patients, especially in those with mild to moderate pain from OA. Acetaminophen is well tolerated and is generally safer than NSAIDs in the elderly, especially in those with cardiovascular disease, renal insufficiency, or a history of acid-peptic disorders.

Mechanism of Action

Acetaminophen produces analgesia through a combination of inhibition of prostaglandin synthesis in the central nervous system and peripheral blockade of pain impulse generation. Acetaminophen is antipyretic but not anti-inflammatory.

Administration

Acetaminophen is available in tablet, liquid, capsule, and rectal suppository forms. The adult dose is 325–1000 mg given every 4–6 h, not to exceed 4 g/day. Chronic use is best avoided in patients with hepatic impairment, who should not receive more than 2 g/day in any circumstance.

Adverse Effects

Adverse effects are uncommon with appropriate dosing. However, hepatotoxicity may occur at proper doses but typically only occurs in patients who consume excessive amounts of alcohol. Analgesic nephropathy may occur in the setting of chronic overdosing.

Monitoring and Patient Education

There are no firmly established guidelines for monitoring of chronic use. Periodic alcohol history and checking of transaminase enzymes would seem reasonable. Care should be taken to educate patients as to the presence of acetaminophen in various over-the-counter cold medicines and other types of prescription analgesics (e.g., Tylenol #3, Vicodin).

OPIOID ANALGESICS

The terms opiate and opioid refer to a group of analgesics that have the properties of morphine. There are naturally occurring opiates, synthetic opiates, and endogenous opioids. These drugs may be indicated for patients who have debilitating arthritic pain in the following circumstances: (1) contraindication to NSAIDs, acetaminophen, or adjuvant analgesics, and (2) failure to respond adequately to nonnarcotic analgesics.

The decision to prescribe opioids should be made in accordance with the patient's wishes, after thorough discussion and consideration of the potential risks of sedation, dependence, constipation, and drug–drug interactions. A graduated, pain intensity–driven approach to the pharmacotherapy of pain is illustrated in Figure 9.1.

Mechanism of Action

Opioids bind to and activate opioid receptors located in the brain, spinal cord, and peripheral sensory nerves. The activation of opioid receptors results in diverse physiological effects, which include analgesia as well as alterations in respiratory, cardiovascular, GI, and neuroendocrine functions. There are a large number of short- and long-acting opioid analgesics (Table 9.3).

Patients who have the most severe and consistent pain levels are best served by using one of the long-acting opioids, sometimes concomitantly with a short-acting opioid for breakthrough pain.

Administration

Except in the case of transdermal fentanyl, the oral route of administration is the preferred one for the outpatient management of arthritis pain. Typical starting doses are listed in Table 9.3, but these should be reduced by 25%–50% in the elderly.

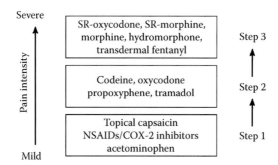

FIGURE 9.1 Stepwise approach to pharmacologic management of pain. Mild pain should be treated with topical capsaicin, acetaminophen, and NSAIDs or COX-2 inhibitors. Low-dose opioids for patients with arthritis who fail these Step 1 measures can be effective. High-dose opioids should be used cautiously as part of a multimodal approach to pain control. (From Klippel, J.H., ed., *Primer on the Rheumatic Diseases*, 13th ed., Figure 39-2. Springer, New York, 2008. With permission.)

TABLE 9.3
Opioid Analgesic Drugs

Drugs	Oral Equivalent (mg)	Starting Dose	Comment
Short acting			
Morphine sulfate (Roxanol)	30	15–30 mg every 4 h	For all, start low and titrate; begin bowel program early; most of these opioids are available in combination with aceta-minophen or aspirin (do not exceed maximum dose). For all, short-acting opioid often is needed for breakthrough pain
Codeine (Fiomal)	120	30–60 mg every 4–6 h	
Hydrocodone (Lortab)	30	5–10 mg every 3–4 h	
Oxycodone (percodan)	20–30	5–10 mg every 3–4 h	
Hydromorphone (Dilaudid)	7.5	1.5 mg every 3–4 h	
Propoxyphene (Darvon)	100	100 mg every 4 h	
Tramadol (Ultram)	120	50–100 mg every 6 h	
Methadone (Dolophine)	—	15–100 mg every 8 h	
Long acting			
SR-Morphine (MS Contin)	30	5–10 mg every 3–4 h	
SR-Oxycodone (Oxycontin)	20–30	10–20 mg every 3–4 h	
Transdermal fentanyl (Duragesic)	Not available	See package insert	

Source: From Klippel, J.H., ed., *Primer on the Rheumatic Diseases*, 13th ed., Table 39-1. Springer, New York, 2008. With permission.

Adverse Effects

Nausea and/or vomiting occur in up to half of patients upon initiation of opioid medicines, although these symptoms typically wane with continued use. Constipation is quite common, especially in the elderly. Sedation and cognitive impairment can be problematic, particularly with initiation and dose escalation. Respiratory depression is the most serious potential adverse effect of opiates, although this is very uncommon with appropriate dose titration. Tolerance commonly develops, both to the analgesic effects of opioids and with the exception of constipation, also to the adverse effects. Dose titration may be necessary over time, the pace of which should be guided by reported pain intensity. Physical dependence, which is different than tolerance, refers to anxiety and vasomotor and other symptoms that may occur when chronic opioid therapy is abruptly discontinued. The term addiction refers to the psychological dependence on the emotional and euphoric effects of opioids. The symptoms of addiction are manifested in aberrant behaviors like prescription forgery, stealing drugs, and the like. Addiction occurs in about 3%–5% of patients taking opiates for noncancer pain. The trend toward increasing medical use of opiates has not been accompanied by an increase in addiction rates.

Monitoring and Patient Education

All patients started on opiates should also be started on a bowel program of increased fiber and stool softeners. A mild stimulant laxative may also be necessary. Most patients eventually develop tolerance to nausea, but antiemetics or antihistamines may be needed initially. Likewise, tolerance usually develops to the soporific effects of opioids; however, it is important to discuss driving and fall precautions with patients, both with initiation of therapy and periodically thereafter. If a decision is made to stop chronic opioid therapy, this must be done with a gradual taper program to avoid or to minimize physical withdrawal symptoms.

DISEASE MODIFICATION IN ARTHRITIS

It has now been recognized that joint destruction from inflammation occurs early in the course of RA and related inflammatory arthritides. It has likewise been recognized that early therapy with DMARD medications can downregulate autoimmune inflammation effectively enough to retard joint destruction and deformity, thereby reducing disability and functional limitation. Such DMARD therapy should be offered to all patients with an established diagnosis of RA. Those patients with more severe disease or with poor prognostic indicators should be treated the most aggressively. A discussion of the currently used DMARDs follows (Saag et al., 2008).

METHOTREXATE

Methotrexate is the mainstay of therapy in RA. It has been used successfully since the 1950s and is usually the "background therapy" in trials of new drugs. It is also frequently used in combination with other DMARDs.

Mechanism of Action

Methotrexate is a folate antimetabolite. It inhibits DNA synthesis by irreversibly binding to dihydrofolate reductase and blocking the enzyme thymidylate synthetase, which results in decreased purine and thymidylic acid synthesis.

Administration

Methotrexate can be given via oral, intramuscular, and subcutaneous routes. It comes in 2.5-mg pills or 25-mg/mL vials. Doses of methotrexate for RA typically start at 7.5–12.5 mg, given on a single day per week, and range up to 25 mg weekly. Slightly higher doses can be given parenterally.

All patients taking methotrexate should also be given folic acid, 1 mg daily. This is thought to prevent hematologic and other side effects.

Adverse Effects

Common adverse effects include nausea and fatigue on the day of methotrexate administration; these generally subside after a few weeks of repeated dosing. Other side effects include oral mucosal ulcers and alopecia; these can occasionally be prevented with the use of folic acid, 1 mg daily.

Rare but serious toxicities include hepatotoxicity, myelosuppression, and pulmonary toxicity. Hepatotoxicity can occur through direct damage to hepatocytes or by augmenting the effects of alcohol use or viral hepatitis. Myelosuppression, including mild anemia with macrocytosis, is common, but pancytopenia can also occur. Hypersensitivity pneumonitis is the most frequent pulmonary complication associated with methotrexate. Patients most frequently present subacutely with complaints of dyspnea, nonproductive cough, and fever within the first year of therapy. Less than 10% of these patients continue on to develop pulmonary fibrosis.

Monitoring and Patient Education

Baseline testing should include CBC, liver and renal function tests, viral hepatitis serologies, and chest x-ray. Patients taking methotrexate should be monitored with CBC, transaminases (alanine aminotransferase and aspartate aminotransferase), albumin, and creatinine every 8–12 weeks. In addition, they should be counseled to drink no more than one serving of alcohol per week. All women of childbearing age should be on a reliable form of contraception because methotrexate is a known teratogen. Women contemplating pregnancy should be informed that they should have a 3- to 6-month "washout period" before conception.

LEFLUNOMIDE

Leflunomide is a newer disease-modifying agent. It can be used instead of methotrexate as a background drug in cases of methotrexate intolerance. It is used independently or in combination with other DMARDs.

Mechanism of Action

Leflunomide is also an antimetabolite. It is converted to teriflunomide, which inhibits pyrimidine synthesis, and results in antiproliferative and anti-inflammatory effects.

Administration

Leflunomide is given orally at a dose of 20 mg daily. If adverse effects occur, the dose can be reduced to 10 mg daily.

Adverse Effects

Common adverse effects include headache, diarrhea, or nausea. GI side effects can sometimes be abated by reducing the dose to 10 mg daily. Elevated liver enzymes occur in 10%–20% of cases. Leflunomide has also been associated with a new-onset hypertension (especially among patients taking NSAIDs) and a reversible peripheral neuropathy.

Monitoring and Patient Education

Baseline studies should include CBC, liver function tests, and blood pressure measurement. These should be monitored every 8–12 weeks. Women of childbearing age should not be prescribed leflunomide because it is teratogenic and has a very large volume of distribution (and thus has a very long washout period). Women who have ever been exposed to leflunomide who become pregnant should be given cholestyramine to accelerate elimination of the drug. Patients taking warfarin should be informed that leflunomide can increase the PTT (partial thromboplastin time).

SULFASALAZINE

Sulfasalazine is a second-line disease-modifying agent and considered less potent than methotrexate or leflunomide. It is frequently used in patients with contraindications to other drugs or in combination with other drugs. Although it has been known to be effective in RA since the 1940s, it became widely used only in the 1970s.

Mechanism of Action

The majority of ingested sulfasalazine enters in the colon unaltered. In the large intestine, the bacterial enzyme azoreductase cleaves the molecule in two: sulfapyridine is the active metabolite, and 5-aminosalicylic acid remains in the colon and is excreted. Coliform bacteria are required for the absorption of sulfapyridine. The mechanism of action of sulfapyridine in RA has not been fully elucidated.

Administration

Sulfasalazine is given orally on a daily basis. Starting doses are usually in the 500- to 1000-mg range. Patients can be titrated by 500 mg weekly up to a maximum of 3000 mg/day in three divided doses.

Adverse Effects

Common adverse effects include nausea, diarrhea, GI distress, and headaches. These can usually be avoided at lower doses or with slow titration from lower to higher doses.

Rare but serious toxicities include megaloblastic anemia, a hypersensitivity reaction that can consist of rash, fever, and elevated liver enzymes, and agranulocytosis. Agranulocytosis is idiopathic, usually observed in the first few months of therapy, and takes 1–2 weeks to resolve after the drug is discontinued.

Monitoring and Patient Education

Because of the risk of agranulocytosis, a CBC should be drawn within 2 weeks after drug initiation and monthly thereafter for 3 months. Subsequently, patients should be monitored every 12 weeks with a CBC and liver transaminases. Patients with a known sulfa allergy or colectomy should avoid sulfasalazine. Sulfasalazine can be used safely in pregnancy.

HYDROXYCHLOROQUINE

Hydroxychloroquine (and chloroquine) is an antimalarial medication also used as second-line agent in the treatment of RA. Like sulfasalazine, hydroxychloroquine is less potent than methotrexate or leflunomide and is often used in combination with other DMARDs.

Mechanism of Action

Hydroxychloroquine reduces lysosomal degradation of hemoglobin, inhibits locomotion of neutrophils and chemotaxis of eosinophils, and impairs complement-dependent antigen–antibody reactions, likely by increasing the pH of lysosomal compartments. A more precise mechanism has not been elucidated.

Administration

Hydroxychloroquine is given orally, usually at a dose of 400 mg daily. Doses should not exceed 6.5 mg/kg, so patients weighting less than 136 lb. should be given 200 or 300 mg daily.

Adverse Effects

Hydroxychloroquine is very safe. Common side effects include headache, rash, and nausea. Within the first 1–2 weeks of therapy, patients can develop difficulty focusing; this is temporary and resolves after 1–2 weeks. Patients receiving long-term therapy can develop a hyperpigmentation, especially on the lower legs.

Rare but serious complications include myopathy and arrhythmias. Retinopathy is extremely rare and tends to occur with long-term use of doses of greater than 6.5 mg/kg in patients with renal failure.

Monitoring and Patient Education

Baseline studies should include CBC, creatinine, liver transaminases, and ophthalmologic examination. These studies should be repeated yearly, although the ophthalmologic examination can be done every 2 years in low-risk (i.e., young, normal renal function) patients. Patients should be counseled that hydroxychloroquine has a large volume of distribution and the onset of its effects can be very slow. Hydroxychloroquine can be used safely in pregnancy.

OTHER NONBIOLOGIC DMARDS

Other nonbiologic DMARDs for RA are less effective or more toxic than those described above. Therefore, they are used rarely in patients with multiple contraindications to more popular drugs. They are listed in Table 9.4.

UPDATE ON DRUG DEVELOPMENT: A NEW GENERATION OF DISEASE-MODIFYING AGENTS

In the late 1990s, biologic DMARDs were developed for the treatment of RA. These drugs are potent anti-inflammatories and generally used in combination with methotrexate. The first class of biologics was the anti–tumor necrosis factor (anti-TNF) antibodies; these are reviewed in detail elsewhere in this text. Since then, a second generation of biologics has been developed (Table 9.5). Some of these continue to target TNF, but others affect other molecules involved in inflammation, including various cytokines, chemokines, and intracellular signal-transduction enzymes. The mechanisms of action involved in these new therapies are described in Figures 9.2 and 9.3.

TABLE 9.4
Disease-Modifying Agents Used in the Treatment of RA

First Line	Second Line	Rarely Used
Methotrexate	Sulfasalazine	Azathioprine
Leflunomide	Hydroxychloroquine	Cyclosporine
	Biologic agents	Tetracyclines
		Cyclophosphamide
		Gold
		Penicillamine
		Staphylococcal protein A

TABLE 9.5
Biologic Disease-Modifying Agents as of 2009

	Available	In Development
TNF-α inhibitors	Infliximab	
	Etanercept	
	Adalimumab	
	Certolizumab pegol	
	Golimumab	
IL-1 inhibitors	Anakinra	
Selective costimulatory inhibitors	Abatacept	
B-cell depletion therapy	Rituximab	Ofatumumab
		Ocrelizumab
IL-6 inhibitors	Tocilizumab	
Cellular kinase inhibitors		Jak kinase inhibitor
		Syk kinase inhibitor
		Apremalast
IL-17 inhibitors		AIN-457
		LY2439821
Anti-BAFF treatments		Atacicept
		LY2127399

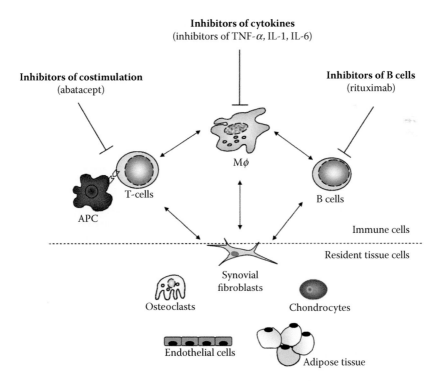

FIGURE 9.2 Regulation of proinflammatory cytokines and immune cells within a joint by currently available biological therapies for RA. Cytokine inhibitors such as TNF-α inhibitors and IL-1 and IL-6 inhibitors have pleiotropic effects. Costimulation inhibitors such as abatacept reduce T-cell activation. B-cell therapies such as rituximab reduce B-cell activation. (From Šenolt, L., et al., *Autoimmun. Rev.*, doi:10.1016/jautrev.2009.03.010, 2009. With permission.)

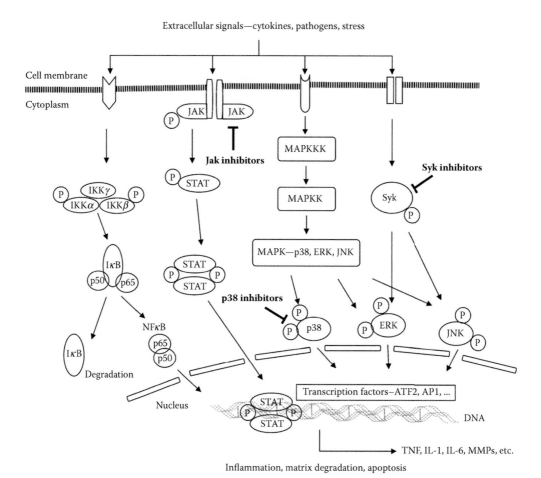

FIGURE 9.3   Schematic drawing of signal transduction pathways and transcription factors, and their potential modulation by drugs currently being developed for the treatment of RA. Upon exposure of a cell to a proinflammatory environment, cytokines or pathogens, several regulatory enzymes are phosphorylated and activated. As a result, an intracellular signaling cascade is activated to transmit the signal from a receptor via MAP and tyrosine kinases to transcription factors, which affect the expression of genes for cytokines, matrix metalloproteinases, apoptosis-regulating molecules, and proliferation. Inhibitors of Syk kinase and Jak3 have been most successful in clinical trials in patients with RA so far. AP1, activator protein 1; ATF2, activating transcription factor 2; ERK, extracellular signal-regulated kinases; IKK, inhibitor IκB; IL, interleukin; JAK, Janus tyrosine kinase; JNK, c-Jun N-terminal kinase; MAPK, mitogen-activated protein kinase; MAPKK, MAPK kinase; MAPKKK, MAPKK kinase; MMPs, matrix metalloproteinases; NF-κB, nuclear factor-κB; STAT, signal transducer and activator of transcription; Syk, spleen tyrosine kinase; TNF, tumor necrosis factor. (From Šenolt, L., et al., *Autoimmun. Rev.*, doi: 10.1016/jautrev.2009.03.010, 2009. With permission.)

REFERENCES

Bajwa ZH, Warfield CA, Wootton RJ. Overview of the treatment of chronic pain. Up to Date. August 2008.

Klippel JH, ed. Primer on the Rheumatic Diseases. 13th ed. New York: Springer; 2008.

Nicholson B. Responsible prescribing of opioids for the management of chronic pain. Drugs 2003;63(1):17–32.

Recommendations for the Medical Management of Osteoarthritis of the Hip and Knee: 2000 Update. American College of Rheumatology Subcommittee on Osteoarthritis Guidelines. Arthritis Rheum 2000;43:1905.

Rostom A, Dube C, Wells G, Tugwell P, Welch V, Jolicoeur E, McGowan J. Prevention of NSAID-induced gastroduodenal ulcers. Cochrane Database Syst Rev 2002;(4):CD002296.

Saag KG, Teng GG, Patkar NM, Anuntiyo J, Finney C, Curtis JR, Paulus HE, et al. American College of Rheumatology 2008 recommendations for the use of nonbiologic and biologic disease-modifying anti-rheumatic drugs in rheumatoid arthritis. Arthritis Care and Research 2008;59(6):762–784.

Singh G, Ramey DR, Morfeld D, Shi H, Hatoum HT, Fries JF. Gastrointestinal tract complications of nonsteroidal anti-inflammatory drug treatment in rheumatoid arthritis: a prospective observational cohort study. Arch Intern Med 1996;156:1530–1536.

Senolt L, Vencovský J, Pavelka K, Ospelt C, Gay S. Prospective new biological therapies for rheumatoid arthritis. Autoimmun Rev 2009. doi:10.1016/jautrev.2009.03.010.

10 Nonsteroidal Anti-Inflammatory Drugs

Anand Lal and Seeta Sharma

CONTENTS

INTRODUCTION

Nonsteroidal anti-inflammatory drugs (NSAIDs) are one of the most commonly prescribed medicines worldwide. In the United States, it is estimated that more than 70 million prescriptions and more than 30 billion over-the-counter tablets of these drugs are sold annually [1]. At lower over-the-counter doses, these drugs are used to treat pain. When given at higher doses, these medicines may also be helpful in reducing inflammation.

HISTORY

Salicylic acid, from the willow bark, had been used to treat inflammation for centuries. Aspirin, the first anti-inflammatory drug, was synthesized more than 100 years ago. The U.S. patent for aspirin was granted to Hoffman of Bayer on August 1, 1898 [2]. Over the next century, several compounds were formulated that share the ability of aspirin to block prostaglandin—these drugs are collectively called NSAIDs.

MECHANISM OF ACTION

Traditionally, NSAIDs have been thought to work by inhibiting the synthesis of prostaglandins, although they may also work by other mechanisms including inhibition of leukotriene synthesis, superoxide scavenging, and control of cytokine production [3].

Prostaglandins are synthesized by cyclooxygenase (COX) enzymes. There are two groups of COX enzymes—COX-1 is a constitutive enzyme and appears to function as a "housekeeping enzyme" in most tissue including the gastric mucosa, the kidneys, and the platelets, whereas COX-2 is induced by inflammatory mediators like interleukin-1 and tumor necrosis factor-alpha. NSAIDs work by blocking COX.

There was considerable excitement in the 1990s that drugs like celecoxib and rofecoxib, which selectively inhibited COX-2, would provide the benefits of NSAIDs without causing gastrointestinal (GI) ulceration or platelet dysfunction. This enthusiasm has been tempered now that there are concerns that the COX-2 inhibitors may be associated with increased cardiac mortality. Rofecoxib and valdecoxib, both COX-2 inhibitors, have been withdrawn from the United States due to these concerns.

PHARMACOLOGY

Most NSAIDs are well absorbed after oral ingestion [3]. Once absorbed, they are >95% bound to plasma proteins, and the amount of free drug is relatively low. This fact has important implications in that the toxicity of NSAIDs may be higher in states where the concentration of albumin is low as in the malnourished and the elderly.

NSAIDs are usually cleared by the liver—the products of the metabolism of NSAIDs are excreted by the kidney and the liver.

Because NSAIDs are metabolized by the hepatic P-450 system, there is a risk of drug interaction with other agents that are metabolized by this system.

CLASSIFICATION OF NSAIDs

There are a number of classes of NSAIDs. Some of the important classes are as follows:

(1) The carboxylic acid groups includes salicylic acid and esters (aspirin and diflunisal), phenylacetic acid (diclofenac), and carbo- and heterocyclic acids (etodolac, indomethacin, sulindac).
(2) The propionic acid group includes naproxen, ibuprofen, and ketoprofen.
(3) The enolic acid group includes meloxicam and piroxicam.
(4) Nabumetone is a nonacidic NSAID.
(5) Celecoxib belongs to the sulfonamide group.
(6) Nonacetylated salicylates include salsalate and choline magnesium trisalicylate.

Although the NSAIDs are all part of one group of medications and there appears to be no difference in their efficacy in large studies, there is considerable individual variability in the response to NSAIDs. Although some patients may respond to drug A, other patients with the same medical indication may not respond to drug A but to drug B. The reason for this discrepancy is not clear.

INDICATIONS FOR THE USE OF NSAIDs

Until the advent of disease-modifying antirheumatic drugs (DMARDs) in rheumatoid arthritis, aspirin and NSAIDs were the primary drugs used to treat this condition. Now DMARDs are the primary drugs used in treatment of inflammatory diseases, although NSAIDs still have an important role in the treatment of pain, especially in the early stages of the disease when the DMARDs have not yet started working.

NSAIDs are also commonly used for treatment of pain and inflammation in diseases like psoriatic arthritis, reactive arthritis, and ankylosing spondylitis. In fact, response to NSAIDs is thought by some to be suggestive of the diagnosis of a spondyloarthropathy. There are also some data to suggest that this group of drugs may prevent joint damage in patients with spondyloarthropathies [4].

In osteoarthritis, these drugs are generally felt to be more efficacious than acetaminophen, although the latter is often used as the first line agent because of its lower toxicity on the GI tract and kidneys.

NSAIDs are also being studied for the prevention of colon cancer. Initially, it was thought that this protective effect was due to patients on NSAIDs developing GI bleeding and therefore more endoscopies leading to increased surveillance for cancer and therefore earlier detection and removal of colonic polyps. However, the expression of COX-2 messenger RNA is enhanced in human colorectal adenomas and adenocarcinomas, and NSAIDs may work by inhibiting COX-2 messenger RNA expression.

There is also interest in the effect of NSAIDs in preventing Alzheimer's disease. There is a wealth of data indicating that aspirin is cardioprotective. Although its role in the secondary protection of coronary artery disease is well established, its role in the primary prevention of coronary artery disease is less clear. Some physicians encourage aspirin use in patients who have strong risk factors for coronary artery disease (like diabetes mellitus) because the risk/benefit of aspirin in these situations appears to be clearly in favor of taking aspirin. There is no evidence that NSAIDs provide cardioprotection. In fact, there appears to be growing evidence that NSAIDs like rofecoxib may actually increase the risk of coronary artery disease.

DRUG INTERACTIONS

NSAIDs are widely considered to reduce the effectiveness of antihypertensive medications. There is a higher risk of renal toxicity if NSAIDs are used with diuretics and angiotensin-converting enzyme inhibitors. Because of their risk of causing ulcers, they should be avoided in patients taking warfarin and steroids.

ADVERSE EFFECTS

NSAIDs are associated with many adverse effects. Severity of side effects may vary with the dose and durations of NSAID use. The benefits of NSAIDs need to be carefully weighed against risk of toxicity. NSAIDs affect multiple systems including GI, renal, hepatic, cardiovascular (CV), central nervous, hematologic, and dermatologic systems.

GROUPS AT INCREASED RISK FOR ADVERSE EFFECTS

The toxicity of NSAIDs appears to be higher in older individuals. There is also an aspirin toxicity syndrome where patients develop asthma and nasal polyps on exposure to aspirin. NSAIDs may increase the risk of gastrochisis and premature closure of ductus arteriosus if used in pregnancy [5].

GI SYSTEM

GI toxicity is common with NSAIDs and sometimes requires stopping the NSAIDs [6]. The most common adverse effects are heartburn, nausea, abdominal pain, diarrhea, ulceration, and bleeding.

In upper endoscopy surveys, 35%–60% of patients on NSAIDs have gastric erosions or submucosal hemorrhage. Older age, female gender and patients with ulcer disease are at higher risk [7]. Other risk factors include use of more than one NSAID, concomitant use of steroids, blood group O, and cigarette smoking [8]. In clinical studies, it has been reported that there is a three- to four-fold increase in severe GI side effects in subjects who use NSAID [9–11]. Prostaglandins E1and E2 are important for gastro-protection [12]. Carson et al. [13] did not find any significant difference between phenylbutazone, tolmetin, ibuprofen, indomethacin, fenoprofen, naproxen, and sulindac. However, Griffin et al. [14] found that users of naproxen, piroxicam, tolmetin, and meclofenamate had greater risk of hemorrhage and ulcer than users of ibuprofen. Laporte et al. [15] conducted a case–control study of 875 cases and 2687 controls and showed that the highest odds ratio for GI tract bleeding was with piroxicam (19.1), followed by diclofenac (7.9), naproxen (6.5), and indomethacin (4.9). Another epidemiological study was conducted in rheumatoid arthritis patients who received 11 different NSAIDs. Symptoms and laboratory abnormalities were evaluated in 2747 patients [16]. Indomethacin, tolmetin, and meclofenamate had more toxic affect compared with aspirin, nonacetylated salicylates, and ibuprofen. In patients with osteoarthritis, oxaproxin had similar GI adverse effects when compared with piroxicam [17].

Newer NSAIDs like etodolac, enteric-coated diclofenac, enteric-coated aspirin, and nabumetone have lesser side effects [18–26]. Enteric-coated aspirin causes less gastric mucosal damage but still causes erosion [18] and bleeding because it decreases the platelet functions and the prostaglandin levels. In a small study ($n = 55$) of patients with rheumatoid arthritis, salsalate had similar efficacy as naproxen but caused lesions in only seven patients [19]. Another study done by Cryer et al. [20] found that salsalate causes minimal mucosal injury in stomach and duodenum compared with aspirin ($p < 0.001$).

One report suggests that 600–1000 mg of etodolac does not cause bleeding compared with piroxicam [21]. Lanza and Arnold [22] conducted a study where risk of short-term bleeding with etodolac was similar to placebo but lower than aspirin, naproxen, ibuprofen, or indomethacin. Endoscopic score of etodolac was similar to placebo and lower than aspirin, naproxen, ibuprofen, and indomethacin in a double-blind controlled study. Studies has also shown that the risk of bleeding with diclofenac and enteric-coated NSAIDs are similar to placebo [22].

Nabumetone has less gastrointestinal adverse effect because it's inactive form is absorbed as a base and therefore does not cause irritation to the gastric mucosa. Roth et al have observed that the frequency of endoscopically detected ulcers with nabumetone was 2%, whereas in the ibuprofen group, the frequency of endoscopically detected ulcers was 14%, which is similar to the incidence found in a number of other endoscopy studies of patients receiving NSAIDs [25].

Serious complications can arise without any prior history of symptoms because of the analgesic effects of these compounds masking ulcer-type symptoms. A study by Lanza et al. [27] found that prostaglandin E_1, misoprostol, cimetidine, and H_2 receptor were better than placebo at protecting gastric mucosa. This 2-week study may not be reliable because patients may have different levels of gastric adaptation, and some of the side effects are not apparent in the first 2 weeks.

RENAL SYSTEM

Prostaglandins have a role in maintaining renal functions in normal healthy individuals but NSAIDs do not impair glomerular infiltration rates in healthy individuals [28]. Renal prostaglandins E_2 and I_2 maintain renal blood flow, regulate water excretion and electrolyte balance, and stimulate rennin secretion [29]. Peripheral edema has been reported with the usage of phenylbutazone and indomethacin. Some NSAIDs may have fewer renal side effects. Sulindac may have renal "sparing" properties because of its inactive sulfone metabolite [30, 31]. Renal functions should be closely monitored in patients with preexisting renal abnormality. Analgesic nephropathy is caused by prolonged use of other NSAIDs such as aspirin and phenacetin [32, 33]. It is advisable to carefully monitor patients in long-term NSAIDs therapy because one study has shown that up to 25% of end-stage renal disease is due to analgesic nephropathy [34].

CV Risks

Farkouh and Greenberg [35] recently analyzed the CV risks of NSAIDs after their exhaustive review of scientific data [35]. According to their review, five key variables appear to determine the CV toxicity of NSAIDs:

1. COX-2 selectivity—higher COX-2 selectivity was associated with greater CV toxicity;
2. Dose responsivity—toxicity of drugs like rofecoxib appeared to be more with increase in dosage;
3. Plasma half-life—long plasma half-life of drugs like rofecoxib and celecoxib may increase CV toxicity;
4. Effect on blood pressure—rofecoxib appeared to increase blood pressure, and this may have accounted for some of its toxicity; and
5. Interaction with aspirin—NSAIDs like ibuprofen, if given along with aspirin, appeared to antagonize the irreversible platelet inhibition induced by aspirin.

Naproxen appears to have lower risk of CV toxicity than nonselective NSAIDs and COX-2-specific agents. Ibuprofen appears to have a slightly higher risk than placebo and comparable with the CV risk of COX-2-selective agents and nonselective NSAIDs. Diclofenac appears to have the highest risk among the nonselective NSAIDs and a risk comparable with celecoxib.

Central Nervous System

Many adverse reactions related to the central nervous system have been reported with NSAIDs. Headache is reported by up to 10% of patients on indomethacin [36]. Dizziness, drowsiness, light-headedness, confusion, and psychosis have also been reported with NSAIDs. These adverse events usually reverse when NSAIDs are stopped. Rare episodes of aseptic meningitis have been reported with NSAIDs. These patients complained of headache, fever, and nuchal rigidity. Cerebrospinal fluid cultures in these patients were abnormal, and these patients recovered when the NSAIDs were stopped [37].

Hematologic System

NSAIDs have been rarely associated with aplastic anemia, agranulocytosis, and related blood dyscrasias. NSAIDs also affect platelet function and can predispose to bleeding in patients.

Hepatic System

Risk factors for liver damage include advanced age, prolonged therapy, large dose, viral infection, and renal function impairment. Diclofenac, piroxicam, phenylbutazone, and sulindac may be more toxic. Liver function tests should be monitored periodically in patients on chronic NSAIDs.

Dermatologic System

NSAIDs like tolmetin, sulindac, meclofenamate sodium, naproxen, and piroxicam have been associated with urticaria, exanthema, pruritus, and photosensitivity [38].

Summary of Strategies to Reduce the Toxicity of NSAIDs

In general, NSAIDs should be used for the least amount of time in the lowest possible dose. They should be avoided in the elderly. Unfortunately, this is not always a viable option. Some of the strategies to reduce the GI toxicity of NSAIDs are using these drugs with misoprostol or a proton pump inhibitor. Some NSAIDs like etodolac and nabumetone may have lower GI toxicity.

In some situations, for example in the case of a patient who has an acute flare of gout who also has renal insufficiency, it may be prudent to use a corticosteroid that does not affect the kidney.

CONCLUSIONS

In summary, NSAIDs are one of the most commonly prescribed drugs. If used appropriately, they are very effective in treating pain and inflammation. However, like any other medicine, they have potential for considerable toxicity, and in each case, risk/benefit of therapy and alternatives to the use of NSAIDs should be carefully evaluated before prescribing these agents.

REFERENCES

1. Wolfe MM, Lichtenstein DR, Singh G. Gastrointestinal toxicity of nonsteroidal anti-inflammatory agents. NEJM 1999;340(24):1888–1899.
2. Schadewaldt H. Historical aspect of pharmacologic research at Bayer 1890–1990. Stroke 1990; 21(Suppl):IV-5–IV-8.
3. Hochberg MC, Silman AJ, Smolen J. Non-steroidal anti-inflammatory drugs in rheumatology. 3rd ed. Elsevier; 2003.
4. Wanders A, van der Heidje D, Landewe R, et al. Nonsteroidal anti-inflammatory drugs reduce radiographic progression in patients with ankylosing spondylitis—a randomized clinical trial. Arthritis Rheum 2005;52:1756–1765.
5. James AH, Brancazio LR, Price T. Aspirin and reproductive outcomes. Obstet Gynecol Surv 2008;63(1):49–57.
6. Ehsanullah RSB, Page MC, Tildesley G, Wood JR. Prevention of gastroduodenal damage induced by nonsteroidal anti-inflammatory drugs: controlled trial of ranitidine. BMJ 1988;297:1017–1021.
7. Simon LS. Toxicity of NSAIDs. Curr Opin Rheumatol 1990;2:481–488.
8. McCarthy DM. Misoprostol. Drug Ther 1989;19:59–69.
9. Henry DA. Side effects of NSAIDs. Baillieres Clin Rheumatol 1988;2:425–454.
10. Summerville K, Faulkner G, Langman M. NSAIDs and bleeding peptic ulcer. Lancet 1986;1:4624.
11. Fries JF, Miller SR, Spitz PA, Williams CA, Hubert HB, Bloch DA. Identification of patients at risk for gastropathy associated with NSAID use. J Rheumatol 1990;17(Suppl 20):12–19.
12. Paulus HE. Nonsteroidal anti-inflammatory drugs: major side effects. J Musculoskel Med 1991;8 (Suppl 4):S29-S33.
13. Carson JL, Strom BL, Soper KA, West SL, Morse ML. The association of non steroidal antiinflammatory drugs with upper gastrointestinal bleeding. Arch Intren Med 1987;147;85–88.
14. Griffin MR, Piper JM, Daugherty JR, Snowden M, Ray WA. Nonsteroidal anti-inflammatory drug use and increased risk for peptic ulcer disease in elderly persons. Ann Intern Med 1991;114:256–263.
15. Laporte JR, Carne X, Vidal X, Moreno V, Juan J. Upper GI bleeding in relation to previous use of analgesics and nonsteroidal anti-inflammatory drugs: Catalan countries study of upper GI bleeding. Lancet 1991;337(8733):8785–8789.
16. Fries JF, Williams CA, Block DA. The relative toxicity of nonsteroidal anti-inflammatory drugs. Arthritis Rheum 1991;34:1353–1360.
17. Osborn TG. Oxaprozin compared with piroxicam for osteoarthritis. J Musculoskel Med 1993;10 (Suppl 3):S33-S37.
18. Hawthorne AB, Mahida YR, Cole AT, Hawkey CJ. Aspirin-induced gastric mucosal damage: prevention by enteric-coating and relation to prostaglandin synthesis. Br J Clin Pharmacol 1991;32:77–83.
19. Roth S, Bennett R, Caldron P, et al. Reduced risk of NSAID gastropathy with nonacetylate salicylate (salsalate): an endoscopic study. Semin Arthritis Rheum 1990:19(Suppl 2):11–19.
20. Cryer B, Goldschmiedt M, Redfern JS, Feldman M. Comparison of salsalate and aspirin on mucosal injury and gastroduodenal mucosal prostaglandins. Gastroenterology 1990;99:1616–1621.
21. Arnold JD. Assessing gastrointestinal safety of anti-inflammatory drugs. J Musculoskel Med 1991; 8(Suppl 4):S54–S59.
22. Lanza FL, Arnold JD. Etodolac, a new nonsteroidal anti-inflammatory drug: gastrointestinal microbleeding and endoscopic studies. Clin Rheumatol 1989;8(Suppl 1):5–15.
23. Sanda M, Jacob G, Stand DB. A study profile of etodolac in arthritis; clinical experience based on 600 patients-year. Today's Ther Trends 1985;3:1–15.

24. Roth SH. Nabumetone: a new NSAID for rheumatoid arthritis and osteo-arthritis. Orthop Rev 1992;21:223–227.

25. Roth SH, Tindall EA, Jain AK, McMahon FG, April PA, Bockow BI, Cohen SB, Fleischmann RM. A controlled study comparing the effects of nabumetone, ibuprofen, and ibuprofen plus misoprostol on the upper gastrointestinal tract mucosa. Arch Intern Med 1993;153(22):2565–2571.

26. Jenner PN. A post-marketing surveillance of nabumetone. Drugs 1990;40(Suppl 5):80–86.

27. Lanza FL, Aspinall RL, Swabb EA, Davis RE, Rack MF, Rubin A. Double-blind placebo-controlled endoscopic comparison of the mucosal protective effects of misoprostol versus cimetidine for tolmetin induced mucosal injury to the stomach and duodenum. Gastroenterology 1988;995:289–294.

28. Haylor J. Prostaglandin synthesis and renal function in man. J Physiol 1980;298:382–396.

29. Hochherg MC. NSAIDs: patterns of uses and side effects. Hosp Pract (Off Ed) 1989;24:167–174.

30. Berg KJ, Talseth T. Acute renal effects of sulindac and indomethacin in chronic renal failure. Clin Pharmacol Ther 1985;37:447–452.

31. Bunning RD, Barth WF. Sulindac: a potentially renal-sparing nonsteroidal anti-inflammatory drug. JAMA 1982;248:2864–2867.

32. Prescott LF. Analgesic nephropathy: a reassessment of the role of phenacetin and other analgesics. Drugs 1982;23:75–149.

33. Shelley JH. Pharmacologic mechanisms of analgesic nephropathy. Kidney Int 1978;13:15–26.

34. Nanna RS, Stuart-Taylor J, DeLeon AM, White KH. Analgesic nephropathy: etiology, clinical syndrome and clinicopathologic correlations in Australia. Kidney Int 1978;13:79–92.

35 Farkouh ME, Greenberg BP. An evidence-based review of the cardiovascular risks of nonsteroidal anti-inflammatory drugs. Am J Cardiol 2009;103:1227–1237.

36. Henry D. Assessing the benefits and risks of drugs: the example of NSAIDs. Aust Fam Physician 1990;19:378–387.

37. American Medical Association. AMA's Drug Evaluations. Chicago, IL: American Medical Association 1990;5:1–42.

38. The International Agranulocytosis and Aplastic Anemia Study. Risks of agranulocytosis and aplastic anemia: a first report of their relation to drug use with special reference to analgesics. JAMA 1986;256:1749–1757.

11 Biologics
Target-Specific Treatment of Systemic and Cutaneous Autoimmune Diseases

Siba P. Raychaudhuri and Smriti K. Raychaudhuri

CONTENTS

INTRODUCTION

In this chapter, we will present an overview of biological agents used in the management autoimmune and inflammatory diseases. The Food and Drug Administration (FDA) considers a biologic to be any therapeutic serum, toxin, antitoxin, vaccine, virus, blood, blood component or derivative, allergenic product or analogous product, or derivatives applicable to the prevention, treatment, or cure of injuries or disease of man. Biologics are designed to "target" specific components of the immune system. The goal is to weaken or immobilize those features of the immune system that are triggering autoimmune diseases without the adverse side effects that can come from broadly weakening the immune system [1, 2]. As the new drugs are capable of targeting disease-causing proteins in a more specific fashion while also carrying lower risks of adverse side effects, they have considerable advantages over traditional treatments. Biologics are having a major impact on the treatment of these diseases for which there has been significant unmet need for decades. Most of these agents are expensive, as is the laboratory monitoring for side effects that may be required. Cost-effectiveness may be a consideration in choosing to use a biological agent and in picking among the available agents.

ANTICYTOKINE THERAPY

Cytokines encompasses a large and diverse family of proteins that are produced by variety of cells. Cytokines are used extensively by cells of immune system for cellular communication and act as intercellular mediators in the generation and control of immune and inflammatory response. Cytokines play a pivotal role in the pathogenesis of inflammatory diseases. In an inflammatory disease, several proinflammatory cytokines (such as tumor necrosis factor α [TNF-α], interleukin [IL]-1, IL-6, IL-8, IL-12, and IL-17) are counterbalanced by anti-inflammatory cytokines (such as IL-4, IL-10, IL-11, and IL-13).

T cells are often described as a specific subpopulation according to their nature or expression of certain specific kinds of cytokines such as Th1, Th2, and Th17. The concept that specific types of immune responses are dominated exclusively by Th1 or Th2 profiles is now recognized as too simplistic to explain any rheumatic disease entirely. However, many biological therapies have been developed for the purpose of targeting either the downregulation of proinflammatory Th1 responses or the upregulation of anti-inflammatory Th2 cytokine production. Thus, the Th1/Th2 paradigm is discussed briefly in the next paragraph.

Th1 cells—Th1 lymphocytes participate in a broad variety of inflammatory responses, including cell-mediated inflammation in rheumatoid arthritis (RA), psoriasis, psoriatic arthritis (PsA), acute allograft rejection, graft-versus-host disease, and others. The list of proinflammatory mediators produced by Th1 cells includes but is not limited to the following [3]:

- IL-2
- Interferon gamma
- TNF
- IL-12
- IL-15
- IL-18

Th2 cells—Th2 lymphocytes stimulate antibody production by B cells and augment eosinophil responses. The activation of Th2 cells contributes to the development of chronic graft-versus-host disease, systemic lupus erythematosus, and systemic sclerosis. The list of mediators produced by Th2 cells includes but is not limited to the following [3]:

- IL-4
- IL-5
- IL-9
- IL-10
- IL-13

Genetic, immunologic, and environmental factors contribute to the pathogenesis of autoimmune disease. HLA phenotypes, cell trafficking mechanisms, nature of T-cell phenotypes, cytokine profiles, and angiogenesis act in an integrated way in various autoimmune diseases. At the disease site, the cytokine networks play a determining role in the outcome of the pathological features of autoimmune diseases. As cytokines and their receptors are expressed outside the cell, they can be targeted by protein-based biologics like monoclonal antibodies and soluble receptor immunoglobulin (Ig) fusion proteins and have become targets for drug development. In general, therapies designed to upregulate or augment the function of Th2 cytokines have been less successful in clinical trials than have interventions that target Th1 cytokine inhibition. To downregulate or to inhibit the effector functions of cytokines *in vivo*, three general approaches have been used: (1) soluble receptor antagonists, (2) monoclonal antibodies to cytokines or their receptors, and (3) cell surface receptor antagonist proteins.

TNF-α, A UNIQUE TARGET MOLECULE FOR THE TREATMENT OF INFLAMMATORY DISEASES

Monocyte/macrophage and cells derived from their lineage are the primary resource of TNF (cachexin or cachectin). However various other cells including activated T cells can secrete adequate amount of TNF. TNF is a cytokine involved in systemic inflammation and is a member of a group of cytokines that all stimulate the acute phase reaction. TNF is synthesized initially as a transmembrane precursor protein. The cytoplasmic tail of this protein is then cleaved to release soluble TNF. TNF's primary role is in the regulation of immune cells. TNF is able to induce apoptotic cell death and inflammation and inhibits tumorigenesis and viral replication. The biological activity of TNF requires the aggregation of three TNF monomers to form trimeric TNF, which then acts by binding to one of two types of receptors: TNF-R1 or TNF-R2 [4]. TNF-R1 and TNF-R2 are also known as p55 and p75, respectively. The trimeric structure of the receptors mimics that of the active cytokine [5]. TNF-R1 is constitutively expressed in most tissues and can be fully activated by both the membrane-bound and soluble trimeric forms of TNF, whereas TNF-R2 is only found in cells of the immune system and respond to the membrane-bound form of the TNF homotrimer. As most information regarding TNF signaling is derived from TNF-R1, the role of TNF-R2 is likely underestimated. This binding causes a conformational change to occur in the receptor, leading to the dissociation of the inhibitory protein SODD from the intracellular death domain. This dissociation enables the adaptor protein TRADD to bind to the death domain, serving as a platform for intracellular signal transduction and activation of nuclear factor-κB and mitogen-activated protein kinase. These transcription factors then translocate to the nucleus and mediate the transcription of a vast array of proteins involved in cell survival and proliferation, inflammatory response, and antiapoptotic factors.

TNF-α along with its receptors (TNF-R1 and TNF-R2) regulates critical cellular and molecular events associated with inflammatory cascades of autoimmune diseases. TNF-α stimulates the release of the inflammatory cytokines IL-1β, IL-6, IL-8, and GM-CSF. It induces the expression of endothelial adhesion molecules (intercellular adhesion molecule-1 [ICAM-1], vascular cell adhesion molecule-1, and E-selectin) and chemokines (monocyte chemoattractant protein-1, macrophage inflammatory protein-2, RANTES, and macrophage inflammatory protein-1α). In addition, at the disease site, TNF-α directly acts on target tissues to induce proliferation or apoptosis and thus participates in remodeling of the connective tissue and epithelial tissue. On the other hand, blocking of TNF-α will also counter these critical processes required for immunosurveillance of pathological microbial agents. Hence, it is not surprising that all anti-TNF-α agents have been associated with a variety of serious and "routine" opportunistic infections because they suppress the inflammatory response [6].

Thus, TNF inhibitors offer a targeted strategy that contrasts with the nonspecific immunosuppressive agents traditionally used to treat most inflammatory diseases. There has been major clinical breakthrough with the use of TNF-α-blocking biologics [7]. TNF-α blockers are being used in a number of immunological diseases like psoriasis, PsA, Crohn's disease, RA, and ankylosing spondylitis (Table 11.1). As of 2010, millions of patients have been treated with TNF-α blockers for the treatment of inflammatory diseases [8–12].

TABLE 11.1
FDA-Approved Clinical Indications for the Use of TNF-α Blockers

Rheumatologic indications
Severe and active RA, refractory to an adequate trial of DMARDs
Active polyarticular juvenile idiopathic arthritis, refractory to one or more
DMARDs
Ankylosing spondylitis
PsA

Gastrointestinal indications
Moderate to severe Crohn's disease (including fistulating Crohn's disease) with
  inadequate response to conventional therapies (TGA approved but not yet PBS listed)

Dermatological indications
Moderate to severe psoriasis

To date, the FDA has approved five TNF-α inhibitors for the treatment of a variety of inflammatory conditions:

(1) Adalimumab—a human monoclonal anti-TNF-α antibody
(2) Certolizumab pegol—a PEGylated Fab fragment of humanized monoclonal TNF-α antibody
(3) Etanercept—a soluble p75 TNF-α receptor fusion protein
(4) Golimumab—a human monoclonal anti-TNF-α antibody
(5) Infliximab—a mouse/human chimeric anti-TNF-α monoclonal antibody

Enbrel is administered by self-injection under the skin once or twice weekly. Marketed by Amgen and Wyeth, it received its first FDA approval in 1998. Etanercept (Enbrel) is currently used to treat plaque psoriasis, PsA, ankylosing spondylitis, RA, and juvenile RA. A randomized trial of etanercept in 652 adult patients with active but stable plaque psoriasis involving at least 10% of the body surface area found three doses of subcutaneous etanercept (25 mg weekly, 25 mg twice weekly, and 50 mg twice weekly) significantly superior to placebo [13]. Results of various clinical trials suggest that one-half of patients experienced a 75% reduction in psoriasis severity (Psoriasis Area and Severity Index [PASI] 75) after 12 weeks of twice weekly treatments.

Remicade (infliximab) first received FDA approval in 1998 for the treatment of Crohn's disease. It is marketed by Centocor. Subsequently, it received approval for use in patients with RA, ulcerative colitis, ankylosing spondylitis, PsA, and in 2006 severe plaque psoriasis. After the Active Controlled Study of Patients Receiving Infliximab for Treatment of RA of Early Onset Study, the FDA has approved infliximab to be used as first line with methotrexate (MTX) in moderate–severe RA. The study group patients on infliximab + MTX with early RA less than 3 years were found to have less new joint erosions after 1 year than control. This emphasized the impact of early intervention in RA. Remicade is administered by intravenous infusion in a physician's office; receipt of a single dose takes 2–4 h. Patients usually receive the first three doses within 10 weeks and then a dose every 8 weeks. Remicade is very effective for psoriasis. As an example, a multicenter randomized trial in 249 patients with severe plaque psoriasis found that compared with placebo, more patients treated with infliximab 3 or 5 mg/kg (given intravenously at weeks 0, 2, and 6) achieved at least a 75% improvement at week 10 (6% vs 72% and 88%, respectively) [14].

Adalimumab (Humira) first won FDA approval in 2002 and is currently used to treat psoriasis, PsA, RA, ankylosing spondylitis, and Crohn's disease. It is marketed by Abbott. Humira is very effective, with more than two-thirds of patients in clinical trials experiencing a 75% reduction in psoriasis severity (PASI 75) after 16 weeks of treatment, including approximately 40% of patients who achieved a 90% reduction in psoriasis severity. Humira is administered by self-injection under the skin, typically once every 2 weeks.

Etanercept is not a monoclonal antibody but a fusion protein that acts as a "decoy receptor" for TNF-α, acts competitively to inhibit the binding of TNF to its cell surface receptor, and also binds to the soluble form of TNF-α, thus making TNF-α biologically inactive by inhibiting their interaction with the cell surface. All three agents block the biological effects of TNF-α, although there are some differences in their structure, pharmacokinetics, and mechanisms of action. Both infliximab and adalimumab are anti-TNF-α monoclonal antibodies that bind specifically to human TNF-α with high affinity and neutralize the biological activity of TNF-α by inhibiting its binding to its receptors. The main difference between these two agents is that infliximab is a chimeric monoclonal antibody composed of both human and murine proteins and given as an intravenous infusion, whereas adalimumab is entirely of human origin given as subcutaneous injections every 2 weeks. MTX can be coadministered with infliximab to prevent the development of neutralizing antibodies to infliximab that could reduce its therapeutic efficacy. Adalimumab contains only human proteins, so chance of development of neutralizing antibodies is much less.

Golimumab (a human monoclonal anti-TNF-α antibody) and certolizumab (a PEGylated Fab fragment of humanized monoclonal TNF-α antibody) are the two latest additions to the anti-TNF regimen. Both of these medicines are approved by the FDA in the early part of 2009 for RA and likely to be used for various other autoimmune diseases.

On the basis of experience gained in cytokine modulation therapy of chronic inflammatory diseases such as RA and psoriasis, the application of TNF inhibitors represents a novel, a more specific, and an effective therapeutic option for distinct chronic inflammatory diseases. Various reports suggest that anti-TNF could be very effective in inflammatory skin diseases like Behcet's disease, pyoderma gangrenosum, cutaneous Chron's disease, and subcorneal pustular dermatitis [15].

Multiple adverse effects of TNF inhibition have been identified through both clinical trials and postmarketing surveillance [16]. Side effects of anti-TNF therapy are mentioned in the Table 11.2. Although TNF-α blockers are generally well tolerated, physicians needs to be extremely cautious about the potential of serious side effects of anti-TNF drugs and should review the indications/contraindications of anti-TNF agents in every patient. The existence of any contraindications to the use of these agents (Table 11.3) needs to be considered before the commencement of therapy.

High incidence of latent tuberculosis is a major hurdle for the successful use of anti-TNF agents in Indian subcontinents. Reactivation of latent tuberculosis infection has been reported with the initiation of anti-TNF-α treatment; appropriate screening of patients with Mantoux test and chest x-ray should be performed before starting therapy. In PPD+ patients, it is preferable that a dermatologist works closely with a chest medicine specialist before prescribing any anti-TNF agent. Various uncommon infections such as listeriosis, disseminated histoplasmosis, and other deep fungal infections are reported among patients treated with anti-TNF agents. Dermatologists using anti-TNF should play an important role in educating their patients regarding the possible side effects of anti-TNF-α therapy and highlight some of the early warning symptoms. Patients should be instructed regarding the rudiments of differentiating simple viral illnesses and minor infections from those

TABLE 11.2
Major Adverse Effects of Anti-TNF Therapy

Injection site reactions

Infusion reactions

Infections

Demyelinating disease

Heart failure

Malignancy

Induction of autoimmunity

TABLE 11.3
Contraindications for the Use of TNF-α Blockers

Absolute

Active infections (including infected prosthesis, severe sepsis)

History of recurrent or chronic infections (e.g., bronchiectasis)

After previous, untreated tuberculosis

Moderate to severe congestive cardiac failure

Multiple sclerosis or optic neuritis

Combination treatment with anakinra (IL-1RA)

Active or recent history (past 10 years) of malignancy except for skin cancer

Relative

Pregnancy

Lactation

HIV, hepatitis B, hepatitis C infection

with the potential to cause serious harm and should be instructed to inform their TNF-α inhibitor prescriber when signs of the more serious infections occur. Although rare, clinicians need to closely monitor for malignancy and induction of autoimmunity in patients receiving anti-TNF agents.

Conventional immunomodulatory agents (e.g., glucocorticoids, MTX, cyclophosphamide, and azathioprine) are not without risks either. Thus, the decision to use an anti-TNF agent must be an individual one on the basis of the risk/benefit profile, the severity of the disease, and the involvement of the vital organs.

IL-1 INHIBITORS

The original members of the IL-1 superfamily are the IL-1α, the IL-1β, and the IL-1 receptor antagonist (IL-1RA). The IL-1RA is a molecule that competes for receptor binding with IL-1α and IL-1β, blocking their role in immune activation. Both IL-1α and IL-1β are produced by macrophages, monocytes, and dendritic cells. They form an important part of the inflammatory response. IL-1 blockers are effective in animal models of RA but less effective than TNF-α in human RA. A variety of approaches to IL-1 inhibition have been used, which includes IL-1Ra gene therapy, IL-1 trap, and Anakinra. The IL-1 trap comprises the extracellular domains of the IL-1 receptor accessory protein and the human IL-1 receptor, arranged inline and fused to the Fc portion of human IgG1. The clinical utility of cytokine traps is under investigation. Among these IL-1 inhibitors, Anakinra is only available for treatment. Anakinra (recombinant form of human IL-1RA) is approved in United States for the treatment of moderate–severe RA with MTX [17]. Combination of anti-TNF and anti-IL-1 therapy could be potentially dangerous. Study of combination of etanercept and anakinra in patient treated unsuccessfully with MTX showed no added benefit but an increase in serious infection (0% in etanercept and 3.7%–7.4% for combination therapy), injection site reaction, and neutropenia [18]. By comparison with the TNF inhibitors, IL-1 inhibitors have had a smaller impact on rheumatic disease.

IL-6 INHIBITOR

IL-6 binds to both soluble and membrane-bound receptors and leads to the transduction of intracellular signals through the interaction of this complex with gp130, mediating gene activation and a wide range of biological activities [19]. IL-6 has the ability to activate T cells, B cells, macrophages, and osteoclasts and is a pivotal mediator of the hepatic acute phase response. Tocilizumab (atlizumab, MRA) is a humanized anti-IL-6 receptor antibody. Tocilizumab competes for both the membrane-bound and the soluble forms of human IL-6 receptor, thereby inhibiting the binding of the native cytokine to its receptor and interfering with the cytokine's effects. It was tested in patients with RA and showed reduced disease activity and dose-dependent improvement in the American College of Rheumatology (ACR) 20 [20].

OTHER IL ANTAGONISTS

AMG714, a human monoclonal IgG1 kappa anti-IL-15 Ab, has shown good response in RA [21, 22]. In the phase 2 study of patients with RA who had failed at least the disease-modifying anti-rheumatic drugs (DMARD), 54% of patients receiving 280 mg of AMG714 achieved ACR 20 compared with 38% in the placebo group. A phase 1 study of new formulation of AMG714 is ongoing.

IL-10 is a cytokine that has anti-inflammatory and immunosuppressant properties. IL-10 plays a crucial role in several immune reactions, including regulatory mechanisms in the skin. In psoriasis, a common cutaneous immune disease, a relative deficiency in cutaneous IL-10 expression is observed. Several lines of evidence suggest that IL-10 could have antipsoriatic abilities. One pilot and two phase 2 trials with subcutaneous IL-10 administration more than 3–7 weeks in patients with moderate to severe psoriasis have supported this hypothesis [23].

IL-18 is involved in the TH1 immune response. Antibodies against IL-18 reduced the severity of colitis in animal models [24]. Clinical trials of a human anti-IL-18 antibody or IL-18 binding protein are anticipated [25].

T-CELL-TARGETED THERAPIES IN THE TREATMENT OF SYSTEMIC AND CUTANEOUS AUTOIMMUNE DISEASES

Activation of T cells by antigen-presenting cells (APCs) requires two distinct signals. First, the tri-molecular complex must be formed, consisting of the T-cell receptor (TCR), antigenic peptide, and major histocompatibility complex class II molecule from the APC. The engagement of costimulatory receptors with its respective ligands provides an essential "second signal" for the optimal activation of T cells. A number of costimulatory molecules have been shown to influence T-cell activation. The most well-characterized T-cell costimulatory ligands are CD28 and cytotoxic T-lymphocyte-associated antigen-4 (CTLA4) (CD152), which engage CD80 and CD86 receptors on APCs [26, 27]. Among these, a principal signal is delivered by engagement of CD28 on T cells with CD80 (B7–1) and CD86 (B7–2) on APCs. This process enhances T-cell activation by stabilization of cytokine mRNA and upregulation of antiapoptotic genes. In contrast, CTLA4-Ig binds to B7–1 and B7–2 molecules on APCs and blocks the CD28-mediated costimulatory signal for T-cell activation. Thus, the B7 family of molecules on APCs regulates T-cell activation by delivering antigen-independent stimulatory signals through CD28 and inhibitory signals through CD152. This unique mechanism of T-cell activation has provided several target molecules for therapeutic manipulation of immune responses. These include the following:

- Inhibition of the "second signal" required for T-cell activation: Targeting the various components of the T-lymphocyte costimulatory systems such as CD28 (an activation receptor), CTLA4 (an inhibitory receptor), and CD80 or CD86 on APCs. Alternative strategy could be to target other costimulatory molecules such as CD40/CD40 ligand system.
- Manipulation of TCR and major histocompatibility complex–antigen interactions: One approach is to identify the specific T cells that cause tissue injury and to produce monoclonal antibodies to the binding site of the TCR. A complementary strategy can be to identify the particular peptide sequence of the antigen molecule that is responsible for the initiation of the disease. A mimic of this peptide, referred to as an altered-peptide ligand, can then

be synthesized, which may block T-cell recognition at the level of the APC. Attempts to prevent immune responses by targeting this approach remain unsuccessful because of the lack of information regarding the specific antigen(s) recognized by pathogenic T cells in autoimmune diseases.

The effectiveness of costimulatory signal blockade as a therapeutic device was shown over a decade by demonstrating that CTLA4-Ig inhibited graft rejection and induced long-term tolerance in mice [28]. Encouraging results in animal models have led to successful clinical trials with CTLA4-Ig in psoriasis and RA [29, 30].

To date, only costimulatory molecule inhibition with CTLA4-Ig (abatacept) has been demonstrated to be effective in the treatment of RA and psoriasis. Abatacept (CTLA4-Ig) is a soluble fusion protein that consists of the CTLA4 and the Fc portion of IgG1. Through its high-affinity binding for CD28, CTLA4-Ig interferes with the binding of CD80 (B7–1) or CD86 (B7–2) to CD28, thereby inhibiting transmission of the second signal required for T-cell activation. Abatacept should not be used concurrently with TNF inhibitors or with the IL-1RA, anakinra, because these combinations cause significant immunosuppression and lead to severe infections. Live vaccines should not be given concurrently or within 3 months of stopping abatacept.

Currently, we are working on an alternative approach to develop immunomodulatory drug by manipulating CD28CD80/86 interactions using a monoclonal anti-CD28 antibody (FR255734) prepared by the Fujisawa Pharmaceutical Co., Ltd. (now Astellas Pharmaceuticals Inc., Tokyo, Japan). FR255734 is a humanized IgG2κ anti-human CD28 antibody that has the complementary determining regions of the mouse anti-human monoclonal antibody TN228 and the Fc domain of human IgG2M3 in which two amino acid mutations (V234A and G237A) have been introduced into the human γ2 chain to eliminate binding of the antibody to FcγR. The original TN228 cell line was generated by immunizing BALB/c mice with human CD28-transfected mouse fibroblast L cells and fusing immune splenocytes with P3 U1 myeloma cells. The purified molecule consists of two heavy chains and two light chains, which are 447 amino acid residues (C2177H3358N575O669S19; MW 48898.64) and 218 amino acid residues (C1043H1628N279O342S7; MW 23772.21) in length, respectively. FR255734 binds to a human CD28– mouse IgG Fc fusion protein ($K_d = 3.72 \times 10^{-8}$) and inhibits proliferation of human T cells stimulated with anti-CD3 and P815/human CD80+ cells in a concentration-dependent manner. FR255734 does not cross-react with mouse CD28 [31].

We have demonstrated by *in vitro* studies that FR255734 effectively inhibits cell activation by blocking CD28/B7 costimulatory interactions [32]. This encouraged us to evaluate the clinical efficacy of FR255734 in T-cell-mediated disease. To evaluate the therapeutic efficacy of FR255734 as a costimulatory antagonist, we have used the SCID mouse model of psoriasis. We noticed significant improvement in the thickness of the epidermis and reduction in infiltrates in the FR255734-treated group ($p < 0.005$ at 10 mg/kg and $p = 0.002$ at 3 mg/kg). In the normal saline-treated group and isotype controls (negative controls), the epidermal thickness and the amount of infiltrates remained unchanged. The results of our study substantiate a novel approach for treatment of T-cell-mediated diseases by specifically manipulating the interaction of CD28 and B7 costimulatory molecules of activated T cells. It is expected FR255734 to be effective in diseases associated with active role of T cells such as psoriasis, RA, and multiple sclerosis.

TARGETING THE EFFECTOR MEMORY T CELLS

It has been reported that most T cells in psoriatic lesions are of the effector memory phenotype (effector memory T cells [T_{EM}]); thus, it would be desirable to selectively inhibit the function of these cells without affecting other T cells. Lymphocyte function associated antigen (LFA)-3/ IgG1 fusion protein (Alefacept) preferentially targets T_{EM} cells and has been used for treatment of psoriasis with partial success [33]. Alefacept binds to CD2, a receptor that is mostly expressed on

T_{EM} cells and is critical for T-cell activation. Alefacept is approved by the FDA for treatment of adult patients with moderate to severe chronic plaque psoriasis who are candidates for systemic therapy or phototherapy. It is administered weekly for 12 weeks as a 15-mg intramuscular injection. CD4 cell counts should be checked every week or every other week while on therapy, and the dose should not be administered if the count is less than $250/\mu L$; Alefacept should be discontinued if the CD4 count remains less than $250/\mu L$ for 1 month. It is contraindicated in patients infected with HIV because of theoretical concerns related to the effects of Alefacept on CD4 cell counts.

K^+ CHANNELS IN THE IMMUNE SYSTEM

K^+ channels in humans are encoded by an extended superfamily of 78 genes and regulate membrane potential and Ca^{2+} signaling in both excitable and nonexcitable cells. Two of these channels, the voltage-gated Kv1.3 and the Ca^{2+}-activated KCa3.1 channel are expressed in human lymphocytes, where they play an important role in the T-cell activation cascade. Engagement of the TCR triggers a Ca^{2+} influx through voltage-independent Ca^{2+} channels, which results in the increase in cytosolic Ca^{2+} concentration necessary for the translocation of nuclear factor of activated T cells to the nucleus and the initiation of new transcription, ultimately resulting in cytokine secretion and T-cell proliferation. However, this crucial Ca^{2+} influx is only possible if the T cell can keep its membrane potential negative by a counterbalancing K^+ efflux through Kv1.3 and/or KCa3.1. Both channels are therefore regarded as attractive new targets for immunotherapy: KCa3.1 for acute immune reactions mediated by naive T cells and Kv1.3 for chronic immune reactions carried by memory T cells. We therefore believe that Kv1.3 blockers constitute a promising new drug candidate for the treatment of T_{EM}-cell-mediated inflammatory skin diseases like allergic contact dermatitis and psoriasis [34]. Because of their different mechanism of action, Kv1.3 blockers might also work in those patients with psoriasis that have no benefit from the existing therapies. For example, long-term therapeutic efficacy (PASI 75) of anti-TNF agents and Alefacept for psoriasis is only 60% and 20%, respectively, and an urgent need for new psoriasis treatments still exists. In addition, topical Kv1.3 blockers might be able to replace topical steroids in patients with moderate psoriasis who are looking for a treatment with less side effects or a different side effect profile.

B-CELL-TARGETED THERAPIES IN THE TREATMENT OF SYSTEMIC AND CUTANEOUS AUTOIMMUNE DISEASES

The major goal of B-cell depletion therapy is to destroy malignant B lineage cells or autoimmune disease-producing B cells in patients with cancers or autoimmune diseases while at the same time retaining protective B-cell immunity. For many years, rheumatologists have debated how B cells contribute to the development of RA and whether depleting B cells in patients might be therapeutic. In a landmark study, Shlomchik et al. [35] showed that autoimmune-prone MRL-lpr/lpr mice lacking B cells do not develop autoimmune kidney destruction, vasculitis, or autoantibodies. They concluded that their "data demonstrate that B cells could be an important target for therapy of systemic autoimmunity" and that "elimination of B cells or B-cell subsets would have distinct advantages over removal of Ig alone." They turned out to be right. In a follow-up study by a different group, it has been shown that MRL-lpr/lpr mice that have B cells but cannot make antibodies still develop autoimmune disease. This suggested that B-cell depletion therapy might be able to work by removing B-cell APCs presenting autoantigens and by removing autoantibody-producing B cells. Thus, B cells have a dual role in the pathogenesis of autoimmune diseases, which include presentation of antigen to the T cells and antibody production. Similar to T cells, various markers of B cells such as CD20, CD22, and B-cell growth factors like BLyS and APRIL have been targeted to develop treatment of autoimmune diseases.

B-CELL-DEPLETING AGENTS

Rituximab—Rituximab is a B-cell-depleting monoclonal anti-CD20 antibody, composed of
both mouse and human portions.

Ofatumumab—Clinical development is reportedly proceeding with fully human anti-CD20
monoclonal antibodies. One such agent, ofatumumab, is undergoing clinical trials to assess
dosing, efficacy, and safety when used in patients with RA.

Belimumab—Belimumab is an anti-BLyS monoclonal antibody (LymphoStat-B) that has
been used in a dose-ranging, phase 2 trial in RA and lupus.

Atacicept—Atacicept is a recombinant fusion protein composed of a portion of the transmembrane activator and calcium modulator and an Ig chain (TACI-Ig or atacicept). Atacicept
targets molecules on the B-cell surface that promote B-cell survival (BLyS and APRIL).

Among all these B-cell-depleting agents, rituximab is only currently in clinical use. Rituximab
is a chimeric monoclonal anti-CD20 antibody that selectively depletes CD20-expressing B cells. It
has been used extensively to treat non-Hodgkin's lymphoma, and it has also received approval in the
United States and Europe to treat RA unresponsive to a TNF blocker [36].

Data suggest that, for patients with severe systemic lupus erythematosus who have failed to
respond to conventional treatment, the combination of rituximab and cyclophosphamide can provide a new therapeutic alternative [37]. There are various other specific uses of rituximab for
cutaneous diseases that are currently in developing stage. Rituximab is highly effective in pemphigus [38]. The dose of rituximab (unlabeled use) for pemphigus vulgaris has been proposed as
375 mg/m^2 once weekly of weeks 1, 2, and 3 of a 4-week cycle, repeat for one additional cycle,
then one dose per month for 4 months (total of 10 doses in 6 months). Rituximab appears to
be of benefit in patients with anti-neutrophil cytoplasmic antibody (ANCA)-positive vasculitis.
Rituximab also has been found to be effective in complicated dermatomyositis.

ANGIOGENESIS FACTOR

Angiogenesis plays an integral role in psoriasis and RA by supplying oxygen and nutrients necessary for cell metabolism and division as well as by bringing in leukocytes and signaling mediators
such as cytokines, chemoattractants, and growth factors. As the synovium/epidermis expands, more
blood vessels are needed to supply poorly perfused and oxygenated areas distant from the preexisting blood vessels. This promotes formation of further blood vessels ("angiogenesis"). A range of different factors can promote angiogenesis, including fibroblast growth factors 1 and 2, angiopoietins,
and vascular endothelial growth factor (VEGF). VEGF inhibition has been shown to be effective in
models of arthritis, including collagen-induced arthritis (CIA) [39, 40]. VEGF inhibition *in vivo* is,
however, associated with side effects, such as impaired wound healing, hemorrhage, and gastrointestinal perforation. As a consequence, other members of this family have been targeted. Placental
growth factor (PlGF), like VEGF, binds to VEGF-R1 (and soluble VEGF-R1), but in contrast to
VEGF, PlGF does not bind VEGF-R2 [41, 42]. PlGF appears not only to induce distinct signaling
events via VEGF-R1 but also to amplify VEGF-driven effects through VEGF-R2 and to complex
with VEGF/VEGF-R2-forming heterodimeric complexes that transphosphorylate each other [43].
Interestingly, PlGF-deficient mice are fertile, viable, and do not display major vascular abnormalities [44]. Instead, PlGF may play a more pronounced role in pathological angiogenesis, as evidenced
by impaired tumor growth and vascularization in mice lacking this molecule. Furthermore, PIGF is
expressed in synovial fluid, making it a potentially important therapeutic target [45].

DRUGS THAT INHIBIT LEUKOCYTE ADHESION

Blockage of leukocyte migration has been proposed as a means of downregulating inflammation.
ICAM-1 is a transmembrane glycoprotein that has multiple functions involving propagation of

inflammatory processes and is upregulated in inflammatory bowel disease. LFA-1 (CD11a) mediates interactions between T cells and mononuclear phagocytes through its ligand, the ICAM-1 (CD54).

Multicenter randomized, controlled trials have shown that efalizumab (Raptiva), a humanized monoclonal antibody to CD11A, has benefit in the treatment of psoriasis [46].

As an example, a randomized trial found that subcutaneous efalizumab (1 or 2 mg/kg/week) was significantly superior to placebo. After 12 weeks, there was at least a 75% improvement in a psoriasis severity index in 22%, 28%, and 5%, respectively. Among patients who initially improved at least 75% after 12 weeks of efalizumab, improvement was maintained through 24 weeks in 77% of those who were randomly assigned to continue efalizumab and in 20% of those switched to placebo, and more patients with lesser degrees of initial improvement showed continued improvement with efalizumab than with placebo. Adverse events including headache, chills, pain, and fever were more common in patients receiving efalizumab, but serious adverse events and infections were no more common than in those receiving placebo.

In April 2009, efalizumab, a monoclonal antibody against CD11—a component of LFA-1 chain—was voluntarily withdrawn from the U.S. market for the treatment of psoriasis because of an association between long-term therapy and the development of progressive multifocal leukoencephalopathy (PML) [47].

NEW GENERATIONS OF BIOLOGICS

GOLIMUMAB AND CERTOLIZUMAB

Golimumab is a fully human anti-TNF-α monoclonal antibody created in specific transgenic mice. Instead of humanizing the mouse antibodies by using phage display technology, recent technologies have allowed for the humanization of the mice. In transgenic mice, the genes coding for the mouse antibody genes can been suppressed and human antibody genes can be inserted [48]. Thus, when the resulting transgenic mouse is immunized with a target antigen, the mouse produces antibodies from the human genes inserted into its genome. Golimumab is made using this technology with a specific aim to make genetically engineered mice that will make human anti-TNF antibody [48, 49]. Golimumab forms high-affinity, stable complexes with human TNF. Action of golimumab is very similar like that of infliximab, adalimumab, and certolizumab, and it acts by neutralizing both circulating and membrane-bound forms of human TNF [49, 50].

Certolizumab is a PEGylated recombinant, humanized antibody Fab' fragment specific for human TNF-α. Certolizumab does not contain an Fc region, unlike infliximab and adalimumab, and it does not fix complement or cause antibody-dependent cell-mediated cytotoxicity *in vitro* [51]. The PEGylation of the antibody delays the elimination and thus provides a longer half-life; as a result, the medication may be administered monthly. Certolizumab is the only TNF inhibitor that uses PEGylated technology.

THERAPEUTIC EFFICACY NOTICED IN CLINICAL TRIALS

THERAPEUTIC EFFICACY OF GOLIMUMAB (SIMPONI)

In several multicenter, randomized, double-blind, controlled trials, efficacy and safety of golimumab have been evaluated [50, 52–57]. Safety and efficacy studies have been carried out in RA, PsA, psoriasis, and ankylosing spondylitis. Majority of the studies have been done in patients with RA, including early onset untreated patients. In a recent phase 3, multicenter, randomized, double-blind, placebo-controlled study, it has also been reported that in RA golimumab can be considered as first-line therapy for early onset RA [52].

In RA, efficacy and safety data of golimumab are available from a series of studies denoted as RA-1, RA-2, and RA-3. RA-1 study is known as GO-AFTER, and RA-2 is known as GO-FORWARD [51, 57]. These studies were performed in 1542 patients of ≥18 years of age with moderately to severely active RA [50, 53, 54]. Double-blind controlled efficacy data were collected and analyzed through week 24. In studies RA-1 and RA-2, patients were allowed to continue low dose of corti-costeroids (equivalent to ≤10 mg of prednisone a day) and/or nonsteroidal anti-inflammatory drugs, and patients may have received oral MTX during the trials.

Study RA-1 evaluated 461 patients who were previously treated (at least 8–12 weeks before administration of study agent) with one or more doses of a biological TNF blocker without a serious adverse reaction. Study RA-2 evaluated 444 patients who had active RA despite a stable dose of at least 15 mg/week of MTX and who had not been previously treated with a biological TNF blocker. Study RA-3 evaluated 637 patients with active RA who were MTX naive and had not previously been treated with a biological TNF blocker.

The primary end point in studies RA-1 and RA-2 was the percentage of patients achieving an ACR 20 response at week 14, and the primary end point in study RA-3 was the percentage of patients achieving an ACR 50 response at week 24 [50, 53, 54]. Golimumab was found to be more effective than the placebo and MTX in these trials. The combination therapy of golimumab and MTX achieved higher percentage ACR responses at week 14 (studies RA-1 and RA-2) and week 24 (studies RA-1, RA-2, and RA-3) versus patients treated with the MTX alone [50]. There was no clear evidence of improved ACR response with the higher golimumab dose group (100 mg) compared with the lower golimumab dose group (50 mg). In study RA-1, the proportion of patients achieving ACR 20, 50, and 70 responses at week 14 were 35%, 16%, and 10%, respectively, in the golimumab 50 mg + MTX group ($n = 103$) compared with 17%, 6%, and 2%, respectively, in the placebo + MTX group ($n = 107$) [50, 54].

The safety and efficacy of golimumab has also been evaluated in a multicenter, randomized, double-blind, placebo-controlled trial in PsA. This study was done in 405 adult patients with moderate to severe forms of active PsA (three or more swollen joints and three or more tender joints) [50, 55]. Patients in this study had PsA with a median duration of 5.1 years and with a qualifying psoriatic skin lesion of at least 2 cm in diameter. Previous treatment with a bio-logical TNF blocker was not allowed; however, patients could receive MTX/oral corticoster-oid/nonsteroidal anti-inflammatory drug. The primary end point was the percentage of patients achieving ACR 20 response at week 14. In this 24-week double-blind, randomized trial, patients were randomly assigned to placebo, golimumab 50 mg, or golimumab 100 mg given subcutane-ously every 4 weeks. ACR 20 responses at week 14 occurred in 9%, 51%, and 45% of the three groups, respectively. At week 14, at least 75% improvement in the PASI scores occurred in 3%, 40%, and 58%, respectively. There was no clear evidence of improved ACR response with the higher golimumab dose group (100 mg) compared with the lower golimumab dose group (50 mg). Similarly, golimumab has been found to be effective in 356 adult patients with active ankylosing spondylitis [50, 56].

CERTOLIZUMAB PEGOL (CIMZIA)

In RA, efficacy and safety data of certolizumab are available from a series of studies denoted as RAPID 1, RAPID 2, and FAST4WARD. Certolizumab has been compared with placebo in 1821 patients with moderate to severe forms of active RA in these multicenter, double-blind, randomized controlled trials. Outcomes of efficacy were determined by the percentage of patients achieving ACR 20 response at week 24. FAST4WARD compared certolizumab 400 mg every 4 weeks with placebo in patients with RA who failed at least one prior DMARD [58]. Patients were randomized into two treatment groups: CIMZIA 400 mg ($n = 111$) every 4 weeks from baseline to week 20 and placebo ($n = 109$) every 4 weeks from baseline to week 20. ACR 20 response rate at week 24 was defined as the primary end point of this study. Other outcomes included ACR 50 and ACR 70 response rates at week 24 and adverse effects. CIMZIA demonstrated a significant therapeutic response at week 24. ACR 20 response rate was higher in patients who received certolizumab 400 mg (45.5% vs 9.3%; $p < 0.001$). Secondary end points of ACR 50 and ACR 70 were superior to placebo (ACR 50: certolizumab, 22.7% vs 3.7% ($p < 0.001$); ACR 70: certolizumab, 5.5% vs 0% ($p \leq 0.05$)). Patient-reported outcomes were also better in the certolizumab arm. Physical function (Health Assessment Questionnaire Disability Index minimal clinically important differences) is defined as a decrease of ≥ 0.22 points from baseline in the Health Assessment Questionnaire Disability Index: More patients in the certolizumab arm reported physical function improvement (49% vs 12%; $p < 0.001$). RAPID 1 compared the combination of MTX and certolizumab with MTX monotherapy in TNF-inhibitor naive patients with active, uncontrolled RA despite treatment with MTX monotherapy. Primary efficacy outcomes included ACR 20 response rate at week 24 and total modified Sharp score at week 52. More patients in the combination treatment arms achieved the primary end point of ACR 20 response rate at week 24. At week 52, there was a smaller mean change from baseline in the modified total Sharp score in patients who received combination treatment compared with MTX monotherapy, which indicates less bone erosion and joint-space narrowing. RAPID 2 compared the combination of certolizumab and MTX with MTX monotherapy in patients with active RA whose symptoms were inadequately controlled with ≥ 6 months of treatment with MTX monotherapy. Patients ($n = 619$) were randomized 2:2:1 to subcutaneous certolizumab pegol (liquid formulation) 400 mg at weeks 0, 2, and 4 followed by 200 or 400 mg plus MTX or placebo plus MTX every 2 weeks for 24 weeks. The results showed that significantly more patients in the certolizumab pegol 200- and 400-mg groups achieved an ACR 20 response versus placebo ($p < 0.001$); rates were 57.3%, 57.6%, and 8.7%, respectively. Certolizumab pegol 200 and 400 mg also significantly inhibited radiographic progression. Most adverse events were mild or moderate, with low incidence of withdrawals because of adverse events. Five patients developed tuberculosis [59].

The efficacy and safety of certolizumab pegol in the treatment of Crohn's disease was evaluated by randomized, double-blind, placebo-controlled trials (also known as PRECiSE1 and PRECiSE2) [60–62]. The results of these studies demonstrated that in moderate to severe Crohn's disease, induction and maintenance therapy with certolizumab pegol was associated with a modest improvement in response rates as compared with placebo.

Another approach is to target IL-23 or IL-6, which is necessary for differentiation and survival of Th17. IL-23-deficient mice are found to be resistant to experimental autoimmune encephalitis, CIA, and inflammatory bowel disease [63–65]. Th17 cells express ROR gamma transcription factor and IL-17A and IL-17F. IL-17 induces TNF-α and IL-6, growth factor (GM-CSF and G-CSF), and chemokines CXCL8, CXCL1, and CXCL10. Blockade of Th17 has been shown to be effective in a number of animal models of disease including CIA [66–68] and hence is a target for psoriasis and RA.

IL-23 induces IL-22 in the Th17 cells. In RA, both IL-22 and its receptor IL-22R1 are expressed in synovial tissues, and IL-22 was shown to increase monocyte chemoattractant protein-1 expression and proliferation of fibroblast *in vitro*, suggesting proinflammatory role. In Crohn's disease, it has a protective role by upregulating LPS binding protein, thereby reducing LPS. Further work needs to be done to find its role in other autoimmune diseases.

The recognition that nerve growth factor (NGF) and its receptor system (NGF-R) have a critical role in the pathomechanisms of inflammation, inflammatory disease, and pain mechanisms has provided unexpected and attractive opportunities to develop a novel class of therapeutics for inflammatory diseases and chronic pain syndromes [69]. We have demonstrated that K252a, a high-affinity receptor inhibitor, and neutralizing NGF antibody are therapeutically effective in psoriasis [70]. Several investigators and pharmaceutical companies are currently in search of anti-NGF therapy for inflammatory diseases, arthritis, and pain control. Pincelli et al. [71] have extended our observations and are currently in the process of preparing a topical preparation of K252a for the treatment of psoriasis. Recently, Shelton et al. [72] from the Rinat Neuroscience Corp. have reported that treatment with anti-NGF antibody is efficacious for autoimmune arthritis of rats. These results encouraged the Rinat Neuroscience Corp. to extend their study in chronic painful human diseases such as osteoarthritis [73].

CONCLUSIONS

Since the late 1990s, the success of biological agents in the treatment of RA has dramatically altered the approach for treating this disease and a variety of other inflammatory illnesses. High cost and potential for serious side effects of biologics are social and clinical challenges to the current generation of physicians. Anti-TNF agents have revolutionized treatment of inflammatory diseases of autoimmune origin. They have considerable advantages over the existing immunomodulators. Anti-TNF agents are designed to target a very specific component of the immune-mediated inflammatory cascades and thus have lower risks of systemic side effects. The development of TNF-α blocker biologics for the treatment of psoriasis, PsA, RA, Crohn's disease, and ankylosing spondylitis is a major breakthrough. In a brief period of 10 years, a growing number of biological therapies are entering the clinical arena, and many more biologics remain on the horizon. On the other side, B-cell depletion therapy has provided a very effective therapeutic option for critical patients of lupus, pemphigus, RA, and ANCA-associated vasculitis. Biological treatments are relatively expensive, and given the widespread patient dissatisfaction with conventional therapy, the demand for them is high. Clinical experience of biological therapies is currently an ongoing process, and still the long-term safety is uncertain. PML is a severe emerging infection in immunocompromised patients. Since the identification of PML in two patients with multiple sclerosis treated with natalizumab in 2005, there has been great interest in this disease in patients treated with immunomodulating agents. Unexpected cases of PML have been reported in patients who received immunomodulatory monoclonal antibodies rituximab, efalizumab, and natalizumab. There is a need to better define which patients should be considered for biological therapy. With time, long-term side effects and efficacies of these individual agents will become clearer and will help to determine which ones are the most suitable for long-term care.

REFERENCES

1. Feldmann M, Steinman L. Design of effective immunotherapy for human autoimmunity. Nature 2005;435:612–619.
2. Raychaudhuri SP, Raychaudhuri SK. Biologics: target-specific treatment of systemic and cutaneous autoimmune diseases. Indian J Dermatol 2009;54(2):100–119.
3. Feldmann M, Brennan FM, Maini R. Cytokines in autoimmune disorders. Int Rev Immunol 1998;17:217.
4. Beutler B, Cerami A. The biology of cachectin/TNF—a primary mediator of the host response. Annu Rev Immunol 1989;7:625.
5. Locksley RM, Killeen N, Lenardo MJ. The TNF and TNF receptor superfamilies: integrating mammalian biology. Cell 2001;104(4):487–501.
6. Raychaudhuri SP, Nguyen CT, Raychaudhuri SK, Gershwin ME. Incidence and nature of infectious disease in patients treated with anti-TNF agents. Autoimmun Rev 2009;9(2):67–81.
7. Hochberg MC, Lebwohl MG, Plevy SE, Hobbs KF, Yocum DE. The benefit/risk profile of TNF-blocking agents: findings of a consensus panel. Semin Arthritis Rheum 2005;34:819–836.
8. Tak PP, Taylor PC, Breedveld FC, Smeets TJ, Daha MR, Kluin PM, Meinders AE, Maini RN. Decrease in cellularity and expression of adhesion molecules by anti-tumor necrosis factor alpha monoclonal antibody treatment in patients with rheumatoid arthritis. Arthritis Rheum 1996;39:1077–1081.
9. Taylor PC, Steuer A, Gruber J, McClinton C, Cosgrove DO, Blomley MJ, Marsters PA, Wagner CL, Maini RN. Ultrasonographic and radiographic results from a two-year controlled trial of immediate or one-year-delayed addition of infliximab to ongoing methotrexate therapy in patients with erosive early rheumatoid arthritis. Arthritis Rheum 2006;54:47–53.
10. Finckh A, Simard JF, Duryea J, Liang MH, Huang J, Daneel S, Forster A, Gabay C, Guerne PA. The effectiveness of anti-tumor necrosis factor therapy in preventing progressive radiographic joint damage in rheumatoid arthritis: a population-based study. Arthritis Rheum 2006;54:54–59.
11. Chaudhari U, Romano P, Mulcahy LD, Dooley LT, Baker DG, Gottlieb AB. Efficacy and safety of infliximab monotherapy for plaque-type psoriasis: a randomised trial. Lancet 2001;357:1842.
12. Gordon KB, Langley RG, Leonardi C, Toth D, Menter MA, Kang S, Heffernan M, et al. Clinical response to adalimumab treatment in patients with moderate to severe psoriasis: double-blind, randomized controlled trial and open-label extension study. J Am Acad Dermatol 2006;55:598.

13. Leonardi CL, Powers JL, Matheson RT, Goffe BS, Zitnik R, Wang A, Gottlieb AB; Etanercept Psoriasis Study Group. Etanercept as monotherapy in patients with psoriasis. N Engl J Med 2003;349:2014.
14. Gottlieb AB, Evans R, Li S, Dooley LT, Guzzo CA, Baker D, Bala M, Marano CW, Menter A. Infliximab induction therapy for patients with severe plaque-type psoriasis: a randomized, double-blind, placebo-controlled trial. J Am Acad Dermatol 2004;51:534.
15. Jacobi A, Mahler V, Schuler G, Hertl M. Treatment of inflammatory dermatoses by tumour necrosis factor antagonists. J Eur Acad Dermatol Venereol 2006;20(10):1171–1187.
16. Day R. Adverse reactions to TNF-alpha inhibitors in rheumatoid arthritis. Lancet 2002;359:540–541.
17. Donahue KE, Gartlehner G, Jonas DE, Lux LJ, Thieda P, Jonas BL, Hansen RA, et al. Systematic review: comparative effectiveness and harms of disease-modifying medications for rheumatoid arthritis. Ann Intern Med 2008;148:124.
18. Genovese MC, Cohen S, Moreland L, Lium D, Robbins S, Newmark R, Bekker P. Combination therapy with etanercept and anakinra in the treatment of patients with rheumatoid arthritis who have been treated unsuccessfully with methotrexate. Arthritis Rheum 2004;50:1412–1419.
19. Hirano T. Interleukin 6 and its receptor: ten years later. Int Rev Immunol 1998;16:249.
20. Nishimoto N, Yoshizaki K, Miyasaka N, Yamamoto K, Kawai S, Takeuchi T, Hashimoto J, Azuma J, Kishimoto T. Treatment of rheumatoid arthritis with humanized anti-interleukin-6 receptor antibody: a multicenter, double-blind, placebo-controlled trial. Arthritis Rheum 2004;50:1761–1769.
21. McInnes I, Martin R, Zimmerman-Gorska I, Nayiager S, Sun G, Patel A, Appleton B. Safety and efficacy of a human monoclonal antibody to IL-15 (AMG 714) in patients with rheumatoid arthritis (RA): results from a multicenter, randomized, double blind, placebo-controlled trial. Arthritis Rheum 2004;50(Suppl 9):Abstract 527.
22. McInnes IB, Gracie JA. Interleukin-15: a new cytokine target for the treatment of inflammatory diseases. Curr Opin Pharmacol 2004;4:392–397.
23. Asadullah K, Döcke WD, Sabat RV, Volk HD, Sterry W. The treatment of psoriasis with IL-10: rationale and review of the first clinical trials. Expert Opin Investig Drugs 2000;9(1):95–102.
24. Siegmund B, Fantuzzi G, Rieder F, Gamboni-Robertson F, Lehr HA, Hartmann G, Dinarello CA, et al. Neutralization of interleukin-18 reduces severity in murine colitis and intestinal IFN-gamma and TNF-alpha production. Am J Physiol Regul Integr Comp Physiol 2001;281:R1264.
25. Holmes S, Abrahamson JA, Al-Mahdi N, Abdel-Meguid SS, Ho YS. Characterization of the in vitro and in vivo activity of monoclonal antibodies to human IL-18. Hybridoma 2000;19:363.
26. Mueller DL, Jenkins MK, Schwartz RH. Clonal expansion versus functional inactivation: a costimulatory signaling pathway determines the outcome of T cell antigen receptor occupancy. Annu Rev Immunol 1989;7:445–480.
27. Linsley PS, Brady W, Grosmaire L, Aruffo A, Damle NK, Ledbetter JA. Binding of the B cell activation antigen B7 to CD28 costimulates T cell proliferation and interleukin 2 mRNA accumulation. J Exp Med 1991;173:721–730.
28. Lenschow DJ, Zeng Y, Thistlethwaite JR, Montag A, Brady W, Gibson MG, Linsley PS, et al. Long-term survival of xenogeneic pancreatic islet grafts induced by CTLA4Ig. Science 1992;257:789–792.
29. Abrams JR, Lebwohl MG, Guzzo CA, Jegasothy BV, Goldfarb MT, Goffe BS, Menter A, et al. CTLA4Ig-mediated blockade of T-cell costimulation in patients with psoriasis vulgaris. J Clin Invest 1999;103:1243–1252.
30. Kremer JM, Westhovens R, Leon M, Di Giorgio E, Alten R, Steinfeld S, Russell A, et al. Treatment of rheumatoid arthritis by selective inhibition of T-cell activation with fusion protein CTLA4Ig. N Engl J Med 2003;349:1907–1915.
31. Shiao SL, McNiff JM, Masunaga T, Tamura K, Kubo K, Pober JS. Immunomodulatory properties of FK734, a humanized anti-CD28 monoclonal antibody with agonistic and antagonistic activities. Transplantation 2007;83(3):304–313.
32. Raychaudhuri SP, Kundu-Raychaudhuri S, Tamura K, Masunaga T, Kubo K, Hanaoka K, Jiang WY, Herzenberg LA, Herzenberg LA. FR255734, a humanized, Fc-silent, anti-CD28 antibody, improves psoriasis in the SCID mouse-psoriasis xenograft model. J Invest Dermatol 2008;128:1969–1976.
33. Krueger GG, Ellis CN. Alefacept therapy produces remission for patients with chronic plaque psoriasis. Br J Dermatol 2003;148(4):784–788.
34. Azam P, Sankaranarayanan A, Homerick D, Griffey S, Wulff H. Targeting effector memory T cells with the small molecule Kv1.3 blocker PAP-1 suppresses allergic contact dermatitis. J Invest Dermatol 2007;127:1419–1429.
35. Shlomchik MJ, Madaio MP, Ni D, Trounstein M, Huszar D. The role of B cells in lpr/lpr-induced autoimmunity. J Exp Med 1994;180:1295–1306.

36. Edwards JC, Szczepanski L, Szechinski J, Filipowicz-Sosnowska A, Emery P, Close DR, Stevens RM, Shaw T. Efficacy of B-cell-targeted therapy with rituximab in patients with rheumatoid arthritis. N Engl J Med 2004;350:2572.

37. Jónsdóttir T, Gunnarsson I, Risselada A, Henriksson EW, Klareskog L, van Vollenhoven RF. Treatment of refractory SLE with rituximab plus cyclophosphamide: clinical effects, serological changes, and predictors of response. Ann Rheum Dis 2008;67(3):330–334.

38. Ahmed AR, Spigelman Z, Cavacini LA, Posner MR. Treatment of pemphigus vulgaris with rituximab and intravenous immune globulin. N Engl J Med 2006;355:521.

39. Miotla J, Maciewicz R, Kendrew J, Feldmann M, Paleolog E. Treatment with soluble VEGF receptor reduces disease severity in murine collagen-induced arthritis. Lab Invest 2000;80:1195–1205.

40. Afuwape AO, Feldmann M, Paleolog EM. Adenoviral delivery of soluble VEGF receptor 1 (sFlt-1) abrogates disease activity in murine collagen-induced arthritis. Gene Ther 2003;10:1950–1960.

41. Autiero M, Luttun A, Tjwa M, Carmeliet P. Placental growth factor and its receptor, vascular endothelial growth factor receptor-1: novel targets for stimulation of ischemic tissue revascularization and inhibition of angiogenic and inflammatory disorders. J Thromb Haemost 2003;1:1356–1370.

42. Tjwa M, Luttun A, Autiero M, Carmeliet P. VEGF and PlGF: two pleiotropic growth factors with distinct roles in development and homeostasis. Cell Tissue Res 2003;314:5–14.

43. Autiero M, Waltenberger J, Communi D, Kranz A, Moons L, Lambrechts D, Kroll J, et al. Role of PlGF in the intra- and intermolecular cross talk between the VEGF receptors Flt1 and Flk1. Nat Med 2003;9:936–943.

44. Oosthuyse B, Moons L, Storkebaum E, Beck H, Nuyens D, Brusselmans K, Van Dorpe J, et al. Deletion of the hypoxia-response element in the vascular endothelial growth factor promoter causes motor neuron degeneration. Nat Genet 2001;28:131–138.

45. Bottomley MJ, Webb NJ, Watson CJ, Holt L, Bukhari M, Denton J, Freemont AJ, Brenchley PE. Placenta growth factor (PlGF) induces vascular endothelial growth factor (VEGF) secretion from mononuclear cells and is co-expressed with VEGF in synovial fluid Clin Exp Immunol 2000;119:182–188.

46. Lebwohl M, Tyring SK, Hamilton TK, Toth D, Glazer S, Tawfik NH, Walicke P, et al. A novel targeted T-cell modulator, efalizumab, for plaque psoriasis. N Engl J Med 2003;349:2004.

47. U.S. Food and Drug Administration. FDA public health advisory: updated safety information about Raptiva (efalizumab) [online]. http://www.fda.gov/Safety/MedWatch/SafetyInformation/SafetyAlertsforHumanMedicalProducts/ucm149675.htm Accessed June 6, 2010.

48. Ishida I, Tomizuka K, Yoshida H, Tahara T, Takahashi N, Ohguma A, Tanaka S. et al. Production of human monoclonal and polyclonal antibodies in TransChromo animals. Cloning Stem Cells 2002;4(1):91–102.

49. Shealy D, Cai A, Lacy E, Nesspor T, Staquet K, Johns L. Characterization of golimumab (CNTO 148), a novel fully human monoclonal antibody specific for TNFalpha (EULAR abstract THU0088). Ann Rheum Dis 2007;66(Suppl II):151.

50. U.S. Food and Drug Administration. FDA labelling information. http://www.accessdata.fda.gov/drugsatfda_docs/label/2009/125289s000lbl.pdf. Acessed June 6, 2010.

51. Melmed GY, Targan SR, Yasothan U, Hanicq D, Kirkpatrick P. Certolizumab pegol. Nat Rev Drug Discov 2008;7(8):641–642.

52. Emery P, Fleischmann RM, Moreland LW, Hsia EC, Strusberg I, Durez P, Nash P, et al. Golimumab, a human anti-tumor necrosis factor alpha monoclonal antibody, injected subcutaneously every four weeks in methotrexate-naive patients with active rheumatoid arthritis: twenty-four-week results of a phase III, multicenter, randomized, double-blind, placebo-controlled study of golimumab before methotrexate as first-line therapy for early-onset rheumatoid arthritis. Arthritis Rheum 2009;60(8):2272–2283.

53. Keystone EC, Genovese MC, Klareskog L, Hsia EC, Hall ST, Miranda PC, Pazdur J, et al. Golimumab, a human antibody to tumour necrosis factor α given by monthly subcutaneous injections, in active rheumatoid arthritis despite methotrexate therapy: the GO-FORWARD study. Ann Rheum Dis 2009;68:789–796.

54. Smolen JS, Kay J, Doyle MK, Landewé R, Matteson EL, Wollenhaupt J, Gaylis N, et al. Golimumab in patients with active rheumatoid arthritis after treatment with tumour necrosis factor α inhibitors (GO-AFTER study): a multicentre, randomised, double-blind, placebo controlled, phase III trial. Lancet 2009;374:210–221.

55. Kavanaugh A, McInnes I, Mease P, Krueger GG, Gladman D, Gomez-Reino J, Papp K, et al. Golimumab, a new human tumor necrosis factor α antibody, administered every four weeks as a subcutaneous injection in psoriatic arthritis: twenty-four-week efficacy and safety results of a randomized, placebo-controlled study. Arthritis Rheum 2009;60:976–986.

56. Inman RD, Davis JC Jr., Heijde D, Diekman L, Sieper J, Kim SI, Mack M, et al. Efficacy and safety of golimumab in patients with ankylosing spondylitis: results of a randomized, double-blind, placebo-controlled, phase III trial. Arthritis Rheum 2008;58:3402–3412.

57. McCluggage LK, Scholtz JM. Golimumab: a tumor necrosis factor alpha inhibitor for the treatment of rheumatoid arthritis. Ann Pharmacother 2010;44(1):135–144.

58. Fleischmann R, Vencovsky J, van Vollenhoven RF, et al. Efficacy and safety of certolizumab pegol monotherapy every 4 weeks in patients with rheumatoid arthritis failing previous disease-modifying antirheumatic therapy: the FAST4WARD study. Ann Rheum Dis 2009;68:805–811.

59. Smolen J, Landewé RB, Mease P, Brzezicki J, Mason D, Luijtens K, van Vollenhoven RF, et al. Efficacy and safety of certolizumab pegol plus methotrexate in active rheumatoid arthritis: the RAPID 2 study. A randomised controlled trial. Ann Rheum Dis 2009;68:797–804.

60. Sandborn WJ, Feagan BG, Stoinov S, Honiball PJ, Rutgeerts P, Mason D, Bloomfield R, et al. and the PRECiSE 1 Study Investigators. Certolizumab pegol for the treatment of Crohn's disease. N Engl J Med 2007;357:228–238.

61. Schreiber S, Khaliq-Kareemi M, Lawrance IC, Thomsen OØ, Hanauer SB, McColm J, Bloomfield R, et al. and the PRECiSE 2 Study Investigators. Maintenance therapy with certolizumab pegol for Crohn's disease. N Engl J Med 2007;357:239–250.

62. Allez M, Vermeire S, Mozziconacci N, Michetti P, Laharie D, Louis E, Bigard MA, et al. Efficacy and safety of a third anti-TNF monoclonal antibody in Crohn's disease after failure of two other anti-TNF. Aliment Pharmacol Ther 2009;31(1):92–101.

63. Cua DJ, Sherlock J, Chen Y, Murphy CA, Joyce B, Seymour B, Lucian L, et al. Interleukin-23 rather than interleukin-12 is the critical cytokine for autoimmune inflammation of the brain. Nature 2003;421:744–748.

64. Murphy CA, Langrish CL, Chen Y, Blumenschein W, McClanahan T, Kastelein RA, Sedgwick JD, Cua DJ. Divergent pro- and antiinflammatory roles for IL-23 and IL-12 in joint autoimmune inflammation. J Exp Med 2003;198:1951–1957.

65. Hue S, Ahern P, Buonocore S, Kullberg MC, Cua DJ, McKenzie BS, Powrie F, Maloy KJ. Interleukin-23 drives innate and T cell-mediated intestinal inflammation. J Exp Med 2006;203:2473–2483.

66. Nakee S, Nambu A, Sudo K, Iwakura Y. Suppression of immune induction of collagen-induced arthritis in IL-17 deficient mice. J Immunol 2003;171:6173–6177.

67. Lubberts E, Joosten LA, Oppers B, van den Bersselaar L, Coenende Roo CJ, Kolls JK, Schwarzenberger P, van de Loo FA, van den Berg WB. IL-1-independent role of IL-17 in synovial inflammation and joint destruction during collagen-induced arthritis. J Immunol 2201;167:1004–1013.

68. Lubberts E, Koenders MI, Oppers-Walgreen B, van den Bresselaar L, Coenen-de Roo CJ, Joosten LA, van den Berg WB. Treatment with a neutralizing anti-murine interleukin-17 antibody after the onset of collagen-induced arthritis reduces joint inflammation, cartilage destruction and bone erosion. Arthritis Rheum 2004;50:650–659.

69. Raychaudhuri SP, Jiang WY, Raychaudhuri SK. Revisiting the Koebner phenomenon: role of NGF and its receptor system in the pathogenesis of psoriasis. Am J Pathol 2008;172(4):961–971.

70. Raychaudhuri SP, Sanyal M, Weltman H, Kundu-Raychaudhuri S. K252a, a high-affinity nerve growth factor receptor blocker, improves psoriasis: an in vivo study using the severe combined immunodeficient mouse–human skin model. J Invest Dermatol 2004;122(3):812–819.

71. Pincelli C, Pignattim M. Keratinocyte-based mechanisms are trendy again in psoriasis-the role of a K252a derivative as a novel treatment. European Dermatology Review 2006;3:13–16.

72. Shelton DL, Zeller J, Ho WH, Pons J, Rosenthal A. Nerve growth factor mediates hyperalgesia and cachexia in auto-immune arthritis. Pain 2005;116(1–2):8–16.

73. Lane N, Webster L, Lu S, Gray M, Hefti F, Walicke P. RN624 (Anti-NGF) improves pain and function in subjects with moderate knee osteoarthritis: a phase 1 study. Arthritis Rheum 2005;52(Suppl):9.

12 Topical Applications for Pain and Arthritic Diseases

Norifumi Tanida, Kotaro Maekawa, and Masaru Nakanishi

CONTENTS

INTRODUCTION

Topical preparations now used for treatment of arthritis in the medical practice include hyaluronic acid, steroid, and nonsteroidal anti-inflammatory drugs (NSAIDs) for topical use.

Intra-articular injection of hyaluronic acid is used for compensation for deficiency of hyaluronic acid, which acts as a cushion or lubricant in joints, so that joint pain may be relieved. Intra-articular injection of a steroid is sometimes used for suppression of severe inflammation in joints. However, intra-articular injection of a steroid sometimes causes adverse reactions such as steroid arthropathy. Intra-articular injections are associated with infection risks, and therefore they should be used very cautiously. In addition, they are undesirable in convenience because self-administration is impossible.

On the other hand, external preparations, being excellent in convenience, have widely been used in various fields. However, steroids for external use in treatment of arthritis are considered to induce adverse reactions frequently after long-term continuous using (skin atrophy, skin infection risk, and influence on pituitary–adrenocortical function). NSAID preparations for external use are recognized to be excellent not only in convenience but also in good balance between safety and effectiveness and are now used widely in treatment of various types of arthritis and periarthritis.

HISTORY OF EXTERNAL PREPARATIONS

The history of external preparations is said to have begun in about 1000 BC in the ancient Babylonian era. Letters "poulitice" and "plaster" are found engraved in the clay tablet, suggesting that patch may have been used already in this era. External preparations were then spread out all over the world and are said to have been introduced to Japan in the late 18th century [1].

Preparations for external use have made unique progress in Japan: Various types of NSAIDs external preparations including ointments, liquid, creams, cataplasms, and tape preparations have been developed and are now used widely in clinical practice. Various topical NSAIDs such as ketoprofen, indomethacin, felbinac, flurbiprofen, diclofenac, and loxoprofen are now on the market (Table 12.1).

Especially patches such as cataplasms and tape preparations have established their positions as traditional medications in Japan because they can easily be applied to the affected area, can provide some relief to the patient because of visible medication, and are generally better in percutaneous absorption than other external preparations.

These patches have scientifically been confirmed in clinical studies to be effective for treatment of various types of arthritis and periarthritis such as osteoarthritis, low back pain, shoulder periarthritis, tenosynovitis, peritendinitis, and humeral epicondylitis (tennis elbow) and have formed a big market at present in Japan.

In the United States, NSAIDs have been used principally as oral preparations, and gel preparations among their preparations for external use have only rarely been used. In 2007, however, Flector® Patch (aqueous cataplasm of diclofenac epolamine) was approved as the first NSAID patch preparation in the United States, and its sales has rapidly increased. In addition, diclofenac tape and ketoprofen tape are being developed in clinical trials in anticipation of being approved as the first NSAID tape preparation in the United States. Thus, the option for additional NSAID patches will be available in the clinical practice in the United States and Japan, and therefore the demand for topical NSAIDs will expand further.

Among the reasons for worldwide expanding demand for topical NSAIDs, especially for patches, the most significant one is avoidance of NSAID-induced gastrointestinal disorders. NSAID oral preparations with potent anti-inflammatory analgesic effects are used very frequently in treatment of arthritis and periarthritis, but it has emerged as a problem in that they may cause gastrointestinal disorders such as gastric ulcer at a high incidence as adverse reactions. Many deaths have been reported in Europe and in the United States that are attributable to hemorrhage or perforation in the event of gastrointestinal disorders. According to an investigation in the United States, as many as 13 million patients took NSAID oral preparations per year, among whom about 100,000 patients had to be hospitalized for treatment of gastrointestinal disorders and about 16,500 patients died [2].

For avoidance of adverse reactions peculiar to NSAIDs, cyclooxygenase (COX)-2-selective inhibitors have been developed. NSAID-induced gastrointestinal disorders are considered to be

TABLE 12.1
The Main Topical NSAIDs Marketed in Japan, United States, and Europe

Japan	United States	Europe
Diclofenac	Diclofenac	Diclofenac
Ketoprofen		Ketoprofen
Indomethacin		Ibuprofen
Flurbiprofen		Piroxicum
Ferbinac		
Loxoprofen		

caused by inhibition of COX-1, which is produced constantly in the body and is said to be involved in the repair of tissues such as gastric mucosa. Because it is theoretically possible to avoid gastrointestinal disorders by selective inhibition of inflammation-induced COX-2, COX-2 inhibitors have actively been developed so far. Concerning COX-2-selective inhibitors, however, cardiovascular risks have become critical issues [3].

On the other hand, topical NSAIDs did not yet gain worldwide use because only insufficient clinical evidence was obtained until recently. Patches containing NSAIDs with good percutaneous permeability and strong activity have been developed, and evidences have been accumulated that they can deliver the drug substance directly to the restricted area in the region, that they are expected to have clinical effectiveness equivalent to that of oral preparations, and that they can relieve gastrointestinal disorders. These evidences suggest that topical NSAIDs will make rapid expansion in near future. In this chapter, evidences about topical NSAIDs are outlined in expectation of promotion of better understanding of topical NSAIDs.

CHARACTERISTICS OF TOPICAL PREPARATIONS

Topical preparations, in general, have the following characteristics as compared with injections and oral preparations and are very desirable from the viewpoint of improvement of patient's compliance and quality of life level.

- They can avoid risks and troubles associated with injection.
- They can be administered to patients in whom oral administration is impossible (patients with aphagia or abnormalities in the gastrointestinal tract).
- They can be administered easily (self-administration is possible).
- Whether or not administration has been performed can be confirmed, and this provides reassurance.
- They can avoid the first-pass effect and show high bioavailability.
- They can maintain a stable tissue concentration.
- Patients' (particularly elderly patients' and pediatric patients') compliance is high.
- Discontinuation of administration is easy.

Topical preparations are classified into paints such as ointments, lotions, and creams and patches such as cataplasms and tape preparations [4].

For administration to joint regions in various types of arthritis and periarthritis, paints that can be applied freely to the affected area are better in usability and in convenience. However, paints have problems in use in that the application site feels tacky when ointments are used and that hands and clothes are stained when paints are applied. In contrast, patches are characterized in that long-term persistence of the effect of the drug can be expected by once or twice daily application to the affected area without requiring repeated application which paints require. Topical patches to be applied to joint regions in the shoulder and knees are prepared by spreading the adhesive polymer containing the active drug substance over the stretch backing cross so that the preparation may be fit to the joint region. Such a preparation, when applied to the joint region, is expected to protect the affected area (acting as a supporter). Cataplasm, retaining a lot of water in the base, is expected to have effects to relieve inflammation based on the cooling effect of water. Topical patches are required to be adhesive enough to prevent detachment or dropout in the application period and at the same time they are required to suppress skin irritation in removal of the preparation. It is known that one of the causes of skin irritation is the stripping of the stratum corneum at removal of a patch. Mohrus tape® containing ketoprofen has excellent adhesiveness and readhesion and has no skin irritation because the stratum corneum is not stripped at removal

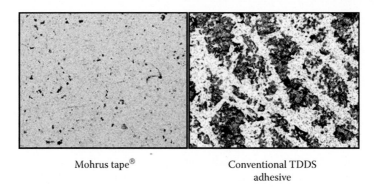

Mohrus tape®   Conventional TDDS
                                                adhesive

FIGURE 12.1   (See color insert.) Optical microscope photograph of the comparison of corneocytes peeling off at patch removal. The corneocytes (stratum corneum) peeling off at patch removal were stained with dye solution (amid black), and stained corneocytes were observed with optical microscopy. (Terahara, unpublished data.)

of a patch (Figure 12.1). The patches should have appropriate adhesiveness in good balance of these two requirements.

PERCUTANEOUS ABSORPTION AND PHARMACOLOGICAL ACTIVITIES OF NSAIDS

PERCUTANEOUS ABSORPTION OF NSAIDS

The most popular active drug substance for topical preparations is NSAIDs, and topical preparations containing indomethacin, ketoprofen, diclofenac sodium, or flurbiprofen are commercially available in Japan.

Yano et al. [5] compared percutaneous absorbability among various NSAIDs. A solution containing an NSAID in acetone was applied onto the skin, the drug remaining on the skin was collected after 4 h, and the amount percutaneously absorbed was calculated from the amount of the drug remaining on the skin. Salicylic acid and ketoprofen were absorbed well, whereas the amount percutaneously absorbed was relatively low for diclofenac and indomethacin. A parabolic relationship was noted between the amount percutaneously absorbed and the n-octanol/water partition coefficient of each drug (Figure 12.2). This result suggests that suitable lipophilicity is need to good percutaneous absorption.

PHARMACOLOGICAL ACTIVITIES OF NSAIDS

NSAIDs are supposed to exert anti-inflammatory action and analgesic action by inhibition of COX, which is involved in production of prostaglandin E_2 (PGE_2). There are two subtypes of COX: the subtype COX-1 occurs constantly in the body, and the subtype COX-2 is induced by inflammation. Cryer et al. [6] studied *in vitro* inhibitory activities of NSAIDs on COX-1 and COX-2 in the whole blood from healthy adults using inhibitory activity on thromboxane synthesis (COX-1 assay) and inhibitory activity on lipopolysaccharide-induced PGE_2 production (COX-2 assay). The results demonstrated that diclofenac had the most potent COX-2 inhibitory activity among the existing NSAIDs (Table 12.2). Ketoprofen was less potent than diclofenac and indomethacin, more potent than flurbiprofen in COX-2 inhibitory activity, and most potent in COX-1 inhibitory activity. As mentioned earlier, COX-2 that is induced by inflammatory reaction is supposed to be deeply involved in the aggravation of inflammatory reaction. However, PGE_2 is constantly produced also by COX-1, and

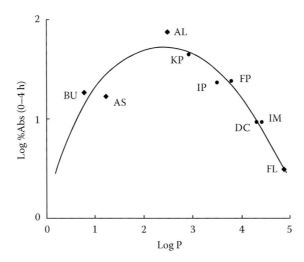

FIGURE 12.2 Relationship between log %Abs and log P of anti-inflammatory drugs. AL, alclofenac; AS, aspirin; BU, bufexamac; DC, diclofenac; FL, flufenamic acid; FP, flurbiprofen; IP, ibuprofen; IM, indomethacin; KP, ketoprofen. (From Yano, T., Nakagawa, A., Tsuji, M., and Noda, K., *Life Sci.,* 39, 1043–1050, 1986.)

therefore it is meaningful for the local area of the site of inflammation that both COX-1 and COX-2 are inhibited so that total PGE_2 production at the local area is reduced. In conclusion, diclofenac which is the most potent in COX-2 inhibitory activity among the existing NSAIDs is assumed to exert a potent anti-inflammatory action even when the drug concentration at the inflammation site is low, and it is a suitable drug for topical preparations. Ketoprofen is not suitable for systemic application because it is potent in COX-1 inhibitory activity but may be suitable for topical application.

PHARMACOKINETIC CHARACTERISTICS, EFFICACY, AND SAFETY OF TOPICAL NSAIDS

DICLOFENAC

Diclofenac is one of the NSAIDs that are most frequently used in the world. Its topical preparations of various dosage forms including lotions, gels, cataplasms, and tape preparations are commercially available in Japan, in the United States, and in Europe. In the United States, a gel (Voltaren Gel®) and a cataplasm (Flector®), in addition to a lotion, were approved by the Food and Drug Administration in 2007 and are now on the market. In Japan, gels, liquid preparations, cataplasms, and tape preparations were approved as over-the-counter drugs in 2009 and are now used not only for prescription by physicians but also widely as nonprescription drugs. Topical diclofenac have gained widespread use because its oral preparations had already been established as standard NSAID preparations. Diclofenac, being scientifically confirmed to have the most potent COX-2-inhibiting activity among the existing NSAIDs, is expected to exert potent pharmacological effects. This potent pharmacological activity may also be one of the factors that have led to widespread use of diclofenac as a drug for percutaneous absorption.

Absorption and Distribution of Topical Diclofenac

Yoshida et al. [7] applied a diclofenac sodium–containing gel (10 mg/g) at the daily dose of 5 or 15 g repeatedly for 6–7 days to patients (12 patients) who were planned to receive joint replacement at the knee or at the hip for treatment of osteoarthritis and determined diclofenac concentrations in plasma, synovial fluid, and various tissues under the application site. High concentrations

TABLE 12.2
Concentration of Drug (IC50) that Inhibited 50% of COX Activity in Blood and in Gastric Mucosa (µM)

Drug	COX-1 in Blood (Rank)	COX-2 in Blood (Rank)	Gastric Mucosa (Rank)
Ketoprofen	0.11 (1)	0.88 (8)	0.08 (2)
Indomethacin	0.21 (2)	0.37 (7)	0.85 (11)
Diclofenac	0.26 (3)	0.01 (1)	0.23 (4)
Ketorolac	0.27 (4)	0.18 (6)	0.33 (6)
Flurbiprofen	0.41 (5)	4.23 (13)	0.23 (5)
Tolmetin	1.08 (6)	2.25 (11)	3.50 (16)
Mefenamic acid	1.94 (7)	0.16 (4)	0.70 (10)
Piroxicam	2.68 (8)	2.11 (10)	0.87 (12)
Fenoprofen	2.73 (9)	14.03 (17)	0.17 (3)
Aspirin	4.45 (10)	13.88 (16)	0.03 (1)
Ibuprofen	5.90 (11)	9.90 (14)	0.70 (9)
Nimesulide	10.48 (12)	0.18 (5)	1.49 (13)
Oxaprosin	14.58 (13)	36.67 (23)	2.62 (14)
Etodolac	19.58 (14)	2.47 (12)	3.20 (15)
NS-398	21.93 (15)	0.92 (9)	100.00 (18)
6-MNA	31.01 (16)	19.84 (19)	0.48 (7)
Naproxen	32.01 (17)	28.19 (22)	0.52 (8)
Valeryl salicylate	32.64 (18)	0.04 (2)	>100.00 (21)
Nabumetone	33.57 (19)	20.83 (20)	20.09 (17)
Sulindac	41.26 (20)	24.94 (21)	>100.00 (19)
Acetaminophen	42.23 (21)	10.69 (15)	>100.00 (23)
Dexamethasone	59.95 (22)	0.13 (3)	>100.00 (25)
Bismuth subsalicylate	75.24 (23)	37.50 (24)	>100.00 (22)
Salicylic acid	>100.00 (24)	14.08 (18)	>100.00 (20)
Salsalate	>100.00 (25)	39.90 (25)	>100.00 (24)

Source: Data from Cryer, B. and Feldman, M., *Am. J. Med.*, 104, 413–421, 1998.
Abbreviation: 6-MNA, 6-methoxy napthalene acetic acid.

of diclofenac were detected in the tissues and were higher than the plasma concentrations (Figure 12.3). The diclofenac concentration in the synovial membrane (5 g dose group: 34.7 ng/g; 15 g dose group: 14.7 ng/g) was remarkably higher than that in the plasma (5 g dose group: 2.2 ng/mL; 15 g dose group: 9.3 ng/mL). Bender et al. [8] administered orally Voltaren SR® (diclofenac sodium sustained release tablet) 75 mg tablet twice daily for 5 days to patients (10 patients) of coxarthrosis who were planned to receive joint replacement and determined diclofenac concentrations in the cartilage and in the synovial membrane to be 3.8 and 2.23 ng/mL, respectively. A mean plasma concentration was 25 ng/mL. The concentrations in the synovial membrane were higher after administration of a diclofenac gel than after oral administration, suggesting that a sufficient amount of the drug may permeate into the inside of the joint and to the surrounding tissues, the site of action, after percutaneous administration of a diclofenac gel. In addition, it is reported that diclofenac may permeate to these tissues after application of cataplasm and tape formulation of diclofenac (Table 12.3).

Efficacy and Safety of Topical Diclofenac

Brühlmann et al. [18] conducted a 2-week placebo-controlled double-blind study in 103 outpatients for the evaluation of efficacy and safety of diclofenac hydroxyethylpyrrolidine (DHEP) patch for osteoarthritis at the knee. The primary end point was Lequesne's Index, an index for

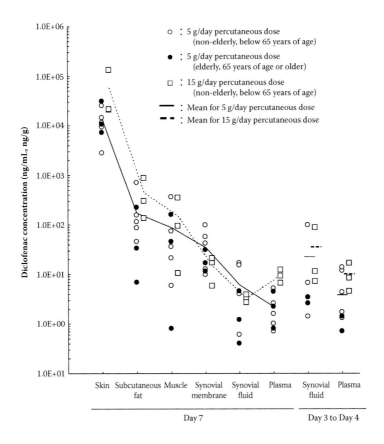

FIGURE 12.3 DF concentrations in plasma, synovial fluid and tissues after 1-week repeated percutaneous dose of TP318 at daily dose of 5 g or 15 g in patients with osteoarthropathy. (From Yoshida, H., Watanabe, H., and Chiba, K., *J. Clin. Ther. Med.*, 16(4), 393–405, 2000.)

evaluation of spontaneous pain and pain and function of the joint. Secondary indices used were duration of walking beyond the standard distance and the amount of an analgesic paracetamol consumed. Significant alleviation of pain was found in the group treated with the active drug in the Lequesne's Index and in the overall evaluation of the patients. There was no intergroup difference in respect of occurrence of adverse drug reactions. These results indicate that topical application of diclofenac patch is effective in relief of pain in osteoarthritis patients and represents a safe therapy.

Aoki et al. [19] also conducted a placebo-controlled double-blind study to investigate efficacy and safety of 1% diclofenac sodium gel (TP318) in knee osteoarthritis patients. TP318 was given to 198 subjects (99 each for the TP318 group and the placebo group). For final global improvement, "moderately improved" or "better" was 61.0% for the TP318 group and 40.5% for the placebo group. TP318 improved significantly ($p < 0.05$) compared with the placebo group. For improvement rate classified by symptom, tenderness was improved at 4 weeks in 75.0% for the TP318 group and 58.0% for the placebo group. TP318 improved significantly ($p < 0.05$) compared with the placebo group. Adverse events were seen in 3.2% and 3.1% for the TP318 and placebo groups, respectively. These results indicated that topical application of diclofenac gel is an effective and safe therapy for improvement of symptoms in osteoarthritis patients.

In addition to those mentioned earlier, there are many reports [20], and it may be concluded that diclofenac topical preparation is effective and safe for treatment of various types of arthritis and periarthritis including osteoarthritis.

TABLE 12.3
Summary of Single and Multiple Dose Topical NSAIDs Application Studies

Dosage	Route	n	Plasma Concentration (ng/mL)	Tissue Concentration (ng/mL or ng/g)	Ref.
Diclofenac					
30 mg of DF-Na tape (30 cm²) Slow-release capsule containing 37.5 mg of DF-Na	Topical application on knee Oral administration	14	Topical: 4.70 ± 1.95 (SD) Oral: 6.63 ± 4.54 (SD) At 12 h after application	Synovial fluid Topical: 1.96 ± 0.68 (SD) Oral: 16.76 ± 12.0 (SD) Synovial membrane Topical: 4.99 ± 3.84 (SD) Oral: 15.07 ± 9.17 (SD) Muscle Topical: 9.29 ± 8.34 (SD) Oral: 0.66 ± 1.11 (SD) At 12 h after application	[9]
180 mg of DHEP cataplasm (150 cm²) bid for 4 days	Topical application on knee	8	3.62 ± 1.05 (SE) At 4 h after application on day 5	Synovial fluid: 1.02 ± 0.38 (SE) At 4 h after application on day 5	[10]
80 mg of DF gel tid for 3 days	Topical application on knee	10	40.6 ± 4.7 (SE) At 4 h after application on day 4	Synovial fluid: 25.5 ± 3.6 (SE) At 4 h after application on day 4	[11]
80 mg of DF foam bid for 7 days	Topical application on thigh	12	C_{max}: 18.75 ± 4.97 (SE)	C_{max} in skeletal muscle: 219.68 ± 66.36 (SE) Microdialysis for 10 h	[12]
Ketoprofen					
30 mg of KP cataplasm once daily for 5 days Capsule containing 50 mg of KP once daily	Topical application on ankle or knee Oral administration	60	Topical: 17.9 (C_{max}) Oral: 2253.1 (C_{max})	Tendon sheath Topical: 5026.3 (C_{max}) Oral: 298.8 (C_{max}) Tendon Topical: 952.8 (C_{max}) Oral: 283.1 (C_{max})	[13]
5-cm-strip of KP gel with and without ultrasound	Topical application on knee	26	Below 4 ng/mL at 120 min after application	Synovial tissue With ultrasound: 28650 Sham: 2000 At 58 min after application	[14]

Drug / Dose	Application	n	Plasma concentration	Tissue concentration	Ref.
Ibuprofen 375 mg of IP gel tid for 3 days 600 mg IP tablet bid for 3 days	Topical application on knee Oral administration	17	Topical:1000 ± 500 (SD) Oral: 1600 ± 1300 (SD) At 15 h after application on day 4	Synovial fluid Topical: 1300 ± 1100 (SD) Oral: 2200 ± 1900 (SD) Fasciae Topical: 2700 ± 1700 (SD) Oral: 2900 ± 2800 (SD) Muscle Topical: 8400 ± 8900 (SD) Oral: 5300 ± 3700 (SD) At 15 h after application on day 4	[15]
400 mg of IP gel tid for 3 days	Topical application on knee	8	91 ± 46 (SD) At 10 h after the last application	Tendon: 8670 ± 1510 (SD) Muscle: 20320 ± 3470 (SD) Joint capsule: 6920 ± 940 (SD)	[16]
Indomethacin 50 mg of IM gel	Topical application on knee, waist, and hip joint	14	ND–194.8	Muscle: 22.2–817.4 Synovial membrane: 64.1–1482.6 Synovial fluid: N.D.–399.5	[17]

Abbreviations: bid, twice daily; DF, diclofenac; DF-Na, diclofenac sodium; DHEP, diclofenac hydroxyethylpyrrolidine; IM, indomethacin; IP, ibuprofen; KP, ketoprofen; ND, not detected; tid, three times daily.

KETOPROFEN

Also topical preparations containing ketoprofen are now on the market in Japan and Europe in various dosage forms such as gel, cataplasm, and tape preparation. Ketoprofen, as mentioned earlier, is excellent in percutaneous absorbability so that much of the dose is delivered to the local action site to exert its effects.

Ketoprofen is used in a gel and a patch in Europe. In Japan, various dosage forms including liquid preparations, creams, cataplasms, and tape preparations have been developed since launching of the gel in 1986. After cataplasms and tape preparations went on sale, the ketoprofen topical preparations, especially the tape preparation, made a huge market and the total sales of the tape preparation (Mohrus tape®) and the cataplasm (Mohrus® pap) grew to be ranked in the top 10 drugs with high sales in Japan. A reason why the ketoprofen tape preparation accomplished such a rapid growth may be that the preparation has the most indications among the NSAID-containing tape preparations. The indications of the tape preparation are as follows: analgesia and anti-inflammation in patients with chronic symptoms (circulatory deficit, muscle spasm, and muscle contracture) of osteoarthropathy, low back pain (muscular/fascial low back pain, spondylosis deformans, disk disease, and back strain), shoulder periarthritis, tendonitis/tenosynovitis, peritendinitis, and humeral epicondylitis (tennis elbow, etc.). Recently Mohrus tape® was approved for an additional indication for chronic rheumatoid arthritis. Ketoprofen, as mentioned earlier, is one of the drugs best in percutaneous absorbability among the existing NSAIDs, and this characteristic is considered to be a factor that made the drug be indicated for various types of arthritis and periarthritis with a variety of pathological aspects.

Absorption and Distribution of Topical Ketoprofen

Yano et al. [21] conducted an absorption test in guinea pigs, where ketoprofen concentrations in fascia, muscle, and plasma were determined after administration of ketoprofen-containing tape and cataplasm, and oral ketoprofen and exposure was compared among tissues. The results demonstrated that tissue exposure and the ratio of tissue to plasma concentration were larger after administration of the tape or the cataplasm than after oral administration, indicating that topical application can deliver Ketoprofen at high concentration to the tissues under the application site (Table 12.4). Comparison between the tape and the cataplasm revealed that the tissue concentration was higher after administration of the tape, indicating that the tape is superior in percutaneous absorption.

It has been demonstrated in Mexican hairless pigs that the drug is delivered to the tissues immediately below the application site [22]. After a 12-h application of 2% ketoprofen-containing tape preparation to the back of Mexican hairless pigs, ketoprofen was detected in the skin, subcutaneous fat, fascia, superficial muscle, and deep muscle (Figure 12.4). The ketoprofen concentration was the lowest in the deep muscle among the tissues but higher than the plasma concentration.

Ballerini et al. [23] applied 2.5% ketoprofen gel (Fastum gel) to around the knee joint once a day repeatedly from 3 days before the operation (70–80 mg on ketoprofen) in patients (six patients) and determined the ketoprofen concentration in the intra-articular adipose tissue, capsular tissue, synovial fluid, and plasma. The ketoprofen concentration was 4.70 μg/g in the intra-articular adipose tissue, 2.35 μg/g in the capsular tissue, and 1.31 μg/g in the synovial fluid, which were about 100-fold higher than the plasma concentration (0.018 μg/g).

Rolf et al. [24] applied ketoprofen cataplasms (containing 30 mg ketoprofen) on one occasion (40 patients) or once a day repeatedly from 5 days before the operation (30 patients) to the knee joint of patients with knee joint disease who were planned to receive knee arthroscopic surgery and determined the ketoprofen concentration in plasma and in the intra-articular tissues (synovial tissue, meniscus, cartilage, and synovial fluid). The same determination was performed also in patients (30 patients) who received single oral administration of 50 mg ketoprofen immediate release tablet. The median C_{max} of the ketoprofen concentration in tissues was compared between the cataplasms percutaneous administration group and the oral administration group: the T/O ratio (the ratio of the concentration after the cataplasms percutaneous administration group to the concentration after the oral administration group)

TABLE 12.4
Elimination Half-Life ($T_{1/2}$) and AUC$_{0-24h}$ of the Radioactivity in Fascia, Muscles, and Plasma After a Single Application of [^{14}C]KPT and [^{14}C] HKP to Intact Skin as well as After Oral Administration of [^{14}C]KP to Guinea Pigs

	$T_{1/2}$ (h)	AUC$_{0-24h}$ (µg eq.*h/g or mL)	Tissue/Plasma AUC
Single topical application of [14C]KPT			
Plasma	32.49	2.41	
Fascia	34.90	27.24	11.30
Muscle	20.03	6.41	2.66
Single topical application of [14C]HKP			
Plasma	12.67	2.10	
Fascia	9.63	7.98	3.80
Muscle	5.06	2.35	1.12
Oral administration of [^{14}C]KP (5 mg/kg)			
Plasma	1.92	5.93	
Fascia	1.61	0.88	0.15
Muscle	1.35	0.59	0.10

Source: Data from Yano, T., Wada, M., Furukawa, K., et al., *Iyukuhin Kenkyu*, 24(7), 727–741, 1993.

Note: [^{14}C]KPT, ketoprofen-containing tape. Ketoprofen content = 1.51 mg; adhesive mass = 76.0 mg; application area = 5.29 cm^2.
[^{14}C]HKP, ketoprofen-containing cataplasm. Ketoprofen content = 1.50 mg; adhesive mass = 500 mg; application area = 7.00 cm^2.

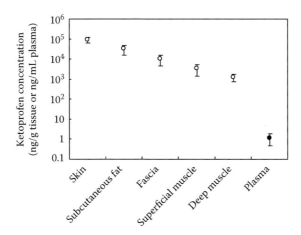

FIGURE 12.4 Ketoprofen concentration in the tissues at 12 h after the ketoprofen patch application to the back of pigs. Mean ± SE are shown (*n* = 4). (From Horie, M., Sekiya, I., Nakamura, T., et al., *Biopharm. Drug Dispos.*, 30(4), 204–208, 2009.)

in plasma was 0.0034, whereas the T/O ratio in the synovial tissue and synovial fluid were 0.2 and 0.036, respectively. This result indicates that percutaneous administration can suppress the systemic exposure to the drug while delivering the drug at a high concentration to the intra-articular tissues.

Osterwalder et al. [25] applied ketoprofen tape preparation (containing 100 mg ketoprofen) once a day repeatedly from 6 days before the operation to patients who were planned to receive operation at the knee joint or at the wrist (5 patients each) and determined ketoprofen concentration in plasma and in tissues immediately below the application site. The ketoprofen concentration in the synovial tissue after application to the knee was about sixfold higher than the plasma concentration. The ketoprofen concentration in the tendon sheath after application to the wrist was about 354-fold higher than the plasma concentration, indicating that the tape preparation can also deliver the drug directly to the joint tissues.

As mentioned so far, percutaneous administration of ketoprofen topical preparations in various dosage forms can deliver the drug directly to the tissue below application site (Table 12.3).

Efficacy and Safety of Topical Ketoprofen

Takagishi et al. [26] applied cataplasm containing 0.3% of ketoprofen (HKP-210) to patients with knee osteoarthritis and obtained the following results. Comparators of HKP-210 were HKP-210 placebo and Papsalon G, an adhesive skin patch containing methyl salicylate, for comparison among three groups consisting of 106, 108, and 104 patients, respectively. The rate of improvement expressed by percentage of patients with moderate or better improvement in the HKP-210 group was significantly higher than that in other groups. Adverse drug reactions were found in five patients in the HKP-210 group, and this incidence was not different from that in other groups. These results indicated that topical application of ketoprofen cataplasm is an effective and safe therapy for alleviation of symptoms in osteoarthritis patients.

Sugioka et al. [27] conducted a double-blind study by the double dummy method for comparison of a tape preparation containing 2% of ketoprofen (KPT -220, the K group hereinafter) with ketoprofen oral preparation (the C group hereinafter) in patients with low back pain. The number of patients included in the analysis was 121 (59 in the K group and 62 in the C group) for evaluation of final overall improvement, 161 (79 in the K group and 82 in the C group) for evaluation of global safety, and 133 (62 in the K group and 71 in the C group) for evaluation of usefulness. As for the final overall improvement, the improvement rate expressed by the percentage of patients who showed "moderate improvement" or "better" improvement was 62.7% (37/59) in the K group and 61.3% (38/62) in the C group; that is, improvement rate was comparable between the two groups (Table 12.5). The incidence of adverse reactions was 8.9% (7/79) in the K group and 20.7% (17/82) in the C group (Table 12.6). No patient in the K group discontinued the treatment because of adverse

---

TABLE 12.5

Final Overall Improvement After Treatment of Ketoprofen-Containing Tape Preparation or Oral Ketoprofen in Patients with Low Back Pain

Drug	Remarkably Improved	Moderately Improved	Mildly Improved	Unchanged	Aggravated	Total	χ^2 test[a]	U test
K group	13 (22.0)	24 (62.7)	17 (91.5)	5 (100.0)	0	59	NS	NS
C group	13 (21.0)	25 (61.3)	17 (88.7)	6 (98.4)	1 (100.0)	62		

Source: Data from Sugioka, Y., Takagishi, N., Inoue, A., and Asano, C., *Jpn. Pharmacol. Ther.*, 22(9), 349–370, 1994.

Note: Values in parentheses are cumulative percentages. A double-blind study by the double dummy method was conducted for comparison of a tape preparation containing 2% of ketoprofen (KPT-220, the K group) with ketoprofen oral preparation (the C group) in patients with low back pain. The tape preparations were topically applied to the affected site once a day for 2 weeks. The oral preparations were administered three times a day for 2 weeks.

[a] The χ^2 test was performed after categorization of the patients into those who showed "moderate or better improvement" and those who showed worse than moderate improvement.

reactions, whereas seven patients in the C group discontinued; the number of discontinued patients was significantly larger in the C group. Stomach pain/stomach discomfort was found in one patient in the K group and in nine patients in the C group. The percentage of patients who were regarded as "safe" in global safety was 91.1% (72/79) in the K group and 79.3% (65/82) in the C group; the safety was significantly higher in the K group. These results indicated that KPT-220 is almost as effective as ketoprofen oral preparation for low back pain and superior to the oral preparation in safety.

There is no report of clinical study for comparison between a topical preparation and an oral preparation using ulcerogenesis in the stomach as the index, whereas in nonclinical studies in animals, there was evident difference in ulcerogenic effects between the two preparations [28]. In male Wistar rats, gastrointestinal disorder in respect of ulcerogenesis in the stomach and in the small intestine was compared between percutaneous application of 1%–10% ketoprofen tape preparation (KPT) and oral administration of ketoprofen. Ulcerogenic effect was hardly found in the groups given KPT of 3% or less and in the groups given oral preparation at 2 mg/kg or less (Table 12.7).

TABLE 12.6
Details of Adverse Reactions After Treatment of Ketoprofen-Containing Tape or Oral Ketoprofen in Patients with Low Back Pain

Item	Drug		χ^2 Test or Fisher's Exact Test[b]
	K Group	C Group	
Number of patients included in analysis	79	82	N.S.
Number of patients with adverse reactions	7 (8.9)	17 (20.7)	$p_0 = 0.015$
Number of discontinued patients because of adverse reactions[a]	0	7	K group < C group
Number of events of adverse reactions	8	23	
Systemic symptoms	7 [6]	16 [14]	NS
Gastrointestinal symptoms	4 [4]	14 [13]	NS
Constipation	2	2	
Stomach pain	1	4	
Abdominal pain	1	1	
Stomach discomfort	0	5	
Heaviness in stomach	0	1	
Feeling sick at the stomach	0	1	
Other symptoms	3 [3]	2 [1]	NS
Facial rash	1	0	
Facial edema	0	1	
General malaise	0	1	
Urticaria	1	0	
Stomatitis	1	0	
Skin symptoms at application site	1 [1]	7 [6]	NS
Small papule	1	0	
Itching	0	1	
Itch	0	2	
Redness	0	1	
Eczema	0	1	
Poisoning rash	0	1	
Skin irritation	0	1	

Source: Data from Sugioka, Y., Takagishi, N., Inoue, A., Asano, C., *Jpn. Pharmacol. Ther.*, 22(9), 349–370, 1994.

Note: Values in brackets are the number of patients with the adverse reaction; values in parentheses, %.

[a] Number of patients where administration of the preparation containing the active substance was discontinued.

[b] Tests were performed on the data of number of patients.

TABLE 12.7
Ulcerogenic Effects of Various KPT (Ketoprofen-Containing Tape) and Oral Ketoprofen on the Stomach in Fasted Rats

Drug	Dose (cm²)	Dose (mg/kg)	Route	Ulcer Index	Ulcer Rate	UD_{50} (ng/kg) (95% CI)
None	–	–	–	0.25 ± 0.16	0/8	49.9 (19.4–126.0)[a]
KPT base	3 × 3	–	Topical	0.75 ± 0.16	0/8	
1% KPT	3 × 3	–	Topical	0.50 ± 0.27	1/8	
2% KPT	3 × 3	–	Topical	0.75 ± 0.25	1/8	
3% KPT	3 × 3	–	Topical	1.13 ± 0.35	2/8	
10% KPT	3 × 3	–	Topical	1.75 ± 0.45	5/8	
Ketoprofen	–	1	Oral	0.75 ± 0.25	1/8	3.6 (2.3–5.6)
	–	2	Oral	1.25 ± 0.53	2/8	
	–	5	Oral	1.75 ± 0.37	5/8	
	–	10	Oral	2.25 ± 0.16	8/8	

Source: Data from Taniguchi, Y., Inui, K., Furuta, K., Saita, M. *Iyukuhin Kenkyu*, 24(8), 831–841, 1993.

Note: Each KPT preparation was topically applied to the dorsal skin for 6 h, and ketoprofen was orally administered. Ulcerogenic activity was evaluated at 6 h after a single administration of each drug. UD_{50} value and 95% confidence interval (CI) were calculated from the number of rats with ulcer. Ulcer index represents the mean ± SE of eight animals.

[a]   Dose as ketoprofen.

Ulcerogenesis in the stomach was clearly found in the group given 10% KPT and in the group given oral preparation at 5 mg/kg. The UD_{50} value (on ketoprofen basis) of KPT was 49.9 mg/kg for the stomach and 48.9 mg/kg for the small intestine, whereas the UD_{50} value of ketoprofen orally administered was 3.6 mg/kg for the stomach and 3.7 mg/kg for the small intestine; thus, the doses for ulcerogenesis in the stomach and in the small intestine were about 13-fold higher with KPT than with ketoprofen orally administered. When the fact is taken into account that 2% KPT was effective enough but caused no ulcer in a different experimental system, it is assumed that ketoprofen tape preparation can clinically bring about great relief of gastrointestinal disorders.

Ketoprofen tape preparation is indicated for treatment of various inflammatory diseases in the musculoskeletal system but not for treatment of rheumatoid arthritis at present. Rheumatoid arthritis, being a systemic inflammatory autoimmune disease, is treated primarily by stabilization of the systemic immune status by an immunosuppressant such as methotrexate or tacrolimus or by a biopharmaceutical such as anti–tumor necrosis factor α antibody. However, the use of a topical anti-inflammatory agent is considered to be meaningful for suppression of symptoms such as pain and inflammation that still persist in some joints even when systemic conditions are stabilized. Rat adjuvant arthritis model and rat collagen arthritis model are experimental chronic inflammation models and were used to evaluate the pharmacological efficacy of the ketoprofen-containing tape preparation [29]: The preparation showed edema-suppressing effect in both chronic inflammation models (Figures 12.5 and 12.6). In the adjuvant arthritis model study, pain threshold was also determined on each day of assessment: The ketoprofen tape preparation was confirmed to show the analgesic effect from day 3 of treatment as observed for the edema-suppressing effect (Figure 12.7). These two different arthritis models are generally regarded as resembling to human rheumatoid arthritis in pathogenesis and established histopathological findings [30, 31]. Therefore, the ketoprofen containing tape preparations is expected to be effective also in human rheumatoid arthritis.

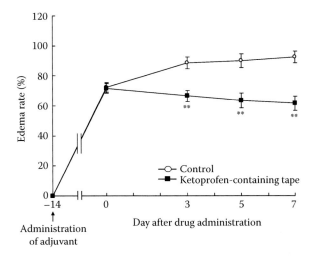

FIGURE 12.5 Anti-inflammatory effects of ketoprofen-containing tape on the adjuvant arthritis model in rats. Mean ± SE are shown ($n = 8$, $**p < 0.01$ vs control group). Arthritis was induced by injecting 1% w/v suspension of *Mycobacterium butyricum* in a volume of 0.1 mL subcutaneously into the left hind paw of male Lewis rats. Ketoprofen-containing tape (1 cm × 1 cm) was applied on the right hind paw for 24 h a day for 7 days continuously from the 14th day after the injection of the inflammatory agent. The volume of the right hind paw was determined on days 0, 3, 5, and 7 after the start of application of the preparation to calculate the edema rate. (Modified from Tanida, N. and Sakurada, S., *Jpn. Pharmacol. Ther.*, 36(12), 1123–1129, 2008.)

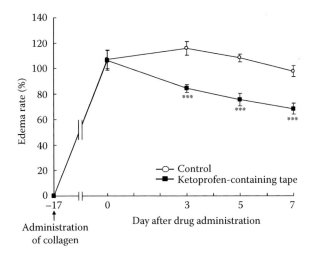

FIGURE 12.6 Anti-inflammatory effects of ketoprofen-containing tape on the collagen-induced arthritis model in rats. Mean ± SE are shown ($n = 10$, $***p < 0.001$ vs control group). Female DA rats were injected intradermally with 300 μg (0.4 mL) of bovine type-II collagen in four sites on the dorsal skin of the rats. Ketoprofen-containing tape (1 cm × 1 cm) was applied on the right hind paw for 24 h a day for 7 days continuously from the 17th day after the injection of the inflammatory agent. The volume of the right hind paw was determined on days 0, 3, 5, and 7 after the start of application of the preparation to calculate the edema rate. (Modified from Tanida, N. and Sakurada, S., *Jpn. Pharmacol. Ther.*, 36(12), 1123–1129, 2008.)

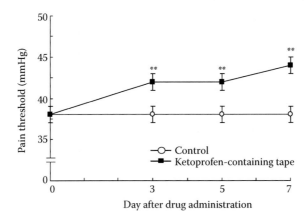

FIGURE 12.7 Analgesic effects of ketoprofen-containing tape on the adjuvant arthritis model in rats. Mean ± SE are shown ($n = 10$, $**p < 0.01$ vs control group). Arthritis was induced by injecting 1% w/v suspension of *Mycobacterium butyricum* in a volume of 0.1 mL subcutaneously into the left hind paw of male Lewis rats. Ketoprofen-containing tape (1 cm × 1 cm) was applied on the right hind paw for 24 h a day for 7 days continuously from the 14th day after the injection of the inflammatory agent. The pain threshold of the right hind paw was determined on days 3, 5, and 7 after the start of application of the preparation. (Terahara, unpublished data.)

As mentioned so far, the ketoprofen tape preparation is expected to be as effective as the oral preparation in treatment of various types of arthritis and periarthritis such as OA and RA and considered to be a preparation that can relieve gastrointestinal disorders associated with NSAIDs.

FUTURE CONSIDERATIONS

Topical NSAIDs are safer than oral preparations in respect of occurrence of systemic adverse reactions such as gastrointestinal disorders, and therefore they may be said to be easily accessible drugs of first choice for treatment of arthritis. The topical preparation may cause adverse reactions because of skin irritation, such as contact dermatitis. Some NSAIDs cause photoallergy contact dermatitis [32–36]. Therefore, after application of the topical NSAIDs to an area exposed to sunlight, the area should be shielded from sunlight. In addition, it is important to pay attention to a skin condition. When a large amount of the drug applied damages the skin, the topical preparation also causes gastrointestinal disorder.

Development of COX-2 inhibitors has slowed down because of cardiovascular adverse reactions. However, if systemic adverse reactions including cardiovascular adverse reactions could be avoided by a topical COX-2 inhibitor, COX-2 inhibitor would be selected as the next candidate for NSAIDs patches. In addition, recently some topical preparations except NSAIDs such as local anesthetics and vasodilators have been investigated as a novel target of topical preparations for arthritis treatments. Galer et al. [37] reported a 2-week, open-label study to evaluate the effectiveness and safety of lidocaine patch 5% monotherapy in adults with osteoarthritis pain of the knee. As a result, the effectiveness and safety of the lidocaine patch for pain relief was confirmed. Thus, topical preparations of drugs other than NSAIDs may be useful for treatment of arthritis in near future.

Oral NSAIDs are useful because of their potent anti-inflammatory and analgesic effect, whereas it is also true that many patients suffer from gastrointestinal disorders. Topical preparations that were developed in Japan have long established their positions as traditional therapies. Use of adhesive patches has gradually increased in the world but adhesive patches have not yet become as popular as in Japan. In the near future, many NSAID adhesive patches will be introduced to the market in many countries, including the United States, like in Japan. We hope that many patients will be relieved from pain of arthritis, and the benefits of treatment by application of a patch preparation will be known to the world.

REFERENCES

1. Ohno M. Cataplasms—drugs and culture grown in Japan [in Japanese]. Japan: Yakuji Nippo Ltd.; 2003.
2. Singh G. Recent considerations in nonsteroidal anti-inflammatory drug gastropathy. Am J Med 1998;105(1B):31S-38S.
3. Kerr DJ, Dunn JA, Langman MJ, Smith JL, Midgley RSJ, Stanley A, Stokes JC, et al. Rofecoxib and cardiovascular adverse events in adjuvant treatment of colorectal cancer. N Engl J Med 2007;357:360–369.
4. Kurata N, Choshi T. Types of non-steroidal anti-inflammatory drugs and its use [in Japanese]. Journal of Pain and Clinical Medicine 2005;5(4):65–72.
5. Yano T, Nakagawa A, Tsuji M, Noda K. Skin permeability of various non-steroidal anti-inflammatory drugs in man. Life Sci 1986;39:1043–1050.
6. Cryer B, Feldman M. Cyclooxygenase-1 and cyclooxygenase-2 selectivity of widely used nonsteroidal anti-inflammatory drugs. Am J Med 1998;104:413–421.
7. Yoshida H, Watanabe H, Chiba K. Percutaneous absorption and tissue distribution of TP318 [in Japanese]. Journal of Clinical Therapeutics and Medicine. 2000;16(4):393–405.
8. Bender T, Schafer M, Bariska J. Tissue concentration of the active substance of Voltaren SR 75 in articular cartilage, synovial membrane and bone. Clin Rheumatol 2000;19:89–91.
9. Miyatake S, Ichiyama H, Kondo E, Yasuda K. Randomized clinical comparisons of diclofenac concentration in the soft tissues and blood plasma between topical and oral applications. Br J Clin Pharmacol 2008;67:125–129.
10. Gallacchi G, Marcolongo R. Pharmacokinetics of diclofenac hydroxyethylpyrrolidine (DHEP) plasters in patients with monolateral knee joint effusion. Drugs Exp Clin Res 1993;XIX(3):97–100.
11. Radermacher J, Jentsch D, Scholl MA, Lustinetz T, Frolich JC. Diclofenac concentrations in synovial fluid and plasma after cutaneous application in inflammatory and degenerative joint disease. Br J Clin Phamacol 1991;31:537–541.
12. Muller M, Rastelli C, Ferri P, Jansen B, Breiteneder H, Eichler HG. Transdermal penetration of diclofenac after multiple epicutaneous administration. J Rheumatol 1998;25:1833–1836.
13. Rolf C, Movin T, Engstrom B, Jacobs LD, Beauchard C, Liboux A. An open, randomized study of ketoprofen in patients in surgery for Achilles or patellar tendinopathy. J Rheumatol 1997;24(8):1595–1598.
14. Cagnie B, Vinck E, Rimbaut S, Vanderstraeten G. Phonophoresis versus topical application of ketoprofen: comparison between tissue and plasma levels. Phys Ther 2003;83(8):707–712.
15. Dominkus M, Nicolakis M, Kotz R, Wilkinson FE, Kaiser RR, Chlud K. Comparison of tissue and plasma levels of ibuprofen after oral and topical administration. Arzeim-Forsch/Drug Res 1996;46(II):1138–1143.
16. Berner G, Engels B, Vogtle-Junkert U. Percutaneous ibuprofen therapy with Trauma-Dolgit gel: bioequivalence studies. Drug Exp Clin Res 1989;XV(11/12):559–564.
17. Sugawara S, Ohno H, Ueda R, Ishigami M, Hashimoto S, Fujiwara E, Sato H, Ymazaki K, Abe H, Suzuki J. Percutaneous absorption and tissue penetration of indomethacin after cutaneous application of indomethacin kowa gel [in Japanese]. Jpn Pharmacol Ther 1987;15(3):1419–1425.
18. Bruhlmann P, Vathaire F, Dreiser RL, Michel BA. Short-term treatment with topical diclofenac epolamine plaster in patients with symptomatic knee osteoarthritis: pooled analysis of two randomised clinical studies. Curr Med Res Opin 2006;22:2429–2438.
19. Aoki T, Imai N, Ooi T, Kawaji W, Kuroki Y, Sugawara S, Fujimaki E, et al. A comparative study of a diclofenac sodium percutaneous agent (TP318) and its base preparation in treating osteoarthrosis of the knee conclusion [in Japanese]. Rinsho Iyaku 2000;16(4):427–443.
20. Banning M. Topical diclofenac: clinical effectiveness and current uses in osteoarthritis of the knee and soft tissue injuries. Expert Opin Pharmacother 2008;9(16):2921–2929.
21. Yano T, Wada M, Furukawa K, Kanetake T, Fukuda K, Ohta J, Hoshi T, Saita M. Absorption, distribution and excretion of ketoprofen after topical application of a [^{14}C]ketoprofen-containing tape preparation to guinea pigs [in Japanese]. Iyukuhin Kenkyu 1993;24(7):727–741.
22. Horie M, Sekiya I, Nakamura T, Tanaka H, Maekawa K, Nakanishi M, Muneta T, Kobayashi E. In vivo pharmacokinetics of ketoprofen after patch application in the Mexican hairless pig. Biopharm Drug Dispos 2009;30(4):204–208.
23. Ballerini R, Casini A, Chinol M, Mannucci C, Giaccai L, Salvi M. Study on the absorption of ketoprofen topically administered in man: comparison between tissue and plasma levels. Int J Clin Pharm Res 1986;VI(1):69–72.

24. Rolf C, Engstrom B, Beauchard C, Jacobs LD, Liboux AL. Intra-articular absorption and distribution of ketoprofen after topical plaster application and oral intake in 100 patients undergoing knee arthroscopy. Rheumatology 1993;38:564–567.

25. Osterwalder A, Reiner V, Reiner G, Lualdi P. Tissue absorption and distribution of ketoprofen after patch application in subjects undergoing knee arthroscopy or endoscopic carpal ligament release. Arzneim-Forsch/Drug Res 2002;52(11):822–827.

26. Takagishi N, Sugioka Y, Inoue A, Asano C, Matsukuma T, Kida H, Ueno A, et al. Clinical evaluation of HKP-210 in knee osteoarthritis. Results of a multicenter 3-group comparison study [in Japanese]. Jpn J Clin Exp Med 1986;63(10):3437–3454.

27. Sugioka Y, Takagishi N, Inoue A, Asano C. Clinical Evaluation of KPT-220 (Ketoprofen Patch) in Lumbago. Double-blind Controlled Trial Using Oral Ketoprofen as Control [in Japanese]. Jpn Pharmacol Ther 1994;22(9):349–370.

28. Taniguchi Y, Inui K, Furuta K, Saita M. Pharmacological studies of ketoprofen tape preparation (II). A study on the anti-inflammatory, analgesic and gastrointestinal damaging actions of tape preparation containing ketoprofen in relation to frequency and number of applications [in Japanese]. Iyukuhin Kenkyu 1993;24(8):831–841.

29. Tanida N, Sakurada S. Skin permeability, anti-inflammatory and analgesic effects of ketoprofen-containing tape and loxoprofen sodium-containing tape [in Japanese]. Jpn Pharmacol Ther 36(12): 1123–1129.

30. Takahashi K, Okumura S, Sato J, Mizumura K. Adjuvant-induced arthritis [in Japanese]. Nippon Rinsho 2005; 63(Suppl 1):51–54.

31. Sekine C. 2005. Collagen-induced arthritis (CIA) [in Japanese]. Nippon Rinsho 63(Suppl 1):35–39.

32. Condorelli G, Costanzo LL, Guidi G, De Guidi G, Giuffrida S, Miano P, Sortino S, Velardita A. Photosensitization induced by non steroidal anti inflammatory drugs: an overview of molecular mechanisms in biological systems. EPA Newsl 1996;58:60–77.

33. Cutaneous reactions of topical NSAIDs. Prescrire Int 2000;9(48):114–115.

34. Kowalzick L, Ziegler H. Photoallergic contact dermatitis from topical diclofenac in Solaraze gel. Contact Dermatitis 2006;54:348–349.

35. Montoro J, Rodriguez M, Diaz M, Bertomeu F. Photoallergic contact dermatitis due to diclofenac. Contact Dermatitis 2003;46:115–119.

36. Sugiura M, Hayakawa R, Kato Y, Sugiura K, Ueda H. 4 cases of photocontact dermatitis due to ketoprofen. Contact Dermatitis 2000;43:16–19.

37. Galer BS, Sheldon E, Patel N, Codding C, Burch F, Gammaitoni AR. Topical lidocaine patch 5% may target a novel underlying pain mechanism in osteoarthritis. Curr Med Res Opin 2004;20(9):1455–1458.

13 Hyaluronic Acid and Arthritis
A Review

Michele Abate

CONTENTS

INTRODUCTION

Osteoarthritis (OA) is a very common disease in the elderly. According to the American College of Rheumatology, nearly 70% of people older than 70 years have x-ray evidence of OA, although only half ever develop symptoms. Notwithstanding, because of the huge amount of persons affected, OA is a frequent cause of disability [1].

Different joints can be damaged by the OA process; among these, glenohumeral and trapezio-metacarpal OA can affect, particularly in the elderly, the activities of daily living (ADL), whereas spine, hip, knee, and ankle OA can influence walking and balance.

Several therapeutic approaches, such as analgesics, nonsteroidal anti-inflammatory drugs (NSAIDs), cyclooxygenase (COX)-2 inhibitors [2], and steroids, have been proposed, with the aim of reducing pain and maintaining and/or improving the joint function, but none of these options has shown to delay the progression of OA or reverse joint damage.

In addition, the incidence of adverse reactions (ADRs) to these drugs increases with age.

Data from epidemiological studies consistently show that the risk of gastrointestinal (GI) complications is very high and that, in the elderly, it is largely dose dependent [3]. Among persons of age >65 years, 20%–30% of all hospitalizations and deaths due to peptic ulcer disease were attributable to therapy with NSAIDs [3–5].

Because it has been firmly established that GI lesions are the result of COX-1 inhibition, more selective COX-2 inhibitors have been developed. These drugs, indeed, have reduced the risk of GI side effects, in comparison with nonselective NSAIDs, but are charged by more relevant cardiovascular complications [6–9].

Moreover, it is well known that NSAIDs as well as selective COX-2 inhibitors may cause renal failure, hypertension, and water retention and have a thrombotic potential, especially for high doses and long-term treatments [10]. Important interactions include those with warfarin, ACE inhibitors, angiotensin II type 1 receptor antagonists, and diuretics, which can result in loss of control of blood pressure and cardiac and renal failure (in hypovolemic conditions). In addition, it must be underlined that NSAIDs may cause negative effects also on cartilage metabolism [11]. Therefore, the pharmacological interactions and the possible impact on comorbidities are a strong limiting factor to the use of NSAIDs and COX-2 inhibitors in the elderly [6–9, 11, 12].

Corticosteroids are provided with relevant ADRs, when given systemically, and therefore are usually administered by intra-articular injection in patients who fail to respond to other conservative measures (decreased activity, physical therapy, topic analgesic, or systemic NSAIDs) [13, 14]. According to literature, patients with joint effusions and local tenderness may have greater benefit from intra-articular steroid injection [15–17].

Although it has been established that corticosteroid injections are relatively safe, there are concerns regarding their possible adverse effects after repeated injections. These adverse effects include local tissue atrophy, particularly when small joints are injected with potent corticosteroids, long-term joint damage due to reduced bone formation, and risk of infection due to suppression of adrenocortical function [18–22]. Rare complications are osteonecrosis [23], skin depigmentation [24], or dysphonia [25]. Indeed, steroid phobia is common among both doctors and patients.

In consideration of the above-reported limits of OA therapies at present available, drugs with minimal side effects are therefore warranted.

Synovial fluid is essential for the normal joint functioning: it acts both as a lubricant during slow movement (e.g., in walking) and as an elastic shock absorber during rapid movement (e.g., in running). It also serves as a medium for delivering nutrition and transmitting cellular signals to articular cartilage.

Hyaluronic acid (HA), produced by synoviocytes, fibroblasts, and chondrocytes, is the major chemical component of synovial fluid. It is essential for the viscoelastic properties of the fluid because of its high viscosity and has a protective effect on articular cartilage and soft tissue surfaces of joints [26, 27].

In OA, the concentration of HA in the joints is reduced: the factors that contribute to the low concentrations of HA are dilutional effects, reduced hyaluronan synthesis, and free radical degradation [28]. When viscoelasticity of synovial fluid is reduced, the transmission of mechanical force to cartilage may increase its susceptibility to mechanical damage.

The restoration of the normal articular homeostasis is therefore the rationale for the administration of HA into the OA joints. Moreover, because HA is a physiological component of the human body, it is very likely that it may be deprived of ADRs, also after repeated administrations.

CHARACTERISTICS OF HA

The native HA has a molecular weight of 4–10 million Da, and it is present in articular fluid in concentration of approximately 0.35 g/100 mL.

The direct injection in the joint space allows to reach a proper concentration with low doses, favoring a longer permanence in the joint and therefore the therapeutic response.

HA preparations have a short half-life; therefore, the long-term effects of viscosupplementation (VS) cannot solely be attributed to the substitution of molecule itself [29]. This suggests that clinical efficacy may be mediated by several different pathways: restoration of joint rheology, anti-inflammatory and antinociceptive effects, normalization of endogenous HA synthesis, and chondroprotection [30].

In experimental rabbit OA, HA inhibits matrix metalloproteinase-3 production [31, 32] and decreases the synovial expression of interleukin 1β [32]. Similarly, the chain of events, from fibronectin fragments via cytokines, that leads to a reduced synthesis of proteoglycans is blocked [32–35].

At present, preparations with different molecular weight are available (low molecular weight [LMW] and high molecular weight [HMW]), which display different pharmaceutical effects because of their different composition.

The enhanced penetration of LMW preparations (0.5–1.5 million Da) through the extracellular matrix of the synovium is thought to maximize its concentration and to facilitate its interaction with target synovial cells, hence reducing the synovial inflammation [36, 37].

However, because of the low elastoviscosity of these hyaluronan solutions compared with native hyaluronan in the synovial fluid, interests were shifted to a VS fluid similar to the native HA.

Recently, an HA cross-linked (Hylan G-F 20) preparation, with HMW (6–7 million Da) similar to native HA, has been developed.

This formulation, by means of its hydrophilic properties, retains higher amounts of fluid in articular space [37], and is provided by a greater anti-inflammatory activity, as shown by studies on migration of inflammatory cells in the joint and on the reduced prostaglandin E_2 and bradykinin concentration [33, 38, 39]. Moreover, HMW HA is considered more effective in relieving pain compared with LMW HA.

A novel HA preparation, non-animal stabilized HA, has been manufactured by a two-stage procedure: biosynthesis of HA by cultured bacteria followed by a mild stabilization process. Stabilization does not change the biochemical properties of HA but creates biocompatible gel with improved viscoelastic properties and longer residence time in the joint compared with non-stabilized HA preparation [40].

Currently, with the aim of favoring a longer presence of HA in the joint, long acting preparations are under study [41, 42].

Hopefully, these compounds, with better rheological and biological properties, could influence positively the natural history of OA disease.

INDICATIONS TO TREATMENT

VS can be considered when the patient has not found pain relief from exercise, physical therapy, weight loss, use of orthotics, and analgesics or NSAIDs. Other indications may be the intolerance to analgesics or NSAIDs or the use of multiple systemic medications, as frequently happens in the elderly.

The treatment, in general, is offered to patients with intermediate Kellgren–Lawrence (K–L) score [43–46] who report better results in terms of function and reduction of pain.

The administration of HA is contraindicated only in patients with known hypersensitivity to egg proteins, whereas patients with absence of any articular space (K–L score IV) or affected by inflammatory musculoskeletal diseases (rheumatoid arthritis, chondrocalcinosis, psoriasis, and gout) may have limited benefit from the treatment.

INFILTRATION TECHNIQUES

GENERAL CONSIDERATIONS

Intra-articular injection of HA must be performed in sterile conditions to minimize the risk of inflammatory complications (i.e., septic arthritis).

Moreover, the use of "image-guided" infiltration techniques is mandatory. When joint infiltration is performed blindly, the failure rate is high, and the drug may be administered in the para-articular space. Indeed, when HA is administered outside the articular space, treatment loses its efficacy and side effects, mainly pain, frequently occur.

The ultrasound-guided injection has several advantages compared with fluoroscopy: it is simple, fast, economic, and safe; it does not require the use of contrast media [47], allowing the infiltration in patients intolerant to iodized contrasts. It can be repeated without limits, allows an easy visualization of fluid in the articular recess (which may be aspirated), and shows how narrow is the articular space. Moreover, it is able to show the position of the needle and, by means of continuous color Doppler monitoring, to evaluate its distance from vessels [47]. Finally, the ultrasound technique allows the visualization of the viscous fluid injected inside the joint [47].

Fluoroscopy offers the advantage of a wider visual field, which may be important for large joints infiltration, and allows a very proper positioning of the needle in joints where the articular space is very narrow. However, fluoroscopy does not show the presence of fluid, which, if left *in situ*, can dilute the HA preparation inside the articular recess (HA partially loses its efficacy), and is associated to the risk of radiation and contrast media use [47]. Moreover, it does not allow identification and avoidance of vascular and nervous structures [47, 48] and must be performed in the radiological setting. Therefore, it is more time consuming and more expensive.

GLENOHUMERAL JOINT

For glenohumeral joint infiltration, the patient is placed in a semiprone position with the shoulder to be injected uppermost. The ipsilateral arm is placed over a pillow to maintain the position and to optimize patient comfort. A broadband 5- to 12-MHz linear array transducer is aligned in the long axis of the musculotendinous junction of the infraspinatus muscle, just inferior to the scapular spine, with the posterior glenoid rim and the posterior glenohumeral joint line centered in the field of view [49].

Then, a 20- to 22-gauge spinal needle (90–120 mm) is introduced and, during real time ultrasound monitoring, its passage into the glenohumeral joint is visualized. After saline injection control, an amount of 2–4 mL of HA is introduced.

CARPOMETACARPAL JOINT

For thumb carpometacarpal (CMC) joint infiltration, with the patient's hand to be injected held in the semiprone position, a preliminary ultrasound investigation of CMC joint is carried out. After the identification of the CMC space, a 27-gauge needle is inserted lateral to the abductor pollicis longus tendon, and an amount of HA ranging from 0.1 to 1 mL is injected (Figure 13.1).

In a recent study, Karalezli et al. [50] point out that CMC infiltration, when performed with no imaging control, is a painful procedure because of para-articular injection or periosteal irritation.

HIP JOINT

For hip joint infiltration, particular care is required to avoid lesions of femoral nerves and vessels because of their frequent anatomic variability [51].

A 20- to 22-gauge spinal needle is used, and 2–4 mLs of HA are administered. When the injection is performed antero-inferiorly, it is possible to inject the HA preparation at the base of the femoral neck and a complete evacuation of intra-articular fluid, if present, is allowed [52, 53] (Figure 13.2). The anterosuperior parasagittal approach allows the injection over the femoral head so that the drug is evenly distributed on the cartilage of both femoral head and acetabulum. Also, a lateral approach is possible, injecting the preparation near to the great trochanter's tuberosity [54].

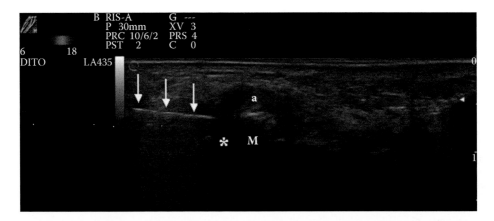

FIGURE 13.1 Ultrasound-guided carpometacarpal infiltration. Note the correct placement of the needle (solid arrows) inside the trapeziometacarpal joint (*). a, articular space; M, I metacarpal bone.

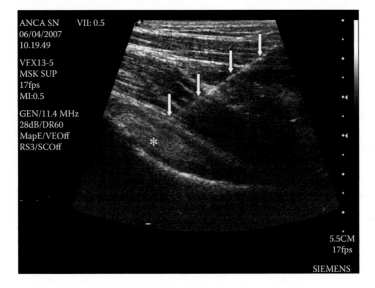

FIGURE 13.2 Ultrasound-guided hip infiltration. Note the correct placement of the needle (solid arrows) inside the articular space. HA is visible as hyperechoic material (*).

KNEE JOINT

Even if the knee joint infiltration is simple and widely performed blinded, the ultrasound-guided procedure is anyhow recommended because ultrasound may make sure about the correct placement of the needle.

A 21-gauge needle (0.8 × 50 mm) is inserted from the lateral aspect of the joint at the superior margin of the patella. In this case, the position of the ultrasound probe is parallel to the needle insertion [55]. The amount of HA varies from 2 to 4 mL.

ANKLE JOINT

For ankle joint infiltration, the patient is placed in the supine position with the ankle relaxed. The articular space is identified between the anterior border of the medial malleolus and the medial border of the tibialis anterior tendon.

To visualize the anterior recess of the tibiotalar joint, a 5- to 12-MHz linear probe is placed in the mid longitudinal plane over the dorsum of the ankle.

A 20- to 22-gauge spinal needle is then introduced, and its course to the articular space is visualized during real time ultrasound monitoring. A small amount of HA (2 mL) is therefore injected.

CLINICAL RESULTS

KNEE OA

In this section, the more relevant studies on the treatment of OA with intra-articular HA in different joints are reported, starting with VS in knee OA, which has been approved by the Food and Drug Administration [56].

Recent guidelines, developed by the Royal College of Physicians [57], are based on a meta-analysis, including 5257 participants of 40 randomized controlled trials (RCT), several of them including a representative sample of elderly patients [58–63]. These studies were performed, single or double blind, with different types of HA (LMW and HMW) against placebo. The number of injections ranged from three to five times weekly, with a maximum of 11 times in 23 weeks, the doses from 15 to 60 mg, and the trials length from 4 weeks to 18 months.

Pain was evaluated by means of the Visual Analogue Scale (VAS) or the Wester Ontario and McMaster Universities Osteoarthritis Index (WOMAC) subscale, at rest or under different load conditions. A minor number of studies evaluated the functional outcomes (WOMAC physical function, Lequesne index, and range of motion), the subjective global assessment, and the quality of life of the patients. The results of the majority of studies are in favor of HA, although in several RCTs no significant differences have been found in comparison with intra-articular placebo. The percentages of improvement from baseline, in all the outcomes measures, were 28%–54% for pain and 9%–32 % for function and were similar in the trials in which LMW HA and HMW HA were used separately and also in the trials specifically designed to assess differences about the preparations [37, 46, 64–66]. However, the number of injection needed was in general lower for HMW HA preparation, and this is not a negligible advantage for the patients.

The benefit, in general, becomes more evident within 3 months and persists in the following months. It should be observed that the benefit is not equally distributed among patients, some of them being non-responders to therapy. Although, at present, all the characteristics of responders have not been clearly identified, some authors claim that a greater benefit may be obtained in patients with low-grade OA [67–69]. On the contrary, age does not influence the therapeutic response [70].

HIP OA

The number of studies about VS of hip OA is limited, when compared with studies in knee OA [71]. The reason for this can be the deeper localization of the hip joint, being closer to femoral vessels and nerves.

The level of evidence for most of these studies is low because they are cohort studies and lack of a reference group [28, 30, 40, 48, 52–54, 72–78], a score I (i.e., the highest level of evidence), according to the Center for Evidence Based Medicine criteria [79], having been assigned only to the studies of Tikiz et al. [80] and Qvistgaard et al. [81].

As for studies in knee OA, several types of HA preparations were used. The number of injections ranged from one to three for each patients, and only in few cases four or five injections were performed. In general, the number of injections was lower for HMW preparations. The length of treatments and the outcome measures were similar to those used in knee RCTs.

The pain relief and the improvement in articular function were significantly greater than that seen after intra-articular injection of placebo in the majority of studies [2, 82–89], but some RCTs failed in demonstrating a superiority of HA against placebo [81, 90].

Ankle OA

The efficacy of HA infiltration has been demonstrated also for the treatment of ankle OA.

After 1 week post-treatment, significant improvements in the VAS pain score as well as in the Ankle Osteoarthritis Scale and in the American Orthopaedic Foot and Ankle Society have been reported [91], with effects lasting from 3 [91, 92] to 12 [93] and 18 months [94].

The patient's global satisfaction was high (86.7% at 6 months) [91], and the analgesics consumption fell from an average of 14 tablets weekly at baseline to 3 after 6 months ($p < 0.001$) [91].

Furthermore, a statistically significant pain decrease was reported in patients who received intra-articular HA after ankle arthroscopy compared with those who underwent only arthroscopy [95].

These positive results have been challenged in two different studies, in which no significant difference was reported at 3 [96] and 6 months [97] between HA and placebo. These discrepancies could be explained by the LMW of HA used in the studies.

Finally, preliminary promising results have been reported also for the treatment of other ankle diseases such as osteochondritis dissecans [98], ankle sprain [99, 100], and comminuted fracture of ankle [101].

Glenohumeral OA

HA is effective and well tolerated for the treatment of OA [102] and persistent shoulder pain refractory to other standard non-operative interventions [103].

Several authors [104, 105] report that intra-articular injections of LMW HA, both three and five times weekly, provide significant improvement in terms of shoulder pain (VAS score on movement). Treatment effects last 7–26 weeks [104].

Similarly, in a 6-month follow-up study [106], a significant reduction in VAS pain score (from 54 to 30, $p < 0.001$) was also provided with three weekly intra-articular HMW HA (Hylan G-F 20) injections. In addition, most of the patients experienced an improvement in the shoulder function score (University of California and Los Angeles (UCLA) from 15.7 to 24, $p < 0.001$; Simple Shoulder Test from 5.7 to 7.6, $p < 0.001$) and in the ADL ($p < 0.001$) [107].

Finally, the efficacy of HA has been recently demonstrated in the treatment of different shoulder diseases, such as subacromial bursitis (Figure 13.3), adhesive capsulitis, and rotator cuff tear [104, 108–111], with positive results on pain, joint mobility, and shoulder function.

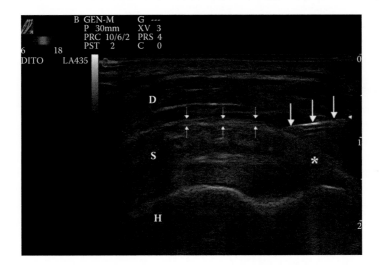

FIGURE 13.3 Ultrasound-guided infiltration of the subacromial bursa. Note the correct placement of the needle (solid arrows) inside the subacromial bursa (broken arrows). D, deltoid muscle; H, humeral head; S, supraspinatus tendon; distal acoustic shadowing (*).

CMC OA

It is well known that CMC OA contributes to hand dysfunction, depending on the severity of OA, pain, and joint involvement [112]. Several conservative treatments have been proposed (corticosteroids, NSAIDs, prolotherapy, and splinting), but none of these have shown to delay the progression of OA or reverse joint damage.

Recent studies, however, have investigated the efficacy of HA in the treatment of CMC OA, and positive results have been reported by most of the authors. In particular, an early improvement in VAS score was already observed after 2 weeks post-treatment [113], with the effects lasting until 1–3 months [114–117]. The long-term effects of hyaluronan are demonstrated only in few studies [113, 118], in which the pain relief was reported at 6 months.

Beside pain reduction, also grip strength improved significantly, although these effects are achieved slowly, with better results observed at 6 months [113, 117, 118]. Moreover, in the mid [114, 115, 117] and long term, most of the patients report significant improvement in the hand function and mobility (Dreiser Functional Index, Purdue Pegboard Test).

OTHER JOINTS

Encouraging results have been reported in the treatment of painful hallux rigidus [119], sacroiliac joint syndrome [120, 121], and nerve root adhesion after lumbar intervertebral disk herniation [122].

In the treatment of elbow OA, the results are inconclusive. Positive effects have been observed only in two small studies [109, 123], whereas in a larger study (18 patients), intra-articular HA was not effective in the treatment of post-traumatic OA of the elbow [124].

Controversial results have been observed also in the treatment of spine OA. Fuchs et al. [125] reported significant pain relief and improved quality of life, also in the long term, in patients affected from facet joints OA with chronic non-radicular pain in the lumbar spine [125]. However, these results are not in agreement with a recent study by Cleary et al. [126], who did not demonstrate any benefit of VS in the management of symptomatic lumbar facet OA.

Finally, there is growing evidence of the benefit of HA in the treatment of temporo-mandibular joint OA. Several studies have shown the efficacy of serial injections of HA in reducing symptoms over time. In particular, a significant early pain relief, both at rest and during mastication, was observed 1–6 months post-injection [127–131], with the effects lasting until 12 months [130].

SIDE EFFECTS

Several factors may contribute to the occurrence of side effects: among them, the characteristics and amount of HA preparation injected, the number of injections, the skill of the operator, the technique used, and the local and systemic tissue reactions.

In quite all the clinical trials, no general side effects were observed, and only few patients reported a sensation of heaviness and pain in their joint after injection [40, 47, 71]. These effects were more frequent in studies performed in blind conditions compared with those performed under imaging guidance. No differences were observed in relation to HA preparation used or to the number of injections [80].

Side effects usually disappeared after 2–7 days without any therapeutic intervention and did not limit basic or instrumental ADL. Neither vascular or nervous complications nor gout was reported; chondrocalcinosis was sometimes observed after OA VS of the knee. Septic arthritis or aseptic synovial effusion occurred in a very limited number of cases [72, 132].

HA VERSUS CORTICOSTEROIDS

Intra-articular corticosteroids are the alternative choice to HA for treatment of OA. Therefore, it is very interesting to evaluate the studies, which compared these treatment modalities. The large majority of comparison studies has been performed between different HA preparations and steroids (methylprednisolone and triamcinolone) [133].

In several studies, better results were observed after HA injection [96, 118, 125]; in other studies, no significant difference was found [81, 132]. Steroids, however, offered the best results on joints with inflammatory effusions.

Only one study compared the clinical efficacy of HA VS versus corticosteroids and placebo in hip OA. This very large trial, including 101 patients, did not show significant differences between the treatments in all the outcome measures after 3 months [81]. However, within this time period, an improvement was found, which resulted clearly evident in the steroid group and moderate in the HA group compared with placebo [81].

Comparison studies between HA and corticosteroid in the treatment of ankle and shoulder OA are lacking, whereas in CMC OA a rapid pain relief was observed after triamcinolone or methylpredniso-lone injections (after 2–4 weeks) [117, 118], although these results disappeared by week 12 [113].

Positive effects were achieved with HA more slowly but were long lasting and persisted 6 months after the end of the treatment period [118].

Also for the treatment of temporo-mandibular joint OA, the comparison between corticosteroids and HA has shown that both the compounds reduce pain and improve articular function.

CONCLUSIONS

On the basis of the published trials, we may affirm that VS therapy with HA is a safe and effective method in the management of OA resistant to conventional therapies. This treatment has been approved by the Food and Drug Administration for knee OA, whereas for the other joints OA, there are promising results but not conclusive evidence.

The use of HA is mainly recommended when NSAIDs are contraindicated or badly tolerated, when NSAIDs or corticosteroids are inefficacious, or in young patients candidate for prosthesis.

VS significantly reduces pain within 3 months, and this beneficial effect is maintained in the long term (12–18 months). The articular function is improved, and therefore patients can rapidly come back to work and to social activities.

Only few trials have shown a very early improvement, which has been related to the lubricating effect of hyaluronate in "dry" joints, as reported in studies of VS in knee OA, and/or to a short-term placebo effect [72].

The reduction in NSAIDs consumption is another important clinical achievement with significant health economic consideration [12]. Not only the direct costs (NSAIDs purchasing) but also the indirect costs associated with management of NSAIDs side effects are saved.

Cost-benefit analysis is difficult in comparison with corticosteroids. Corticosteroid doses are cheaper than HA preparation, but the efficacy of these drugs seems to last less longer than HA preparations, with more relevant side effects, which can offset the initial saving [81].

Patients with mild morphological alterations and with preserved articular space are more responsive to treatment [28, 72, 134]; the results are less encouraging in patients with severe OA (K-L score IV), only few studies reporting a good therapeutic effects [28, 76, 134].

Articular effusion usually is associated to a reduced therapeutic efficacy because of the "dilution effect" of the drug [81]. In this situation, a better therapeutic response is observed with intra-articular corticosteroids, probably linked to their anti-inflammatory activity [81].

The better biological activity, shown by HMW HA preparations *in vitro*, has not been confirmed in clinical trials [80]. In fact, the percentage of improvement in all the outcomes measures is similar with LMW HA and HMW HA preparations [54]. An advantage of HMW HA may be the reduced number of the injections needed to obtain the therapeutic effect.

When the therapy is delivered by appropriately trained doctors, under strict imaging guidance, VS is a safe procedure, without any systemic or local side effect, excluding the pain of the injection and a sensation of heaviness for few hours/days after treatment. It is likely that persistent pain and joint swelling or major complications, such as septic arthritis, may occur when injection is not properly performed. Even experienced clinicians can miss intra-articular placement of the drug, especially in small joints [135, 136].

The very high tolerability of the preparation allows the contemporary use of other drugs, which is very important in elderly patients with comorbid conditions and polypharmaceutically treated.

Although these are promising results, these questions are still opened:

1. Inclusion and exclusion criteria vary largely in different studies, and therefore the characteristics of patients who are better responsive to treatment are not clearly defined. Therefore, the identification of these patients is strongly recommended.
2. No consensus exist about the doses of HA, the interval between doses, and the number of injections, which are more effective in the different clinical situations. A three- to five-dose regimen is usually recommended, but studies that compare different treatment schedules are lacking [80].
3. It is also debated whether HMW HA has to be preferred to LMW HA. The better biological activity, shown by HMW HA preparations *in vitro*, has not been confirmed in clinical trials [80]. Some authors prefer to use HMW HA because these preparations have a longer half-life time so that the number of the injections needed to obtain the therapeutic effect may be reduced.
4. Interpretation of result is made difficult by the different degree of severity of OA, by the genetic and biological characteristics of patients enrolled in the studies, and by the concurrent therapies with other drugs and rehabilitation treatments [30, 52, 53, 72, 80].
5. Finally, it must be remembered that there is a strong placebo effect from joint injection, which may cause a nearly 30% reduction in pain relief during the first 2 weeks [72, 80, 137–139].

REFERENCES

1. Lawrence RC, Helmick CG, Arnett FC, Deyo RA, Felson DT, Giannini EH, Heyse SP, et al. Estimates of the prevalence of arthritis and selected musculoskeletal disorders in the United States. Arthritis Rheum 1998;41(5):778–799.
2. Altman R, Alarcon G, Appelrouth D, Bloch D, Borenstein D, Brandt K, Brown C, et al. The American College of Rheumatology criteria for the classification and reporting of osteoarthritis of the hip. Arthritis Rheum 1991;34(5):505–514.
3. Smalley WE, Griffin MR. The risks and costs of upper gastrointestinal disease attributable to NSAIDs. Gastroenterol Clin North Am 1996;25(2):373–396.
4. Griffin MR, Ray WA, Schaffner W. Nonsteroidal anti-inflammatory drug use and death from peptic ulcer in elderly persons. Ann Intern Med 1988;109(5):359–363.
5. Griffin MR, Piper JM, Daugherty JR, Snowden M, Ray WA. Nonsteroidal anti-inflammatory drug use and increased risk for peptic ulcer disease in elderly persons. Ann Intern Med 1991;114(4):257–263.
6. Hochberg MC, Altman RD, Brandt KD, Clark BM, Dieppe PA, Griffin MR, Moskowitz RW, Schnitzer TJ. Guidelines for the medical management of osteoarthritis. Part I. Osteoarthritis of the hip. American College of Rheumatology. Arthritis Rheum 1995;38(11):1535–1540.
7. Motsko SP, Rascati KL, Busti AJ, Wilson JP, Barner JC, Lawson KA, Worchel J. Temporal relationship between use of NSAIDs, including selective COX-2 inhibitors, and cardiovascular risk. Drug Saf 2006;29(7):621–632.
8. Roughead EE, Ramsay E, Pratt N, Gilbert AL. NSAID use in individuals at risk of renal adverse events: an observational study to investigate trends in Australian veterans. Drug Saf 2008;31(11):997–1003.
9. Savage R. Cyclo-oxygenase-2 inhibitors: when should they be used in the elderly? Drugs Aging 2005;22(3):185–200.
10. Page J, Henry D. Consumption of NSAIDs and the development of congestive heart failure in elderly patients: an underrecognized public health problem. Arch Intern Med 2000;160(6):777–784.
11. Rashad S, Revell P, Hemingway A, Low F, Rainsford K, Walker F. Effect of non-steroidal anti-inflammatory drugs on the course of osteoarthritis. Lancet 1989;2(8662):519–522.

12. Sturkenboom MC, Romano F, Simon G, Correa-Leite ML, Villa M, Nicolosi A, Borgnolo G, Bianchi-Porro G, Mannino S. The iatrogenic costs of NSAID therapy: a population study. Arthritis Rheum 2002;47(2):132–140.

13Flanagan J, Casale FF, Thomas TL, Desai KB. Intra-articular injection for pain relief in patients awaiting hip replacement. Ann R Coll Surg Engl 1988;70(3):156–157.

14. Plant MJ, Borg AA, Dziedzic K, Saklatvala J, Dawes PT. Radiographic patterns and response to corticosteroid hip injection. Ann Rheum Dis 1997;56(8):476–480.

15. Menkes CJ. Intraarticular treatment of osteoarthritis and guidelines to its assessment. J Rheumatol Suppl 1994;41:74–76.

16. Pyne D, Ioannou Y, Mootoo R, Bhanji A. Intra-articular steroids in knee osteoarthritis: a comparative study of triamcinolone hexacetonide and methylprednisolone acetate. Clin Rheumatol 2004;23(2):116–120.

17. Srinivasan A, Amos M, Webley M. The effects of joint washout and steroid injection compared with either joint washout or steroid injection alone in rheumatoid knee effusion. Br J Rheumatol 1995;34(8):771–773.

18. Creamer P. Intra-articular corticosteroid treatment in osteoarthritis. Curr Opin Rheumatol 1999;11(5):417–421.

19. Lazarevic MB, Skosey JL, Djordjevic-Denic G, Swedler WI, Zgradic I, Myones BL. Reduction of cortisol levels after single intra-articular and intramuscular steroid injection. Am J Med 1995;99(4):370–373.

20. Mader R, Lavi I, Luboshitzky R. Evaluation of the pituitary-adrenal axis function following single intraarticular injection of methylprednisolone. Arthritis Rheum 2005;52(3):924–928.

21. Weitoft T, Larsson A, Saxne T, Ronnblom L. Changes of cartilage and bone markers after intra-articular glucocorticoid treatment with and without postinjection rest in patients with rheumatoid arthritis. Ann Rheum Dis 2005;64(12):1750–1753.

22. Weitoft T, Larsson A, Ronnblom L. Serum levels of sex steroid hormones and matrix metalloproteinases after intra-articular glucocorticoid treatment in female patients with rheumatoid arthritis. Ann Rheum Dis 2008;67(3):422–424.

23. Yamamoto T, Schneider R, Iwamoto Y, Bullough PG. Rapid destruction of the femoral head after a single intraarticular injection of corticosteroid into the hip joint. J Rheumatol 2006;33(8):1701–1704.

24. Rogojan C, Hetland ML. Depigmentation—a rare side effect to intra-articular glucocorticoid treatment. Clin Rheumatol 2004;23(4):373–375.

25. Zaman FM, Wong M, Slipman CW, Ellen MI. Dysphonia associated with shoulder steroid injection. Am J Phys Med Rehabil 2005;84(4):307–309.

26. O'Regan M, Martini I, Crescenzi F, De Luca C, Lansing M. Molecular mechanisms and genetics of hyaluronan biosynthesis. Int J Biol Macromol 1994;16(6):283–286.

27. van den Bekerom MP, Lamme B, Sermon A, Mulier M. What is the evidence for viscosupplementation in the treatment of patients with hip osteoarthritis? Systematic review of the literature. Arch Orthop Trauma Surg 2008;128(8):815–823.

28. van den Bekerom MP, Mylle G, Rys B, Mulier M. Viscosupplementation in symptomatic severe hip osteoarthritis: a review of the literature and report on 60 patients. Acta Orthop Belg 2006;72(5):560–568.

29. Kikuchi T, Yamada H, Fujikawa K. Effects of high molecular weight hyaluronan on the distribution and movement of proteoglycan around chondrocytes cultured in alginate beads. Osteoarthritis Cartilage 2001;9(4):351–356.

30. Vad VB, Sakalkale D, Sculco TP, Wickiewicz TL. Role of hylan G-F 20 in treatment of osteoarthritis of the hip joint. Arch Phys Med Rehabil 2003;84(8):1224–1226.

31. Han F, Ishiguro N, Ito T, Sakai T, Iwata H. Effects of sodium hyaluronate on experimental osteoarthritis in rabbit knee joints. Nagoya J Med Sci 1999;62(3–4):115–126.

32. Takahashi K, Goomer RS, Harwood F, Kubo T, Hirasawa Y, Amiel D. The effects of hyaluronan on matrix metalloproteinase-3 (MMP-3), interleukin-1beta (IL-1beta), and tissue inhibitor of metalloproteinase-1 (TIMP-1) gene expression during the development of osteoarthritis. Osteoarthritis Cartilage 1999;7(2):182–190.

33. Goto H, Onodera T, Hirano H, Shimamura T. Hyaluronic acid suppresses the reduction of alpha2(VI) collagen gene expression caused by interleukin-1beta in cultured rabbit articular chondrocytes. Tohoku J Exp Med 1999;187(1):1–13.

34. Homandberg GA, Hui F, Wen C, Kuettner KE, Williams JM. Hyaluronic acid suppresses fibronectin fragment mediated cartilage chondrolysis: I. In vitro. Osteoarthritis Cartilage 1997;5(5):309–319.

35. Williams JM, Plaza V, Hui F, Wen C, Kuettner KE, Homandberg GA. Hyaluronic acid suppresses fibronectin fragment mediated cartilage chondrolysis: II. In vivo. Osteoarthritis Cartilage 1997;5(4):235–240.

36. Bagga H, Burkhardt D, Sambrook P, March L. Longterm effects of intraarticular hyaluronan on synovial fluid in osteoarthritis of the knee. J Rheumatol 2006;33(5):946–950.
37. Ghosh P, Guidolin D. Potential mechanism of action of intra-articular hyaluronan therapy in osteoarthritis: are the effects molecular weight dependent? Semin Arthritis Rheum 2002;32(1):10–37.
38. Aihara S, Murakami N, Ishii R, Kariya K, Azuma Y, Hamada K, Umemoto J, Maeda S. Effects of sodium hyaluronate on the nociceptive response of rats with experimentally induced arthritis. Nippon Yakurigaku Zasshi 1992;100(4):359–365.
39. Forrester JV, Balazs EA. Inhibition of phagocytosis by high molecular weight hyaluronate. Immunology 1980;40(3):435–446.
40. Berg P, Olsson U. Intra-articular injection of non-animal stabilised hyaluronic acid (NASHA) for osteoarthritis of the hip: a pilot study. Clin Exp Rheumatol 2004;22(3):300–306.
41. Larsen NE, Leshchiner EA, Parent EG, Hendrikson-Aho J, Balazs EA, Hilal SK. Hylan gel composition for percutaneous embolization. J Biomed Mater Res 1991;25(6):699–710.
42. Weiss C, Band P. Musculoskeletal applications of hyaluronan and hylan. Potential uses in the foot and ankle. Clin Podiatr Med Surg 1995;12(3):497–517.
43. Kellgren JH, Lawrence JS. Radiological assessment of osteo-arthrosis. Ann Rheum Dis 1957;16(4):494–502.
44. Brzusek D, Petron D. Treating knee osteoarthritis with intra-articular hyaluronans. Curr Med Res Opin 2008;24(12):3307–3322.
45. Kemper F, Gebhardt U, Meng T, Murray C. Tolerability and short-term effectiveness of hylan G-F 20 in 4253 patients with osteoarthritis of the knee in clinical practice. Curr Med Res Opin 2005;21(8):1261–1269.
46. Waddell DD. Viscosupplementation with hyaluronans for osteoarthritis of the knee: clinical efficacy and economic implications. Drugs Aging 2007;24(8):629–642.
47. Migliore A, Tormenta S, Martin Martin LS, Valente C, Massafra U, Latini A, Alimonti A. Safety profile of 185 ultrasound-guided intra-articular injections for treatment of rheumatic diseases of the hip. Reumatismo 2004;56(2):104–109.
48. Pourbagher MA, Ozalay M, Pourbagher A. Accuracy and outcome of sonographically guided intra-articular sodium hyaluronate injections in patients with osteoarthritis of the hip. J Ultrasound Med 2005;24(10):1391–1395.
49. Zwar RB, Read JW, Noakes JB. Sonographically guided glenohumeral joint injection. AJR Am J Roentgenol 2004;183(1):48–50.
50. Karalezli N, Ogun TC, Kartal S, Saracgil SN, Yel M, Tuncay I. The pain associated with intraarticular hyaluronic acid injections for trapeziometacarpal osteoarthritis. Clin Rheumatol 2007;26(4):569–571.
51. Leopold SS, Battista V, Oliverio JA. Safety and efficacy of intraarticular hip injection using anatomic landmarks. Clin Orthop Relat Res 2001;391:192–197.
52. Conrozier T, Bertin P, Mathieu P, Charlot J, Bailleul F, Treves R, Vignon E, Chevalier X. Intra-articular injections of hylan G-F 20 in patients with symptomatic hip osteoarthritis: an open-label, multicentre, pilot study. Clin Exp Rheumatol 2003;21(5):605–610.
53. Migliore A, Martin LS, Alimonti A, Valente C, Tormenta S. Efficacy and safety of viscosupplementation by ultrasound-guided intra-articular injection in osteoarthritis of the hip. Osteoarthritis Cartilage 2003;11(4):305–306.
54. Caglar-Yagci H, Unsal S, Yagci I, Dulgeroglu D, Ozel S. Safety and efficacy of ultrasound-guided intra-articular hylan G-F 20 injection in osteoarthritis of the hip: a pilot study. Rheumatol Int 2005;25(5):341–344.
55. Qvistgaard E, Kristoffersen H, Terslev L, Danneskiold-Samsoe B, Torp-Pedersen S, Bliddal H. Guidance by ultrasound of intra-articular injections in the knee and hip joints. Osteoarthritis Cartilage 2001;9(6):512–517.
56. Hunter DJ, Lo GH. The management of osteoarthritis: an overview and call to appropriate conservative treatment. Rheum Dis Clin North Am 2008;34(3):689–712.
57 National Collaborating Centre for Chronic Conditions at the Royal College of Physicians. Osteoarthritis: national clinical guideline for care and management in adults. London, UK: Royal College of Physicians; 2008.
58. Bellamy N. Hyaluronic acid and knee osteoarthritis. J Fam Pract 2006;55(11):967–968.
59. Bellamy N, Campbell J, Robinson V, Gee T, Bourne R, Wells G. Intraarticular corticosteroid for treatment of osteoarthritis of the knee. Cochrane Database Syst Rev 2006;(2):CD005328.
60. Bellamy N. Hyaluronic acid and knee osteoarthritis. J Fam Pract 2006;55(11):967–968.

61. Flanagan J, Casale FF, Thomas TL, Desai KB. Intra-articular injection for pain relief in patients awaiting hip replacement. Ann R Coll Surg Engl 1988;70(3):156–157.

62. Meenagh GK, Patton J, Kynes C, Wright GD. A randomised controlled trial of intra-articular corticosteroid injection of the carpometacarpal joint of the thumb in osteoarthritis. Ann Rheum Dis 2004;63(10):1260–1263.

63. Petrella RJ, Petrella M. A prospective, randomized, double-blind, placebo controlled study to evaluate the efficacy of intraarticular hyaluronic acid for osteoarthritis of the knee. J Rheumatol 2006;33(5):951–956.

64. Aggarwal A, Sempowski IP. Hyaluronic acid injections for knee osteoarthritis. Systematic review of the literature. Can Fam Physician 2004;50:249–256.

65. Belo JN, Berger MY, Reijman M, Koes BW, Bierma-Zeinstra SM. Prognostic factors of progression of osteoarthritis of the knee: a systematic review of observational studies. Arthritis Rheum 2007;57(1):13–26.

66. Divine JG, Zazulak BT, Hewett TE. Viscosupplementation for knee osteoarthritis: a systematic review. Clin Orthop Relat Res 2007;455:113–122.

67. Campbell J, Bellamy N, Gee T. Differences between systematic reviews/meta-analyses of hyaluronic acid/hyaluronan/hylan in osteoarthritis of the knee. Osteoarthritis Cartilage 2007;15(12):1424–1436.

68. Dagenais S. Intra-articular hyaluronic acid (viscosupplementation) for knee osteoarthritis. Issues Emerg Health Technol 2006;(94):1–4.

69. Hamburger MI, Lakhanpal S, Mooar PA, Oster D. Intra-articular hyaluronans: a review of product-specific safety profiles. Semin Arthritis Rheum 2003;32(5):296–309.

70. Chua SD, Jr., Messier SP, Legault C, Lenz ME, Thonar EJ, Loeser RF. Effect of an exercise and dietary intervention on serum biomarkers in overweight and obese adults with osteoarthritis of the knee. Osteoarthritis Cartilage 2008;16(9):1047–1053.

71. Abate M, Pelotti P, De Amicis D, Di Iorio A, Galletti S, Salini V. Viscosupplementation with hyaluronic acid in hip osteoarthritis (a review). Ups J Med Sci 2008;113(3):261–277.

72. Brocq O, Tran G, Breuil V, Grisot C, Flory P, Euller-Ziegler L. Hip osteoarthritis: short-term efficacy and safety of viscosupplementation by hylan G-F 20. An open-label study in 22 patients. Joint Bone Spine 2002;69(4):388–391.

73. Migliore A, Tormenta S, Valente C, Massafra U, Martin Martin LS, Carmenini E, Bernardini A, Alimonti A. Intra-articular treatment with Hylan G-F 20 under ultrasound guidance in hip osteoarthritis. Clinical results after 12 months follow-up. Reumatismo 2005;57(1):36–43.

74. Migliore A, Tormenta S, Martin LS, Valente C, Massafra U, Granata M, Alimonti A. Open pilot study of ultrasound-guided intra-articular injection of hylan G-F 20 (Synvisc) in the treatment of symptomatic hip osteoarthritis. Clin Rheumatol 2005;24(3):285–289.

75. Migliore A, Tormenta S, Massafra U, Carloni E, Padalino C, Iannessi F, Alimonti A, Martin LS, Granata M. Repeated ultrasound-guided intra-articular injections of 40 mg of Hyalgan may be useful in symptomatic relief of hip osteoarthritis. Osteoarthritis Cartilage 2005;13(12):1126–1127.

76. Migliore A, Tormenta S, Martin Martin LS, Iannessi F, Massafra U, Carloni E, Monno D, Alimonti A, Granata M. The symptomatic effects of intra-articular administration of hylan G-F 20 on osteoarthritis of the hip: clinical data of 6 months follow-up. Clin Rheumatol 2006;25(3):389–393.

77. Migliore A, Tormenta S, Massafra U, Martin Martin LS, Carloni E, Padalino C, Alimonti A, Granata M.18-month observational study on efficacy of intraarticular hyaluronic acid (Hylan G-F 20) injections under ultrasound guidance in hip osteoarthritis. Reumatismo 2006;58(1):39–49.

78. van den Bekerom MP, Rys B, Mulier M. Viscosupplementation in the hip: evaluation of hyaluronic acid formulations. Arch Orthop Trauma Surg 2008;128(3):275–280.

79. Fletcher B, Sackett D. Canadian task force on the periodic health examination: the Periodic Health Examination. CMAJ 1979;121:1193–1254.

80. Tikiz C, Unlu Z, Sener A, Efe M, Tuzun C. Comparison of the efficacy of lower and higher molecular weight viscosupplementation in the treatment of hip osteoarthritis. Clin Rheumatol 2005;24(3):244–250.

81. Qvistgaard E, Christensen R, Torp-Pedersen S, Bliddal H. Intra-articular treatment of hip osteoarthritis: a randomized trial of hyaluronic acid, corticosteroid, and isotonic saline. Osteoarthritis Cartilage 2006;14(2):163–170.

82. Adams ME, Atkinson MH, Lussier AJ, Schulz JI, Siminovitch KA, Wade JP, Zummer M. The role of viscosupplementation with hylan G-F 20 (Synvisc) in the treatment of osteoarthritis of the knee: a Canadian multicenter trial comparing hylan G-F 20 alone, hylan G-F 20 with non-steroidal anti-inflammatory drugs (NSAIDs) and NSAIDs alone. Osteoarthritis Cartilage 1995;3(4):213–225.

83. Felson DT, Anderson JJ. Hyaluronate sodium injections for osteoarthritis: hope, hype, and hard truths. Arch Intern Med 2002;162(3):245–247.

84. Kirwan JR, Rankin E. Intra-articular therapy in osteoarthritis. Baillieres Clin Rheumatol 1997;11(4):769–794.

85. Lo GH, LaValley M, McAlindon T, Felson DT. Intra-articular hyaluronic acid in treatment of knee osteoarthritis: a meta-analysis. JAMA 2003;290(23):3115–3121.

86. Lohmander LS, Dalen N, Englund G, Hamalainen M, Jensen EM, Karlsson K, Odensten M, et al. Intra-articular hyaluronan injections in the treatment of osteoarthritis of the knee: a randomised, double blind, placebo controlled multicentre trial. Hyaluronan Multicentre Trial Group. Ann Rheum Dis 1996;55(7): 424–431.

87. Maheu E, Dreiser RL, Lequesne M. Methodology of clinical trials in hand osteoarthritis. Issues and proposals. Rev Rhum Engl Ed 1995;62(6 Suppl 1):55S-62S.

88. Puhl W, Bernau A, Greiling H, Kopcke W, Pforringer W, Steck KJ, Zacher J, Scharf HP. Intra-articular sodium hyaluronate in osteoarthritis of the knee: a multicenter, double-blind study. Osteoarthritis Cartilage 1993;1(4):233–241.

89. Raynauld JP, Torrance GW, Band PA, Goldsmith CH, Tugwell P, Walker V, Schultz M, Bellamy N; Canadian Knee OA Study Group. A prospective, randomized, pragmatic, health outcomes trial evaluating the incorporation of hylan G-F 20 into the treatment paradigm for patients with knee osteoarthritis (part 1 of 2): clinical results. Osteoarthritis Cartilage 2002;10(7):506–517.

90. Richette P, Ravaud P, Conrozier T, Euller-Ziegler L, Mazieres B, Maugars Y, Mulleman D, Clerson P, Chevalier X. Effect of hyaluronic acid in symptomatic hip osteoarthritis: a multicenter, randomized, placebo-controlled trial. Arthritis Rheum 2009;60(3):824–830.

91. Sun SF, Chou YJ, Hsu CW, Hwang CW, Hsu PT, Wang JL, Hsu YW, Chou MC. Efficacy of intra-articular hyaluronic acid in patients with osteoarthritis of the ankle: a prospective study. Osteoarthritis Cartilage 2006;14(9):867–874.

92. Witteveen AG, Giannini S, Guido G, Jerosch J, Lohrer H, Vannini F, Donati L, et al. A prospective multi-centre, open study of the safety and efficacy of hylan G-F 20 (Synvisc) in patients with symptomatic ankle (talo-crural) osteoarthritis. Foot Ankle Surg 2008;14(3):145–152.

93. Karatosun V, Unver B, Ozden A, Ozay Z, Gunal I. Intra-articular hyaluronic acid compared to exercise therapy in osteoarthritis of the ankle. A prospective randomized trial with long-term follow-up. Clin Exp Rheumatol 2008;26(2):288–294.

94. Luciani D, Cadossi M, Tesei F, Chiarello E, Giannini S. Viscosupplementation for grade II osteoarthritis of the ankle: a prospective study at 18 months' follow-up. Chir Organi Mov 2008;92(3):155–160.

95. Carpenter B, Motley T. The role of viscosupplementation in the ankle using hylan G-F 20. J Foot Ankle Surg 2008;47(5):377–384.

96. Cohen MM, Altman RD, Hollstrom R, Hollstrom C, Sun C, Gipson B. Safety and efficacy of intra-articular sodium hyaluronate (Hyalgan) in a randomized, double-blind study for osteoarthritis of the ankle. Foot Ankle Int 2008;29(7):657–663.

97. Salk RS, Chang TJ, D'Costa WF, Soomekh DJ, Grogan KA. Sodium hyaluronate in the treatment of osteoarthritis of the ankle: a controlled, randomized, double-blind pilot study. J Bone Joint Surg Am 2006;88(2):295–302.

98. Mei-Dan O, Maoz G, Swartzon M, Onel E, Kish B, Nyska M, Mann G. Treatment of osteochondritis dissecans of the ankle with hyaluronic acid injections: a prospective study. Foot Ankle Int 2008;29(12):1171–1178.

99. Gregory AJ. Periarticular hyaluronic acid as an adjunct to standard care for acute ankle sprain. Clin J Sport Med 2008;18(5):474–475.

100. Petrella RJ, Petrella MJ, Cogliano A. Periarticular hyaluronic acid in acute ankle sprain. Clin J Sport Med 2007;17(4):251–257.

101. Wang CW, Gao LH, Jin XY, Chen PB, Zhang GM. Clinical study of sodium hyaluronate in supplementary treatment of comminuted fracture of ankle. Zhongguo Xiu Fu Chong Jian Wai Ke Za Zhi 2002;16(1):21–22.

102. Moskowitz RW, Blaine TA. An overview of treatment options for persistent shoulder pain. Am J Orthop 2005;34(12 Suppl):10–15.

103. Andrews JR. Diagnosis and treatment of chronic painful shoulder: review of nonsurgical interventions. Arthroscopy 2005;21(3):333–347.

104. Blaine T, Moskowitz R, Udell J, Skyhar M, Levin R, Friedlander J, Daley M, Altman R. Treatment of persistent shoulder pain with sodium hyaluronate: a randomized, controlled trial. A multicenter study. J Bone Joint Surg Am 2008;90(5):970–979.

105. Leardini G, Perbellini A, Franceschini M, Mattara L. Intra-articular injections of hyaluronic acid in the treatment of painful shoulder. Clin Ther 1988;10(5):521–526.

106. Silverstein E, Leger R, Shea KP. The use of intra-articular hylan G-F 20 in the treatment of symptomatic osteoarthritis of the shoulder: a preliminary study. Am J Sports Med 2007;35(6):979–985.

107. Itokazu M, Matsunaga T. Clinical evaluation of high-molecular-weight sodium hyaluronate for the treatment of patients with periarthritis of the shoulder. Clin Ther 1995;17(5):946–955.

108. Calis M, Demir H, Ulker S, Kirnap M, Duygulu F, Calis HT. Is intraarticular sodium hyaluronate injection an alternative treatment in patients with adhesive capsulitis? Rheumatol Int 2006;26(6):536–540.

109. Fernandez-Palazzi F, Viso R, Boadas A, Ruiz-Saez A, Caviglia H, De Bosch NB. Intra-articular hyaluronic acid in the treatment of haemophilic chronic arthropathy. Haemophilia 2002;8(3):375–381.

110. Rovetta G, Monteforte P. Intraarticular injection of sodium hyaluronate plus steroid versus steroid in adhesive capsulitis of the shoulder. Int J Tissue React 1998;20(4):125–130.

111. Tamai K, Mashitori H, Ohno W, Hamada J, Sakai H, Saotome K. Synovial response to intraarticular injections of hyaluronate in frozen shoulder: a quantitative assessment with dynamic magnetic resonance imaging. J Orthop Sci 2004;9(3):230–234.

112. Bagis S, Sahin G, Yapici Y, Cimen OB, Erdogan C. The effect of hand osteoarthritis on grip and pinch strength and hand function in postmenopausal women. Clin Rheumatol 2003;22(6):420–424.

113. Heyworth BE, Lee JH, Kim PD, Lipton CB, Strauch RJ, Rosenwasser MP. Hylan versus corticosteroid versus placebo for treatment of basal joint arthritis: a prospective, randomized, double-blinded clinical trial. J Hand Surg [Am] 2008;33(1):40–48.

114. Coaccioli S, Pinoca F, Puxeddu A. Short term efficacy of intra-articular injection of hyaluronic acid in osteoarthritis of the first carpometacarpal joint in a preliminary open pilot study. Clin Ter 2006;157(4):321–325.

115. Roux C, Fontas E, Breuil V, Brocq O, Albert C, Euller-Ziegler L. Injection of intra-articular sodium hyaluronidate (Sinovial) into the carpometacarpal joint of the thumb (CMC1) in osteoarthritis. A prospective evaluation of efficacy. Joint Bone Spine 2007;74(4):368–372.

116. Schumacher HR, Meador R, Sieck M, Mohammed Y. Pilot Investigation of hyaluronate injections for first metacarpal-carpal (MC-C) osteoarthritis. J Clin Rheumatol 2004;10(2):59–62.

117. Salini V, De Amicis D, Abate M, Natale MA, Di Iorio A. Ultrasound-guided hyaluronic acid injection in carpometacarpal osteoarthritis: short-term results. Int J Immunopathol Pharmacol 2009;22 (2):455–460.

118. Fuchs S, Monikes R, Wohlmeiner A, Heyse T. Intra-articular hyaluronic acid compared with corticoid injections for the treatment of rhizarthrosis. Osteoarthritis Cartilage 2006;14(1):82–88.

119. Pons M, Alvarez F, Solana J, Viladot R, Varela L. Sodium hyaluronate in the treatment of hallux rigidus. A single-blind, randomized study. Foot Ankle Int 2007;28(1):38–42.

120. Calvillo O, Skaribas I, Turnipseed J. Anatomy and pathophysiology of the sacroiliac joint. Curr Rev Pain 2000;4(5):356–361.

121. Srejic U, Calvillo O, Kabakibou K. Viscosupplementation: a new concept in the treatment of sacroiliac joint syndrome: a preliminary report of four cases. Reg Anesth Pain Med 1999;24(1):84–88.

122. Wang W, Li P, Zhang YL, Yang Y, Wang FL, Zhang Y. The clinical effects of percutaneous lumbar discectomy combined with sodium hyaluronate in the treatment of lumbar intervertebral disc herniation. Zhongguo Xiu Fu Chong Jian Wai Ke Za Zhi 2002;16(1):23–25.

123. Hanson EC. Sodium hyaluronate—application in a community practice. Am J Orthop 1999;28(Suppl 11):11–12.

124. van Brakel RW, Eygendaal D. Intra-articular injection of hyaluronic acid is not effective for the treatment of posttraumatic osteoarthritis of the elbow. Arthroscopy 2006;22(11):1199–1203.

125. Fuchs S, Erbe T, Fischer HL, Tibesku CO. Intraarticular hyaluronic acid versus glucocorticoid injections for nonradicular pain in the lumbar spine. J Vasc Interv Radiol 2005;16(11):1493–1498.

126. Cleary M, Keating C, Poynton AR. Viscosupplementation in lumbar facet joint arthropathy: a pilot study. J Spinal Disord Tech 2008;21(1):29–32.

127. Bertolami CN, Gay T, Clark GT, Rendell J, Shetty V, Liu C, Swann DA. Use of sodium hyaluronate in treating temporomandibular joint disorders: a randomized, double-blind, placebo-controlled clinical trial. J Oral Maxillofac Surg 1993;51(3):232–242.

128. Bjornland T, Gjaerum AA, Moystad A. Osteoarthritis of the temporomandibular joint: an evaluation of the effects and complications of corticosteroid injection compared with injection with sodium hyaluronate. J Oral Rehabil 2007;34(8):583–589.

129. Guarda-Nardini L, Masiero S, Marioni G. Conservative treatment of temporomandibular joint osteoarthrosis: intra-articular injection of sodium hyaluronate. J Oral Rehabil 2005;32(10):729–734.

130. Guarda-Nardini L, Stifano M, Brombin C, Salmaso L, Manfredini D. A one-year case series of arthrocentesis with hyaluronic acid injections for temporomandibular joint osteoarthritis. Oral Surg Oral Med Oral Pathol Oral Radiol Endod 2007;103(6):e14–e22.

131. Guarda NL, Oliviero F, Ramonda R, Ferronato G. Influence of intra-articular injections of sodium hyaluronate on clinical features and synovial fluid nitric oxide levels of temporomandibular osteoarthritis. Reumatismo 2004;56(4):272–277.

132. Chazerain P, Rolland D, Cordonnier C, Ziza JM. Septic hip arthritis after multiple injections into the joint of hyaluronate and glucocorticoid. Rev Rhum Engl Ed 1999;66(7–9):436.

133. Bellamy N, Campbell J, Robinson V, Gee T, Bourne R, Wells G. Viscosupplementation for the treatment of osteoarthritis of the knee. Cochrane Database Syst Rev 2006;(2):CD005321.

134. Gaston MS, Tiemessen CH, Philips JE. Intra-articular hip viscosupplementation with synthetic hyaluronic acid for osteoarthritis: efficacy, safety and relation to pre-injection radiographs. Arch Orthop Trauma Surg 2007;127(10):899–903.

135. Gaffney K, Ledingham J, Perry JD. Intra-articular triamcinolone hexacetonide in knee osteoarthritis: factors influencing the clinical response. Ann Rheum Dis 1995;54(5):379–381.

136. Jones A, Regan M, Ledingham J, Pattrick M, Manhire A, Doherty M. Importance of placement of intra-articular steroid injections. BMJ 1993;307(6915):1329–1330.

137. Egsmose C, Lund B, Bach AR. Hip joint distension in osteoarthrosis. A triple-blind controlled study comparing the effect of intra-articular indoprofen with placebo. Scand J Rheumatol 1984;13(3):238–242.

138. Kirwan J. Is there a place for intra-articular hyaluronate in osteoarthritis of the knee? Knee 2001;8(2):93–101.

139. Ravaud P, Moulinier L, Giraudeau B, Ayral X, Guerin C, Noel E, Thomas P, Fautrel B, Mazieres B, Dougados M. Effects of joint lavage and steroid injection in patients with osteoarthritis of the knee: results of a multicenter, randomized, controlled trial. Arthritis Rheum 1999;42(3):475–482.

14 Hyaluronan for the Treatment of Osteoarthritis and Rheumatoid Arthritis

Toshiaki Nakano and Yasufumi Takahashi

CONTENTS

INTRODUCTION

Osteoarthritis (OA) is one of the most commonly diagnosed joint disorders characterized by slowly progressing degeneration and erosion of the articular cartilage matrix. OA most affects middle-aged and older populations and is generally present in weight-bearing joints such as the knees, hips, feet, and back. OA can hamper activities of daily living and decrease quality of life. It remains an important lifestyle-related and life-shortening disease, with the estimated number of people having latent OA reaching 24 million and those suffering from the manifest disease reaching 8.2 million [1] in Japan. Hyaluronan (HA) is present in all vertebrates and is also present in the capsule of some strains of streptococci. HA is also an essential component in many extracellular matrices in mature tissues. HA's high capacity for holding water and high viscoelasticity give it a unique profile among biological materials and make it suitable for various medical applications.

HAs in the synovial fluid (SF) of the knee in patients with OA are degraded into small molecules compared with those of healthy subjects as a result of synovial inflammation. Currently, palliation

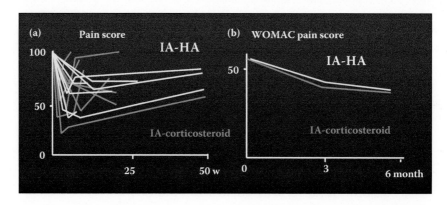

FIGURE 14.1 **(See color insert.)** Effect of intra-articular HA and intra-articular corticosteroid on OA. (a) Pain source. (From Kirwan J. Is there a place for intra-articular hyaluronate in osteoarthritis of the knee? The Knee 2001;8:93–101.) (b) WOMAC pain source. (From Leopold SS, Redd BB, Warme WJ, Wehrle PA, Pettis PD, Shott S. Corticosteroid compared with hyaluronic acid injections for the treatment of osteoarthritis of the knee: a prospective, randomized trial. J Bone Joint Surg Am 2003;85-A:1197–1203.)

of pain is the main goal of pharmacological treatment in OA, and the therapeutic armamentarium includes analgesics, nonsteroidal anti-inflammatory drugs (NSAIDs), intra-articular therapies with corticosteroids, and HA as well as topical treatments [2].

The effects of intra-articular HA injection, as compared with intra-articular corticosteroid injections, have more delayed onset and prolonged duration, although the strength of both pharmacological agents differs in degree but not in kind. This was also proven by 6-month long-term studies on the basis of measurements of the Western Ontario and MacMaster Universities Osteoarthritis Index, which did not demonstrate any significant differences in pain palliation or improvement of joint function between corticosteroid and HA intra-articular injections [3] (Figure 14.1). Accumulating evidence on the effectiveness and safety of intra-articular HA injections from many clinical trials around the globe has been recognized in the OA treatment guidelines published by the Osteoarthritis Research Society International (OARSI), an authoritative scientific committee composed of OA experts from the United States, Canada, and Europe. In the newest edition of the guidelines, indications for intra-articular HA injections are not only limited to cases presenting with insufficient effects of a corticosteroid therapy, but regardless of corticosteroid usage, intra-articular HA injection is treated as an important active treatment choice ranked with the highest level of evidence (Ia) among six available grades (Ia, Ib, IIa, IIb, III, and IV) [4].

HISTORY OF THE RESEARCH AND DEVELOPMENT OF THE 2700-kDa HA IN JAPAN

The original development of HA in clinical medicine is entirely due to Endre Balazs. In 1971, Rydell and Balazs [5] reported that injected HA in arthritic joints showed a dramatic positive effect on the clinical symptoms in truck horses. In 1974, J.G. Peyron [6] first reported the efficacy of HA in treating human OA. In 1987, HAs with a molecular weight (MW) of 500–1200 kDa named Hyalgan and Artz were marketed in Italy and Japan, respectively. Suvenyl (Chugai Pharmaceutical Co., Ltd., Tokyo) is a nonanimal, non-cross-linked, high-molecular-weight HA produced by a bacterial fermentation process, with a weight-average MW of 2700 kDa, determined by multiangle laser light scattering. Suvenyl has been reported to improve joint fluid viscoelasticity and lubrication and to inhibit articular cartilage degeneration and inflammatory synovial proliferation in MW in an HA-dependent manner since 1987.

In 1991, nationwide large-scale clinical studies of intra-articular 2700-kDa HA injection were initiated in patients with knee OA, periarthritis of the shoulder (PS), and knee rheumatoid arthritis

(RA) in Japan. It has been demonstrated that Suvenyl was more effective than the HA product, with an MW of 800 kDa, in the treatment of knee OA and PS [7, 8]. Furthermore, Suvenyl was shown to be effective in the treatment of knee RA as well [9]. Suvenyl was first approved for knee RA in addition to knee OA and PS in 2000.

THERAPEUTIC POSITIONING OF INTRA-ARTICULAR HA FOR OA IN EUROPE, THE UNITED STATES, AND JAPAN

In Japan, intra-articular HA injections have been registered as pharmaceuticals through the approval process of the regulatory authorities. Intra-articular HA injection is one of the most common treatments for knee OA. Intra-articular HA injection has so far established its position, selling 20 million syringes each year against 120 million people with an estimated 20 million OA patients in Japan. Most orthopedic surgeons in Japan are in consensus regarding the early use of HA in treating patients with OA. The clinical goal of intra-articular HA injection in Japan is to aid viscoelasticity and lubrication of the joint fluid, to prevent the pain associated with arthritis, and to prolong the duration until total joint replacement is needed.

In 1997, the U.S. Food and Drug Administration approved intra-articular HA injection as a medical device for the treatment of OA. Intra-articular HA injections have been exclusively used as medical devices in the United States and are used mostly as medical devices and partially as pharmaceuticals in the EU.

The question centers on whether intra-articular HA injection should be considered as a medical device or as a drug. As it is still being debated whether the effects of intra-articular HA injection were exhibited on the basis of the actual pharmacological effects or the mechanical effects, controversial argument on this issue is continuing.

At present, there are three kinds of intra-articular HA injection on the market as formulations of animal, cross-linked, nonanimal, and non-cross-linked products. The most important difference between medical devices and drugs is the manner of the reimbursement system. Gaining approval for use of reimbursed medical devices is usually much more difficult than that for drugs in Europe and in the United States. In the case of intra-articular HA injections, the process of determining the classification of reimbursement is quite complicated and different from country to country. The prices of intra-articular HA devices in Europe and in the United States are 9–14 times higher than that of intra-articular HA drugs in Japan.

That is why most orthopedists/rheumatologists hesitate in the greater use of intra-articular HA injections. At present, the therapeutic target of intra-articular HA injection seems to be relatively limited mainly only to increasing viscoelasticity and lubrication of joint fluid and relieving pain and a long-term perspective lacking. In Japan, more efficient clinical use of intra-articular HA injection that leads to prolongation of the duration until total knee replacement (TKR) is needed has been executed on the basis of its variety of pharmacological effects such as its chondroprotective and anti-inflammatory effects.

OARSI RECOMMENDATION FOR THE MANAGEMENT OF HIP AND KNEE OA

OA is the most common type of arthritis and the major cause of chronic musculoskeletal pain and mobility disability in elderly populations worldwide. Knee and hip pain are the major causes of difficulty in walking and climbing stairs in the elderly, and as many as 40% of people older than 65 years in Europe and in the United States suffer symptoms associated with knee or hip OA. Treatment of OA of the knee and hip is directed toward the following:

- Reducing joint pain and stiffness
- Maintaining and improving joint mobility
- Reducing physical disability and handicap
- Improving health-related quality of life

- Limiting the progression of joint damage
- Educating patients about the nature of the disorder and its management.

More than 50 modalities of nonpharmacological, pharmacological, and surgical therapy for knee and hip OA are described in the medical literature. Over the years, a number of national and regional guidelines have been developed to assist physicians, allied health professionals, and patients in their choice of therapy for the management of knee and hip OA, but internationally agreed and universally applicable guidelines for the management of these global disorders are lacking.

In September 2005, OARSI appointed an international, multidisciplinary committee of experts with a remit to produce up-to-date, evidence-based, globally relevant consensus recommendations for the management of knee and/or hip OA in 2007–2008. The draft guidelines were finally reached by OARSI members in 25 carefully worded recommendations. Optimal management of patients with OA hip or knee requires a combination of nonpharmacological and pharmacological modalities of therapy [4]. The recommendations cover the use of 12 nonpharmacological modalities: education and self-management; regular telephone contact; referral to a physical therapist; aerobic exercise; muscle strengthening and water-based exercises; weight reduction; walking aids; knee braces; footwear and insoles; thermal modalities; transcutaneous electrical nerve stimulation; and acupuncture. Eight recommendations cover the pharmacological modalities of treatment, including acetaminophen; cyclooxygenase-2 (COX-2) nonselective and selective oral NSAIDs; topical NSAIDs and capsaicin; intra-articular injections of corticosteroids and hyaluronates; glucosamine and/or chondroitin sulfate for symptom relief; glucosamine sulfate, chondroitin sulfate, and diacerein for possible structure-modifying effects; and the use of opioid analgesics for the treatment of refractory pain. There are recommendations covering five surgical modalities: total joint replacement, unicompartmental knee replacement, osteotomy and joint-preserving surgical procedures, joint lavage and arthroscopic debridement in knee OA, and joint fusion as a salvage procedure when joint replacement has failed. Strengths of recommendation and 95% confidence intervals (CIs) are provided.

Twenty-five carefully worded recommendations have been generated on the basis of a critical appraisal of existing guidelines, a systematic review of research evidence, and the consensus opinions of an international, multidisciplinary group of experts. The recommendations may be adapted for use in different countries or regions according to the availability of treatment modalities and strength of recommendation (SOR) for each modality of therapy.

STRENGTH OF RECOMMENDATION

The SOR for each treatment proposition was based on the opinions of the guideline development group after taking into consideration the research evidence for efficacy, safety, and cost-effectiveness of each treatment proposed and the clinical expertise of the members of the guideline committee, including such considerations as the experts' experience and perception of patient tolerance, acceptability, and adherence to the treatment in question and their expert knowledge on any logistical issues involved in the administration of the treatment.

LEVEL OF EVIDENCE

Level of Evidence	Type of Evidence
Ia	Meta-analysis of randomized controlled trials
Ib	At least one randomized controlled trial
IIa	At least one well-designed controlled study, but without randomization
IIb	At least one well-designed quasi-experimental study
III	At least one nonexperimental descriptive study (e.g., comparative, correlation, or case-controlled study)
IV	Expert committee reports, opinions, and/or experience of respected authorities

In the newest edition of the OARSI 2008 Guidelines, the indication for intra-articular HA injection is treated as an important active treatment choice ranked with the highest level of evidence (Ia) among six available grades.

Two propositions about intra-articular injections from eight pharmacological modalities of treatment in the OARSI 2008 OA Guidelines are as follows.

Intra-articular Corticosteroid Injections

Intra-articular injections with corticosteroids can be used in the treatment of hip or knee OA and should be particularly considered when patients have moderate to severe pain not responding satisfactorily to oral analgesic/anti-inflammatory agents and in patients with symptomatic knee OA with effusions or other physical signs of local inflammation (SOR = 78%, 95% CI = 61–95).

Intra-articular injections of corticosteroids have been widely used as adjunctive therapy in the treatment of patients with knee OA. The efficacy of intra-articular corticosteroid injections in patients with knee OA is well supported by more than 50 years of evidence. Potential side effects of intra-articular corticosteroid injections include postinjection flares of pain, crystal synovitis, and steroid articular cartilage atrophy.

Most experts recommend caution regarding too-frequent use of intra-articular corticosteroid injections to patients with OA hip or knee; repeat injections more than four times annually are not generally recommended.

Intra-articular HA Injections

Injections of intra-articular hyaluronate may be useful in patients with knee or hip OA. They are characterized by delayed onset but prolonged duration of symptomatic benefit when compared with intra-articular injections of corticosteroids (SOR = 64%, 95% CI = 43–85).

HA is a high-molecular-weight glycosaminoglycan, which is a constituent of SF in normal and osteoarthritic joints. Intra-articular injections of HA, with relatively high and low MW averages, are widely used and are recommended in most existing guidelines as a useful therapeutic modality for treating patients with OA knee as a viscosupplement or pharmaceutical. Most systematic reviews of intra-articular injections of HA in patients with OA knee suggest that the higher MW HA preparations may be more effective.

In 10 trials comparing intra-articular HA injections with intra-articular corticosteroid injections, there were no significant differences 4 weeks after injection, but intra-articular HA injection was shown to be more effective 5–13 weeks postinjection for one or more of a number of outcome variables (Western Ontario and MacMaster Universities Osteoarthritis Index, Lequesne Index, pain, range of flexion, and number of responders).

VISCOELASTICITY AND LUBRICATING EFFECTS OF HA

SF has interesting rheological properties. The MW of HA present in the SF of healthy individuals equals 3.5 to 5 × 1000 kDa [10]. Table 14.1 shows a comparison between viscosity, HA content, and MW in normal SF and those in pathological SFs. The viscosities of OA and RA remarkably decreased as compared with those of normal SF. The concentrations and MW of HA also decreased in the SFs in OA and RA [11].

The friction coefficient of a living joint is approximately 0.005, which is one tenth of the friction coefficient in skating or skiing. It indicates that an excellent lubrication mechanism exists for the joint (Figure 14.2).

Figure 14.3 shows the dynamic viscoelasticity of HA with different MWs. Two metal balls with the same weight were dropped into low- and high-molecular-weight HA solutions at the same time. The ball fell more slowly in high-molecular-weight HA solutions. This shows the higher viscosity of high-molecular-weight HA compared with that of low-molecular-weight HA (left-hand figure).

TABLE 14.1
Comparison of Viscosity, Hyaluronan (HA) Content, and Molecular Weight in Normal Synovial Fluid (SF) with Those in Pathological SFs

	Viscosity centi Poise (3.84/s)	HA Content (mg/mL)	Molecular Weight of HA ($\times 10^6$)
Osteoarthritis (OA)	219.6	1.7	2.7
Rhematoid arthritis (RA)	47.8	1.0	1.6
Normal	1992.0	3.6	3.7

Note: The viscosities of OA and RA remarkably decreased as compared with that of normal SF. The concentrations of HA also decreased in the SFs of OA and RA. The molecular weights of HA also decreased in OA and RA.

Source: Adapted from Kondo, H. *Kitasato Igaku* (Japan), 10, 485, 1980.

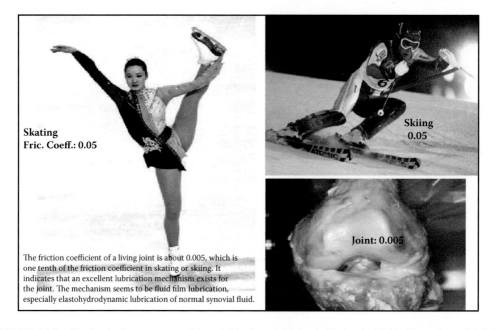

The friction coefficient of a living joint is about 0.005, which is one tenth of the friction coefficient in skating or skiing. It indicates that an excellent lubrication mechanism exists for the joint. The mechanism seems to be fluid film lubrication, especially elastohydrodynamic lubrication of normal synovial fluid.

FIGURE 14.2 Sizuka Arakawa won a gold medal in figure skating in Torino in 2006. (From Leopold, S.S., Redd, B.B., Warme, J.W., Wehrle, A.P., Pettis, D.P., and Shott, S., *J. Bone Joint Surg. Am.*, 85, 1197–1203, 2003.)

Two metal balls with the same weight were dropped from the same height into dishes with low- and high-molecular-weight HA solutions. The ball bounced against the high-molecular-weight HA solutions but not the low-molecular-weight HA. This shows the higher elasticity of high-molecular-weight HA compared with low-molecular-weight HA (right-hand figure).

Intra-articular HA restores the SF biorheologic characteristics and retards progression of degenerative changes within the articular cartilage.

Figure 14.4 shows the time course of liquid film formation of HA. In this figure, Oka et al. [12] reported that the 2700-kDa HA maintains a liquid film formation for a significantly longer period than the physiological saline and the 800-kDa HA.

They also showed that in OA and RA SFs, the reduction rate of the coefficient of friction obtained by adding the 2700-kDa HA was statistically significantly larger than that obtained by adding the 800-kDa HA (Figure 14.5) [13]. These results indicate that the 2700-kDa HA is superior to the 800-kDa HA in terms of both fluid film and boundary lubrication.

2700-kDa HA   800-kDa HA

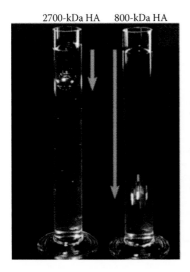
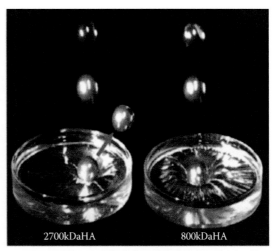

FIGURE 14.3   Viscoelasticity of HA with different MWs. (From Yamamoto M. The world of the articular cartilage supporting the locomotion. Sakura Video Library, Tokyo, 1996.)

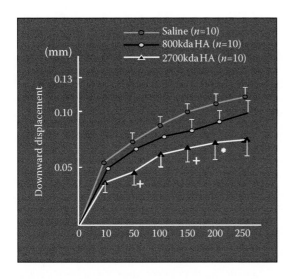

2700-KDa HA maintains a liquid film formation for significantly longer than physiological saline.

⟨Downward Displacement =
Chages in distance between cartilagesarface
& glass plate
⟨MEAN± S.E.⟩
⟨+: $p < 0.10$, *: $p < 0.05$, paired t-test⟩

FIGURE 14.4   (See color insert.) Time course of liquid film formation of HA. (From Oka, M., Nakamura, T., and Kitsugi, T., *Nihon Riumachi Kansetsu Geka*, 12, 259–266, 1993.)

EFFECT OF HA ON JOINT PAIN

The analgesic effect of HA was first demonstrated in race horses with traumatic arthritis [14]. In those studies, it was also discovered that the analgesic effect lasted much longer than expected from the residence time of injected HA in the joint. It was indicated that the analgesic effect was exerted by the elastoviscous properties existing in higher-molecular-weight HA because the lower-molecular-weight HA was unable to exhibit a long-lasting analgesic effect [15]. Thereafter, Gotoh et al. [16] reported that the pain induced by the injection of bradykinin in rat knee joints treated with hyaluronidase was suppressed by simultaneous injection of HA.

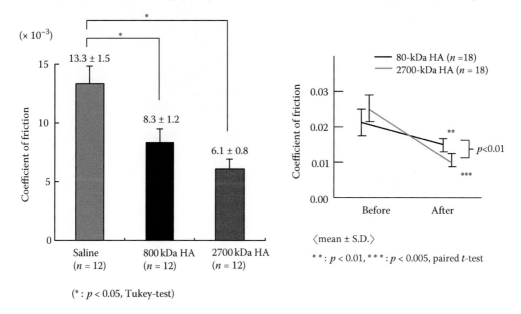

Effect on coefficient of friction in physiological saline   Effect on coefficient of friction in diseae joint fluid

FIGURE 14.5 (See color insert.) Boundary-lubricating effect of HA. (From Oka, M., Nakamura, T., Matsusue, Y., Akagi, M., and Horiguchi, M., *Seikei Saigai Geka*, 40, 77–84, 1997.)

Oda et al. [17] injected either the 800- or the 2700-kDa HA into the joint cavity in beagle dogs, where arthralgia was induced by monosodium urate crystals. The results suggested that the analgesic effect of HA became stronger in an MW- and a concentration-dependent manner.

Recently, Mihara et al. [18] demonstrated the analgesic effect of intra-articularly injected HA with an MW of 2700 kDa against an arthralgia model using partial meniscectomized rabbit.

In the mid-1990s, electrophysiological studies were conducted by Balazs [19] using cat knee joints to demonstrate the analgesic effect of high-average-molecular-weight HA such as hylan G-F 20 cross-linked by chemical modification. Hylan G-F 20 had a desensitizing effect on the nociceptive sensory receptor by reducing the frequency and intensity of nerve impulses.

ANTI-INFLAMMATORY EFFECTS OF HA

In the synovium of patients with OA or RA, prostaglandin E_2 (PGE_2) production is elevated and proliferation of synovial cells is observed. Enhancement of PGE_2 production and proliferation of synovial cells are implicated in the progression of proliferative inflammation in RA or OA.

Tamoto et al. [20] examined the inhibitory effects of the 300-, the 800-, and the 2700-kDa HA preparations on PGE_2 production by RA synovial cells. HA with an MW of 2700 kDa had the most significant inhibitory effect on production in the presence or absence of interleukin-1 (IL-1) (Figure 14.6).

They also studied the mechanism of the inhibitory effect and showed the most potent inhibitory effect of the 2700-kDa HA against the expression of COX-2 in RA synovial cells induced by IL-1. Because COX-2 expression is blocked by p38 MAP kinase inhibitors, HA with an MW of 2700 kDa is anticipated to exert its anti-inflammatory effects by binding firmly to HA receptors on the synovial cells, by inhibiting activation of p38 MAP kinase, and by blocking transcription of the COX-2 gene [21].

Yasui et al. [22] also reported that HA suppressed IL-1-induced PGE_2 production in human osteoarthritic synovial cells. From their results, it is suggested that HA suppresses the vicious cycle

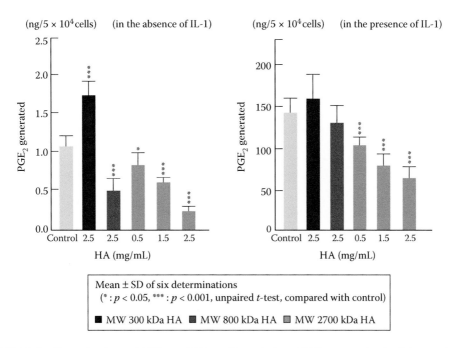

FIGURE 14.6 **(See color insert.)** Effects of HA on IL-1α-induced PGE$_2$ generation by RA synovial cells. (From Tamoto, K., Nochi, H., and Tokumitsu, Y., *Jpn. J. Rheumatol.*, 5, 227–236, 1994.)

of inflammation induced by stimulatory factors such as IL-1 and PGE$_2$ and exhibits efficacy against arthralgia in RA or OA. HA also inhibited the expression of urokinase-type plasminogen activator and plasminogen activator inhibitor-1 as well as urokinase-type plasminogen activator receptor in human synovial fibroblasts in OA and RA [23].

Angiogenesis is observed in the synovium of patients with RA and implicated in the progression and chronicity of synovitis. Saegusa et al. [24] reported that HA with a high MW more than 2000 kDa suppressed the proliferation of human endothelial cells but that lower-molecular-weight HA did not.

Among the cytokines that play a central role in chronic inflammation and joint destruction in RA joint pathology, there are IL-1, tumor necrosis factor α (TNF-α), and IL-6, which are predominantly produced by macrophages and synovial fibroblasts.

To investigate the therapeutic effect on RA, HA with an MW of 2700 kDa was injected into the proximal interphalangeal joints of monkeys with collagen-induced arthritis, an experimental RA model. HA reduced the degeneration of the articular cartilage and inflammatory proliferation of the synovial tissue, preserved the hyaline cartilage matrix, and blocked the expression of inflammatory cytokines such as IL-1 and TNF-α as well as matrix metalloproteinase 3 (MMP-3) in the cartilages and synovial cells compared with joints not treated with HA, as detected by an immunohistochemical study [25].

Goldberg and Toole [26] demonstrated that HA suppressed the proliferation of synovial cells in an MW-dependent manner and suggested that HA suppressed pannus formation in RA.

Yasuda [27] investigated the inhibitory mechanism of HA on lipopolysaccharide (LPS)-stimulated production of proinflammatory cytokines in U937 macrophages. HA with an MW of 2700 kDa at a concentration of 1 mg/mL significantly suppressed LPS-stimulated production of TNF-α, IL-1β, and IL-6 in U937 macrophages. In contrast to the 2700-kDa HA, the 800-kDa HA had no significant inhibitory effects on the production of these cytokines even at 3 mg/mL (Figure 14.7). The concentrations used in this study are within a range of physiological concentration (<4 mg/mL).

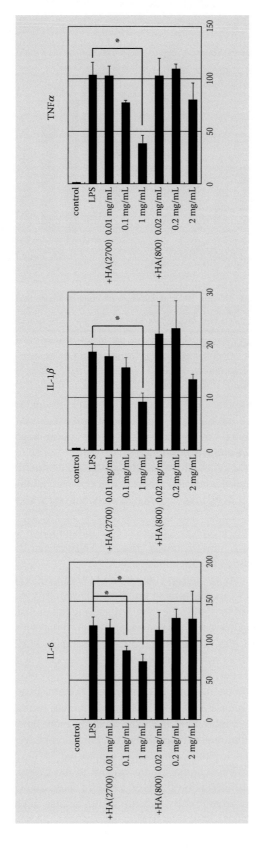

FIGURE 14.7 Inhibition by the 2700-kDa HA of proinflammatory cytokine production in LPS-stimulated U937 cells. (From Yasuda, T., *Inflamm. Res.*, 56, 246–253, 2007.)

Yasuda also demonstrated that the inhibitory effects of the 2700-kDa HA on the production of these cytokines were significantly reversed by the preincubation of the U937 macrophages with anti–intercellular adhesion molecule-1 (ICAM-1) antibody.

LPS also induces many intracellular responses, including the activation of NF-κB and the MAPK family (ERK, p38, and JNK). Therefore, they investigated whether the 2700-kDa HA affected the intracellular signaling pathways in LPS-stimulated U937 macrophages. When U937 macrophages were preincubated with the 2700-kDa HA, the LPS-induced levels of phosphorylated p65 NF-κB and IκBα were significantly downregulated. Pretreatment with the 2700-kDa HA at 1 mg/mL significantly reduced the nuclear accumulation of NF-κB by LPS. The necessity of NF-κB for proinflammatory cytokine production by LPS was confirmed using the NF-κB inhibitors, APDC, and BAY11–7085.

From these results, it was indicated that the 2700-kDa HA suppressed LPS-stimulated production of proinflammatory cytokines via ICAM-1 through downregulation of NF-κB and IκB. From these results, HA was strongly suggested to exhibit an inhibitory effect on the production of proinflammatory cytokines in the macrophages via the HA receptor, ICAM-1.

EFFECTS OF HA ON ARTICULAR CARTILAGE

In OA, the degeneration of articular cartilage is widely observed. Aggrecan degradation and subsequent decomposition of collagen fibrils play the central role in the destruction of cartilage in OA.

Shimazu et al. [28] reported that the inhibitory effect of HA on proteoglycan release by chondrocyte culture in the presence and absence of cytokines was dependent on the concentration and MW of HA.

Kikuchi et al. [29] investigated the effect of HA on cartilage degeneration in a partial meniscectomy model of OA prepared in rabbit knees. Intra-articular injection of HA (2700- or 800-kDa HA, 0.1 mg/kg) or PBS was conducted immediately after surgery and repeated twice weekly. The injection of HA suppressed the erosion and fibrillation of the cartilage matrix surface often observed in early degenerative OA in both the femoral condyle and the tibial plateau. The protective effect against early cartilage degeneration in the rabbit OA model with the 2700-kDa HA was more effective than that with the 800-kDa HA [29] (Figure 14.8).

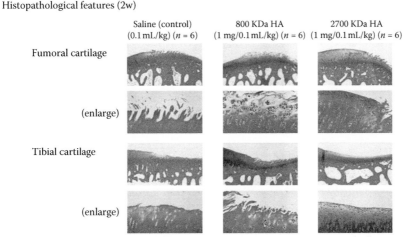

Histopathological features (2w)

Cartilage degeneration was inhibited by HA in a molecular weight-dependent manner   (saffrain Ostaining)

FIGURE 14.8   Effect of HAs in cartilage degeneration in a partial meniscectomy model of OA in the rabbit knee. (From Kikuchi, T., Yamada, H., and Shimmei, M., *Osteoarthritis Cartilage*, 4, 99–110, 1996.)

Fukuda et al. [30] showed that HA can penetrate the cartilage after IL-1 treatment. Recently, Kato et al. [31] demonstrated that HA can already penetrate synovial tissue and surface-damaged cartilage in partially meniscectomized OA model rabbits 3 h after intra-articular injection and might access and affect the synovial cells and the chondrocytes directly.

The MW-dependent effects of the 2700-kDa HA on the development of early degenerative OA changes observed by Kikuchi et al. [29] suggest that higher-molecular-weight HA is clinically more efficacious in the treatment of OA than lower-molecular-weight HA.

MMPs are considered to play an important role in the degradative process of cartilage matrix that leads to a degenerative change in OA cartilage. Kikuchi et al. [32] showed that the activity of MMP-3 in a chondrocyte culture medium was decreased by the addition of HA with an MW more than 2700 kDa.

Kang et al. [33] indicated that by blocking the penetration of fibronectin fragment into the cartilage at the cartilage surface, HA suppressed fibronectin fragment-mediated MMP production and degradation of cartilage in human cartilage explant cultures by enhancing proteoglycan synthesis.

Julovi et al. [34] reported that HA suppressed production of MMPs such as MMP-1, 13, and 3 in IL-1β-stimulated articular cartilage. They also demonstrated that the suppressive effect of HA on MMP production was mediated by CD44 as indicated by using anti-CD44 antibody.

Tanaka et al. [35] also indicated that HA suppressed MMP-1 and RANTES (regulated upon activation, normal T cell expressed, and secreted) production in IL-1β-stimulated OA chondrocytes, partly via the CD44 receptor in an MW-dependent manner (Figure 14.9). The recent study of Naito et al. [36] suggests that ADAMTS4 is a major aggrecanase and plays an essential role in aggrecan degradation in human osteoarthritic cartilage.

Yatabe et al. [37] recently reported the suppressive mechanism of HA on the expression of ADAMTS4 in chondrocytes via the signaling cascade (Figure 14.10). They first demonstrated that the suppressive effect of the 2700-kDa HA on the expression of ADAMTS4 in OA articular chondrocytes is mediated via CD44 and ICAM-1 expressed on the chondrocyte plasma membrane.

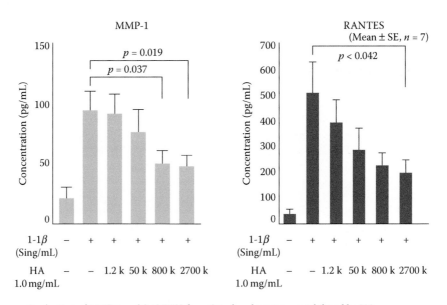

Production of MMP-1 and RANTES from OA chondrocytes was irhibited by HA in a molecular weight dependent manner.

FIGURE 14.9 Suppressive effects of HA on MMP-1 and RANTES production from OA chondrocytes. (From Tanaka M, Masuko-Hongo K, Kato T, Nishioka K, Nakamura H. Suppressive effects of hyaluronan on MMP-1 and RANTES production from chondrocytes. Rheumatol Int 2006;26:185–190.)

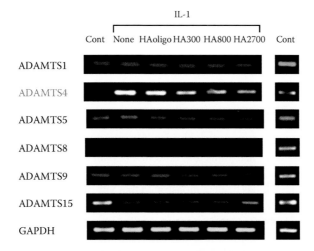

(HAoligo, 1.2-kDa HA; HA300, 300-kDa HA; HA800, 800-kDa HA; HA2700, 2700-kDa HA)

FIGURE 14.10 HA inhibits IL-1α-induced expression in OA chondrocytes in MW of HA-dependent manner. (Yatabe T, Mochizuki S, Takizawa M, Chijiiwa M, Okada A, Kimura T, Fujita Y, Matsumoto T, Toyama Y, Okada Y. Hyaluronan inhibits expression of ADAMTR4 (aggrecanase-1) in human osteoarthritic chondrocytes. Ann Rheum Dis 2009;68:1051–1058.)

In a study on the accessibility of the articular cartilage and synovium to the 2700-kDa HA, Kato et al. [31] also reported that higher-molecular-weight HA exhibits longer-term residence in the articular cartilage after penetration into the cartilage.

In relation to their report, Uzuki and Sawai [38] reported interesting results showing high affinity to degenerative cartilage of high-molecular-weight HA of 2700 kDa compared with low-molecular-weight HA less than 1000 kDa.

Kato et al. [31] also investigated the interaction between proteoglycan or chondroitin sulfate and HA of various MWs using bovine cartilage (300, 800, 1200, and 2700 kDa).

They showed that the interaction between HA and proteoglycan or chondroitin sulfate becomes stronger in high-molecular-weight HA of 2700 kDa compared with lower-molecular-weight HA less than 1200 kDa [39].

From these results, it is suggested that the 2700-kDa HA penetrating the degenerative cartilage might protect the cartilage from progression of degeneration by strong direct interaction with the cartilage matrix, aggrecan.

EFFECTS OF HA ON THE SUBCHONDRAL BONE

In OA, hypertrophic change of the subchondral bone with osteophyte formation and subchondral plate thickening are also observed, as is cartilage degeneration [40]. Recent studies suggest that subchondral bone sclerosis may be more closely involved in the progression or onset of OA than merely being a consequence of this disease [41]. Pelletier et al. [42] also showed that abnormal metabolism of osteoblasts in the subchondral bone may lead to osteophyte formation and sclerotic change in OA. They reported that HA inhibited the production of IL-6 and PGE_2 by osteoblasts in the subchondral bone in OA in an MW-dependent manner.

EFFECTS OF HA ON THE PROPERTIES OF JOINT FLUID

As a result of inflammation and destruction of articular cartilage, protein content and concentrations of chondroitin 4-sulfate and chondroitin 6-sulfate increase in the SF of patients with RA.

Viscosity decreases in the SF of patients with RA. HA with an MW of 2700 kDa significantly decreased the concentration of protein and chondroitin 4- and 6-sulfate and increased the viscosity in SF after intra-articular injection [43]. These results strongly suggest that a higher MW of HA exhibits efficacy in patients with RA and improves the properties of SF via anti-inflammatory and chondroprotective actions.

CLINICAL EFFECTIVENESS OF HA

In a phase III randomized controlled trial, 52.5-mL intra-articular injections of 1% Suvenyl were administered into OA and RA knee joints and PS joints of patients at intervals of 1 week. Efficacy was finally evaluated at 1 week after five injections by measuring the change in the pain score and the overall improvement rate. It has been demonstrated that Suvenyl was more effective than the HA product, with an MW of 800 kDa, in the treatment of knee OA and PS.

Comparing 1% Suvenyl (2700 kDa) with the 800-kDa HA, the overall improvement rate of 1% Suvenyl (2700 kDa) was higher (72.6%) than that of the 800-kDa HA (58.6%) for OA, as 1% Suvenyl was higher (65.7%) than that of the 800-kDa HA (50.5%) for PS [7, 8].

Comparison of 1% Suvenyl with a placebo (0.01% Suvenyl) revealed that the overall improvement rate of 1% Suvenyl was higher (65%) than that of 0.01% Suvenyl for knee RA [9] (Table 14.2).

Furthermore, a long-term study for knee RA showing a CRP value of less than 10 mg/dl and assigned Larsen's knee x-ray grades I to III also confirmed that Suvenyl provides symptomatic and structural efficacy in patients with knee RA [44] (Figure 14.11).

CONCLUSIONS

Since the 1980s, we have been tackling two questions: (1) Why is a higher MW of HA effective in the treatment of inflammatory disease? (2) Do the therapeutic effects of HA vary with its MW? Worldwide research groups have reported that the viscoelastic properties and analgesic,

TABLE 14.2
Results of Phase III Randomized Controlled Trials (RA, OA, and PS) Overall Improvement Rate

	Drug	Markedly Improved	Moderately Improved	Mildly Improved	Unchanged/ Aggravated	Total	Comparison between Groups*
RA[1]	Suvenyl (2700 kDa)	13 (19.1)	31 (64.7)	13	11	68	$z = 6.780$ $p = 0.0001$
	Placebo (0.01% Suvenyl)	0	4 (5.7)	29	37	70	
OA[2]	Suvenyl (2700 kDa)	20 (21.1)	49 (72.6)	18	8	95	$z = 2.521$ $p = 0.0117$
	Artz (800 kDa)	8 (9.2)	43 (58.6)	24	12	87	
PS[3]	Suvenyl (2700 kDa)	10 (10.1)	55 (65.7)	26	8	99	$z = 2.047$ $p = 0.041$
	Artz (800 kDa)	8 (8.1)	42 (50.5)	36	13	99	

( ), cumulative %; *Wilcoxon's rank sum test.

Abbreviations: OA, osteoarthritis; PS, periarthritis scapulohumeralis; RA, rheumatoid arthritis.

Sources: 1) S. Tanaka et al. *Clinical Rheumatol.* 12, 179, 2000; 2) M. Yamamoto et al. *Jpn Pharmacol. Ther.* 22, 4059, 1994; 3) R. Yamamoto et al. *Jpn Pharmacol. Ther.* 22, 4029, 1994.

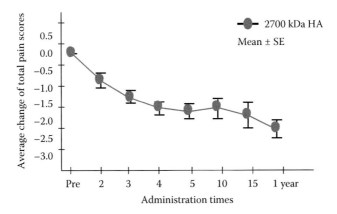

Intra-articular Suvenyl (2700-kDa HA) provides symptomatic efficacy in patients with knee RA for 1 year.

Severity of pain/inflammation symptoms were scored (Severe: 3, moderate: 2, mild: 1, absent: 0) and total pain score was evaluated as the difference in the score before and after administration (score after-score before)

FIGURE 14.11   Changes in total pain scores in knee RA.

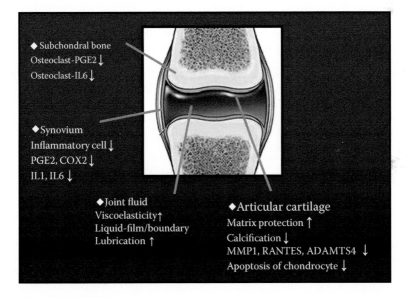

FIGURE 14.12   (See color insert.) Possible mechanisms of intra-articular HA for arthritis. (From Tanaka S, Fujii K, Nishioka K. Possible mechanism of intra-articular hyaluronan injections for arthritis. In "Intra-articular injection of high molecular weight hyaluronan" Medical Tribune, Tokyo, Japan 2003.)

anti-inflammatory, and chondroprotective effects of HA become stronger in an MW-dependent manner. A higher MW of HA is a substance quite unique that simultaneously suppresses inflammation of the synovial membranes, protects the articular cartilage and subchondral bone, and normalizes the properties of the joint fluid (Figure 14.12).

Today, there is no doubt about the inhibitory effect of a higher MW of HA on local inflammation of joints.

In 2000, a 2700-kDa HA product, Suvenyl, was first approved for knee RA in addition to knee OA and PS in Japan. Although Suvenyl has been well known to be effective in the treatment of knee RA and OA, it will be able to reduce or eliminate corticosteroid therapy and be able to retard arthroplasty for as long as possible in some advanced patients with OA and RA. In the newest OARSI 2008 Guidelines, indications for intra-articular HA are treated as an important active treatment choice ranked with the highest level of evidence for knee and hip OA.

REFERENCES

1. Muraki S, Oka H, Akune T, Mabuchi A, En-yo Y, Yoshida M, Saika A, et al. Prevalence of radiographic knee osteoarthritis and its association with knee pain in the elderly of Japanese population-based cohorts: the ROAD study. Osteoarthritis Cartilage 2009;17(19):1137–1143.
2. American College of Rheumatology Subcommittee on Osteoarthritis Guidelines. Recommendation for the medical management of osteoarthritis of the hip and knee. Arthritis Rheum 2000;43:1905–1915.
3. Leopold SS, Redd BB, Warme JW, Wehrle AP, Pettis DP, Shott S. Corticosteroid compared with hyaluronic acid injections for the treatment of osteoarthritis of the knee: a prospective, randomized trial. J Bone Joint Surg Am 2003;85:1197–1203.
4. Zhang W, Moskowitz RW, Nuki G, Abramson S, Altman RD, Arden N, Bierma-Zeinstra S, et al. OARSI recommendation for the management of hip and knee osteoarthritis. Part II: OARSI evidence-based, expert consensus guidelines. Osteoarthritis Cartilage 2008;16:137–162.
5. Rydell WN, Balazs AE. Effect of intra-articular injection of hyaluronic acid on the clinical symptoms of osteoarthritis and on granulation tissue formation. Clin Orthop 1971;80:25–32.
6. Peyron GJ, Balazs AE. Preliminary clinical assessment of Na-hyaluronate injection into human arthritic joints. Pathol Biol 1974;22:731–736.
7. Yamamoto M, Sugawara S, Tsukamoto Y, Motegi M, Iwata H, Ryu J, Takagishi K, Nakashima M. Clinical evaluation of high molecular weight sodium hyaluronate (NRD101) on osteoarthritis of the knee: a phase III comparative clinical study with ARTZ® as a control drug. Jpn Pharmacol Ther 1994;22:4059–4087.
8. Yamamoto R, Tabata S, Mikasa M, Takagishi K, Nakashima M. Phase III comparative clinical study of high molecular weight sodium hyaluronate (NRD101) with ARTZ® on periarthritis scapulohumeralis. Jpn Pharmacol Ther 1994;22:4029–4057.
9. Tanaka S, Yamamoto M, Komatsubara Y, Sugawara S, Sohen S, Matsubara T. Additional analysis for multi-center, long-term clinical study of high molecular weight hyaluronic acid (NRD101) on rheumatoid arthritis. Clin Rheumatol 2000;12:213–240.
10. Neustadt HD, Altman DR. Intra-articular therapy. In: Moskowitz WR, Altman DR, Hochberg CM, Buckwalter AJ, Goldberg MV, eds. Osteoarthritis diagnosis and medical/ surgical management. 4th ed. Philadelphia: Wolters Kluwer Lippincott Williams & Wilkins 2007;287–301.
11. Balazs AE, Watson D, Duff FI, Roseman S. Hyaluronic acid in synovial fluid. I. Molecular parameters of hyaluronic acid in normal and arthritic human fluids. Arthritis Rheum 1967;10:57–376.
12. Oka M, Nakamura T, Kitsugi T. Effect of high molecular weight hyaluronic acid on joint lubrication [in Japanese]. Nihon Riumachi Kansetsu Geka 1993;12:259–266.
13. Oka M, Nakamura T, Matsusue Y, Akagi M, Horiguchi M. Effects of high-molecular weight hyaluronate on joint disorders [in Japanese]. Seikei Saigai Geka 1997;40:77–84.
14. Balazs AE, Denlinger LJ. Sodium hyaluronate and joint function. Equine Vet Sci 1985;5:217–228.
15. Gomis A, Pawlak M, Balazs AE, Schmidt FR, Belmonte C. Effects of different molecular weight elastoviscous hyaluronan solutions on articular nociceptive afferents. Arthritis Rheum 2004;50:314–326.
16. Gotoh S, Miyazaki K, Onaya J, Sakamoto T, Tokuyasu K, Namiki O. Experimental knee pain model in rats and analgesic effect of sodium hyaluronate (SPH). Folia Pharmacol Jpn 1988;92:17–27.
17. Oda Y, Nomaki H, Arakawa H, Nakajima A, Ishihara R, Komatsu S, Hayashi T, Fujihira E. Analgesic effects of high molecular weight sodium hyaluronate (NRD101) upon monosodium urate-induced arthralgia in beagle dogs. Prog Med 1996;16:84–91.
18. Mihara M, Higo S, Uchiyama Y, Tanabe K, Saito K. Different effects of high molecular weight sodium hyaluronate and NSAID on the progression of the cartilage degeneration in rabbit OA model. Osteoarthritis Cartilage 2007;15:543–549.
19. Balazs AE. Analgesic effects of elastoviscous hyaluronan solutions and the treatment of arthritic pain. Cells Tissues Organs 2003;174:49–62.
20. Tamoto K, Nochi H, Tokumitsu Y. High molecular weight hyaluronic acids inhibit interleukin1-induced prostaglandin E_2 generation and prostaglandin E_2-elicited cyclic AMP accumulation in human rheumatoid arthritic synovial cells. Jpn J Rheumatol 1994;5:227–236.
21. Nochi H, Tanaka N, Tamoto K. Anti-inflammatory and analgesic effects of high-molecular-weight hyaluronic acids: action mechanism which control interleukin1-induced cyclooxygenase-2 expression in articular synovial cells. Clin Rheumatol 2004;16:383–394.

22. Yasui T, Akatsuka M, Tobetto K, Hayashi M, and Ando. The effect of hyaluronan on interleukin-1-alpha-induced prostaglandin E_2 production in human osteoarthritic synovial cells. Agents Actions 1992;37:155–156.

23. Nonaka T, Kikuchi H, Ikeda T, Okamoto Y, Hamanishi C, Tanaka S. Hyaluronic acid inhibits the expression of u-PA, PAI-1, and u-PAR in human synovial fibroblasts of osteoarthritis and rheumatoid arthritis. J Rheumatol 2000;27:997–1004.

24. Saegusa Y, Hirata S, Matsubara T, Hirohata K. Inhibition of human endothelial cell proliferation by hyaluronic acid. Clin Rheumatol 1989;2:127–131.

25. Ukari Y, Fujii K, Murota K. Therapeutic effect of high molecular weight hyaluronate on rheumatoid arthritis: experimental study on monkey with collagen-induced arthritis. Nihon Riumachi Kansetsu Geka 1993;12:351–366.

26. Goldberg LR, Toole PB. Hyaluronate inhibition of cell proliferation. Arthritis Rheum 1987;30: 769–778.

27. Yasuda T. Hyaluronan inhibits cytokine production by lipopolysaccharide-stimulated U937 macrophages through down-regulation of NF-κB via ICAM-1. Inflammation Res 2007;56:246–253.

28. Shimazu A, Jikko A, Iwamoto M, Koike T, Yan W, Okada Y, Shimmei M, Nakamura S, Kato Y. Effects of hyaluronic acid on the release of proteoglycan from the cell matrix in rabbit chondrocyte cultures in the presence and absence of cytokines. Arthritis Rheum 1993;36:247–253.

29. Kikuchi T, Yamada H, Shimmei M. Effect of high molecular weight hyaluronan on cartilage degeneration in a rabbit model of osteoarthritis. Osteoarthritis Cartilage 1996;4:99–110.

30. Fukuda K, Dan H, Takayama M, Kumano F, Saitoh M, Tanaka S. Hyaluronic acid increase proteoglycan synthesis in bovine articular cartilage in the presence of interleukin-1. J Pharmacol Exp Ther 1996;277:1672–1675.

31. Kato Y, Nishimura M, Kikuchi T, Sawai T. Accessibility of high molecular weight hyaluronan to articular cartilage and synovium. Clin Rheumatol 2009;21:20–31.

32. Kikuchi T, Shimmei M. Effects of hyaluronan on proteoglycan metabolism of rabbit articular chondrocytes in culture. Japanese J Rheumatol 1994;5:207–215.

33. Kang Y, Eger W, Koepp H, Williams J, Kuettner K, Homandberg AG. Hyaluronan suppresses fibronectin fragment-mediated damage to human cartilage explants cultures by enhancing proteoglycan synthesis. J Orthop Res 1999;17:858–869.

34. Julovi MS, Yasuda T, Shimizu M, Hiramitsu T, Nakamura T. Inhibition of interleukin-1β-stimulated production of matrix metalloproteases by hyaluronan via CD44 in human articular cartilage. Arthritis Rheum 2004;50:516–525.

35. Tanaka M, Masuko-Hongo K, Kato T, Nishioka K, Nakamura H. Suppressive effects of hyaluronan on MMP-1 and RANTES production from chondrocytes. Rheumatol Int 2006;26:185–190.

36. Naito S, Shiomi T, Okada A, Kimura T, Chijiiwa M, and Fujita Y, Yatabe T, Komiya K, Enomoto H, Fujikawa K, Okada Y. Expression of ADAMTS4 (aggrecanase-1) in human osteoarthritic cartilage. Pathol Int 2007;57:703–711.

37. Yatabe T, Mochizuki S, Takizawa M, Chijiiwa M, Okada A, Kimura T, Fujita Y, Matsumoto T, Toyama Y, Okada Y. Hyaluronan inhibits expression of ADAMTR4 (aggrecanase-1) in human osteoarthritic chondrocytes. Ann Rheum Dis 2009;68:1051–1058.

38. Uzuki M, Sawai T. Comparative studies of hyaluronan affinity among variable molecular weight on deteriorated cartilage. Japanese J Inflammation 1994;14:129–136.

39. Nishimura M, Yan Y, Mukudai Y, Nakamura S, Nakamasu K, Kawata M, Kawamoto T, et al. Role of chondroitin sulfate-hyaluronan interactions in the viscoelastic properties of extracellular matrices and fluids. Biochim Biophys Acta 1998;1380:1–9.

40. Pelletier PJ, Martel-Pelletier J, Howell SD. Etiopathogenesis of osteoarthritis. In: Koopman JW, ed. Arthritis & allied conditions. A textbook of rheumatology. 14th ed. Baltimore: Williams & Wilkins; 2001:2195–2245.

41. Hilal G, Martel-Pelletier J, Pelletier PJ, Ranger P and Lajeunesse D. Osteoblast-like cells from human subchondral osteoarthritic bone demonstrate an altered phenotype *in vitro*: possible role in subchondral bone sclerosis. Arthritis Rheum 1998;41:891–899.

42. Lajeunesse D, Delalandre A, Martel-Pelletier J, Pelletier PJ. Hyaluronic acid reverses the abnormal synthetic activity of human osteoarthritic subchondral bone osteoblasts. Bone 2003;33:703–710.

43. Matsuno H, Yudoh K, Kondo M, Goto M, Kimura T. Biochemical effect of intra-articular injections of high molecular weight hyaluronate in rheumatoid arthritis patients. Inflamm Res 1999;48:154–159.

44. Komatsubara Y, Inoue K, Sohen S, Murata N, Goto M, Minota S, Tanaka S. Long-term study of the effect of high molecular weight hyaluronic acid (Suvenyl®) on knee pain in rheumatoid arthritis. Clin Rheumatol 2004;16:314–337.

Section IV

Natural Therapeutic Interventions

15 Immunomodulatory Activities of Japanese Traditional Medicines in Rheumatoid Arthritis

Toshiaki Kogure

CONTENTS

INTRODUCTION

TRADITIONAL HERBAL (KAMPO) MEDICINE IN JAPAN

The Japanese traditional herbal (Kampo) medicine, which is covered by a national health insurance in Japan, is often prescribed in the primary care field and is also applied as an alternative remedy for serious diseases such as rheumatoid arthritis (RA). Since ancient times, many kinds of Kampo formulas have been used traditionally and found to be clinically effective for RA treatment. These formulas usually contain components from several medicinal plants that are thought to exert anti-inflammation and immune-regulator effects and contributed effective for treating chronic diseases [1–3].

Characteristics of Japanese Traditional Herbal (Kampo) Medicines

Kampo medicine has two features that differ from Western medicine: (1) the Kampo formula is composed of crude drugs, not purified chemical products, and (2) the diagnostic system in Kampo medicine is different from that in Western medicine. Kampo formulas are generally composed of several herbal components; therefore, it is considered that these remedies are safe. However, pseudoaldosteronism by licorice root is a well-known adverse effect of Traditional Herbal Medicines (THM), and there are also allergic effects, such as skin eruptions and liver injury, that can be induced by crude drugs. It is also thought that Kampo diagnosis may not be easy for readers to understand. When we treat RA patients with Kampo medicine, it is necessary to make a Kampo diagnosis as well as a diagnosis by Western medicine. This issue makes it difficult to perform controlled clinical trials. Therefore, there is very little evidence supporting Kampo formula for RA, although Kampo formulas are often prescribed for RA in Japan.

In this chapter, we described the immunomodulatory activities and clinical effects on RA as well as the characteristics of Kampo responders among the patients with RA.

IMMUNOMODULATORY ACTIVITIES

In a Mouse Arthritis Model

Collagen-induced Arthritis

Collagen-induced arthritis (CIA) has been considered a useful animal model for studying pathological mechanisms and therapeutic agents of RA. This experimental model shows many features that mimic those of RA in humans. For example, RA, synovitis, and erosion of cartilage and bone are hallmarks of CIA, and susceptibility to both RA and CIA is linked to the expression of specific MHC class II molecules. Although CIA is not identical to RA, the features of CIA clearly indicate that an autoimmune reaction to a cartilage component can lead to chronic, destructive polyarthritis. CIA can be induced in susceptible strains of rodents and primates by immunization with heterologous type II collagen (CII) [4–6], and it is the autoreactive component of the immune response that leads to disease [7]. CIA development has been shown to involve both cellular and humoral immunity to collagen type II, and passive transfer of T lymphocytes sensitized with collagen type II [8] or transfer of type II collagen-reactive sera [9] can also induce the disease in DBA/1 mice.

Immunomodulatory Activities of Hochu-ekki-to

Hochu-ekki-to (HET; Japanese name), a herbal formula, also known as Bu-Zhong-Yi-Qi-Tang (Chinese name), is composed of 10 species of medicinal plants and used for chronic diseases or weakness after illness [10]. HET has been widely used to treat patients with certain immune-related diseases. Recent studies have shown that HET formula also exhibits immunopharmacological activities such as increased protection against tumors [11, 12] and protection against bacterial infection [13] and viral infection [14]. Our previous report showed that HET caused a reduction of soluble CD23, a marker of activated B cells in a patient with RA, as well as improvement in joint symptoms [15].

Suppressive Effect of HET on the Development of CIA in Mouse

HET treatment resulted in a significant reduction in the incidence of CIA. On day 20 after the boost, only 66.7% (10/15) of mice in the 0.1-g/kg HET-treated group and 57.1% (24/42) of mice in the 0.5-g kg HET-treated group developed CIA in contrast to 92.8% (26/28) in the control (CONT) group.

We observed a delay in the onset of CIA symptoms by HET treatment. The first symptoms of CIA (onset) appeared around day 6 after the second CII injection in the CONT group. The 0.5-g/kg

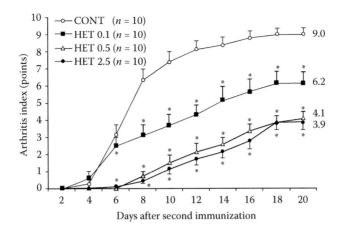

FIGURE 15.1　Suppressive effect of HET treatment on the progression of CIA. CIA was induced in DBA/1J mice by two injections of CII. Mice were orally treated from the day of the first injection with HET 0.1 g/kg (HET 0.1), 0.5 g/kg (HET 0.5), and 2.5 g/kg (HET 2.5) or untreated (CONT). The arthritis index in each group is presented as mean ± SE values. *$p < 0.05$ versus CONT, Mann–Whitney U test. (From Kogure, T., *J. Rheumatol.*, 29(8), 1601–1608, 2002.)

HET treatment from the day of the first CII injection significantly delayed the onset of CIA, until day 10 after the boost (*$p < 0.05$, Mann–Whitney U test). However, at a low dose of HET (0.1 g/kg), there was no delay in onset.

In addition, we observed a dose-dependent suppression of the clinical progression of CIA by HET treatment (Figure 15.1). In this experiment, HET treatment was performed at 0.1, 0.5, and 2.5 g/kg. In the CONT group, the arthritis severity was significantly more serious than that in the HET-treated groups at all indicated time points. The arthritic inflammation in the CONT group showed rather severe swelling of the entire paw in most mice. Fewer mice had swelling of the entire paw in the HET-treated groups. Figure 15.1 also shows that the suppressive effect of HET on the progression of CIA was dose dependent. HET treatment at 0.5 and 2.5 g/kg was clearly more effective than that at 0.1 g/kg.

The Suppression of B-Cell Activation in CIA by HET

Suppressive effect of HET on the development of CIA may have resulted from modulation of the immune response to CII. Although we do not yet completely understand the mechanism of the anti-RA activity of HET, these laboratory findings facilitate a partial explanation of these activities. The serum level of specific anti-CII IgG was reduced in the HET-treated group, indicating that HET treatment can inhibit the production of IgG specific for CII. This observation is very interesting because the production of anti-CII antibodies is thought to be important for the induction of arthritis and because the disease can be transferred by injection of antibodies specific for CII [9] and anti-CII antibodies cause deposition of immune complexes in the synovium or cartilage [16]. In addition, it is known that the production of anti-CII antibodies is associated with B-cell activation as well as cellular immunity. In CIA, blocking B-cell activation by treatment with anti-CD40 ligand leads to protection against the disease and a total block of the antibody response [17]. Thus, B-cell activation in the introduction phase plays a critical role in the development of CIA. It has been observed that oral administration of HET reduced the serum concentration of anti-CII antibody [18] (Figure 15.2). This reduction seems likely because of the result from the suppression of B-cell activation, and this effect might contribute to the suppression of CIA development.

With regard to change in serum interleukin-6 (IL-6) and tumor necrosis factor α (TNF-α) levels, in the CONT group, the serum levels of IL-6 and TNF-α dramatically increased. HET treatment significantly reduced the IL-6 serum level from 45.07 pg/mL in the CONT group to 8.45 pg/mL in the HET-treated mice. HET also reduced the serum TNF-α level. HET treatment also significantly decreased the concentration of circulating TNF-α from 16.73 pg/mL in untreated mice (CONT) to

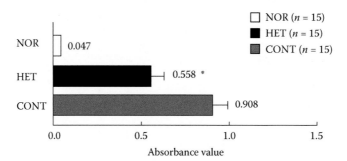

FIGURE 15.2 Suppressive effect of HET treatment on serum level of specific anti-CII antibody. Mice were injected with type II collagen twice to induce CIA and treated with HET or water only. Blood samples were collected on day 21 after boost. Specific anti-CII IgG Ab concentrations are presented as mean ± SE absorbance values. NOR, normal unimmunized mice; HET, mice treated with 0.5 g/kg Hochu-ekki-to; CONT: untreated mice. *$p < 0.005$ versus CONT, Mann–Whitney U test. (From Kogure, T., *J. Rheumatol.*, 29(8), 1601–1608, 2002.)

12.39 pg/mL in HET-treated mice. These results suggest that the modulation of IL-6 and TNF-α synthesis might contribute to the therapeutic effect of HET.

Lymphocyte Subset Partition Change in Lymphatic Tissues

Several investigators have shown an increase in B cells and a decrease in CD4/8-positive cells in blood and lymph nodes from CIA mice. In HET-treated mice, the proportions of CD8+,CD4+ T cells as well as B220+ cells were significantly restored toward normal levels. These observations indicated that the CIA-suppressing effect of HET might be due to modulation of the immune response to CII. In addition, regarding lymphocyte subpopulations in the thymus in both no-treated CIA mice and HET-treated mice, the subpopulation of thymic T cells did not change, suggesting that thymic T cell differentiation might not be associated with the action of HET.

As described earlier, the importance of CD40–CD40L ligation in the development of autoimmune disease has been illustrated in several murine models of autoimmunity by applying blocking antibodies [17, 19]. In CIA, blocking B-cell activation by treatment with anti-CD40 ligand leads to protection against the disease and a total block of the antibody response [17]. Other investigators demonstrated that the administration of stimulatory anti-CD40 monoclonal antibody resulted in earlier onset and more severe disease using CIA mice [20]. These observations suggest that the level of CD40 activation during the induction of an autoimmune response may determine the severity of the resulting disease. In our experiments, the populations of both CD40L+ cells and CD4+CD40L+ T cells in the lymphocytes obtained from lymph nodes and spleen tended to be decreased in HET mice compared with those in CONT mice, although the difference was not significant. We speculate that these effects, the suppression of T cell activation, may partially contribute to the improvement in joint damage [21].

Antirheumatic Drug: Fun-boi, Single Herb Medicine

RA is a chronic inflammatory disease associated with immune system abnormalities, the origins of which are not known, and there is still no complete cure. Conventional therapy for RA includes administration of nonsteroidal anti-inflammatory drugs, followed by disease-modifying antirheumatic drugs (DMARDs) such as methotrexate (MTX), hydroxychloroquine, sulfasalazine, or gold in patients who have persistent active disease. However, not a few patients discontinue therapy because of drug toxicity [22–24]. By contrast, traditional herbal medicine (Kampo), which has been in clinical use for thousands of years, is so safe that it can be administered continuously over several years. A crude preparation of Fun-boi (Fen-fan-ji in Chinese), which is the tuberous root of the creeper *Stephania tetrandra*, has been used for rheumatic diseases for thousands of years in rural areas of China. Its principle active ingredient, tetrandrine [25], is a bisbenzylisoquinoline alkaloid first isolated in 1935 and has been shown to have anti-inflammatory [26–31] and immunosuppressive [1, 32, 33] properties *in vitro* and in experimental animals.

The Immunomodulatory Effects of Fun-boi, a Herbal Medicine, on CIA *In Vivo*

Fun-boi therapy markedly reduced the severity of arthritis ($p < 0.001$) and tended to reduce the serum anti-CII antibody level ($p = 0.06$). Whereas CII immunization of DBA/1J mice caused a significant redistribution of CD3/CD8 lymphocytes from blood or lymph nodes, Fun-boi therapy caused significant normalization of the same types of lymphocyte subsets from lymph nodes but did not affect the CD4 or CD4/CD40L lymphocyte subsets.

These observations demonstrated that Fun-boi has therapeutic effects in CIA mice that may be induced through immunomodulation of secondary lymphocyte organs via redistribution of CD3/CD8 T lymphocytes from the blood or lymph nodes in response to local immunization of DBA/1J mice against CII. The treatment of CIA mice with Fun-boi extract prevented the development of arthritis and promoted normalization of the levels of these molecules in the lymph nodes only. The production of anti-CII antibody tended to be decreased in Fun-boi-treated mice [34].

IN HUMAN RA PATIENTS

Immunomodulatory Activities of Fun-boi, a Herbal Medicine, in RA

We undertook a prospective open label trial for 12 weeks using a decoction of Fun-boi to determine whether this remedy (1) is effective for RA, and (2) affects the peripheral blood lymphocyte subpopulations [35].

Efficacy and Adverse Reactions

Among clinical variables, there were significant improvements in the swollen joint counts, patient's and physician's global assessment, and patient's assessment of pain. There was no significant difference, but there was a tendency toward improvement in tender joint counts ($p = 0.07$). Among laboratory variables, there was a significant decrease in IgM–rheumatoid factor (RF) concentration. There was no significant improvement in C-reactive protein (CRP). According to the American College of Rheumatology definition of improvement in RA criteria [36], seven (24%) of the subjects enrolled in the trial showed 20% improvement and three (10%) showed 50% improvement at 12 weeks. There were no adverse reaction reported except by the two patients described earlier, nor did the laboratory tests demonstrate significant toxicity.

With regard to lymphocyte subpopulations in peripheral blood mononuclear cells, the numbers of CD19+ B cells and CD3+CD8$^+$ T cells were significantly increased, whereas the numbers of total peripheral lymphocytes, CD3+ T cells, and CD3+CD4$^+$ T cells were not changed. There was a significant decrease in the CD4-to-CD8 ratio. The number of natural killer cells was not changed by treatment with Fun-boi.

RA therapy with a decoction of Fun-boi may be effective in some patients and is remarkably safe. The therapeutic effect may be the result of immunomodulation, which seems to be similar to the mode of action shown by some types of DMARDs. This herbal medicine might be a useful alternative agent for the treatment of RA in conjunction with DMARDs.

CLINICAL EFFICACY FOR RA

CASE STUDY: RESPONDER TO KAMPO THERAPY IN RA

At present, clinical efficacy of drug should be proven through randomized controlled trials (RCT). However, it has been difficult to carry out the RCT in Kampo medicine because herbal medicine is a crude drug, and Kampo diagnosis is different from that in Western medicine. When there is the difference in drug efficacy among individuals, it is pointed out the case report written objectively is important [37]. Therefore, we described two patients with RA who were successfully treated with Kampo medicine and demonstrated a decrease in serum levels of anti-cyclic citrullinated peptide (anti-CCP) antibody, which is a useful marker in the diagnosis and prediction of joint damage [38, 39].

REPRESENTATIVE KAMPO FORMULA FOR RA: KEISHINIEPPIITTO-KA-RYOJUTSUBU

Keishinieppiitto-ka-ryojutsubu (KER; decoction), one of the Kampo formula, is often used as an adjunctive treatment for RA. The components of KER, which is a crude drug, are shown in Table 15.1. Some of the 12 herbs composing KER are pseudoephedrine (*Ephedrae herba*), paeoniflorin (*Paeoniae radix*), and tetrandrine (*Sinomeni caulis et rhizoma*). These components have anti-inflammatory or immunomodulatory effects. The clinical effects of KER on RA are thought to be at least partially due to the effects of each of these herbs. In addition, there are probably some interactions between each ingredient and the other components.

KER is usually administered following traditional diagnosis (Kampo diagnosis), in addition to diagnosis by Western medicine. The traditional target group for KER comprises patients with thirst, sweating, coldness in the extremities, and swollen joints as well as polyarthralgia in patients lacking physical strength [10]. If RA patients are outside this target group, other Kampo formulas such as Daibofuto or Boiogito are prescribed. We previously demonstrated that KER decreased the serum levels of IgM-RF as well as the Lansbury articular index [40]. There have not been any reports of toxic effects, although pseudoaldosteronism induced by licorice root is known. Therefore, KER is considered safe.

CASE REPORT

CASE 1

In 200X, a 61-year-old woman developed pain, swelling, and stiffness of the bilateral wrist joints and was diagnosed as having RA at a local hospital. She was treated with bucillamine (100 mg/day), and her condition remained in remission for approximately one year. In 200X + 1, she developed polyarthralgia again and was additionally treated with MTX and salazosulphapyridine (SASP), however, SASP was discontinued due to eczema. Polyarthralgia persisted, and the patient discontinued administration of MTX and bucillamine by herself in August 200X + 3. Thereafter, she consulted our hospital with a request for herbal medicine in September 200X + 3. At the first

TABLE 15.1
Herbs Composed of Keishinieppiitto-ka-ryojutsubu (KER)

Component (Herb)	Weight (g)
Atractylodis lanceae rhizome	10.0
Hoelen	5.0
Gypsum fibrosum	5.0
Zizyphi fructus	4.0
Cinnamomi cortex	3.0
Ephedrae herba	3.0
Paeoniae radix	3.0
Glycyrrhizae radix	3.0
Zingiberis rhizome	1.0
Aconiti tuber	1.5
Sinomeni caulis et rhizoma	5.0
Astragali radix	5.0

Note: Twelve herbs were mixed with 600 mL of water and boiled down to 300 mL, then the aqueous extract was filtered through a sieve. The extract, called a decoction, was administered twice a day in the morning and evening.

medical examination, she had severe polyarthralgia. There were no significant findings on physical examination of the neck, chest, and abdomen. Laboratory data were as follows: hemoglobin, 9.9 g/dL; erythrocyte sedimentation rate, 114 mm/h; CRP, 13.2 mg/dL; RF, 242 IU/mL; matrix metalloproteinase-3, 1839.5 ng/mL; and negative antinuclear antibody. Hepatic, renal, and thyroid functions were normal. Under informed consent, KER (decoction; Uchida Co. Ltd., Tokyo, Japan) alone was prescribed per mouth daily without DMARDs treatment according to the diagnosis by THM. After 3 months, treatment with KER alone resulted in improvement of her symptoms as well as a decrease in the serum levels of a series of serological markers (Figure 15.3). This patient was categorized as showing a good response (5.21–2.90) according to the DAS28; CRP(3) method (DAS28) [41]. Furthermore, her serum level of anti-CCP also decreased.

Case 2

In 200X, a 68-year-old woman developed pain at the bilateral metacarpophalangeal joint and wrist joints. She consulted a local hospital and was diagnosed as having RA. She was treated with gold sodium thiomalate 10 mg i.m./month and actarit 300 mg/day. Although her condition remained in remission for approximately 3 years, she then developed arthralgia in the bilateral wrists and shoulders. Therefore, she consulted our hospital with a request for herbal medicine in July 200X + 4. At the first medical examination, she demonstrated mild deformity in the bilateral metacarpophalangeal and wrist joints. There were no significant findings on physical examination of the neck, chest, and abdomen. Laboratory data were as follows: hemoglobin, 12.1 g/dL; erythrocyte sedimentation rate, 66 mm/h; CRP, 3.5 mg/dL; RF, 119 IU/mL, and negative antinuclear antibody. Hepatic, renal, and thyroid functions were normal. The administration of actarit was continued, but treatment with gold sodium thiomalate was stopped. In addition, KER was prescribed per mouth daily as an adjunctive to actarit. Three months later, joint symptoms have improved, and the serum levels of serological markers as well as anti-CCP had considerably decreased (Figure 15.4). This patient was also categorized as showing a good response (4.95–2.60) according to DAS28.

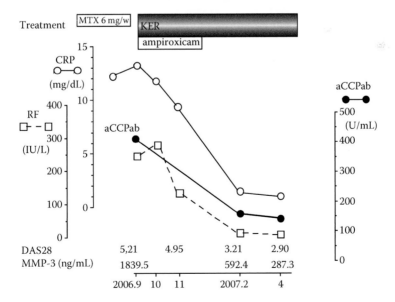

FIGURE 15.3 Clinical course (Case 1: a 61-year-old woman). The treatment with traditional herbal medicine resulted in good response according to DAS28 as well as the considerable decrease in serum level of aCCPab titer. aCCPab, anti-CCP antibodies; CRP, C-reactive protein; KER, Keishinieppiitto-ka-ryojutsubu (Kampo formula); MMP-3, matrix metalloproteinase-3; MTX, methotrexate; RF, IgM rheumatoid factor. (From Kogure, T., et al., *Clin Med. Arthritis Musculoskelet. Diord.*, 2, 22–28, 2009.)

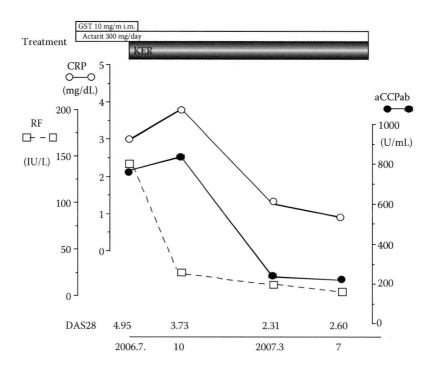

FIGURE 15.4 Clinical course (Case 2: a 68-year-old woman). GST, gold sodium thiomalate; KER, Keishinieppiitto-ka-ryojutsubu (Kampo formula). (From Kogure, T., et al., *Clin Med. Arthritis Musculoskelet. Diord.*, 2, 22–28, 2009.)

Two patients with RA were successfully treated with Kampo medicine and demonstrated a decrease in their serum levels of anti-CCP and RF. These measurements may be a useful adjunct in assessing the efficacy of this kind of treatment [42].

CASE SERIES STUDY

Clinical Efficacy of KER for RA

Study design is as follows: RA patients were treated with KER (decoction) according to the traditional diagnostic system [10]. Some patients were also treated with nonsteroidal anti-inflammatory drugs, bucillamine, SASP, prednisolone (PSL), and MTX at the start of treatment. These concomitant drugs were continued without changing the drugs or dosages during the 3 months before or during the observation period of this study. Every three months, joint symptoms were examined, and routine blood analysis and general serological tests were performed. Furthermore, we monitored the serum levels of anti-CCP every 6 months.

Baseline demographic and clinical characteristics of 34 patients receiving KER therapy are as follows: age 57.5 ± 10.3 years, duration 7.3 ± 6.1 years, RF 174.1 ± 154.7IU/mL, and DAS28-CRP 3.60 ± 0.98. Fourteen patients were classified in the responder group, and 13 patients were classified in the nonresponder group on the basis of DAS28-CRP findings. Patients with low activity (DAS28 < 2.7) from the start of KER treatment until 12 months after treatment was started were excluded; these patients were described as the out-of-assessment group. On comparison of the responder group and nonresponder group, there was no significant difference with regard to age or disease duration. Furthermore, the dosages of concomitant PSL at baseline did not vary between two groups.

Serum Levels of Anti-CCP in Patients with a Beneficial Response to Kampo Medicine

KER responders showed lower levels of anti-CCP at baseline than nonresponders (mean ± SD = 281.0 ± 113.3 vs 573.3 ± 235.7 U/mL, respectively, $p = 0.042$, Mann–Whitney U test). Other

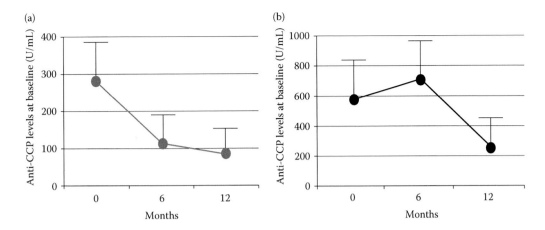

FIGURE 15.5 Changes in anti-CCP levels were assessed in each group. (a) Responder group: the levels of anti-CCP were significantly decreased after 6 months of treatment compared with the baseline values. (b) Nonresponder group: there was no significant decrease in anti-CCP levels at 6 months. It was thought that the decrease in anti-CCP levels after 6 months was due to additional medications other than KER. Importantly, there was a significant difference in the change in anti-CCP levels between the responder group and the nonresponder group when baseline values were compared with those after 6 months ($p < 0.048$, repeated-measures ANOVA). (From Kogure, T., et al., *Rheulmatol.Int.*, 29(12), 1441–1447, 2009.)

univariate analyses did not show any significant differences in baseline clinical measures of anatomical stage, functional class, DAS28-CRP, or RF levels between the two groups.

There have been recent reports focusing on anti-CCP changes induced by biologics targeting TNF or MTX and other DMARDs [43]. In our clinical findings, there was no significant difference in the levels of anti-CCP between the baseline and after 6 months of treatment in any of the patients receiving KER, although anti-CCP titers showed a tendency to decrease. Furthermore, the changes in anti-CCP titers were separately assessed in the responder group and nonresponder group (Figure 15.5). First, in responders to KER, the serum levels of anti-CCP were significantly decreased after 6 months compared with those at baseline. Subsequently, anti-CCP levels gradually decreased further by 12 months, although there was no significant difference between findings after 6 and 12 months in responders. In addition, the serum levels of RF were also decreased significantly in responders. In contrast, nonresponders did not show any decrease in anti-CCP levels after 6 months. In addition, there was a significant difference in the change in anti-CCP levels between the responder group and the nonresponder group. After 6 months, the serum levels of anti-CCP decreased in nonresponders because of additional medications other than KER as described earlier.

These findings demonstrate that pretreatment serum levels of anti-CCP are a useful predictor of a good response to treatment with KER and that a decrease in serum levels of anti-CCP may be an adjunctive indicator predicting the efficacy of this kind of treatment. These considerations may promote the establishment of evidence-based complementary and alternative medicine [44].

Furthermore, of the 12 patients with RA receiving concomitant MTX, 5 patients (41.7%) were defined as responders to KER treatment and 7 patients (58.3%) were classified as nonresponders to KER treatment based on DAS28-CRP findings. Responders to KER showed a significant decrease in the serum levels of anti-CCP. The annual cost of KER treatment is much less than that of other new drugs [45].

CONCLUSIONS

I have described the characteristics of the immunomodulatory effects of the Japanese traditional herbal (Kampo) medicine on CIA mice model and patients with RA and presented case series studies. It is difficult to perform an RCT in Kampo medicine because the diagnosis required by Kampo medicine is different from that performed in Western medicine. However, it is clear that there are responders to Kampo medicine among RA patients treated with Kampo medicine. Therefore, it is considered important to demonstrate the characteristics of responders.

REFERENCES

1. Chang DM, Chang WY, Kuo SY, Chang ML. The effects of traditional antirheumatic herbal medicines on immune response cells. J Rheumatol 1997;24:436–441.
2. Asano K, Matsuishi J, Yu Y, Kasahara T, Hisamitsu T. Suppressive effects of *Tripterygium wilfordii* Hook f., a traditional Chinese medicine, on collagen arthritis in mice. Immunopharmacol 1998;39:117–126.
3. Kobayashi S, Kobayashi H, Matsuno H, Kimura I, Kimura M. Inhibitory effects of anti-rheumatic drugs containing magnosalin, a compound from "Shin-I" (Flos magnoliae), on the proliferation of synovial cells in rheumatoid arthritis models. Immunopharmacol 1998;39:139–147.
4. Trentham DE, Towner AS, Kang AH. Autoimmunity to type II collagen: an experimental model of arthritis. J Exp Med 1977;46:857–868.
5. Courtenay JS, Dallman MJ, Dayan AD, Martin A, Mosedale B. Immunization against heterologous type II collagen induces arthritis in mice. Nature 1980;283:666–668.
6. Holmdahl R, Jansson L, Gullberg D, Rubin K, Forsberg PO, Klareskog L. Incidence of arthritis and auto-reactivity of anti-collagen antibodies after immunization of DBA/1 mice with heterologous and autologous collagen II. Clin Exp Immunol 1985;62:639–646.
7. Myers LK, Rosloniec EF, Cremer MA, Kang AH. Collagen-induced arthritis, an animal model of autoimmunity. Life Science 1997;61:1861–1878.
8. Holmdahl R, Klareskog L, Rubin K, Larsson E, Wigzell H. T lymphocytes in collagen II-induced arthritis in mice. Characterization of arthritogenic collagen II-specific T-cell lines and clones. Scand J Immunol 1985;22:295–306.
9. Stuart JM, Dixon FJ. Serum transfer of collagen-induced arthritis in mice. J Exp Med 1983;158:378–392.
10. Terasawa K. Kampo Japanese-Oriental Medicine, Insights from clinical cases. Hong Kong: K. K. Standard McIntyre publishing; 1993:249.
11. Onishi Y, Yamaura T, Tauchi K, Sakamoto T, Tsukada K, Nunome S, Komatsu Y, Saiki I. Expression of the anti-metastatic effect induced by Juzen-taiho-to based on the content of Shimotsu-to constituents. Biol Pharm Bull 1998;21:761–765.
12. Li T, Tamada K, Abe K, Tada H, Onoe Y, Tatsugami K, Harada M, Kubo C, Nomoto K. The restoration of the antitumor T cell response from stress-induced suppression using a traditional Chinese herbal medicine Hochu-ekki-to (TJ-41:Bu-Zhong-Yi- Qi-Tang). Immunopharmacol 1999;43:11–21.
13. Yamaoka Y, Kwakita T, Kishihara K, Nomoto K. Effect of a traditional Chinese medicine, Bu-Zhong-Yi-Qi-Tang on the protection against an oral infection with Listeria monocytogenes. Immunopharmacol 1998;39:215–223.
14. Hossain MS, Takimoto H, Hamano S, Yoshida H, Ninomiya T, Minamishima Y, Kimura G, Nomoto K. Protective effects of Hochu-ekki-to, a Chinese traditional herbal medicine against murine cytomegalovirus infection. Immunopharmacol 1999;41:169–181.
15. Kogure T, Nizawa A, Fujinaga H, Sakai S, Hai LX, Shimada Y, Terasawa K. A case of rheumatoid arthritis with a decrease in the serum concentration of soluble CD 23 by traditional herbal medicine. J Traditional Medicine 1999;16:190–195.
16. Kerwar SS, Englert ME, McReynolds RA, Landes MJ, Lloyd JM, Oronsky AL, Wilson FJ. Type II collagen-induced arthritis. Studies with purified anticollagen immunoglobulin. Arthritis Rheum 1983;26:1120–1131.
17. Durie FH, Fava RA, Foy TM, Aruffo A, Ledbetter JA, Noelle RJ. Prevention of collagen-induced arthritis with an antibody to gp39 the ligand for CD 40 Science 1993;261:1328–1330.
18. Hai le X, Kogure T, Niizawa A, Fujinaga H, Sakakibara I, Shimada Y, Watanabe H, Terasawa K. Suppressive effect of Hochu-ekki-to on collagen induced arthritis in DBA 1 mice. J Rheumatol 2002;29: 1601–1608.
19. Carayanniotis G, Masters SR, Noelle RJ. Suppression of murine thyroiditis via blockade of the CD40–CD 40 interaction. Immunology 1997;90:421–426.
20. Tellander AC, Michaelsson E, Brunmark C, Andersson M. Potent adjuvant effect by anti-CD4 in collagen-induced arthritis. Enhanced disease is accompanied by increased production of collagen type-II reactive IgG 2 and IFN-gamma. J Autoimmunity 2000;14:295–302.

21. Kogure T, Tatsumi T, Niizawa A, Fujinaga H, Shimada Y, Terasawa K. Population of CD40L-expressing cells was slightly but not significantly decreased in lymphoid tissues of collagen-induced arthritic mice treated with Hochu-ekki-to. Yakugaku Zasshi 2007;127:547–550.

22. Pincus T, Marcum SB, Callahan LF. Longterm drug therapy for rheumatoid arthritis in seven rheumatology private practices: II. Second line drugs and prednisone. J Rheumatol 1992;19:1885–1894.

23. Wolfe F, Hawley DJ, Cathey MA. Termination of slow acting antirheumatic therapy in rheumatoid arthritis: a 14-year prospective evaluation of 101 consecutive starts. J Rheumatol 1990;17:994–1002.

24. Wilske KR, Healey LA. Remodeling the pyramid—a concept whose time has come. J Rheumatol 1989;16:565–567.

25. Chen KK, Chen AL. The alkaloids of Han-Fang-Chi. J Biol Chem 1935;109:681–685.

26. Whitehouse MW, Fairlie DP, Thong YH. Anti-inflammatory activity of the isoquinoline alkaloid, tetrandrine, against established adjuvant arthritis in rats. Agents Actions 1994;42:123–127.

27. Chen F, Sun S, Kuhn DC, Lu Y, Gaydos LJ, Shi X, Demers LM. Tetrandrine inhibits signal-induced NF-kappa B activation in rat alveolar macrophages. Biochem Biophys Res Commun 1997;231:99–102.

28. Li SY, Ling LH, Teh BS, Seow WK, Thong YH. Anti-inflammatory and immunosuppressive properties of the *bis*-benzylisoquinolines: *in vitro* comparisons of tetrandrine and berbamine. Int J Immunopharmacol 1989;11:395–401.

29. Teh BS, Seow WK, Li SY, Thong YH. Inhibition of prostaglandin and leukotriene generation by the plant alkaloids tetrandrine and berbamine. Int J Immunopharmacol 1990;12:321–326.

30. Seow WK, Ferrante A, Li SY, Thong YH. Suppression of human monocyte interleukin 1 production by the plant alkaloid tetrandrine. Clin Exp Immunol 1989;75:47–51.

31. Ferrante A, Seow WK, Rowan KB, Thong YH. Tetrandrine, a plant alkaloid, inhibits the production of tumor necrosis factor-alpha (cachectin) by human monocytes. Clin Exp Immunol 1990;80:232–235.

32. Seow WK, Ferrante A, Goh DB, Chalmers AH, Li SY, Thong YH. *In vitro* immunosuppressive properties of the plant alkaloid tetrandrine. Int Arch Allergy Appl Immunol 1988;85:410–415.

33. Kondo Y, Imai Y, Hojo H, Hashimoto Y, Nozoe S. Selective inhibition of T-cell-dependent immune responses by bisbenzylisoquinoline alkaloids *in vivo*. Int J Immunopharmacol 1992;14:1181–1186.

34. Niizawa A, Kogure T, Hai LX, Fujinaga H, Takahashi K, Shimada Y, Terasawa K. Clinical and immunomodulatory effects of fun-boi, an herbal medicine, on collagen-induced arthritis *in vivo*. Clin Exp Rheumatol 2003;21:57–62.

35. Niizawa A, Kogure T, Fujinaga H, Takahashi K, Shimada Y, Terasawa K. Clinical and immunomodulatory effect of fun-boi, an herbal medicine, in rheumatoid arthritis. J Clin Rheumatol 2000;6:244–249.

36. Felson DT, Anderson JJ, Boers M. American collage of rheumatology preliminary definition of improvement in rheumatoid arthritis. Arthritis Rheum 1995;38:727–735.

37. Jenicek M. Clinical case reporting in evidence-based medicine. Boston: Butterworth-Heinmann 1999.

38. Kogure T, Tatsumi T, Fujinaga H, Niizawa A, Terasawa K. Insights to clinical use of serial determination in titers of cyclic citrullinated peptide autoantibodies. Mediators Inflamm 2007;12367. Epub.

39. Meyer O, Nicaise-Roland P, Santos MD, et al. Serial determination of cyclic citrullinated peptide autoantibodies predicted five-year radiological outcomes in a prospective cohort of patients with early rheumatoid arthritis. Arthritis Res Ther 2006;8:R40.

40. Kogure T, Itoh T, Shimada Y, Takahashi K, Terasawa K. The influence of a traditional herbal medicine on the disease activity in patients with rheumatoid arthritis. Clin Rheumatol Relat Res 1996;8:233–241.

41. Yamanaka H, Tanaka Y, Sekiguchi N, Inoue E, Saito K, Kameda H, Iikuni N, et al. retrospective clinical study on the notable efficacy and related factors of infliximab therapy in a rheumatoid arthritis management group in Japan. Mod Rheumatol 2007;17:28–32.

42. Kogure T, Oku Y, Kishi D, Ito T, Tatsumi T. The influence of traditional herbal medicine (Kampo) on anti–cyclic citrullinated peptide antibody levels. Clin Med Arthritis Musculoskelet Disord 2009;2;22–28.

43. Papadopoulos NG, Tsiaousis GZ, Pavlitou-Tsiontsi A, Giannakou A, Galanopoulou VK. Does the presence of anti-CCP autoantibodies and their serum levels influence the severity and activity in rheumatoid arthritis patients? Clin Rev Allergy Immunol 2008;34:11–15.

44. Kogure T, Sato H, Kishi D, Ito T, Tatsumi T. Serum levels of anti–cyclic citrullinated peptide antibodies are associated with a beneficial response to traditional herbal medicine (Kampo) in rheumatoid arthritis. Rheumatol Int 2009;29:1441–1447.

45. Kogure T, Tatsumi T, Sato H, Oku Y, Kishi D, Ito T. Traditional herbal medicines (Kampo) for patients with rheumatoid arthritis receiving concomitant methotrexate: a preliminary study. Altern Ther Health Med 2010;16:46–51.

16 An Overview on Natural Therapeutic Interventions

Stanley Naguwa

CONTENTS

INTRODUCTION

Natural therapeutic interventions, also termed complementary and natural health products or herbal medicines, are a diverse group of treatments [1] used in addition to or instead of conventional/allopathic treatment of diseases and health conditions. It has been long used, and recently there has been a resurgence of its use despite the advances in modern/Western medicine [2]. It has been extensively developed in China with traditional Chinese medicine and in India with Ayurveda. Its use presently in rheumatology may be driven by the unsatisfactory control or lack of a disease-modifying antirheumatic drug (DMARD), for example, osteoarthritis (OA) and low back pain (LBP); unacceptable adverse drug reactions, for example, DMARD treatment of rheumatoid arthritis (RA); or the desire to exert a greater degree of control of the risks/benefits/cost of treatment. Patients with unsatisfactory control of a disease may have an expectation of remission of the chronic arthritis, and when that is not possible with conventional treatment, they turn to complementary and alternative medicine (CAM) treatment in the hopes of a "miracle cure."

The cost issue is significant in the United States, where there is no national health care. In 2009, Himmelstein et al. [3] reported that in 2007, 62% of bankruptcy was due to medical issues; 92% of the 2314 bankruptcy filings were due to medical debt. CAM treatment costs are perceived to be lower, particularly as their advertisements are less well scrutinized than allopathic medication. However, the data for the true cost-effectiveness of CAM treatment are sparse [4].

EPIDEMIOLOGY

The use of CAM for all conditions ranges from 6% to 73%, depending on the survey tool used [5]. In the United States, the 2007 National Health Interview Survey of 23,393 adults revealed that 38% of adults used CAM (CAM1) at the cost of $34 billion [1, 6]. Natural products were the most commonly used CAM, of which fish oil or omega 3 fatty acid was most commonly used at 37%. Arthritic diseases/symptoms were the first four most common conditions in which CAM was used: back pain 17%, neck pain 6%, joint pain 5%, and arthritis 3.5% [1]. The use of CAM has increased from 2002 (prior survey) from 36% to 38%. In 2003, in a survey in California, a state with a diverse population, having a chronic condition (i.e., cancer, asthma/lung disease, arthritis/rheumatism, back or neck pain, stroke, diabetes, hypertension, and anxiety/depression) increased CAM use [7]. Being female, being older (but not older than 65 years), and having higher income and higher education increased the use of CAM; different race/ethnic group increased specific but not overall CAM use.

THE CHALLENGE

In the United States, natural therapeutic interventions are regulated as dietary supplements under the Dietary Supplement Health and Education Act (DSHEA) of 1994. The supplements derived from plant, animal, or mineral sources may be sold to reduce the risk of a disease/condition (health claim), to emphasize the relative amount of a nutrient (nutrient content claim), or to describe how a product affects an organ system but not disease (structure function claim) [3], whereas drugs, but not dietary supplements, may claim to diagnose, cure, investigate, treat, or prevent a disease.

Although labeling of dietary supplements must (according to DSHEA) contain a list of ingredients, amount, and source, there is no standardization, and until 2010, specified good manufacturing practices will not need to be met by all producers of dietary supplements [8]. It is common knowledge that allopathic drugs in the United States must have approval of the Food and Drug Administration (FDA) before they are marketed. Comprehensive studies of risk/benefit must be submitted, and postmarketing surveillance for side effects is necessary. For dietary supplements, per the DSHEA, supplements on the market before October 15, 1994, are presumed safe by history and not required to be reviewed by the FDA. For removal of a CAM already marketed, the FDA must prove that it is not safe, which is difficult as postmarketing surveillance is not required.

In the case of allopathic drugs, the substrates from which a drug is made must be of specific purity. In the case of dietary supplements, the substrate (plant/animal) is subject to variations of growing conditions (environment, soil, etc.), active ingredient content (e.g., part of plant), different cultivar and species, whole plant versus extract, variation in extraction, country of origin, and so forth [9]. No standardization is required for a dietary supplement. Advertising for allopathic drugs is strictly regulated by the FDA, with penalties for claims of efficacy not approved by the FDA. CAM advertising is monitored by the Federal Trade Commission.

Given the aforementioned, the challenge is to find rational, evidence-based medicine for the use of CAM therapies. The CAM data for four rheumatologic conditions and the data for exercise will be summarized.

OSTEOARTHRITIS

Many CAM therapies have been used for the management of OA, the most commonly experienced arthritis, for which a DMARD is not yet available. The CAM therapy that has recently received attention is glucosamine, of which there were 25 studies that were analyzed in a *Cochrane Review* by Towheed et al. [10]. The review demonstrated that the variation in products influenced the glucosamine treatment efficacy. In total, glucosamine did not show efficacy in pain and function improvement; however, if the Rotta brand glucosamine was analyzed separately, glucosamine use was superior to control. Glucosamine and chondroitin combination therapy was studied in a nonindustry, National Institutes of Health–sponsored evaluation of its use in knee OA. Clegg et al. [11]

reported that the combination did not help knee OA except in a smaller subgroup of patients with moderate to severe pain.

Other herbal CAM therapies were reviewed by Little et al. [12]. In their evaluation of 2,500 citations, only 24 met the inclusion criteria for review. However, only seven meet the full inclusion criteria and only five reported on, including treatment with Reumalex (a combination of biological supplements), capsaicin, avocado-soybean unsaponifiable oil fraction, and tipi tea of Petiveria alliacea. Except for the Tipi study, with a small number of subjects, these CAM therapies appear to have some efficacy. In a meta-analysis of dimethyl sulfoxide/methylsulfonylmethane use in OA by Brien et al. [13], their use did not show efficacy, with the notation that an inadequate dosing period may have been a potential confounding factor.

Instinctively, decreases in muscle strength should increase arthritis symptoms, and this was studied by Verweij et al. [14]. They confirmed that low muscle strength activities increased the risk of knee OA. The data with regard to exercise helping existing OA were evaluated by Fransen and McConnell [15] and showed short-term benefit equal to the use of nonsteroidal anti-inflammatory drugs. Aquatic exercise, with less strain on the joints, has been shown to be useful [16]. The data supporting the benefit of exercise for hip OA are sparse [17].

RHEUMATOID ARTHRITIS

RA is the most common inflammatory arthritis, with an approximately 1% prevalence in the United States. Although there are now very effective DMARDs, in particular the biologic response modifiers (BRM), with which remission is a reachable goal of treatment, the use of BRM DMARDs comes with significant risks, notably serious infections and non-B-cell lymphoma. Non-BRM DMARDs can cause bone marrow suppression, lung disease, and liver dysfunction; nonsteroidal anti-inflammatory drugs cause peptic ulcer, liver, and renal dysfunction; and corticosteroids increase the risk of infection, diabetes, hypertension, and vascular necrosis. Thus, RA patients are tempted to use CAM treatment to decrease the risk of adverse reactions. An excellent review of CAM therapies in RA can be found in the research report of the National Center for Complementary and Alternative Medicine [18]. Herbal therapy for RA was analyzed by Little and Parson [19], where 11 studies met inclusion criteria out of 2,500 citations. Gamma linoleic acid studies were 7 of the 11 studies and were felt to show improvement of joint scores, with the higher gamma linoleic doses better than doses less than 1.4 g/day. Feverfew had no benefit; *Tripterygium wilfordii* Hook F (TWHF) showed improvement of subjective and objective measures of disease activity, but there were adverse reactions; capsaicin topical was helpful in decreasing pains; and Reumalex (combination also used in OA) RA data were combined with OA. A recent study of *T. wilfordii* Hook F by Goldbach-Mansky et al. [20] showed benefits, but there were high dropout rates in both the treatment and the sulfasalazine control group. Dietary manipulations are an attractive CAM therapy, with theoretical benefits such as anti-inflammatory effects, increased antioxidants, or elimination of disease-triggering or disease-aggravating foods. A meta-analysis by Hagen et al. [21] analyzed 1029 studies, of which 15 fulfilled the study criteria. Although pain may decrease with diet manipulation, other outcomes such as function did not change, and the conclusion was with the caveat that there was a moderate risk of bias in the results.

Nutritional deprivation is immunosuppressive, and with weight loss a common factor in the active diet versus placebo diet studies, diets conferring weight loss may be of benefit [22].

Exercises that maintain muscle strength and joint mobility should have an adjunctive role in the management of RA. However, data to support its benefit are modest because of the quality of the studies [23]. Exercise helps with symptoms and may decrease the erythrocyte sedimentation rate [24], but it is not disease modifying [25]. Tai chi exercises, which have been used in China for centuries, was reviewed by Han et al. [26], who concluded that except for ankle range of motion, tai chi did not have a clinical impact on activities of daily living, tender/swollen joints, or patients' global assessment.

LOW BACK PAIN

LBP is a common complaint, with high prevalence and incidence of disability, for which CAM therapy is frequently used [27]. In a review of herbal medicines used in the management of LBP by Gagnier et al. in 2006, only 10 studies met the stringent criteria for review. The quality of the studies on three preparations varied. There were data for efficacy for the treatment of acute LBP with devil's claw (*Harpagophytum procumbens*), willow bark (*Salix alba*), and topical capsicum (*Capsium frutescens*). The data on the benefit of exercise in LBP were more robust, with 61 trials meeting the inclusion criteria for review by Hayden et al. [28]. They found that the cumulative pain scores decreased by 7 points (out of 100) and function improved by 2.5 points (out of 100).

FIBROMYALGIA

Fibromyalgia syndrome (FMS) is a condition of generalized musculoskeletal pain with hyperpathia. As with many rheumatologic conditions, the precise pathophysiology is not known, and there is an American College of Rheumatology classification criteria of 1990 so as to facilitate its study [29]. The most current hypothesis of its pathophysiology involves "the centrally mediated augmentation of pain and sensory process" [30]. As such, an estimated 90% of FMS patients use CAM therapies [31].

There appears limited evidence that magnesium, S-adenosyl-L-methionine, and Chlorella have efficacy in FMS, although more data are needed [32]. Dietary manipulation is notable for one study with good methodology, which showed that a vegetarian diet is less effective than amitriptyline [33].

Exercise/physical fitness as a significant factor in the pathology of FMS was noted in the seminal study by Moldofsky et al. [34]. Exercise in the management of FMS has a "good level of evidence" of benefit in the review by Busch et al. [35].

THE FUTURE

At present, there appears to be a disconnect between the need of CAM therapies by patients and the use and understanding of CAM therapies by allopathic physicians. In a Mayo Clinic study in 2006, 62% of physicians felt it was difficult to find reliable information of CAM therapies, in general, and 79% found it difficult to find reliable information on herbal therapies [36]. Although half felt that CAM treatments have a "true impact" on disease management, 70% also felt that the current practice of CAM represents a "threat to the health of the public." There is a geographic variation in such opinions, but the many *Cochrane Reviews* [12] would underscore the need for more and better data; <1% citations met the inclusion criteria.

To that end, efforts are ongoing to secure such data. A standardized checklist for reporting clinical trials has been proposed [37]. In addition to improving the reporting of the trial, if the checklist is consulted during the design stage, it will improve the quality of the study. As most rheumatologists would like to know the biologic/immunologic basis of CAM therapies in the treatment of arthritis, data are becoming available [38, 39].

If one prescribes a drug or advises on dietary supplements, it would be prudent to know the composition of the substance, its therapeutic dose, and the potential adverse reactions including substance-to-substance interactions. There has to be greater oversight of the CAM products because extreme variations in content have been documented [40]. A more detailed analysis of the composition effect of a CAM therapeutic may be useful as proposed in an article by Chavan et al. [41].

The challenge of providing patients with a safe therapeutic with established benefit and providing physicians with data to better counsel their patients is an immediate priority. In Germany, Commission E performs that difficult task; in England, the National Institute for Clinical Excellence; and in the United States, the National Center for Complementary and Alternative Medicine. Engel and Straus [42] have proposed a scheme that may be very helpful.

Useful Sources of CAM Therapy

Natural Medicines Comprehensive Database. http://naturaldatabase.therapeuticresearch. com.

International Bibliographic Information on Dietary Supplements (IBIDS) database. http://ods. od.nih.gov/health_information/ibids.aspx

REFERENCES

1. Barnes PM, Bloom B, Nahin RL. Complementary and alternative medicine use among adults and children: United States, 2007. Natl Health Stat Report 2008:1–23.
2. Chiappelli F, Prolo P, Cajulis OS. Evidence-based research in complementary and alternative medicine I: history. Evid Based Complement Alternat Med 2005;2:453–458.
3. Himmelstein DU, Thorne D, Warren E, Woolhandler S. Medical bankruptcy in the United States, 2007: results of a national study. Am J Med 2009;122:741–746.
4. Canter PH, Coon JT, Ernst E. Cost-effectiveness of complementary therapies in the United Kingdom—a systematic review. Evid Based Complement Alternat Med 2006;3:425–432.
5. Ramos-Remus C, Raut A. Complementary and alternative practices in rheumatology. Best Pract Res Clin Rheumatol 2008;22:741–757.
6. Nahim R, Barnes P, Stussman B, Bloom B. Costs of complementary and alternative medicine (CAM) in frequency of visits to CAM practitioners: United States, 2007. Natl Health Stat Report 2009;(18):1–14.
7. Goldstein MS, Brown ER, Ballard-Barbash R, Morgenstern H, Bastani R, Lee J, Gatto N, Ambs A. The use of complementary and alternative medicine among California adults with and without cancer. Evid Based Complement Alternat Med 2005;2:557–565.
8. Dietary Supplements: Background Information. http://ods.nih.gov/factsheets/DietarySupplements_pf.asp
9. Biologic Based Practices: An overview. 2007. http://nccam.nih.gov/health/BiologicBasedPractice
10. Towheed TE, Maxwell L, Anastassiades TP, Shea B, Houpt J, Robinson V, Hochberg MC, Wells G. Glucosamine therapy for treating osteoarthritis. Cochrane Database Syst Rev 2005;2:CD002946.
11. Sawitzke A, Shi H, Finco M, Dunlopp D, Bingham C, Harris C, Singer N, et al. The effect of glucosamine and/or chondroitin sulfate on the prognosis if knee osteoarthritis: a report from the glucosamine/chondroitin arthritis intervention trial. Arthritis Rheum 2008;58:3183–3191.
12. Little C, Parsons I, Logan S. Herbal therapy for treating osteoarthritis. Cochrane Database Syst Rev 2000:CD002947.
13. Brien S, Prescott P, Lewith G. Meta-analysis of the related nutritional supplements dimethyl sulfoxide and methylsulfonylmethane in the treatment of osteoarthritis of the knee. Evid Based Complement Alternat Med 2009 doi: 10.1093/ecom/nep045.
14. Verweij LM, van Schoor NM, Deeg DJ, Dekker J, Visser M. Physical activity and incident clinical knee osteoarthritis in older adults. Arthritis Rheum 2009;61:152–157.
15. Fransen F, McConnell S. Exercise for osteoarthritis of the knee. Cochrane Database Syst Rev 2008;4:CD004376.
16. Bartels EM, Lund H, Hagen KB, Dagfinrud H, Christensen R, Danneskiold-Samsoe B. Aquatic exercise for the treatment of knee and hip osteoarthritis. Cochrane Database Syst Rev 2007:CD005523.
17. Fransen M, McConnell S, Hernandez-Molina G, Reichenbach S. Exercise for osteoarthritis of the hip. Cochrane Database Syst Rev 2009:CD007912.
18. Rheumatoid Arthritis and Complementary and Alternative Medicine. NCCAM Publications 2005. http://nccam.nih.gov/health/RA/RA.pdf
19. Little C, Parsons T. Herbal therapy for treating rheumatoid arthritis. Cochrane Database Syst Rev 2000;4:CD002948.
20. Goldbach-Mansky R, Wilson M, Fleischmann R, Olsen N, Silverfield J, Kempf P, Kivitz A, et al. Comparison of *Tripterygium wilfordii* Hook F versus sulfasalazine in the treatment of rheumatoid arthritis: a randomized trial. Ann Intern Med 2009;151:229–240, W249–251.
21. Hagen KB, Byfuglien MG, Falzon L, Olsen SU, Smedslund G. Dietary interventions for rheumatoid arthritis. Cochrane Database Syst Rev 2009;1:CD006400.
22. Lord GM, Matarese G, Howard JK, Baker RJ, Bloom SR, Lechler RI. Leptin modulates the T-cell immune response and reverses starvation-induced immunosuppression. Nature 1998;394:897–901.
23. Cairns AP, McVeigh JG. A systematic review of the effects of dynamic exercise in rheumatoid arthritis. Rheumatol Int 2009;30(2)147–158.

24. Lundberg IE, Nader GA. Molecular effects of exercise in patients with inflammatory rheumatic disease. Nat Clin Pract Rheumatol 2008;4:597–604.

25. Oldfield V, Felson DT. Exercise therapy and orthotic devices in rheumatoid arthritis: evidence-based review. Curr Opin Rheumatol 2008;20:353–359.

26. Han A, Robinson V, Judd M, Taixiang W, Wells G, Tugwell P. Tai chi for treating rheumatoid arthritis. Cochrane Database Syst Rev 2004;3:CD004849.

27. Gagnier JJ, van Tulder M, Berman B, Bombardier C. Herbal medicine for low back pain. Cochrane Database Syst Rev 2006;2:CD004504.

28. Hayden JA, van Tulder MW, Malmivaara A, Koes BW. Exercise therapy for treatment of non-specific low back pain. Cochrane Database Syst Rev 2005;3:CD000335.

29. Wolfe F, Smythe HA, Yunus MB, Bennett RM, Bombardier C, Goldenberg DL, Tugwell P, et al. The American College of Rheumatology 1990 Criteria for the Classification of Fibromyalgia. Report of the Multicenter Criteria Committee. Arthritis Rheum 1990;33:160–172.

30. Williams DA, Clauw DJ. Understanding fibromyalgia: lessons from the broader pain research community. J Pain 2009;10:777–791.

31. CAM and Fibromyalgia: at a Glance. http://nccam.nih.gov/health/pain/fibromyalgia.htm

32. Holdcraft LC, Assefi N, Buchwald D. Complementary and alternative medicine in fibromyalgia and related syndromes. Best Pract Res Clin Rheumatol 2003;17:667–683.

33. Baranowsky J, Klose P, Musial F, Haeuser W, Dobos G, Langhorst J. Qualitative systemic review of randomized controlled trials on complementary and alternative medicine treatments in fibromyalgia. Rheumatol Int 2009;30(1):1–21.

34. Moldofsky H, Scarisbrick P, England R, Smythe H. Musculoskeletal symptoms and non-REM sleep disturbance in patients with "fibrositis syndrome" and healthy subjects. Psychosom Med 1975;37:341–351.

35. Busch AJ, Barber KA, Overend TJ, Peloso PM, Schachter CL. Exercise for treating fibromyalgia syndrome. Cochrane Database Syst Rev 2007;4:CD003786.

36. Wahner-Roedler DL, Vincent A, Elkin PL, Loehrer LL, Cha SS, Bauer BA. Physicians' attitudes toward complementary and alternative medicine and their knowledge of specific therapies: a survey at an academic medical center. Evid Based Complement Alternat Med 2006;3:495–501.

37. Gagnier JJ, Boon H, Rochon P, Moher D, Barnes J, Bombardier C. Reporting randomized, controlled trials of herbal interventions: an elaborated CONSORT statement. Ann Intern Med 2006;144:364–367.

38. Ahmed S, Anuntiyo J, Malemud CJ, Haqqi TM. Biological basis for the use of botanicals in osteoarthritis and rheumatoid arthritis: a review. Evid Based Complement Alternat Med 2005;2:301–308.

39. Setty AR, Sigal LH. Herbal medications commonly used in the practice of rheumatology: mechanisms of action, efficacy, and side effects. Semin Arthritis Rheum 2005;34:773–784.

40. Krochmal R, Hardy M, Bowerman S, Lu QY, Wang HJ, Elashoff R, Heber D. Phytochemical assays of commercial botanical dietary supplements. Evid Based Complement Alternat Med 2004;1:305–313.

41. Chavan P, Joshi K, Patwardhan B. DNA microarrays in herbal drug research. Evid Based Complement Alternat Med 2006;3:447–457.

42. Engel LW, Straus SE. Development of therapeutics: opportunities within complementary and alternative medicine. Nat Rev Drug Discov 2002;1:229–237.

17 Potential Health Benefits from Nutrition and Dietary Supplements in the Prevention of Osteoarthritis and Rheumatoid Arthritis

Cathy Creger Rosenbaum

CONTENTS

INTRODUCTION

Although more than 100 types of arthritis are known, this chapter will focus on osteoarthritis (OA) and rheumatoid arthritis (RA). Healthy knee, hip, and hand joints require proper nutrients (i.e., calcium, phosphorus, protein, vitamin C, vitamin D, vitamin E, and zinc) to regenerate new tissue including collagen. Typically, foods that promote collagen formation are rich in antioxidant and anti-inflammatory value (i.e., monounsaturated fatty acids like extra-virgin olive oil and polyunsaturated fatty acids like omega 3 fatty acids). Although prudent options for general health, proper nutrition, and use of dietary supplements alone cannot cure, reverse, or halt the progression of OA or RA.

Primary strategies to prevent OA and RA as well as secondary strategies that have disease-modifying effects on cartilage or decrease progression of joint symptoms in people with known disease (e.g., pain, reduced mobility, inflammation) will be reviewed from *in vitro,* animal, and human clinical studies when available. Ideally, when interpreting clinical study results focused on disease-modifying activity secondary to use of dietary supplements, well-designed models should include standardized radiological techniques for diagnosing disease as well as measuring changes in knee joint width. Validated pain scales (e.g., the Western Ontario and McMaster University Osteoarthritis Index visual analog scale [WOMAC]) are key for objective interpretation of primary outcome measures focused on joint pain, and validated range of motion tools are included to study effects on joint mobility.

Topical remedies (i.e., ZingiberRx Cream, Traumeel Cream, and Arnica Montana Gel), methyl sulfonyl methane, an oral analgesic and a muscle-related anti-inflammatory agent, and injectable dietary supplements (i.e., intramuscular or intra-articular glucosamine, chondroitin, dimethyl sulfoxide, or resveratrol) have been reviewed elsewhere (Elmali et al., 2005; Widrig et a., 2007; Rosenbaum et al., 2010) and are not included in this review. For perspective, some dietary supplements may cause unwanted effects and interactions with other supplements and prescription or over-the-counter medications used to treat OA and RA, all of which should be managed by a trained health care professional.

OSTEOARTHRITIS

With increased life expectancy come the greater incidence and prevalence of OA. OA is a complex disease associated with multifactorial risks. More research is needed regarding epidemiology, pathophysiology (e.g., including inflammatory and oxidative biomarkers of disease activity), and clinical diagnosis. One intervention that helps maintain healthy joints is weight management through exercise and good nutrition to reduce the risk of developing active disease. Excess caloric intake may cause oxidative stress and joint inflammation. Degenerative joint disease over time is associated with obesity, and obesity is the strongest modifiable risk factor for OA primary prevention. OA may also be prevented by moving, maintaining good posture, engaging in a variety of physical activities, and avoiding injury to the joints.

NUTRITION

People with antioxidant deficiencies in their diet may be at increased risk for OA. No standard nutritional regimen can be recommended for primary or secondary OA prevention, yet the Mediterranean diet with foods high in antioxidant and anti-inflammatory value is an appealing starting point for general health (Cleland et al., 1995; McAlindon 1966b; McAlindon 2005).

DIETARY SUPPLEMENTS

The Osteoarthritis Research Society International (OARSI) has no official position on the value of dietary supplements for the primary prevention of OA (Diann Stern, Executive Director, April 16, 2010, personal communication). The use of dietary supplements (i.e., vitamin C, vitamin D, green tea, glucosamine, chondroitin, SAMe, avocado oil/soybean unsaponifiable residues [ASU], and cat's claw) to manage symptoms and/or to modify disease in people with OA is reviewed.

Vitamin C

Vitamin C is an antioxidant. In theory, antioxidants may help prevent free radicals and reactive oxygen species from destroying cartilage. Yudol et al. (2005) compared human chondrocytes under oxidative stress from articular cartilage in patients with knee OA and human chondrocytes in the presence of vitamin C. Low antioxidative capacity in the chondrocyte correlated with histologic cartilage damage. Vitamin C is needed for collagen synthesis in joint cartilage, and high vitamin C intake may reduce risk of developing OA (primary prevention) as well as reduce joint symptoms in people with OA (secondary prevention). Multiple antioxidant supplements were studied in prevention of knee OA in the prospective observational Framingham Osteoarthritis Cohort Study (McAlindon et al., 1996a). Authors reported that high intake of vitamin C (mean of 430 mg daily), β-carotene (mean of 14,800 IU daily), and vitamin E (126 mg of α-tocopherol equivalents daily) reduced disease progression in people with OA but did not offer protection in healthy individuals. For perspective, well-designed human clinical trials with antioxidants should stratify for diets containing antioxidant foods and antioxidant dietary supplements as well as endogenous oxidative stress–related biomarkers in the blood (assays: lipid hydroperoxides, 4-HNE, F2-isoprostanes, protein thiol oxidation, oxidized amino acids, 8OhdG, and Comet) to accurately interpret outcome measures.

Green Tea

Green tea is another antioxidant available in the form of a dietary supplement or as a tea. Green tea constituents include polyphenolic compounds (e.g., catechins: epigallocatehin 3-gallate [EGCG], and epicatechin 3-gallate) that are known to prevent collagen-induced arthritis in mice (Goggs et al., 2005). EGCG inhibits interleukin (IL)-1-induced proteoglycan release in cartilage explants in a bovine *in vitro* model. EGCG inhibits IL-1B-induced activity of cyclooxygenase-2 and iNOS mRNA in human chondrocytes from OA cartilage *in vitro* (Ahmed et al., 2002). Green tea catechins exhibit anti-inflammatory and chondroprotective effects *in vitro*. More research is needed to determine if consumption of oral green tea dietary supplements or green tea will offer high enough joint concentrations of antioxidant catechins to match results seen *in vitro*.

Vitamin D

There may be as much as a threefold increase in the risk for knee OA disease progression in people with low vitamin C and vitamin D blood levels. Yet, low vitamin D blood levels are not associated with risk for developing OA in people with healthy knees. Vitamin D plays a role in articular cartilage turnover. Bone in addition to joints may be structurally changed in people with OA. However, observational studies demonstrate conflicting results of the role of vitamin D in OA progression in patients with knee OA (McAlindon et al., 1996a). In the Framingham study, low vitamin D intake and low vitamin D blood levels were associated with increased progression of knee OA but not with incidence of newly diagnosed OA (McAlindon et al., 1996a). However, in another prospective study in people 65 years or older, lower blood 25-hydroxyvitamin D levels were associated with increased risk of developing hip OA (Lane et al., 1999). More human clinical research is warranted to quantify the dose of vitamin D necessary to prevent or retard symptom progression.

Glucosamine and Chondroitin

The aminosaccharide dietary supplement glucosamine is available as sulfate, hydrochloride, *N*-acetyl, or chlorhydrate salt. In articular cartilage, glucosamine is acetylated, sulfated, and built into keratin sulfate, heparan sulfate, and hyaluronan. Keratan sulfate and hyaluronan maintain structural and functional integrity of articular cartilage by binding water in joint tissue. Interestingly, glucosamine may suppress T-lymphoblast activation *in vitro* in a dose-dependent manner (e.g., immunosuppression). Chondroitin is a glycosaminoglycan polysaccharide. Both glucosamine and chondroitin are naturally occurring constituents in cartilage proteoglycans yet have not been proven to prevent OA from occurring in healthy individuals. Chondroitin sulfate and glucosamine sulfate have shown modest improvements in pain and mobility in osteoarthritic knee and hip joints. However, study results may not be transferable to finger, spine, and ankle joints in individuals with OA (Towheed et al., 2009).

The Glucosamine/Chondroitin Arthritis Intervention Trial funded by the National Institutes of Health studied patients with knee OA and compared 1500 mg of glucosamine sulfate with 1200 mg of sodium chondroitin sulfate daily. Both supplements combined, Celebrex 200 mg daily, and placebo for 24 weeks. Rescue analgesia with up to 4000 mg acetaminophen daily was permitted. The primary outcome measure was a 20% decrease in knee pain from baseline at 24 weeks of therapy. Clegg et al. (2006) found that neither glucosamine nor chondroitin, nor both supplements combined reduced knee pain with statistical significance more effectively than placebo. Celebrex pain relief was significantly higher than placebo ($p = 0.008$) (Towheed et al., 2009).

The potential structure-modifying effects of glucosamine on knee cartilage are not as consistent as the symptomatic benefit of pain relief according to the OARSI. The OARSI recommends that glucosamine be discontinued if no apparent response is seen within 6 months of treatment. Glucosamine sulfate may contain sodium in the formulation and should be avoided by people with hypertension. Glucosamine may cause a reaction to people allergic to shellfish chitin or insect, algae, or mushroom chitin (European products) and may slightly increase blood sugar (e.g., insulin resistance) in diabetics.

Chondroitin

Chondroitin sulfate is manufactured from shark and bovine cartilage, and merely 10% is bioavailable to synovial fluid, cartilage, or bone when taken by mouth. Chondroitin stimulates synthesis of proteoglycans by chondrocytes *in vitro* (Leeb et al., 2000). Morreale et al. studied 46 patients with knee OA and randomized them into two groups (Morreale 1996). One group received Voltaren 50 mg three times daily for 1 month, followed by placebo for 2 months, and the other group received 3 months' worth of chondroitin sulfate 400 mg three times daily. Both groups received placebo for an additional 3 months. Clinical efficacy was evaluated by the Lesquesne Index, pain scores, and acetaminophen use. Authors reported that chondroitin was statistically significantly more effective than placebo in all measured parameters, and efficacy continued to increase over time while participants were taking chondroitin. Benefits from chondroitin reversed upon discontinuation. No significant side effects were reported.

Leeb et al. conducted a meta-analysis of seven clinical trials using chondroitin sulfate to treat OA, permitting background analgesics and nonsteroidal anti-inflammatory drugs (NSAIDs; i.e., Motrin). Authors reported that chondroitin sulfate was significantly superior to placebo as evaluated by Lesquesne Index and a visual analogue pain scale at 120 days of therapy or greater. Pooled study results indicated a 50% improvement in outcome measures with chondroitin compared to placebo. However, chondroitin is generally thought to be less effective than glucosamine regarding secondary prevention for OA. Sodium chondroitin sulfate should be avoided in people with hypertension as well as at risk for bruising or bleeding.

S-Adenosyl-L-Methionine

S-Adenosyl-L-methionine (SAMe) is a natural constituent in the body and a metabolite of the amino acid methionine. SAMe promotes synthesis of proteoglycans by articular chondrocytes *in vitro* and may reduce joint inflammation in people with OA. SAMe dietary supplements degrade upon exposure to heat or moisture so the enteric coated tablets (from Europe) are preferred.

Konig et al. (1987) randomized people with knee, hip, or spine OA in an open trial to receive 600 mg SAM by mouth daily for 2 weeks, then 400 mg by mouth daily for 2 years. Clinical improvement was noted after 2 weeks and continued up to the sixth month and beyond. Nineteen percent of participants who completed 2 years of treatment experienced total remission of symptoms by the end of the study. Common side effects reported by participants included gastrointestinal upset, which subsided through the 2-year period.

Najm et al. (2004) compared SAMe 1200 mg daily with Celebrex 200 mg daily for 16 weeks in patients with knee OA and reported SAMe to be nonsuperior, although SAMe was shown to have a slower onset than Celebrex. More research is needed to determine long-term efficacy, optimal SAM dosing regimen, and its safety profile.

Avocado Oil/Soybean Unsaponifiable Residues (ASU)

The compound ASU, marketed as Piascledine in France, is classed as a slow-acting product for OA known to stimulate articular chondrocyte collagen synthesis *in vitro* (Pavelka et al., 2010). ASU has shown anti-inflammatory chondroprotective effects in articular cartilage (i.e., metalloproteinase, IL-6 and IL-8, nitric oxide synthase, and prostaglandin E_2 inhibition). Blotman et al. (1997) conducted a prospective randomized double-blind multicenter parallel group trial with ASU 300 mg daily versus placebo for 3 months in people with knee or hip OA and requiring NSAIDs during the first half of the study to control their pain. Acetaminophen was allowed in the first half of the study for reasons other than OA (maximum 3000 mg daily). Mean cumulative dose of NSAID use was significantly less in the ASU group versus placebo posttreatment. Pain scores were similar in the two groups over time. The algofunctional index score fell more in the ASU group. Adverse events reported were similar in both groups.

Cat's Claw

Cat's claw (*Unicaria tomentosa*) is a dietary supplement with antioxidant and anti-inflammatory properties. *In vitro* OA models demonstrate that cat's claw has an inhibitory action on IL-1, tumor necrosis factor α, and nuclear factor κB. Piscoya et al. (2001) randomized men with knee OA to 100 mg cat's claw extract (Vincaria) daily or placebo in a double-blind study for 4 weeks. Researchers reported significant improvement with Vincaria in pain on activity and patient and physician pain assessments after 1 week and again at 2 and 4 weeks of therapy ($p < 0.001$). The long-term safety profile of cat's claw is unknown.

RHEUMATOID ARTHRITIS

Oxidative stress and inflammation play an important role in joint disease. Thus, as with OA primary prevention, an important primary RA prevention strategy for healthy joints is weight management through proper nutrition, including antioxidant and anti-inflammatory foods. No particular food groups have been definitively associated with triggering symptoms of RA in otherwise healthy individuals, and no formal nutrition-based secondary prevention recommendations in people with RA can be made at this time (Panush, 1991).

The authors have speculated that dairy products (i.e., milk, cheese) and nightshade family foods (i.e., tomatoes, peppers, potatoes, eggplant) increase risk of joint symptom development (Panush et al., 1986; Childers and Margoles, 1993) and recommend removal of offending food groups in patients with active disease. Conversely, brewer's yeast, apple cider, wheat germ molasses, honey, ginger, and garlic are reported to reduce arthritis symptoms. We are not aware of randomized controlled clinical trials to support the latter claim.

According to the American College of Rheumatology, elimination diets and fasting do not have a place in mainstream RA prevention. Physician supervised fasting for 7–10 days may be associated with a short-term reduction in inflammatory symptoms related to people with RA, but relapse is typically seen on the reintroduction of the same food groups (Kjeldsen-Kragh et al., 1991; Danao-Camara and Shintani, 1999).

Smedlund et al. (2010) systematically reviewed smaller clinical trials regarding the effectiveness and safety of specialized diets (e.g., 7–10 days with fasting followed by vegetarian diet, Mediterranean diet, elemental diet, and elimination diet) on joints in people with RA. Researchers reported that fasting followed by vegetarian nutrition or Mediterranean diet nutrition may reduce pain but did not affect joint function or joint stiffness. Fasting is not without risk and needs to be conducted with the advice and consent of a physician to avoid nutrient deficiencies and other problems. People with RA may be a greater risk to adverse outcomes from dietary restrictions than the general population. No definitive recommendations could be made from these small trials because of high dropout rates from adverse effects related to the diets. Larger trials with long-term follow-up measurements and emphasis on adverse effects are warranted.

Nenonen et al. (1998) studied a vegan diet rich in lactobacilli and reported that Finnish individuals with RA in the intervention group subjectively reported less joint symptoms than those in the control group for 8 weeks. Seven-day dietary records were reviewed by a dietician before diet intervention, in the middle of diet intervention, and at the end of the study. Objective measures for disease activity (e.g., Health Assessment Questionnaire, duration of morning stiffness, pain on movement, and pain at rest) were not statistically different between groups, nor were markers for rheumatic disease activity different. Nearly 50% of patients reported nausea or diarrhea during the diet and ended up withdrawing from the study.

DIETARY SUPPLEMENTS FOR RA

Dietary supplements for the management of symptoms in people with RA have been reviewed in the literature (Cameron et al., 2009; Darlington and Stone, 2001; Rosenbaum et al., 2010). When analyzing well-designed clinical trials for secondary prevention in people with RA, it is important to look for the Rheumatoid Arthritis Disease Activity Index (European League Against Rheumatism), the Ritchie Articular Index, the American College of Rheumatology Index or objective measures of disease activity. Further, well-designed trials should include results of erythrocyte sedimentation rate, C-reactive protein, and other inflammatory markers at baseline and postintervention.

Diets rich in omega 3 fatty acids may reduce the need for NSAIDs (i.e., Celebrex) as secondary prevention. Foods containing omega 3 fatty acids include salmon, walnuts, herring, light tuna, mackerel, and sardines.

FISH OIL DIETARY SUPPLEMENTS

Multiple studies with the dietary supplement fish oil demonstrate improvement in the number of tender joints, duration of morning stiffness, and pain assessment scores. High-dose omega 3 fatty acids in fish oil (e.g., docosahexaenoic acid [DHA] and eicosapentaenoic acid [EPA]) may suppress joint inflammation in people with RA. Total EPA plus DHA combined daily doses ranged from 1 to 7 g (mean = 3 g) (Rosenbaum et al., 2010). Fish oil may cause a fishy aftertaste and increased risk of bruising and bleeding in doses higher than 3 g of EPA plus DHA combined daily. High-quality fish oil capsules may have a role in secondary prevention of symptoms in people with RA.

Goldberg and Katz (2007) conducted a meta-analysis of 17 randomized controlled trials comparing omega 3 fatty acids to placebo adjunctive to NSAIDs (i.e., Motrin) in patients with RA or joint pain secondary to inflammatory bowel disease for at least 3 months. Researchers reported that most outcome measures were positively impacted by omega 3, including patient-assessed joint pain, physician-assessed joint pain, duration of morning stiffness, number of painful and tender joints, and NSAID consumption.

CONCLUSIONS

More well-designed clinical studies are needed to establish place in therapy for both primary and secondary prevention of OA and RA using nutrition or dietary supplement interventions or both. Study methodologies should include objective measurements of radiographically diagnosed disease and the width of joint spaces, patient assessed pain, physician assessed pain via WOMAC scales, joint and muscle function through validated range of motion scales, other blood markers as indicated throughout this text, intention-to-treat analysis, and quality of life measures.

REFERENCES

Ahmed S, Rahman A, Hasnain A, et al. Green tea-polyphenol epigallocatechin-3-gallate inhibits the IL-1 beta induced activity and expression cyclooxygenase-2 and nitric oxide synthase-2 in human chondrocytes. Free Radic Biol Med 2002;33:1097–1105.

Blotman F, Maheu E, Wulwik A, et al. Efficacy and safety of avocado/soybean unsaponifiables in the treatment of symptomatic osteoarthritis of the knee and hip. A prospective, multicenter, three month, randomized, double blind, placebo controlled trial. Rev Rhum Engl Ed 1997;64:825–834.

Cameron M, Gagnier JJ, Little CV, et al. Evidence of effectiveness of herbal medicinal products in the treatment of arthritis. Part 2: rheumatoid arthritis. Phytotherapy Res 2009;23:1647–1662.

Childers NF, Margoles MS. An apparent relation of nightshades (Solanaceae) to arthritis. J Neuro Ortho Med Surgery 1993;12:227–231.

Clegg DO, et al. Glucosamine, chondroitin sulfate, and the two in combination for painful knee osteoarthritis. New Engl J Med 2006;354:795–808.

Cleland LG, Hill CL, James MJ. Diet and arthritis. Baillieres Clin Rheumatology 1995;9(4):771–785.

Danao-Camara TC, Shintani TT. The dietary treatment of inflammatory arthritis: case reports and review of the literature. Haw Med J 1999;58(5):126–131.

Darlington LG, Stone TW. Antioxidants and fatty acids in the amelioration of rheumatoid arthritis and related disorders. Br J Nutr 2001;85:251–269.

Elmali N, Esenkaya I, Harma A, et al. Effect of resveratrol in experimental osteoarthritis in rabbits. Inflamm Res 2005;54:158–162.

Goggs R, Vaughan-Thomas A, Clegg PD, et al. Nutraceutical therapies for degenerative joint diseases: a critical review. Crit Rev Food Sci Nutr 2005;45:145–164.

Goldberg RJ, Katz J. A meta-analysis of the analgesic effects of omega-3 polyunsaturated fatty acid supplementation for inflammatory joint pain. Pain 2007;129:210–223.

Kjeldsen-Kragh J, Haugen M, Borchgrevink CF, et al. Controlled trial of fasting and one year vegetarian diet in rheumatoid arthritis. Lancet 1991;338:899–902.

Konig B. A long term (two years) clinical trial with S-adenosylmethionine for the treatment of osteoarthritis. Am J Med 1987;83:89–94.

Lane NE, Gore LR, Cummings SR, et al. Serum vitamin D levels and incident changes of radiographic hip osteoarthritis: a longitudinal study. Arthritis Rheum 1999;42:854–860.

Leeb BF, Schweitzer H, Montag K, Smolen JS. A meta-analysis of chondroitin sulfate in the treatment of osteoarthritis. J Rheum 2000;27:205–211.

McAlindon TE, Felson DT, Zhang Y, et al. Relation of dietary intake and serum levels of vitamin D to progression of osteoarthritis of the knee among participants in the Framingham Study. Ann Intern Med 1996a;125:353–359.

McAlindon TE, Jacques P, Zhang Y, et al. Do antioxidant micronutrients protect against the development and progression of knee osteoarthritis? Arthritis Rheum 1996b;39:648–656.

McAlindon TE, Biggee BA. Nutritional factors and osteoarthritis: recent developments. Curr Opin Rheum 2005;17:647–652.

Morreale P, Manopulo R, Galati M, et al. Comparison of the anti-inflammatory efficacy of chondroitin sulfate and diclofenac sodium in patients with knee osteoarthritis. J Rheumatol 1996;23:1385–1391.

Najm WI, Reinsch S, Hoehler F, et al. S-adenosyl methionine (SAMe) versus celecoxib for the treatment of osteoarthritis symptoms: a double-blind cross-over trial. BMC Musculoskelet Disord 2004;5:6.

Nenonen MT, Helve TA, Rauma AL, et al. Uncooked, lactobacilli-rich, vegan food and rheumatoid arthritis. Br J Rheumatology 1998;57:274–281.

Panush RS. American college of rheumatology position statement: diet and arthritis. Nutr Rheum Dis 1991;17:443–444.

Panush RS, Stroud RM, Webster EM. Food-induced (allergic) arthritis. Inflammatory arthritis exacerbated by milk. Arthritis Rheum 1986;29(2):220–226.

Pavelka K, Coste P, Geher P, et al. Efficacy and safety of piascledine 300 versus chondroitin sulfate in a 6 months treatment plus 2 months observation in patients with osteoarthritis of the knee. Clin Rheumatol 2010;29:659–670.

Piscoya J, Rodriguez Z, Bustamante SA, et al. Efficacy and safety of freeze-dried cat's claw in osteoarthritis of the knee: mechanisms of action of the species *Unicaria guianensis*. Inflamm Res 2001;50:442–448.

Rosenbaum CC, O'Mathuna DP, Chavez M, et al. Antioxidants and anti-inflammatory dietary supplements for osteoarthritis and rheumatoid arthritis. Altern Therapies 2010;16:32–40.

Smedlund G, Byfuglien MG, Olsen SU, et al. Effectiveness and safety of dietary interventions for rheumatoid arthritis: a systematic review of randomized controlled trials. J Am Diet Assoc 2010;10:727–735.

Towheed T, Maxwell L, Anastassiades TP, et al. Glucosamine therapy for treating osteoarthritis (review). Coch Library 2009;4:1–75.

Widrig R, Suter A, Saller R, et al. Choosing between NSAID and arnica for topical treatment of hand osteoarthritis in a randomized, double blind study. Rheumatol Int 2007;27:585–591.

Yudol K, Nguyen T, Nakamura H, et al. Potential involvement of oxidative stress in cartilage senescence and development of osteoarthritis: oxidative stress induces chondrocyte telomere instability and down regulation of chondrocyte function. Arth Res Ther 2005;7:R380–R391.

18 Antiarthritic Potential of Glucosamine and Chondroitin
An Overview

Michael W. Orth and Pooi-See Chan

CONTENTS

INTRODUCTION

Glucosamine and chondroitin sulfate (CS) are by far the most popular products sold for providing relief from joint pain. In addition, many products include them as major ingredients in their cocktail. They are often referred to as nutraceuticals because they have both nutritional and pharmaceutical characteristics. For the most part, they are considered safe to use long term at the typical doses of 1500 mg/day for glucosamine and 1200 mg/day for CS (Jordan et al., 2003; Hathcock and Shao, 2007).

GLUCOSAMINE

Glucosamine is a naturally occurring amino monosaccharide formed by the transfer of the amide nitrogen of glutamine to fructose on the carbon 2 position. It is a precursor molecule for components in cartilage matrix, synovial fluid, and other tissues. As the principal building block and intermediate substrate used in the synthesis of *N*- and O-linked glycosaminoglycans (GAGs), it can be rate limiting for proteoglycan production. Once glucosamine gets acetylated to *N*-acetylglucosamine, it becomes a component of GAGs such as keratan sulfate and hyaluronic acid. Glucosamine can also be converted to galactosamine via isomerization to become precursors of CS and dermatan sulfate. Radioligand studies have shown that it is incorporated into cartilage on the GAG chains via the hexosamine pathway (Noyszewski et al., 2001; Setnikar and Rovati, 2001). Glucosamine has relatively low molecular weight (179.2 kDa). This nutraceutical is normally extracted from exoskeletons of shellfish, although recently vegetarian and kosher sources have been developed. Commercially marketed derivatives include glucosamine hydrochloride, glucosamine sulfate, or N-acetylglucosamine.

CHONDROITIN SULFATE

Chondroitin sulfate is a complex GAG that is a major component of aggrecan. It is a heteropolymer consisting of disaccharide units of sulfated N-acetylgalactosamine and glucuronic acid. Sulfation of CS can occur either at carbon 4 or 6 of N-acetylgalactosamine producing chondroitin-4-sulfate or chondroitin-6 sulfate, respectively. Chondroitin sulfate is typically obtained from bovine tracheal cartilage, although it has also been isolated from many types of connective tissue such as the nasal cartilage, articular cartilage, bones, sclera, leukocytes, blood platelets, skin, umbilical cord, and cardiac valves. The CS found in products can vary greatly because of variations in chain length, degree of sulfation, and the location of sulfate ions on N-acetylglucosamine.

SUGGESTED MECHANISMS OF ACTION

Both glucosamine and CS are considered structure-modifying agents with the ability to retard the pathology of osteoarthritis (OA). They have been claimed to possess chondroprotective, anti-inflammatory, antiarthritic, and antirheumatic properties providing symptomatic relief, particularly in ameliorating joint pain. However, the mechanism(s) of action underlying the properties of these compounds in providing joint pain relief is unclear. Outcomes from laboratories exploring the mechanistic aspect of these nutraceuticals by mostly employing concentrations between 0.1 and 10 mg/mL indicate that these agents are capable of supporting anabolic events and arresting catabolic activities of chondrocytes. Both glucosamine and CS have chondroprotective properties *in vivo* and *in vitro* evident by their ability to stimulate proteoglycan synthesis and increase hyaluronic acid content and GAG synthesis in synovial fluid (McCarty et al., 2000; Lippiello et al., 2000; Johnson et al., 2001). An *in vivo* study suggested that glucosamine and CS may be synergistic in improving cartilage lesions (Lippiello, 2003). *In vitro*, the two had complementary effects in regulating the synthesis of catabolic mediators (Schlueter and Orth, 2004; Chan et al., 2006, 2007). In gene expression studies, the combination of the two was optimal with regard to mitigating the synthesis of inflammatory molecules and matrix metalloproteinases (MMPs) in interleukin-1 (IL-1)-stimulated cartilage explants (Chan et al., 2005a, b). Both compounds enhanced the metabolic response of chondrocytes to stress *in vitro* (Lippiello, 2003). The structure-modifying effects of glucosamine and CS were also confirmed through histological studies in rats and dogs used as experimental models (Beren et al., 2001; Johnson et al., 2001).

GLUCOSAMINE

The anabolic activity of glucosamine is supported by the fact that OA chondrocytes treated with the hexosamine sugar demonstrated a dose-dependent increase in proteoglycan synthesis, expression of aggrecan, GAG content, and elevated synovial hyaluronic acid production (Muller-Fassbender et al., 1994; Bassleer et al., 1998; McCarty, 1998; Dodge and Jimenez, 2003). Glucosamine was a preferential precursor for the galactosamine moieties of CS in cartilage explants (Noyszewski et al., 2001). This was contradicted by a study with human chondrocytes (Mroz and Silbert, 2004), possibly because of a lack of stress on the cells. Glucosamine prevented the inhibition of glucurono-syltransferase I gene expression and activity in IL-1-stimulated chondrocytes, suggesting it may mitigate IL-1's impact on proteoglycan synthesis (Gouze et al., 2001).

Aggrecan degradation was suppressed over a long-term culture supplemented with glucosamine (Ilic et al., 2003). Glucosamine was effective in attenuating proteoglycan release slowing OA progression (Fenton et al., 2000). The anticatabolic activity of glucosamine treatment that halts cartilage breakdown is potentially mediated by inhibition of proteolytic enzymes. Glucosamine inhibited aggrecanase and MMPs *in vitro* (Sandy et al., 1998; Piperno et al., 2000; Fenton et al., 2002; Dodge and Jimenez, 2003). Glucosamine was also capable of pretranslational and translational regulation of matrix-degrading enzymes by repressing mRNA expression of aggrecanases, MMP-1, MMP-3, and MMP-13, by reducing MMP-3 protein synthesis, and by decreasing MMP-13 activity (Byron et al., 2003; Dodge and Jimenez, 2003; Chan et al., 2006).

Pain amelioration with glucosamine may be attributed to a reduction in inflammatory mediators possibly via regulation of IL-1 signaling pathways such as nuclear factor κB (NF-κB) and mitogen-activated protein kinases (Mendis et al., 2008; Hong et al., 2009). Glucosamine increased the expression of IL-1RII, a decoy receptor that is unable to generate the IL-1 signaling pathway in chondrocytes (Gouze et al., 2002). Explant cultures treated with glucosamine demonstrated a decline in nitric oxide release into the media (Fenton et al., 2000; Gouze et al., 2001). Cytokine-stimulated nitric oxide release was also depressed in synoviocyte and chondrocyte cocultures (Gouze et al., 2004). The inducible nitric oxide synthase transcript and protein in cartilage stimulated with IL-1 was suppressed by glucosamine (Meininger et al., 2000; Shikhman et al., 2001). Glucosamine also inhibited NF-κB activity and translocation, cyclooxygenase-2 messenger RNA, and protein expression in a dose-dependent manner coupled with an increase in the inhibitor of NF-κB in IL-1-induced articular cartilage (Gouze et al., 2002; Largo et al., 2003). Parallel with the inhibition of cyclooxygenase-2, prostaglandin E_2 production and release were also inhibited with glucosamine (Gouze et al., 2001; Fenton et al., 2002; Nakamura et al., 2004). The anti-inflammatory properties of glucosamine may also be mediated by inhibitory actions on neutrophils and p38 mitogen-activated protein kinase phosphorylation, although this study was conducted with a relatively high glucosamine concentration of about 6 mg/mL (Hua et al., 2002).

CHONDROITIN SULFATE

Chondroitin sulfate can regulate cartilage metabolism *in vitro* and *in vivo*; it increased RNA synthesis that correlates with increases in synthesis of proteoglycan and collagen (Vacha et al., 1984; Bassleer et al., 1998). It also reversed IL-1 inhibition of proteoglycan synthesis (Bassleer et al., 1998; Nerucci et al., 2000). The chondroprotective property of this GAG also includes cartilage repair by increasing hyaluronic acid production (Pipitone, 1991; Ronca et al., 1998). Oral administration of CS reduced proteoglycan loss from articular cartilage in humans and rats (Uebelhart et al., 1998; Omata et al., 1999). In addition, it inhibited cartilage damage by suppressing aggrecanase, elastase, lysosomal enzymes, and collagenolytic activity (Baici and Bradamante, 1984; Pipitone, 1991; Sugimoto et al., 1999). Chondroitin sulfate possesses anti-inflammatory properties by mechanisms involving the reduction of prostaglandin E_2, reactive oxygen species, and free radical release (Ronca et al., 1998; Campo et al., 2003; Chan et al., 2005a).

HUMAN TRIALS

GLUCOSAMINE

The first clinical trial with glucosamine as a therapeutic agent in humans was conducted in Germany in 1969. It was followed by a number of short-term double-blind studies in Europe, Asia, and the

United States in the 1980s and 1990s. The findings indicated that glucosamine was beneficial in modifying OA symptoms and possessed chondroprotective properties while maintaining a good safety profile. Glucosamine can reduce joint tenderness and swelling, decrease pain, and improve joint mobility, gait functions, and quality of life. In double-blind placebo-controlled studies, patients treated with glucosamine for at least 30 days experienced improvement in pain, tenderness, and overall joint function (Drovanti et al., 1980; Pujalte et al., 1980). Alleviation of symptoms with glucosamine occurred faster than patients on placebo. Trials comparing glucosamine with ibuprofen showed that it was at least equal in potency to ibuprofen in reducing pain, but safer and more tolerable (Rovati, 1992; Muller-Fassbender et al., 1994; Qiu et al., 1998). This amino sugar has also demonstrated improvement in structural joint changes where joint space narrowing declined profoundly as assessed by radiological methods (Reginster et al., 2001). The therapeutic effects of glucosamine were also conserved even well after the therapy was discontinued (Tapadinhas et al., 1982; Bassleer et al., 1998; Qiu et al., 1998).

Some subsequent and longer clinical trials, comparative studies, and meta-analyses substantiated previous findings (Delafuente, 2000; Braham et al., 2003; Bruyere et al., 2003; Richy et al., 2003). In a meta-analysis, patients with hip or knee OA who consumed glucosamine experienced about a 40% decline in pain and improvement in mobility (McAlindon et al., 2000). Two hundred twelve patients with knee OA given glucosamine sulfate for 3 years had reduction in pain and no loss in joint space compared with placebo (Reginster et al., 2001). However, in the Glucosamine/Chondroitin Arthritis Intervention Trial (GAIT), the largest U.S. government–sponsored trial done to date, glucosamine did not reduce pain relative to placebo for patients with OA in the knee (Clegg et al., 2006). In addition, in a 2-year study glucosamine sulfate did not reduce either the symptoms or the progression of OA in the hip (Rozendaal et al., 2008). An even more recent study concluded that after 1 year, patients taking glucosamine sulfate did not experience significant reduction in lumbar joint pain relative to placebo (Wilkins et al., 2010). Thus, in some of the more recent studies, glucosamine has not had the same level of success in helping patients with OA.

CHONDROITIN SULFATE

Although initial clinical trials with CS, similar to glucosamine, were relatively short term, CS was effective in alleviating OA symptoms. Patients with knee, hip, and finger OA taking low molecular weight CS used significantly less nonsteroidal anti-inflammatory drugs or other analgesics and experienced pain relief (Morreale et al., 1996; Uebelhart et al., 1998; Bucsi and Poor, 1998). The residual effects of CS also persisted longer than the nonsteroidal anti-inflammatory drugs therapy, where patients experienced positive response up to 3 months after discontinuation of the compound (Morreale et al., 1996). Other beneficial effects of CS include improvement in joint mobility, joint space narrowing, and reduction of erosive OA (Bourgeois et al., 1998; Verbruggen et al., 1998; Rovetta et al., 2002). The results of the GAIT study suggest that CS may improve joint swelling in patients with mild knee OA (Hochberg and Clegg, 2008). Chondroitin sulfate was also advantageous in demonstrating an overall cost-lowering effect for treating OA (Conrozier, 1998). A recent meta-analysis led to the conclusion that CS can be effective for slowing cartilage loss in patients with knee OA (Hochberg, 2010).

COMBINATION

The combination of glucosamine and CS has been suggested to enhance their efficacy in the treatment of OA. The beneficial results seen in several animal studies have been summarized (Neil et al., 2005). Although the number of studies performed with the combination is low, it was efficacious in reducing pain, improving joint function, and halting or reversing joint degeneration in humans with mild to moderate OA of the knee (Leffler et al., 1999; Das and Hammad, 2000). In the GAIT study, the combination did provide significant pain relief relative to control for those with moderate to severe knee OA (Clegg et al., 2006).

ISSUES

Study Designs

Although human trials have been conducted for more than 30 years, results, especially in the last 10 years, have yielded conflicting conclusions. Initially, reviews of trials suggested that glucosamine was beneficial, although the authors did point out concerns in experimental design, such as the length of the trials and potential bias from sponsors (da Camara and Dowless, 1998; Delafuente, 2000; McAlindon et al., 2000). As more studies were conducted, especially longer-term trials from various funding sources, the results began to differ and specifically two of the bigger trials concluded that glucosamine provided no benefit relative to placebo (Clegg et al., 2006; Rozendaal et al., 2008). More recent analyses of the trials do not provide strong support for the benefits of glucosamine (Vlad et al., 2007; Felson, 2008). Issues considered to impact the results include the type of glucosamine used (hydrochloride vs sulfate), the number of subjects used in the study, and the industry bias. Specifically with regard to CS, the results of human trials led some to conclude that CS is beneficial (Kubo et al., 2009; Hochberg, 2010). However, relatively fewer studies of smaller scope have been conducted with CS as compared with glucosamine. Various types of trials continue to be conducted and will likely not settle the debate. Despite the conflicting evidence, some do consider them a viable initial treatment for many who suffer from arthritic pain (Vangsness et al., 2009).

Absorption and Bioavailability

Glucosamine is rapidly absorbed by the small intestine via glucose transporters (Tesoriere et al., 1972). At least 90% of orally administered glucosamine is absorbed in both human and animals (Setnikar et al., 1986; Setnikar and Rovati, 2001). However, much of it is likely metabolized in the liver. The tissue distribution of a single dose of glucosamine after an oral and intravenous administration is prompt, and it has an affinity for cartilage in rats as shown in autoradiographic studies (Setnikar et al., 1984). However, concentrations of glucosamine in the plasma after oral dosing are less than 1 µg/mL (Setnikar and Rovati, 2001; Jackson et al., 2010). The concentrations are well below those seen to have an anti-inflammatory effect *in vitro* (Chan et al., 2005a).

There is no consensus regarding the absorption of CS after oral administration. The absorption of CS is thought to vary depending on molecular weight, chain length, location of the sulfate groups, charge density, and the source of CS. Initially, detection methods lacked sensitivity and specificity to differentiate between constituents of CS disaccharides. However, techniques to detect CS disaccharides are now available. In dogs, CS is absorbed as disaccharide metabolites with low molecular weight and low charge density CS being preferentially absorbed (Du and Eddington, 2002). In humans, CS taken orally was approximately 13% bioavailable (Conte et al., 1991). Peak plasma concentrations of orally administered CS ranged from approximately 5 to 11 µg/mL and reached a climax at about 8 h (Conte et al., 1991; Volpi, 2002, 2003). More recently, researchers using different analytical techniques did not find appreciable increases in plasma CS after oral administration (Jackson et al., 2010).

Regulation of Products

In the United States, glucosamine and CS are not considered pharmaceuticals and thus are not well regulated. Only a few of the commercial products have actually been used in clinical trials. However, many of the untested products claim the benefits found in the tested products. Especially with CS, extrapolation of results cannot be assumed since its purity, molecular weight, and degree of sulfation, which are likely important for its biological activity, are bound to differ between all the commercial products. Different sources of CS can function differently in *in vitro* experiments (Tat et al., 2010). In addition, the amount of active ingredients may not match up with what is stated on the labels of products containing glucosamine (Russell et al., 2002). The same problem has also been found with products containing CS (Adebowale et al., 2001; Volpi, 2009). Generalized statements regarding their chondroprotective benefits cannot be articulated because of such variability in the products.

CONCLUSIONS

Despite the tremendous amount of research concerning glucosamine and CS, coupled with the elucidation of their potential chondroprotective properties, many questions still exist (Block et al., 2010). For example, on the basis of research using animal models, would they be more effective if they are taken right after a traumatic joint injury to prevent or mitigate joint pain in the future? Would they be more effective if they are coupled with omega-3 fatty acids or avocado soybean unsaponifiables? Should they be incorporated into functional foods? Do they have some type of systemic anti-inflammatory effect? Do genetics or other health conditions impact their potential benefits? Definitive statements regarding their efficacy may no longer be possible because of their popularity and easy access. The percentage of health professionals (for both humans and animals) who recommend glucosamine and CS to their clients could easily be around 50%. These nutraceuticals have been beneficial for many people and animals suffering from the debilitating effects of OA. Because of this and their apparent lack of adverse affects, glucosamine and CS will continue to be a reasonable first option to deal with chronic joint pain.

REFERENCES

Adebowale AO, Cox DS, Liang Z, Eddington N. Analysis of glucosamine and chondroitin sulfate content in marketed products and the caco-2 permeability of chondroitin sulfate raw materials. J Am Nutraceut Assoc 2001;3(1):37–44.

Baici A, Bradamante P. Interaction between human leukocyte elastase and chondroitin sulfate. Chem Biol Interact 1984;51(1):1–11.

Bassleer C, Rovati L, Franchimont P. Stimulation of proteoglycan production by glucosamine sulfate in chondrocytes isolated from human osteoarthritic articular cartilage in vitro. Osteoarthritis Cartilage 1998;6(6):427–434.

Beren J, Hill SL, Diener-West M, Rose NR. Effect of pre-loading oral glucosamine HCl/chondroitin sulfate/manganese ascorbate combination on experimental arthritis in rats. Exp Biol Med 2001;226(2):144–151.

Block JA, Oegema TR, Sandy DJ, Plaas A. The effects of oral glucosamine on joint health: is a change in research approach needed? Osteoarthritis Cartilage 2010;18(1):5–11.

Bourgeois P, Chales G, Dehais J, Delcambre B, Kuntz JL, Rozenberg S. Efficacy and tolerability of chondroitin sulfate 1200 mg/day vs chondroitin sulfate 3 × 400 mg/day vs placebo. Osteoarthritis Cartilage 1998;6(Suppl A):25–30.

Braham R, Dawson B, Goodman C. The effect of glucosamine supplementation on people experiencing regular knee pain. Br J Sports Med 2003;37(1):45–49.

Bruyere O, Honore A, Ethgen O, Rovati LC, Giacovelli G, Henrotin YE, Seidel L, Reginster JY. Correlation between radiographic severity of knee osteoarthritis and future disease progression. Results from a 3-year prospective, placebo-controlled study evaluating the effect of glucosamine sulfate. Osteoarthritis Cartilage 2003;11(1):1–5.

Bucsi L, Poor G. Efficacy and tolerability of oral chondroitin sulfate as a symptomatic slow-acting drug for osteoarthritis (SYSADOA) in the treatment of knee osteoarthritis. Osteoarthritis Cartilage 1998;6(Suppl A):31–36.

Byron CR, Orth MW, Venta PJ, Lloyd JW, Caron JP. Influence of glucosamine on matrix metalloproteinase expression and activity in lipopolysaccharide-stimulated equine chondrocytes. Am J Vet Res 2003;64(6):666–671.

Campo GM, Avenoso A, Campo S, Ferlazzo A, Altavilla D, Micali C, Calatroni A. Aromatic trap analysis of free radicals production in experimental collagen-induced arthritis in the rat: protective effect of glycosaminoglycans treatment. Free Radic Res 2003;37(3):257–268.

Chan PS, Caron JP, Orth MW. Effect of glucosamine and chondroitin sulfate on regulation of gene expression of proteolytic enzymes and their inhibitors in interleukin-1-challenged bovine articular cartilage explants. Am J Vet Res 2005b;66(11):1870–1876.

Chan PS, Caron JP, Orth MW. Short-term gene expression changes in cartilage explants stimulated with inter-leukin beta plus glucosamine and chondroitin sulfate. J Rheumatol 2006;33(7):1329–1340.

Chan PS, Caron JP, Orth MW. Effects of glucosamine and chondroitin sulfate on bovine cartilage explants under long-term culture conditions. Am J Vet Res 2007;68(7):709–715.

Chan PS, Caron JP, Rosa GJ, Orth MW. Glucosamine and chondroitin sulfate regulate gene expression and synthesis of nitric oxide and prostaglandin E(2) in articular cartilage explants. Osteoarthritis Cartilage 2005a;13(5):387–394.

Clegg DO, Reda DJ, Harris CL, Klein MA, O JR'Dell, Hooper MM, Bradley JD. Glucosamine, chondroitin sulfate, and the two in combination for painful knee osteoarthritis. N Engl J Med 2006;354(8):795–808.

Conrozier T. Chondroitin sulfates (CS 4&6): practical applications and economic impact. Presse Med 1998;27(36):1866–1868.

Conte A, de Bernardi M, Palmieri L, Lualdi P, Mautone G, Ronca G. Metabolic fate of exogenous chondroitin sulfate in man. Arzneimittelforschung 1991;41(7):768–772.

da Camara CC, Dowless GV. Glucosamine sulfate for osteoarthritis. Ann Pharmacother 1998;32(5):580–587.

Das A, Jr., Hammad TA. Efficacy of a combination of FCHG49 glucosamine hydrochloride, TRH122 low molecular weight sodium chondroitin sulfate and manganese ascorbate in the management of knee osteoarthritis. Osteoarthritis Cartilage 2000;8(5):343–350.

Delafuente JC. Glucosamine in the treatment of osteoarthritis. Rheum Dis Clin North Am 2000;26(1):1–11, vii.

Dodge GR, Jimenez SA. Glucosamine sulfate modulates the levels of aggrecan and matrix metalloprotei-nase-3 synthesized by cultured human osteoarthritis articular chondrocytes. Osteoarthritis Cartilage 2003;11(6):424–432.

Drovanti A, Bignamini AA, Rovati AL. Therapeutic activity of oral glucosamine sulfate in osteoarthrosis: a placebo-controlled double-blind investigation. Clin Ther 1980;3(4):260–272.

Du J, Eddington N. Determination of the chondroitin sulfate disaccharides in dog and horse plasma by HPLC using chondroitinase digestion, precolumn derivatization, and fluorescence detection. Anal Biochem 2002;306(2):252–258.

Felson DT. Glucosamine sulfate might have no effect on pain or structural changes associated with osteoarthri-tis. Nat Clin Pract Rheumatol 2008;4(10):518–519.

Fenton JI, Chlebek KA-Brown, Caron JP, Orth MW. Effect of glucosamine on interleukin-1-conditioned articu-lar cartilage. Equine Vet J Suppl 2002;(34):219–223.

Fenton JI. Chlebek KA-Brown, Peters TL, Caron JP, Orth MW. Glucosamine HCl reduces equine articular cartilage degradation in explant culture. Osteoarthritis Cartilage 2000;8(4):258–265.

Gouze JN, Bianchi A, Becuwe P, Dauca M, Netter P, Magdalou J, Terlain B, Bordji K. Glucosamine modulates IL-1-induced activation of rat chondrocytes at a receptor level, and by inhibiting the NF-kappa B path-way. FEBS Lett 2002;510(3):166–170.

Gouze JN, Bordji K, Gulberti S, Terlain B, Netter P, Magdalou J, Fournel-Gigleux S, Ouzzine M. Interleukin-1beta down-regulates the expression of glucuronosyltransferase I, a key enzyme priming glycosamino-glycan biosynthesis: influence of glucosamine on interleukin-1beta-mediated effects in rat chondrocytes. Arthritis Rheum 2001;44(2):351–360.

Gouze JN, Gouze E, Palmer GD, Kaneto H, Ghivizzani SC, Grodzinsky AJ, Evans CH. Adenovirus-mediated gene transfer of glutamine: fructose-6-phosphate amidotransferase antagonizes the effects of interleukin-1beta on rat chondrocytes. Osteoarthritis Cartilage 2004;12(3):217–224.

Hathcock JN, Shao A. Risk assessment for glucosamine and chondroitin sulfate. Regul Toxicol Pharmacol 2007;47(1):78–83.

Hochberg MC. Structure-modifying effects of chondroitin sulfate in knee osteoarthritis: an updated meta-anal-ysis of randomized placebo-controlled trials of 2-year duration. Osteoarthritis Cartilage 2010;18(Suppl 1):S28-S31.

Hochberg MC, Clegg DO. Potential effects of chondroitin sulfate on joint swelling: a GAIT report. Osteoarthritis Cartilage 2008;16(Suppl 3):S22-S24.

Hong H, Park YK, Choi MS, Ryu NH, Song DK, Suh SI, Nam KY, Park GY, Jang BC. Differential down-regulation of COX-2 and MMP-13 in human skin fibroblasts by glucosamine-hydrochloride. J Dermatol Sci 2009;56(1):43–50.

Hua J, Sakamoto K, Nagaoka I. Inhibitory actions of glucosamine, a therapeutic agent for osteoarthritis, on the functions of neutrophils. J Leukoc Biol 2002;71(4):632–640.

Ilic MZ, Martinac B, Handley CJ. Effects of long-term exposure to glucosamine and mannosamine on aggrecan degradation in articular cartilage. Osteoarthritis Cartilage 2003;11(8):613–622.

Jackson CG, Plaas AH, Sandy JD, Hua C, Kim-Rolands S, Barnhill JG, Harris CL, Clegg DO. The human pharmacokinetics of oral ingestion of glucosamine and chondroitin sulfate taken separately or in combination. Osteoarthritis Cartilage 2010;18(3):297–302.

Johnson KA, Hulse DA, Hart RC, Kochevar D, Chu Q. Effects of an orally administered mixture of chondroitin sulfate, glucosamine hydrochloride and manganese ascorbate on synovial fluid chondroitin sulfate 3B3 and 7D4 epitope in a canine cruciate ligament transection model of osteoarthritis. Osteoarthritis Cartilage 2001;9(1):14–21.

Jordan KM, Arden NK, Doherty M, Bannwarth B, Bijlsma JW, Dieppe P, Gunther K. EULAR Recommendations 2003: an evidence based approach to the management of knee osteoarthritis: report of a Task Force of the Standing Committee for International Clinical Studies Including Therapeutic Trials (ESCISIT). Ann Rheum Dis 2003;62(12):1145–1155.

Kubo M, Ando K, Mimura T, Matsusue Y, Mori K. Chondroitin sulfate for the treatment of hip and knee osteoarthritis: current status and future trends. Life Sci 2009;85(13–14):477–483.

Largo R, Alvarez-Soria MA, Diez-Ortego I, Calvo E, Sanchez-Pernaute O, Egido J, Herrero-Beaumont G. Glucosamine inhibits IL-1beta-induced NFkappaB activation in human osteoarthritic chondrocytes. Osteoarthritis Cartilage 2003;11(4):290–298.

Leffler CT, Philippi AF, Leffler SG, Mosure JC, Kim PD. Glucosamine, chondroitin, and manganese ascorbate for degenerative joint disease of the knee or low back: a randomized, double-blind, placebo-controlled pilot study. Mil Med 1999;164(2):85–91.

Lippiello L. Glucosamine and chondroitin sulfate: biological response modifiers of chondrocytes under simulated conditions of joint stress. Osteoarthritis Cartilage 2003;11(5):335–342.

Lippiello L, Woodward J, R. Karpman, Hammad TA. In vivo chondroprotection and metabolic synergy of glucosamine and chondroitin sulfate. Clin Orthop Relat Res 2000;(381):229–240.

McAlindon TE, LaValley MP, Gulin JP, Felson DT. Glucosamine and chondroitin for treatment of osteoarthritis: a systematic quality assessment and meta-analysis. JAMA 2000;283(11):1469–1475.

McCarty MF. Enhanced synovial production of hyaluronic acid may explain rapid clinical response to high-dose glucosamine in osteoarthritis. Med Hypotheses 1998;50(6):507–510.

McCarty MF, Russell AL, Seed MP. Sulfated glycosaminoglycans and glucosamine may synergize in promoting synovial hyaluronic acid synthesis. Med Hypotheses 2000;54(5):798–802.

Meininger CJ, Kelly KA, Li H, Haynes TE, Wu G. Glucosamine inhibits inducible nitric oxide synthesis. Biochem Biophys Res Commun 2000;279(1):234–239.

Mendis E, Kim MM, Rajapakse N, Kim SK. Suppression of cytokine production in lipopolysaccharide-stimulated mouse macrophages by novel cationic glucosamine derivative involves down-regulation of NF-kappaB and MAPK expressions. Bioorg Med Chem 2008;16(18):8390–8396.

Morreale P, Manopulo R, Galati M, Boccanera L, Saponati G, Bocchi L. Comparison of the antiinflammatory efficacy of chondroitin sulfate and diclofenac sodium in patients with knee osteoarthritis. J Rheumatol 1996;23(8):1385–1391.

Mroz PJ, Silbert JE. Use of 3H-glucosamine and 35S-sulfate with cultured human chondrocytes to determine the effect of glucosamine concentration on formation of chondroitin sulfate. Arthritis Rheum 2004;50(11):3574–3579.

Muller-Fassbender H, Bach GL, Haase W, Rovati LC, Setnikar I. Glucosamine sulfate compared to ibuprofen in osteoarthritis of the knee. Osteoarthritis Cartilage 1994;2(1):61–69.

Nakamura H, Shibakawa A, Tanaka M, Kato T, Nishioka K. Effects of glucosamine hydrochloride on the production of prostaglandin E_2, nitric oxide and metalloproteases by chondrocytes and synoviocytes in osteoarthritis. Clin Exp Rheumatol 2004;22(3):293–299.

Neil KM, Caron JP, Orth MW. The role of glucosamine and chondroitin sulfate in treatment for and prevention of osteoarthritis in animals. J Am Vet Med Assoc 2005;226(7):1079–1088.

Nerucci F, Fioravanti A, Cicero MR, Collodel G, Marcolongo R. Effects of chondroitin sulfate and interleukin-1beta on human chondrocyte cultures exposed to pressurization: a biochemical and morphological study. Osteoarthritis Cartilage 2000;8(4):279–287.

Noyszewski EA, Wroblewski K, Dodge GR, Kudchodkar S, Beers J, Sarma AV, Reddy R. Preferential incorporation of glucosamine into the galactosamine moieties of chondroitin sulfates in articular cartilage explants. Arthritis Rheum 2001;44(5):1089–1095.

Omata T, Segawa Y, Itokazu Y, Inoue N, Tanaka Y. Effects of chondroitin sulfate-C on bradykinin-induced proteoglycan depletion in rats. Arzneimittelforschung 1999;49(7):577–581.

Piperno M, Reboul P, Hellio MP Le Graverand, Peschard MJ, Annefeld M, Richard M, Vignon E. Glucosamine sulfate modulates dysregulated activities of human osteoarthritic chondrocytes in vitro. Osteoarthritis Cartilage 2000;8(3):207–212.

Pipitone VR. Chondroprotection with chondroitin sulfate. Drugs Exp Clin Res 1991;17(1):3–7.

Pujalte JM, Llavore EP, Ylescupidez FR. Double-blind clinical evaluation of oral glucosamine sulphate in the basic treatment of osteoarthrosis. Curr Med Res Opin 1980;7(2):110–114.

Qiu GX, Gao SN, Giacovelli G, Rovati L, Setnikar I. Efficacy and safety of glucosamine sulfate versus ibuprofen in patients with knee osteoarthritis. Arzneimittelforschung 1998;48(5):469–474.

Reginster JY, Deroisy R, Rovati LC, Lee RL, Lejeune E, Bruyere O, Giacovelli G, Henrotin Y, Dacre JE, Gossett C. Long-term effects of glucosamine sulphate on osteoarthritis progression: a randomised, placebo-controlled clinical trial. Lancet 2001;357(9252):251–256.

Richy F, Bruyere O, Ethgen O, Cucherat M, Henrotin Y, Reginster JY. Structural and symptomatic efficacy of glucosamine and chondroitin in knee osteoarthritis: a comprehensive meta-analysis. Arch Intern Med 2003;163(13):1514–1522.

Ronca F, Palmieri L, Panicucci P, Ronca G. Anti-inflammatory activity of chondroitin sulfate. Osteoarthritis Cartilage 1998;6(Suppl A):14–21.

Rovati LC. Clinical research in osteoarthritis: design and results of short-term and long-term trials with disease-modifying drugs. Int J Tissue React 1992;14(5):243–251.

Rovetta G, Monteforte P, Molfetta G, Balestra V. Chondroitin sulfate in erosive osteoarthritis of the hands. Int J Tissue React 2002;24(1):29–32.

Rozendaal RM, Koes BW, van Osch GJ, Uitterlinden EJ, Garling EH, Willemsen SP, Ginai AZ, Verhaar JA, Weinans H, Bierma-Zeinstra SM. Effect of glucosamine sulfate on hip osteoarthritis: a randomized trial. Ann Intern Med 2008;148(4):268–277.

Russell AS, Aghazadeh A-Habashi, Jamali F. Active ingredient consistency of commercially available glucosamine sulfate products. J Rheumatol 2002;29(11):2407–2409.

Sandy JD, Gamett D, Thompson V, Verscharen C. Chondrocyte-mediated catabolism of aggrecan: aggrecanase-dependent cleavage induced by interleukin-1 or retinoic acid can be inhibited by glucosamine. Biochem J 1998;335(Pt 1):59–66.

Schlueter AE, Orth MW. Further studies on the ability of glucosamine and chondroitin sulphate to regulate catabolic mediators in vitro. Equine Vet J 2004;36(7):634–636.

Setnikar I, Giacchetti C, Zanolo G. Pharmacokinetics of glucosamine in the dog and in man. Arzneimittelforschung 1986;36(4):729–735.

Setnikar I, Giachetti C, Zanolo G. Absorption, distribution and excretion of radioactivity after a single intravenous or oral administration of [14C] glucosamine to the rat. Pharmatherapeutica 1984;3(8):538–550.

Setnikar I, Rovati LC. Absorption, distribution, metabolism and excretion of glucosamine sulfate. A review. Arzneimittelforschung 2001;51(9):699–725.

Shikhman AR, Kuhn K, Alaaeddine N, Lotz M. N-acetylglucosamine prevents IL-1 beta-mediated activation of human chondrocytes. J Immunol 2001;166(8):5155–5160.

Sugimoto K, Takahashi M, Yamamoto Y, Shimada K, Tanzawa K. Identification of aggrecanase activity in medium of cartilage culture. J Biochem 1999;126(2):449–455.

Tapadinhas MJ, Rivera IC, Bignamini AA. Oral glucosamine sulphate in the management of arthrosis: report on a multi-centre open investigation in Portugal. Pharmatherapeutica 1982;3(3):157–168.

Tat SK, Pelletier JP, Mineau F, Duval N, Martel-Pelletier J. Variable effects of 3 different chondroitin sulfate compounds on human osteoarthritic cartilage/chondrocytes: relevance of purity and production process. J Rheumatol 2010;37(3):656–664.

Tesoriere G, Dones F, Magistro D, Castagnetta L. Intestinal absorption of glucosamine and N-acetylglucosamine. Experientia 1972;28(7):770–771.

Uebelhart, D, Thonar EJ, Delmas PD, Chantraine A, Vignon E. Effects of oral chondroitin sulfate on the progression of knee osteoarthritis: a pilot study. Osteoarthritis Cartilage 1998;6(Suppl A):39–46.

Vacha J, Pesakova V, Krajickova J, Adam M. Effect of glycosaminoglycan polysulphate on the metabolism of cartilage ribonucleic acid. Arzneimittelforschung 1984;34(5):607–609.

Vangsness CT, Jr., Spiker W, Erickson J. A review of evidence-based medicine for glucosamine and chondroitin sulfate use in knee osteoarthritis. Arthroscopy 2009;25(1):86–94.

Verbruggen G, Goemaere S, Veys EM. Chondroitin sulfate: S/DMOAD (structure/disease modifying anti-osteoarthritis drug) in the treatment of finger joint OA. Osteoarthritis Cartilage 1998;6(Suppl A):37–38.

Vlad SC, LaValley MP, McAlindon TE, Felson DT. Glucosamine for pain in osteoarthritis: why do trial results differ? Arthritis Rheum 2007;56(7):2267–2277.

Volpi N. Oral bioavailability of chondroitin sulfate (Condrosulf) and its constituents in healthy male volunteers. Osteoarthritis Cartilage 2002;10(10):768–777.

Volpi N. Oral absorption and bioavailability of ichthyic origin chondroitin sulfate in healthy male volunteers. Osteoarthritis Cartilage 2003;11(6):433–441.

Volpi N. Quality of different chondroitin sulfate preparations in relation to their therapeutic activity. J Pharm Pharmacol 2009;61(10):1271–1280.

Wilkins P, Scheel IB, Grundnes O, Hellum C, Storheim K. effect of glucosamine on pain-related disability in patients with chronic low back pain and degenerative lumbar osteoarthritis. JAMA 2010;304(1):45–52.

19 An Overview on N-Acetylglucosamine and Arthritis

Daiki Kubomura, Uzuka Naoaki, and Yoshiharu Matahira

CONTENTS

WHAT IS *N*-ACETYLGLUCOSAMINE?

N-acetylglucosamine (NAG) is an amino sugar and the minimum unit of configuration of chitin, a natural polysaccharide present in crustaceans, insects, and fungi. In animals, it is often found in the skin and cartilage in the form of glycosaminoglycans such as hyaluronan and keratan sulfate. In addition, they are universally present as the main component of cell-surface sugar chains, particularly *N*-glycoproteins, and free NAG is also present in breast milk (Hoff, 1963).

NAG and glucosamine are derivative of glucose. The hydroxyl group of glucose at position 2 is replaced with an acetamide group in NAG, whereas glucosamine has the amino group (Figure 19.1). Therefore, NAG is more stable than glucosamine. NAG is commercially produced by two methods: the *N*-acetylation of glucosamine and the enzymatic hydrolyzation of chitin oligosaccharide, partially hydrolyzed chitin of crustaceans. However, the environmental load of the chemosynthetic method is heavier than that of the enzymatic method, and a number of countries such as Japan do not approve to use the chemosynthetic NAG for food ingredient.

ABSORPTION, DISTRIBUTION, METABOLIZATION, AND EXCRETION OF NAG

NAG is mainly used for food ingredient as well as glucosamine. Therefore, several studies were examined to estimate human oral bioavailability from the absorption, distribution, metabolization, and excretion of data in animals and blood data in humans.

The metabolic distribution after oral ingestion of NAG was assessed by radiolabeled NAG in animal experiments (Shoji et al., 1999). Food-deprived 6-week-old Wistar rats (male, $n = 3$) were orally administered [$1–^{14}$C]NAG. Then, over a 7-day period, samples of expired air, urine, feces, blood, and various organs were collected, and the radioactivity levels were measured. Autoradiograms were also prepared. The results indicated that the radiation dose in the blood peaked at 4 h after

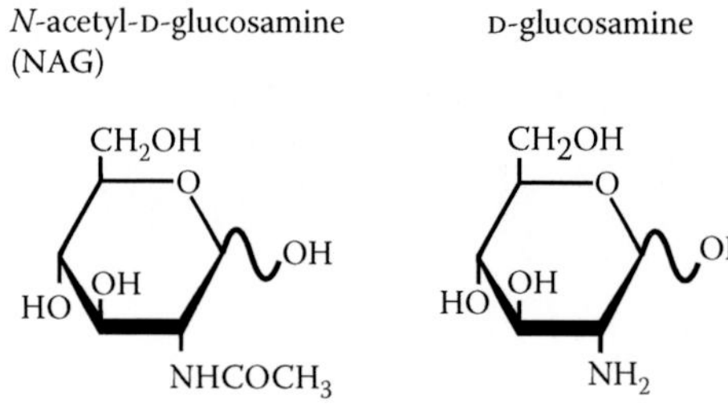

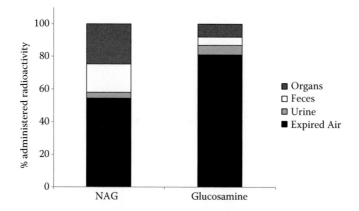

N-acetyl-D-glucosamine
(NAG)

D-glucosamine

FIGURE 19.1   Chemical structures of NAG and glucosamine.

FIGURE 19.2   Cumulative excretion of radioactivity with expired air, urine, feces, and organs after oral administration of [1–¹⁴C]NAG and [1–¹⁴C]glucosamine sulfate. Values represent mean percentages of administered radioactivity from three and four rats.

administration and then rapidly attenuated. However, beginning at 24 h after administration, the decrease became more gradual, and residual radiation was present even at 168 h after administration. At 168 h, 21.0% of the radioactivity in the dose had been excreted in urine and feces, and 54.4% was present in expired air whereas 24.7% remained in the body. Autoradiograms showed residual radioactivity in tissues containing large quantities of glycosaminoglycans, such as the skin, the cartilage, and the eyes, which suggests that the administered NAG was used in the biosynthesis of glycosaminoglycans. On the other hand, in the similar experiment with glucosamine hydrosulfate (Setnikar et al., 1984), 92% of the radiation dose had been excreted in the urine, feces, and expired air by 144 h after ingestion, indicating that a higher percentage was consumed as energy when compared with NAG (Figure 19.2).

In humans, two studies reported blood absorption and clearance after oral administration of NAG (Rubin et al., 2001; Liu et al., 2008). Liu et al. (2008) discussed the results of oral administration of NAG in eight healthy Chinese men (mean ± SD: age = 24.0 ± 3.2 years, body weight = 62.2 ± 8.3 kg). After fasting overnight, the subjects took 100 mg of NAG with 200 mL of water, and blood samples were collected periodically over a 12-h period. The results of LC/MS/MS analyses indicated that blood concentrations reached a maximum of 162.7 ± 125.2 ng/mL after 1.56 ± 1.23 h. After 4 h, levels decreased gradually, and after 10 h, they had returned to the approximate levels before ingestion. Although large individual differences were observed, the results confirmed that uptake into the blood stream was consistent with the animal study.

EFFECT OF NAG ON OSTEOARTHRITIS

Glucosamine is one of the key substrates of articular cartilage, containing polymers such as chondroitin sulfate and hyaluronan, and is believed to play a role in the formation of cartilage and has been used in the treatment of osteoarthritis for more than 30 years. The multiple studies discussed in the next paragraph have indicated that NAG also alleviates osteoarthritis as well as glucosamine.

The therapeutic effects of NAG ingestion were reported in two rabbit models: a stifle joint hole model (Tamai et al., 2003) and an anterior cruciate ligament transaction model (Shikhman et al., 2005). In former study, using 3 male rabbits and 12 female rabbits (age = 12 weeks), a puncture injury was made in the left stifle joint under anesthesia. Nine of the female rabbits were divided into three groups (*n* = 3) and administered water containing 1.0 g/day/head glucose, glucuronic acid, or NAG for 3 weeks. The remaining six animals were used as controls and were administered water alone. After treatment was terminated, the injury sites were histologically assessed. The macroscopic observations were digitized and evaluated. The results showed that the injuries were significantly repaired in the glucuronic acid and NAG groups as compared with controls. Image analyses after Alcian blue and safranin O staining in the groups administered glucuronic acid or NAG revealed significant staining at all sites observed, thus suggesting that cartilage tissue, which largely comprises proteoglycans, had been regenerated.

Oral administration of NAG was also shown to be effective against symptoms of osteoarthritis without producing any adverse drug reactions in human clinical studies.

Kajimoto et al. (2003) conducted a randomized double-blind comparative study in patients diagnosed with osteoarthritis on the basis of clinical symptoms and compared the effects of NAG and placebo. In this study, 31 subjects were assigned to each treatment group and for 8 weeks were administered once-daily bottles (125 mL) of low-fat milk containing 1000, 500, or 0 mg (placebo) of added NAG. In this study, a physician evaluated results before the start of treatment and after 4 and 8 weeks of treatment on the basis of assessments of activities of daily living, spontaneous night pain, and tenderness symptoms, in addition to the four items of the "Criteria for assessing treatment results in patients with osteoarthritis" established by the Japanese Orthopaedic Association (JOA score). The results showed improvements in pain on ascending and descending stairs and tenderness from week 4 in the group administered 1000 mg of NAG and from week 8 in the group administered 500 mg of NAG.

Hatano et al. (2006) conducted a randomized double-blind comparative study to evaluate the effects of NAG on osteoarthritis in 67 untreated patients with mild pain and discomfort in the knee. In this study, subjects were divided into groups and given a bottle containing 200 mL of normal soy milk or soy milk with 1250 mg of added NAG once-daily for 12 weeks. The study period was 20 weeks in total, including a 4-week observation period before treatment and a 4-week period after the conclusion of treatment. Evaluations were performed every week and consisted of assessment of subjective symptoms (visual analog scale), range of motion of the knee, x-ray examination (Kellgren Lawrence Grade), palpation, and blood tests. The results showed significant improvement in knee joint pain during rest and ascending or descending stairs as well as in the range of motion of the knee, beginning after 8 weeks of treatment in the group taking NAG. In the two clinical studies described earlier, adverse events for which a causal relationship with NAG treatment could not be overruled consisted of only cases of mild loose stools, and no other subjective or objective symptoms or abnormal changes in laboratory values were seen.

As a pharmacological effect, NAG was shown to be involved in the intracellular matrix as well as glucosamine. The addition of NAG dose-dependently stimulated hyaluronan synthesis by human epidermal keratinocyte (Sayo et al., 2004) and human dermal fibroblasts (Tu et al., 2009). Hyaluronan synthesis was increased as a result of supplementation-deficient NAG levels in the cutis cells and not by an increase in the activity of hyaluronan synthetase 1–3. On the other hand, in human cartilage cells, NAG stimulated hyaluronan synthetase 2 and glucose transport, resulting in upregulation of hyaluronan production and sulfated glycosaminoglycan (Shikhman et al., 2009). In addition, NAG inhibited the inflammatory response from IL-1β in human cartilage cells (Shikhman et al., 2001). These data represent a cell-type-specific phenomenon of NAG.

SAFETY OF NAG

NAG is an amino sugar that is naturally produced by the human body, and, in the form of polysaccharides such as chitin and free sugars in cow's milk, has been consumed for a long period of time, providing empirical evidence of its safety. Experimental techniques have also demonstrated NAG to be highly safe.

NAG was confirmed that no acute oral toxicity was seen at a dose of 5 g/kg (Yamamoto, 1999). Six-week-old Wistar rats (five of each sex) were administered 5 g/kg NAG, and observations were conducted for 14 days. With the exception of soft stools occurring between 1 and 24 h after administration, no abnormalities were observed, and body weight gain was confirmed. Necropsies conducted at the termination of the study revealed no abnormalities. In addition, long-term ingestion of NAG was judged to have no toxic effects in F344 rats (Takahashi et al., 2009). In that study, F344/DuCrj rats were allocated to four groups, each consisting of 10 males and 10 females, and given pelleted diet containing 0%, 1.25%, 2.5%, or 5% NAG for 52 weeks. Body weight and food consumption were measured every week until week 8 and every 4 weeks thereafter. Hematology and blood chemistry tests were also performed. At the end of the study, histopathological examinations were conducted. The results revealed no abnormalities in any areas, and the no observable effect level was calculated as being 2476 mg/kg/day for males and 2834 mg/kg/day for females.

NAG was also identified as no carcinogenic by multiple studies. The reverse mutation assay was performed using *Salmonella typhimurium* TA100, TA98, and TA1537 strains and *Escherichia coli* WP2 uvrA (Masumori, 2000). The results showed that there was no increase in the number of revertant colonies at NAG concentrations of 8.19 to 5000 µg/plate in comparison with negative controls, with or without the addition of rat liver microsomes. The micronucleus study was conducted in male Crj:CD1 (ICR) SPF mice (Ishii, 2007). NAG was administered orally twice at 24-h intervals to mice at dose levels of 500, 1000, and 2000 mg/kg/day. In this study, the proportion of micronucleated polychromatic erythrocytes was not significantly higher in any test article administration group than that in the negative control group, nor was there any dose-related increase. Takahashi (2009) administered 2.5% or 5% of NAG in the diet to groups of 50 rats of each sex for 104 weeks. As a result, there were no carcinogenic effects of NAG in F344 rats.

In regard to NAG, none of the concerns that have arisen for glucosamine on insulin levels and blood glucose control (Holmäng et al., 1999; Monauni et al., 2000) are applicable. It is due to the following data (Figure 19.3): (1) the cellular uptake of NAG is not mediated by glucose transporter (Shikhman et al., 2009), (2) NAG is phosphorylated by different enzymes because it has a low affinity for glucokinase (Miwa et al., 1994–1995; Virkamaki and Yki-Jarvinen, 1999), and (3) no allosteric effects have been observed for the metabolite NAG-6-phosphate (Shikhman et al., 2001). Rather, NAG supplementation suggested suppressing type 1 diabetes and multiple sclerosis (Grigorian et al., 2007). In fact, the results of a study in which 1250 mg/day NAG was consumed for 12 weeks showed no significant variations in blood glucose and HbA$_{1c}$ (Hatano et al., 2006). In other continuous feeding studies, with the exception of loose stools, no serious adverse events have been reported. On the other hand, glucosamine competitively reacts with glucose transporters, which perform glucose uptake, and glucokinase, which is involved with metabolism, and the fact that it inhibits glucose-induced insulin secretion. It has also been suggested that glucosamine-6-phosphate, a metabolite, allosterically inhibits glucokinase.

OTHER PHYSIOLOGICAL FUNCTIONS AND APPLICATIONS OF NAG

As stated in the previous section, it has been reported that NAG acts on glycosaminoglycan-producing cells and increases the production of mucopolysaccharides such as hyaluronan and

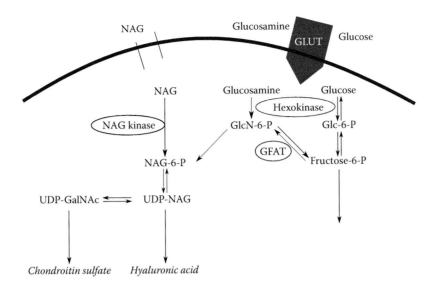

FIGURE 19.3 Simplified summary of the central role of NAG and glucosamine in the metabolism of the synthesis of hyaluronic acid. GalNAc, *N*-acetyl-D-galactosamine; GFAT, L-glutamine:D-fructose-6-phosphate amidotransferase; GlcN, D-glucosamine; GLUT, glucose transporter; P, phosphate; UDP, uridine diphosphate.

chondroitin sulfate. In addition to cartilage, the skin has also been named as a site containing large quantities of mucopolysaccharides. Hyaluronan decreases with age, as does the ability of the skin to retain moisture, producing symptoms such as wrinkles. NAG is reported to improve these symptoms; thus, NAG is used for the cosmetic food ingredient and is also blended into skin care cosmetics. Shibata et al. (2008) investigated the beneficial effects of NAG on dry skin by conducting a placebo-controlled double-blind clinical study in 39 female subjects afflicted by chronic dry skin. Subjects were divided into three groups and ingested a milk beverage containing NAG (500 mg/day), hyaluronan (50 mg/day), or none (placebo) for 8 weeks. Evaluations were performed immediately before the start of the study and after 4 and 8 weeks of treatment on the basis of mechanical measurements of skin moisture, subjective symptoms, and diagnosis by examination of photographs. The results revealed significant improvements in the moisture content of the lower eyelid and the cheek in the NAG group after 8 weeks of treatment, whereas these improvements were not observed in the placebo and the hyaluronan groups. Clinical evaluation of photographs of the face also indicated that the level of improvement in rash and skin dryness was highest in the NAG group. These results suggest that ingestion of 500 mg of NAG is effective in retaining skin moisture in women with dry skin. Similar effects were reported by Kajimoto et al. (2000).

Unlike glucosamine hydrochloride and sulfate, which do not have a pleasant taste and unstable under industrial processing, NAG is a stable substance with a pleasant sweet taste and is widely used in general food products within Japan. NAG (trade name Hyalurogluco), which is sold by Kaneka Nutrients L.P. in the United States, received GRAS recognition in 2008 (maximum use: 2.4 g/day). In the future, as the physiological functions of this substance come to be understood in greater detail, its use is expected to expand.

REFERENCES

Grigorian A, Lee SU, Tian W, et al. Control of T cell-mediated autoimmunity by metabolite flux to N-glycan biosynthesis. J Biol Chem 2007;282:20027–20035.

Hatano K, Hayashida K, Nakagawa S, Miyakuni Y. Effects and safety of soymilk beverage containing *N*-acetyl glucosamine on osteoarthritis [in Japanese with English abstract]. Jpn Pharmacol Ther 2006;34:149–165.

Hoff JE. Determination of *N*-acetylglucosamine-L-phosphate and *N*-acetylglucosamine in milk. J Dairy Sci 1963;46:573–574.

Holmäng A, Nilsson C, Niklasson M, Larsson BM, Lönroth P. Induction of insulin resistance by glucosamine reduces blood flow but not interstitial levels of either glucose or insulin. Diabetes 1999;48:106–111.

Ishii T. A Micronucleus Test of *N*-Acetyl-D-Glucosamine in Mice. Shizuoka, Japan: Bozo Research Center Inc.; 2007.

Kajimoto O, Matahira Y, Kikuchi K, Sakamoto A, Kajitani Y, Hirata H. Effects of milk containing *N*-acetylglucosamine on osteoarthritis [in Japanese]. J New Remedies Clin 2003;52:301–312.

Kajimoto O, Ohiso N, Matahira Y, Kikuchi K, Takahashi T. Clinical effects of *N*-acetylglucosamine on human skin-objective evaluation by 3D diagnostic imaging (in Japanese). J New Remedies Clin 2000;49:539–548.

Liu Y, Li Z, Liu G, Jia J, Li S, Yu C. Liquid chromatography-tandem mass spectrometry method for determination of *N*-acetylglucosamine concentration in human plasma. J Chromatogr B Analyt Technol Biomed Life Sci 2008;862:150–154.

Masumori S. Bacterial Reversion Assay with Marine Sweet (*N*-Acetyl-Glucosamine). Shizuoka, Japan: Biosafety Research Center, Foods, Drugs and Pesticides; 2000.

Miwa I, Mita Y, Murata T, et al. Utility of 3-*O*-methyl-*N*-acetyl-D-glucosamine, an *N*-acetylglucosamine kinase inhibitor, for accurate assay of glucokinase in pancreatic islets and liver. Enzyme Protein 1994–1995;48:135–142.

Monauni T, Zenti MG, Cretti A, et al. Effects of glucosamine infusion on insulin secretion and insulin action in humans. Diabetes 2000;49:926–935.

Rubin BR, Talent JM, Kongtawelert P, Pertusi RM, Forman MD, Gracy RW. Oral polymeric *N*-acetyl-D-glucosamine and osteoarthritis. J Am Osteopath Assoc 2001;101:339–344.

Sayo T, Sakai S, Inoue S. Synergistic effect of *N*-acetylglucosamine and retinoids on hyaluronan production in human keratinocytes. Skin Pharmacol Physiol 2004;17:77–83.

Setnikar I, Giachetti C, Zanolo G. Absorption, distribution and excretion of radioactivity after a single intravenous or oral administration of [^{14}C] glucosamine to the rat. Pharmatherapeutica 1984;3:538–550.

Shibata N, Tsubouchi E. Clinical effects of *N*-acetylglucosamine supplementation on dry skin [in Japanese with English abstract]. Aesthetic Dermatol 2008;18:91–99.

Shikhman AR, Amiel D, D'Lima D, et al. Chondroprotective activity of *N*-acetylglucosamine in rabbits with experimental osteoarthritis. Ann Rheum Dis 2005;64:89–94.

Shikhman AR, Brinson DC, Valbracht J, Lotz MK. Differential metabolic effects of glucosamine and *N*-acetylglucosamine in human articular chondrocytes. Osteoarthritis Cartilage 2009;17(8):1022–1028.

Shikhman AR, Kuhn K, Alaaeddine N, Lotz M. *N*-acetylglucosamine prevents IL-1 beta-mediated activation of human chondrocytes. J Immunol 2001;166:5155–5160.

Shoji A, Iga T, Inagaki S, Kobayashi K, Matahira Y, Sakai K. Metabolic Deposition of [^{14}C] *N*-Acetylglucosamine in Rats [in Japanese with English abstract and figure/table captions]. Chitin Chitosan Res 1999; 5:34–42.

Takahashi M, Inoue K, Yoshida M, Morikawa T, Shibutani M, Nishikawa A. Lack of chronic toxicity or carcinogenicity of dietary *N*-acetylglucosamine in F344 rats. Food Chem Toxicol 2009;47:462–471.

Tamai Y, Miyatake K, Okamoto Y, Takamori Y, Sakamoto K, Minami S. Enhanced healing of cartilaginous injuries by *N*-acetyl-D-glucosamine and glucuronic acid. Carbohydr Polym 2003;54:251–262.

Tu CX, Zhang RX, Zhang XJ, Huang T. Exogenous *N*-acetylglucosamine increases hyaluronan production in cultured human dermal fibroblasts. Arch Dermatol Res 2009;301(7):549–551.

Virkamaki A, Yki-Jarvinen H. Allosteric regulation of glycogen synthase and hexokinase by glucosamine-6-phosphate during glucosamine-induced insulin resistance in skeletal muscle and heart. Diabetes 1999;48:1101–1107.

Yamamoto T. Acute Oral Dose Toxicity Study of Marine Sweet in Rats. Shizuoka, Japan: Biosafety Research Center, Foods, Drugs and Pesticides; 1999.

20 Hexosamine Flux and the Efficacy and Safety of Glucosamine in the Treatment of Osteoarthritis

Akhtar Afshan Ali, William Salminen, and Julian E. Leakey

CONTENTS

INTRODUCTION

Osteoarthritis (OA), also known as degenerative arthritis or degenerative joint disease of articular (joint) cartilage, is primarily due to the breakdown of articular cartilage, resulting in pain and stiffness. OA commonly affects the joints of the hips, knees, spine, and fingers. Other joints affected less frequently include the wrists, the elbows, the shoulders, and the ankles. Although the exact cause of OA is unknown, it has been shown that heredity factors, obesity, injury, and repeated overuse of certain joints are all risk factors. It is also known as the "wear-and-tear" kind of arthritis. Rheumatoid arthritis, which is primarily an autoimmune inflammatory disease of the synovial membrane and fluid, can also result in degeneration of articular cartilage [1].

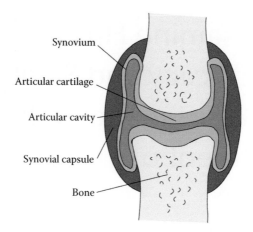

FIGURE 20.1 Structure of a joint. Cartilage covers the end of each bone. The joint is enclosed in a cavity called articular cavity covered with synovial fluid and synovial membrane.

In normal joints, articular cartilage covers the end of each bone, providing a cushion that is typically 2–5 mm thick [2]. The joint is enclosed by the synovial membrane of the articular cavity and is bathed in synovial fluid (Figure 20.1), which supplies oxygen and nutrients to the cartilage. The breakdown of a joint begins when the cartilage surface becomes damaged and loses its elasticity [3]. The cartilage continues to wear over time by injury or excessive use. Inflammatory cells invade the synovial fluid and can stimulate more cartilage breakdown. Deterioration of cartilage can affect the shape and makeup of the joint so that it fails to function smoothly. Fragments of bone and cartilage will float in the joint's fluid, causing irritation and pain. Also, bones can eventually rub together, and as a result, bony spurs, called osteophytes, and cysts may develop near the bones' ends. All of these changes create pain and discomfort when the joint is used.

STRUCTURE AND MAINTENANCE OF CARTILAGE

There are three basic forms of cartilage: elastic, fibrous, and articular (hyaline). Elastic cartilage is found in the pinna of the ear, in the walls of the eustachian tube, and in the epiglottis. This cartilage maintains the specific shape of these organs and is important for proper function. Its principal components are elastic fibers, but type II collagen is also present. Chondrocytes, the cells found in the cartilage and responsible for maintaining cartilaginous matrices, are more tightly packed together in elastic cartilage than in fibrous or articular cartilage [4].

In fibrous cartilage, the fibrous component (which is collagen, not elastic fiber) is predominant, and the matrix is minimal. Nevertheless, the cells are in *lacunae*, small spaces typically containing a single chondrocyte, although often a lacuna may be incomplete. Fibrous cartilage has a very limited distribution in the body. It is only found between the intervertebral disks and in the pubic symphysis [4].

Articular cartilage forms a protective layer of firm, flexible cartilage over the articulating ends of bones and is an avascular, aneural, alymphatic connective tissue [3, 5]. Its primary functions are to distribute loads over the bone surfaces and to provide a low-friction surface over which bones can move. It also helps to absorb shock and distribute forces. Articular cartilage is a porous, highly hydrated material, with 70%–80% water content by volume. The solid component of cartilage consists of an extracellular matrix (ECM) and a sparse population of chondrocytes, present in a concentration of approximately $10–100 \times 10^6$ cells/mm^3. The cartilage matrix is composed primarily of hydrated collagen fibrils, highly charged proteoglycan molecules, and other glycoproteins (Figure 20.2). It has a proteinaceous backbone, to which complex carbohydrate chains of sugars

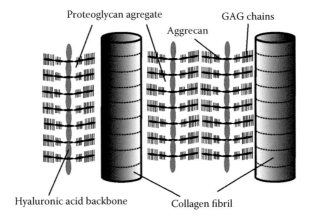

FIGURE 20.2 Schematic representation of cartilage ECM, showing collagen fibrils and highly charged, hydrated proteoglycan molecules.

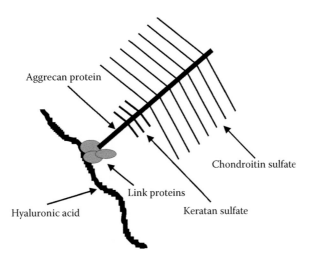

FIGURE 20.3 Detailed structure of cartilage proteoglycan aggregate.

called glycosaminoglycans (GAGs) are attached. The GAGs radiate from the protein core like the bristles of a bottle brush. Cartilage proteoglycan aggregate is shown in more detail in Figure 20.3. These aggregates can be up to 4 μm long and are composed of a hyaluronic acid backbone on which a structural core protein (aggrecan) is attached by linker proteins. Hyaluronic acid is a gelatinous mucopolysaccharide that binds the proteoglycans together into large aggregates. GAG chains (predominantly chondroitin sulfates and keratan sulfate) are attached to serine residues on the aggrecan chain. The GAG chains contain highly negatively charged carboxyl and sulfate groups, which provide them with a high affinity for water. The fibrillar component of hyaline cartilage consists primarily of type II collagen (10–20 nm diameter). The osmotically swollen matrix and the high water content are mainly responsible for the complex mechanical behavior that characterizes the response of the tissue to physiologic loads [3].

Chondroitin sulfate, hyaluronic acid, and keratan sulfate, as major components of cartilage proteoglycan aggregates, are critical for maintaining cartilage structure and function. Hyaluronic acid and keratan sulfate both contain glucosamine, and this contributed to the original rationale for the use of both glucosamine and chondroitin sulfate as dietary supplements for maintaining cartilage health [6].

Because of its durability, articular cartilage can withstand a large amount of repetitive concussion and straining throughout a lifetime. Chondrocytes orchestrate a balance between matrix synthesis and breakdown that facilitates normal tissue metabolism. This process is influenced by several competing factors, including composition of the surrounding matrix, mechanical load, hormones, local growth factors, cytokines, aging, and injury [7]. The major anabolic factors controlling chondrocyte proliferation and ECM production include profibrotic growth factors, transforming growth factor $\beta1$ (TGF-$\beta1$), TGF-$\beta3$, connective tissue growth factor (CTGF, also known as CCN2), insulin-like growth factor 1, and plasminogen activator inhibitor 1 [8–14]. Major catabolic factors include proinflammatory cytokines, such as interleukin-1β (IL-1β) and tumor necrosis factor α, and ECM dissolving proteases, which are the matrix metalloproteinases (MMPs) [8, 15].

The MMPs are a family of at least 12 zinc- and calcium-dependent endopeptidases, which collectively can degrade all ECM constituents. They are divided into three main classes: collagenases, gelatinases, and stromelysins [15]. MMPs that play a major role in cartilage degradation include interstitial collagenase (MMP-1), which is known to degrade collagen types II and X [16], stromelysin-1 (MMP-3), which has been shown to degrade aggrecan and collagen types II, IX, X, and XI [17, 18], and gelatinase-B (MMP-9) [19]. These MMPs are synthesized as zymogens within chondrocytes and synovial fibroblasts. They are exported into the ECM and activated by plasminogen activating proteases such as urokinase [8, 19–22]. They are present in elevated levels in cartilage and synovial fluid of patients with degenerative OA [8, 22] as well as in animal models of OA [23].

GLUCOSAMINE

Glucosamine was first used as a topical medication for treating OA pain in Germany in the late 1960s [24, 25]. Subsequently, it was developed as an oral preparation available on prescription in Europe [26, 27]. Glucosamine is defined under the U.S. Dietary Supplement Health and Education Act of 1994 as a dietary/nutritional supplement and therefore is freely available in the United States without prescription. It is heavily marketed as a dietary supplement to alleviate arthritic pain and as a prophylactic agent against joint damage [28]. Typically in the United States, glucosamine, as either sulfate or hydrochloride salt, is combined with chondroitin sulfate in capsules of 500 mg of glucosamine salt and 400 mg chondroitin sulfate, with a recommended daily dose of three capsules per day. Glucosamine and chondroitin sulfate have been ranked as the third best selling dietary supplements in the United States [29].

Glucosamine is an important constituent of all glycoproteins including those in the cartilage and is a principal component of several O-linked and N-linked GAGs, including hyaluronate, keratan sulfate, and heparan sulfate [6]. However, under normal physiological conditions, glucosamine itself plays only a minor role in the synthesis of GAG chains or glycoproteins. The major precursor of glucosamine residues in GAGs and glycoproteins is UDP-N-acetyl glucosamine (UDP-GlcNAc), which is derived from fructose-6-phosphate and glutamine, not glucosamine [30]. Nevertheless, it is generally believed that supplying extra dietary glucosamine helps maintain the synthesis of aggrecan glycoproteins and GAG, particularly in disease conditions such as OA.

Chemical Properties

Glucosamine is an amino monosaccharide and is a component of almost all animal tissues including cartilage. Like most hexose molecules, glucosamine exists in two anomeric pyranose ring forms, α and β. Both forms coexist in aqueous solution, interconverting via their linear form (Figure 20.4). This and its weak ultraviolet absorbance have made direct quantitative measurements of glucosamine in biological tissues by high-performance liquid chromatography (HPLC) difficult [31, 32]. Glucosamine sulfate has a lower biological equivalency than glucosamine HCl because of its higher molecular weight [6]. Glucosamine is readily soluble in water and boiling methanol and has a

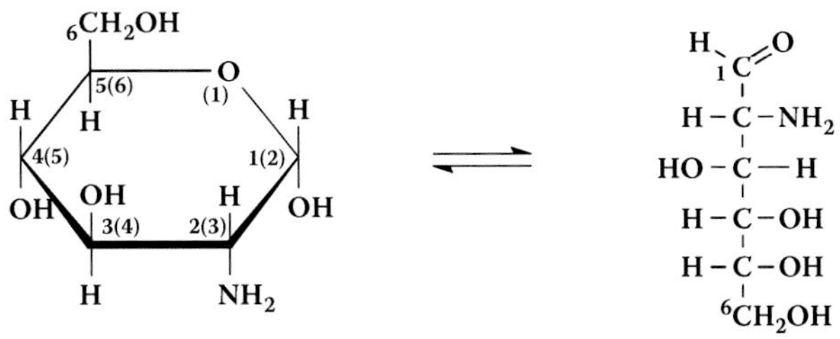

FIGURE 20.4 Structure of glucosamine. [(*3R,4R,5S,6R*)-3-Amino-6-(hydroxymethyl)oxane-2,4,5-triol; 2-amino-2-deoxy-D-glucose] showing both the α (*2S*) ring (oxane ring numbers in parentheses) and linear structures (in the β (*2R*) ring form the H and OH at C_1 are inverted).

melting point of 88°C [33]. It is manufactured usually by the hydrolysis of chitin, which is extracted from the shells of Crustacea [34].

PHARMACOKINETICS AND METABOLISM

Both intracellular and extracellular concentrations of glucosamine are negligible (<1 μM) under normal physiological conditions. Exogenous glucosamine is rapidly taken up by cells via glucose transporter proteins and is phosphorylated to produce glucosamine-6-phosphate and other hexosamines.

Early *in vivo* studies on the absorption, disposition, metabolism, and excretion of glucosamine salts have been conducted in animals and humans by Setnikar et al. [35–37] using ^{14}C-labeled glucosamine and in some cases isolation of radioactive metabolites by ion exchange chromatography. Their findings are summarized in the succeeding paragraphs.

In humans, after single bolus intravenous injection of 1005 mg of glucosamine sulfate (628 mg of glucosamine), the parent glucosamine disappeared from plasma with an apparent $t_{1/2}$ of 1.11 h. The urinary excretion in 24 h of glucosamine (determined by ion exchange chromatography) was 38% of the administered dose, mostly during the first 8 h after administration. Investigations with uniformly ^{14}C-labeled glucosamine administered with 502 mg of glucosamine sulfate indicate that the disappearance of glucosamine is due to an incorporation of glucosamine into the plasma globulins, which occurs with a lag time of 0.45 h and a rate of 0.26 per h. The radioactivity into the plasma globulins reached a peak after 10 h and was eliminated with a $t_{1/2}$ of 95 h. Urinary excretion more than 120 h accounted for 29% of the administered dose. A single intramuscular injection of 502 mg glucosamine sulfate gave results similar to those after intravenous administration. Studies with rats and dogs that were administered intravenous ^{14}C-glucosamine sulfate were consistent with the human findings. In addition, the radioactivity rapidly appeared in liver, kidneys, and other tissues, including the articular cartilage. The excretion of radioactivity in feces was insignificant. In rats, the elimination of radioactivity with the expired air measured as $[^{14}C]$-CO_2 amounted to 49% of the administered dose more than 144 h after administration, 16% of which occurred during the first 6 h after administration.

In humans, after a single oral dose of 7.5 g of glucosamine sulfate, glucosamine in plasma was below the limit of detection (3 μg/mL or 17 μM) for the ion exchange chromatography method used. After a single dose of 314 mg ^{14}C-glucosamine sulfate, radioactivity was incorporated in plasma globulins with a lag time of 1.5 h and increasing with a rate of 0.24 per h. The radioactivity reached its maximum level at 9 h and was eliminated with a $t_{1/2}$ of 58 h. The absolute oral bioavailability evaluated on the AUCs of the globulin-incorporated radioactivity was 44%. The fecal excretion in 120 h was 11.3% of the administered dose showing that at least 88.7% of the administered dose was absorbed through the gastrointestinal (GI) tract. The urinary elimination in humans of the parent glucosamine in 24 h determined with ion exchange chromatography after a single dose of 7.5 g of glucosamine sulfate was 1.19% of the administered dose, occurring mostly in the first 8 h after administration. After administration of 1884 mg/day for 7 days, the daily urinary excretion of glucosamine increased from 1.60% of the daily dose during the first 24 h to 2.22% of the daily dose in the last 24 h. The steady state in urine was reached after the second day. The urinary excretion at steady state by repeated administration suggested that doses of 1884 mg glucosamine sulfate administered either thrice daily in sugar-coated tablets or once a day in oral solution were bioequivalent.

In the rat, when oral doses of ^{14}C-glucosamine sulfate ranging from 126 to 3768 mg/kg of glucosamine sulfate were administered, a linear relationship was found between doses and both the AUCs and the C_{max} of radioactivity in both total and deproteinized plasma. The elimination of radioactivity as expired [^{14}C]-CO_2 measured in rats was 82% of the administered dose more than 144 h after administration, 61% of which occurred in the first 6 h after administration.

With the advent of more sensitive HPLC techniques for quantitating micromolar concentrations of glucosamine in biological samples, more recent studies have directly measured glucosamine in peripheral plasma and synovial fluid of humans and animals after oral dosing. Aghazadeh-Habashi et al. [38] measured glucosamine pharmacokinetics in rat plasma using derivatization with naphthylisothiocyanate and HPLC. They observed plasma glucosamine concentrations with apparent C_{max} of 18.8 μg/mL (105 μM) after a 350-mg/kg oral dose of glucosamine HCl with an apparent $t_{1/2}$ of 2.2 h.

Roda et al. [39] developed a sensitive HPLC-MS method that determined plasma glucosamine concentration values in healthy human volunteers as 64.3 ± 47.2 ng/mL (0.36 ± 0.26 μM). After a single oral bolus dose of 1.5 g of glucosamine sulfate, peak serum concentrations of 5.5 ± 1.5 μM were recorded 3 h after the dose, and their data suggested plasma $t_{1/2}$ values of approximately 8 h so that 24-h values were close to background concentrations. Interestingly, peak concentrations increased to 8.4 ± 2.7 μM after 3 days of daily dosing, suggesting that plasma concentrations rise after repeated exposure. Using HPLC-MS techniques, Persiani et al. [40] measured glucosamine concentrations in plasma and synovial fluid in 12 osteoarthritic patients being treated with 1.5 g bolus doses of glucosamine sulfate for 14 days. The median posttreatment value was 1282 ng/mL (7.17 μM) and ranged from 600 to 4061 ng/mL (3.35–22.7 μM). The median posttreatment synovial glucosamine concentration was 777 ng/mL (4.34 μM), which is significantly lower than in plasma ($p < 0.001$), and ranged from 577 to 3248 ng/mL (3.22–18.1 μM). Plasma and synovial glucosamine concentrations were highly correlated with each other.

Biggee et al. [41] measured glucosamine concentrations using high-performance ion exchange chromatography with amperometric detection in serum from 18 patients with OA after ingestion of a 1.5-g bolus dose of glucosamine sulfate. There was a large variation in peak concentrations that did not relate to sex or body mass index of the patient. However, subjects who had previously taken glucosamine products tended to have higher glucosamine levels. Glucosamine levels of all seven participants who had been using glucosamine began to rise by 15–30 min. In contrast, two of those who had not been taking glucosamine showed no increase until 45 min, two showed no increase until 1.5 h, and one showed no increase at all. The seven patients who had been taking glucosamine had maximum serum levels from 3.2 to 11.5 μM (mean ± SD = 6.6 ± 2.8 μM) in comparison ($p = 0.03$), with the maximum levels from 0 to 6.4 μM (mean ± SD = 3.6 ± 1.8 μM) for the 11 participants who had not been taking glucosamine.

Jackson et al. [42] examined the pharmacokinetics of glucosamine HCl and chondroitin sulfate when taken separately or in combination either as a single dose in normal individuals (1.5 g of glucosamine HCl and/or 1.2 g of chondroitin sulfate in capsules) or after 3 months of daily dosing in patients with symptomatic knee pain (0.5 g of glucosamine HCl and/or 0.4 g of chondroitin sulfate taken three times per day in capsules). Plasma glucosamine concentrations were determined using fluorophore-assisted carbohydrate electrophoresis. For glucosamine HCl alone, a C_{max} value of 492 ± 163 ng/mL (2.75 ± 0.9 μM) was obtained after the single 1.5-g dose, with a $t_{1/2}$ value of 2.5 h. For patients receiving glucosamine HCl alone for 3 months, a C_{max} value of 211 ± 98 ng/mL (1.18 ± 0.5 μM) was obtained after the single 1.5-g dose, with a $t_{1/2}$ value of 3.9 h. Coadministration of chondroitin sulfate reduced the C_{max} value for glucosamine in the individuals receiving the single combination doses, but not significantly in the patients dosed for 3 months.

Taken together, these studies suggest that although intravenous doses of glucosamine salts result in significant plasma concentrations of glucosamine itself, oral doses are predominantly consumed by intestinal flora and enteric tissues where they are incorporated into plasma proteins, degraded to carbon dioxide or urea, or used in biosynthetic processes such as the production of GAGs and glycoproteins. Although tissues connected to the enterohepatic portal circulation in rats may be exposed to significant glucosamine concentrations after oral dosing, other tissues such as articular cartilage would be exposed to much lower concentrations. For humans taking oral glucosamine, concentrations in plasma and synovial fluid can increase from baseline levels of <1 µM up to a maximum of 10–20 µM. Despite early data showing bioequivalence of urinary output, greater C_{max} values are achieved with bolus doses of solubilized glucosamine salts than with multiple doses of capsules or tablets.

TOXICITY

Glucosamine exhibits little or no acute toxicity in humans [43]. It has been studied clinically since the early 1980s and has been used safely by people for more than 20 years. Most glucosamine is derived from shellfish (a few manufacturers offer it derived from corn). Glucosamine derived from shellfish will not contain allergens if it is purified to USP-grade quality under GMP guidelines.

Glucosamine's safety and effects on glucose metabolism were critically evaluated by Anderson et al. [44]. Oral administration of glucosamine at very large doses (5,000–15,000 mg/kg body weight) is well tolerated without any toxicity. The LD_{50} for glucosamine for rats, mice, and rabbits exceeds 5000 mg/kg with a median value of >8000 mg/kg [44]. Echard et al. [45] examined the effects of oral administration of glucosamine hydrochloride compared with the baseline diet in eight male spontaneously hypertensive rats and eight male Sprague–Dawley rats for 9 weeks. They fed 0.5% w/w in the diet or 300 mg/kg body weight. They concluded that there were no consistent effects on blood chemical parameters and organ histology, suggesting no overall toxicity of glucosamine in their study conditions. Unfortunately, there are no published long-term toxicity evaluations of glucosamine currently available.

Pregnant women should avoid glucosamine because there are insufficient long-term studies supporting the safety of glucosamine on the developing fetus. However, one recent study [46] suggests that risk could be minimal. Glucosamine use is discouraged for diabetics because of potential interactions with hexosamine metabolism and insulin resistance (see the next section).

Evidence as to whether clinically relevant doses of glucosamine do affect insulin resistance in man remains equivocal. Muniyappa et al. [47] reported that oral glucosamine HCl given in capsules at 500 g three times per day for 6 weeks did not cause or significantly worsen insulin resistance or endothelial dysfunction in either 20 lean or 20 obese subjects. However, Biggee et al. [48] performed glucose tolerance tests on 16 patients with OA after ingestion of 1.5 g of glucosamine sulfate. Three participants who were found to have previously undiagnosed abnormalities of glucose tolerance demonstrated significant ($p = 0.04$) incremental elevations in glucose levels after ingestion of glucosamine sulfate. The other 13 participants also had mean incremental elevations that were not significant ($p = 0.20$). Glucosamine sulfate ingestion had no effect on insulin levels. This suggested that glucosamine ingestion may affect glucose levels and consequent glucose uptake in patients who have untreated diabetes or glucose intolerance. This has been supported by other studies [49].

Extremely high levels of glucosamine (many times the typical daily dose) can cause gastric disturbance such as soft stools, diarrhea, or nausea, but except for extreme overdoses, glucosamine is generally considered to have a long track record of being safe [43, 44]. This is in contrast to another common class of drugs used in OA, the nonsteroidal anti-inflammatory drugs (NSAIDs), which include COX-2-specific inhibitors. Even at therapeutic doses, prolonged administration of NSAIDs can be associated with life-threatening effects such as GI ulceration and perforation and kidney damage. Although the later generation COX-2 inhibitors such as Vioxx or Celebrex are less likely to affect the GI tract, they are associated with an increase in adverse cardiovascular effects [50].

Glucosamine does not appear to be genotoxic. It did not induce DNA repair in an *Escherichia coli* WP2 strain, but a 0.1% solution of glucosamine hydrochloride injected intraperitoneally into Swiss albino mice at 10 mg/kg body weight did induce chromosomal aberrations in bone marrow cells [33]. However, in Tilapia fish (*Oreochromis mossambica*), glucosamine hydrochloride injected intraperitoneally at a concentration of 0.1%, 10 mg/kg body weight, induced micronuclei in red blood cells. The authors felt, however, that further critical evaluation of the micronucleus assay in fish needed to be done to assess the relevance of these data [33].

BIOLOGICAL EFFECTS *IN VITRO*

Glucosamine was investigated as a cytotoxic chemotherapeutic agent in the 1970s. For example, glucosamine HCl (10–100 mM) inhibited DNA synthesis, RNA synthesis, and protein synthesis in L5178Y mouse leukemic cells and in fibroblasts [51]. Intravenous infusion of high concentrations of glucosamine into rats or mice was also reported to cause regression of implanted tumors and to increase survival of the host animals [52, 53]. Both *in vitro* and *in vivo* effects of high concentration (more than 10 mM) of glucosamine are most likely related to intracellular depletion of ATP and UTP due to excessive synthesis of UDP-GlcNAc [54].

Glucosamine has also been reported to exhibit anti-inflammatory properties in cultured tissues and cells. For example, glucosamine infusion during resuscitation after trauma-hemorrhage in rats has been shown to improve cardiac function and to reduce circulating levels of inflammatory cytokines [55]. Glucosamine mediates these effects by attenuating the activation of the nuclear factor κB signaling pathway in the heart via an increase in protein glycation. Glucosamine also attenuated the LPS-induced activation of nuclear factor κB *in vitro* in a macrophage cell line, RAW 264.7, when added to the culture medium at a final concentration of 5 mM [55].

Other *in vitro* studies have demonstrated that glucosamine can inhibit cartilage degradation and inflammation in cultured chondrocytes or cartilage explants [56, 57] and can stimulate ECM production in both cultured chondrocytes [58, 59] or human synovial explants [60], but these effects also only occur at concentrations in the culture media that are significantly greater than those observed *in vivo*.

EFFECTS ON HEXOSAMINE FLUX

Glucosamine is frequently used in millimolar concentrations in cultured cell systems as an experimental tool to stimulate hexosamine flux and UDP-GlcNAc synthesis. As a result, it is able to bypass the rate limiting enzyme of the hexosamine pathway, glutamine–fructose-6-phosphate amidotransferase [30, 61–65]. This enzyme is under allosteric negative-feedback control by UDP-GlcNAc (Figure 20.5). The hexosamine biosynthetic pathway, which in general consumes only 2%–3% of total glucose entering the cell, has been proposed to be a key component of a regulatory mechanism controlling intracellular glucose and nutrient homeostasis [66, 67]. The metabolic flux through this pathway, the hexosamine flux, and the resultant synthesis and turnover of UDP-GlcNAc are dependent on the intracellular concentrations of fructose-6-phosphate, which is in turn dependent on the relationship between the rate of its utilization via glycolysis and glycogen syntheses and the rate of glucose entry into the cell. In addition to providing substrate for the synthesis of glycoproteins and GAG, UDP-GlcNAc is used by the enzyme UDP-GlcNAc transferase (UDP-GlcNAc–polypeptide β-*N*-acetylglucosaminyl transferase [OGT]) to glycosylate several nucleocytoplasmic proteins and transcription factors [66–68]. These regulatory proteins, which include Sp1 and AKT/PKB, are activated or inactivated via *O*-GlcNAcylation at specific serine or threonine residues adjacent or identical to phosphorylation sites [69]. Evidence suggests that OGT is highly sensitive to UDP-GlcNAc concentrations and exhibits different apparent affinity (K_m) for different *O*-GlcNAcylation sites so that as UDP-GlcNAc concentrations rise because of increased hexosamine flux, different proteins are GlcNAcylated at different rates [68]. UDP-GlcNAc-dependent *O*-GlcNAcylation after increased hexosamine flux has been implicated in the onset of insulin resistance via inhibition of PKB phosphorylation [70] and the induction of HSP70 via direct *O*-GlcNAcylation of Sp1 [71]. Activation of

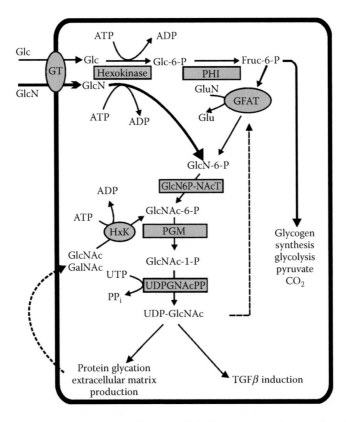

FIGURE 20.5 Hexosamine pathway. Fruc, fructose; GalNAc, N-acetylgalactosamine; GFAT, glutamine-fructose-6-phosphate amidotransferase; Glc, glucose; GlcN, glucosamine; GlcN6P-NAcT, GlcN-6-P-N-acetyltransferase; GlcNAc, N-acetylglucosamine; Glu, glutamate; GluN, glutamine; HxK, hexokinase; P, phosphate; PGM, phosphoglucomutase; PHI, phospho-hexose isomerase; PP$_i$, pyrophosphate; UDPGNAcPP, UDP-GlucNAc pyrophosphatase.

Sp1 is also required for collagen II synthesis in chondrocytes [72]. One of the major consequences on increased hexosamine flux and increased UDP-GlcNAc production is the induction of TGF-β gene expression. In cultured adipocytes and several other cell types, exposure to high glucose concentrations, millimolar concentrations of glucosamine, or overexpression of glutamine–fructose-6-phosphate amidotransferase results in increased expression of TGF-β1 and to a lesser extent TGF-β3 messenger RNA (mRNA) [73–75]. Although the promotor region of the TGF-β1 gene contains Sp1 activating sequences and Sp1 can activate the TGF-β1 promotor in reporter gene assays [76], the primary activating pathway for TGF-β expression is reported to be via AP-1-activating sequences and a p38 MAPKinase signal transduction system [77]. Evidence suggests that the p38 MAPKinase protein is activated by a protein kinase C isoform, PKCβ, and PKCβ is also O-GlcNAcylated OGT [67, 78, 79]. TGF-β mediates many prosclerotic and anti-inflammatory effects in tissues, including induction of CTGF [80–82].

CHONDROITIN SULFATE

Chondroitin sulfate, frequently consumed with glucosamine, occurs in animal tissues usually as proteoglycans, in which the polysaccharide chains are covalently attached to a core protein. The total molecular weight of a proteoglycan monomer is 1.5–2.5 × 10^6 [83, 84]. Chondroitin sulfate biosynthesis is initiated by the addition of xylose to serine residues in the core protein (i.e., aggrecan; Figure 20.3), followed by sequential addition of two galactose residues and one glucuronic

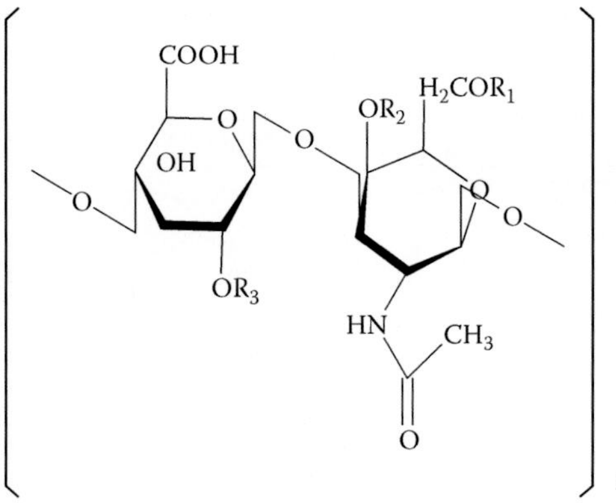

FIGURE 20.6 Disaccharide monomer units for chondroitin sulfates A and C. For chondroitin sulfate A, R_1 & R_2 = H and R_2 = SO_3H. For chondroitin sulfate C, R_1 = SO_3H and R2 & R_3 = H.

acid residue. Chondroitin polymerization then takes place by alternating *N*-acetylgalactosamine and glucuronic acid, forming the repeating disaccharide region (Figure 20.6). Finally, sulfotransferases transfer sulfate residues to the different positions of the repeating unit [85].

CHEMICAL PROPERTIES

Chondroitin sulfates are GAG polymers of molecular weights ranging between 10,000 and 100,000 Da. They occur naturally as mixtures. The two most common forms are chondroitin sulfate A (chondroitin 4-sulfate) and chondroitin sulfate C (chondroitin 6-sulfate). Their monomeric structures are shown in Figure 20.6. Most commercial preparations contain mixtures of the A and C forms [34]. Both forms are present in cartilage proteoglycan aggregate structures, but the ratio of the two forms can differ with the species source of the cartilage [86] and age and health of the cartilage donor [9]. Chondroitin sulfate is usually extracted from animal cartilage. The major commercially available source is bovine. Other animal sources are pork and shark. The latter contains significant amounts of multisulfated disaccharide units [86].

BIOSYNTHESIS, PHARMACOKINETICS, AND METABOLISM

Chondroitin sulfates are present in normal human plasma, accounting for 77%–80% of the total serum GAG content. The major site of metabolism for circulating chondroitin sulfate is the liver, where it may be partially degraded to oligosaccharides and inorganic sulfate. Inorganic sulfate and intact chondroitin sulfate are excreted in the urine [87].

Cartilage proteoglycan aggregates are initially catabolized *in situ* by MMPs [3, 88, 89]. After this digestion, the chondroitin sulfate chains, which are still attached to protein fragments, are degraded by glycosidases. In articular cartilage, hexosamidase was reported to be the major active enzyme and is upregulated during synovial inflammation [90]. Partially depolymerized chondroitin sulfate chains are absorbed or phagocytized into cells and further catabolized by lysosomal enzymes [91, 92]. Chondroitin sulfate polymers are also excreted in urine [93].

Several studies have investigated the absorption of chondroitin sulfate after oral administration in animals and humans. The data reported are somewhat contradictory [87]. Baici et al. [87] reported that oral consumption of 2 g of chondroitin sulfate (64% chondroitin sulfate A and 32% chondroitin sulfate C) by 18 subjects did not produce measurable changes in the total serum concentration of total GAGs, assayed by a spectrophotometric method specific for sulfated hexoses. This led them to suggest that chondroitin sulfate is not absorbed in humans. The possibility that low molecular weight, desulfated oligomers, and monomers may be produced and absorbed could not be ruled out. However, other studies suggest that partially depolymerized chondroitin sulfate may be absorbed from the GI tract [94]. *In vitro* studies have demonstrated that extracts of rat gastric mucosa are highly active in desulfating chondroitin sulfate and that both perfused rat liver and liver extracts degrade chondroitin sulfate to its hexosamine monomers [95, 96]. Jackson et al. [42] analyzed chondroitin sulfate and its breakdown products in plasma from 10 human subjects before and after ingestion of 1.2 g of chondroitin sulfate in capsules alone (10 subjects) or in combination with 1.5 g of glucosamine HCl (11 subjects). Both the size distribution of the chondroitin sulfate polymers and the concentration of digested disaccharide units were evaluated using a combination of gel filtration and fluorophore-assisted carbohydrate electrophoresis. They reported that no detectable changes in either chondroitin sulfate concentration or size distribution were evident at any time point between 1 and 36 h after dosing. Baseline concentrations of chondroitin sulfate were maintained at approximately 20 µg/mL throughout the evaluation period. However, when plasma of patients with OA who had consumed either 1.2 g/day chondroitin sulfate, alone or in combination with 1.5 g/day of glucosamine HCl for 3 months, was evaluated, a small statistically insignificant increase in baseline plasma chondroitin sulfate concentrations (25–30 µg/mL) was observed. It is not known whether this increase in baseline concentrations is due to chronic dosing or to increased cartilage breakdown.

Taken together, these studies suggest that although intact chondroitin sulfate is only poorly absorbed, small amounts possibly do cross the upper regions of the GI tract. However, the bulk of orally ingested material will undergo partial depolymerization and desulfation by both endogenous enzymes and intestinal bacteria in the GI tract, where significant amounts of the digested products may be absorbed. These products would be further catabolized by hepatic lysosomal enzymes, which are responsible for clearing endogenous chondroitin sulfate from the plasma [91, 97]. Large oral doses of high molecular weight chondroitin sulfate are therefore expected to have only a marginal effect on plasma chondroitin sulfate concentrations but may expose the liver to high concentrations of *N*-acetylgalactosamine, which could influence flux through the hexosamine pathway via phosphorylation and conversion to UDP-GlcNAc (Figure 20.5).

TOXICITY AND BIOLOGICAL ACTIVITY

Chondroitin sulfate exhibited low acute toxicity in rodents; the LD_{50} values for intravenous infusion are reported to be 3.1 and 5.0 g/kg for rats and mice, respectively, whereas the oral LD_{50} values were reported to be >10 g/kg for both species [98]. Chondroitin sulfate showed no mutagenicity, and it did not induce chromosomal aberrations in a Chinese hamster fibroblast cell line at concentrations up to 3 mg/mL [99].

High doses of chondroitin sulfate appear to exhibit mild anti-inflammatory and antioxidant activity *in vivo* [85]. *In vitro* studies have also demonstrated anti-inflammatory effects of chondroitin sulfate. For example, Bassleer et al. [100] investigated the effects of chondroitin sulfate (100–1000 µg/mL), with and without IL-1β, on human articular chondrocytes, cultivated in clusters for up to 32 days. They reported that chondroitin sulfate decreased prostaglandin E_2 (PGE_2) synthesis, increased total proteoglycan production, but had no effect on collagen II synthesis. IL-1β decreased proteoglycan and collagen II production and increased PGE_2 synthesis. Chondroitin sulfate inhibited all three effects of IL-1β, suggesting that *in vitro* chondroitin sulfate is able to increase matrix component production by human chondrocytes and to inhibit the inflammatory effects of IL-1β.

Thus, it is possible that if oral chondroitin sulfate is consumed in sufficient doses to increase GAG concentration in peripheral blood, it could augment the effects of glucosamine by providing hexosamine precursors and by reducing the effects of inflammatory cytokines.

EFFICACY OF GLUCOSAMINE AND CHONDROITIN SULFATE

More clinical efficacy trials have been performed on glucosamine than any other over-the-counter supplements, and yet its efficacy remains controversial [101–103]. Towheed et al. [104] reviewed 20 randomized clinical trials conducted between 1966 and 2005 on the effectiveness and toxicity of glucosamine sulfate and glucosamine HCl in the treatment of OA. These 20 studies included a total of 2570 adult patients with a mean age of 61.1 years (67% female), most of whom had OA of the knee. All of the studies were double-blind, randomized, parallel-group trials. Most of the studies were 2–3 months in duration with the exception of two more recent trials that lasted 3 years [105, 106].

Study participants were given placebo, NSAIDs, or glucosamine administered by oral, intra-articular, intramuscular, and intravenous routs. The dosage of glucosamine also varied among studies with oral doses of either 1.5 g/day or 500 mg three times per day and parenteral administration of 400 mg daily or biweekly. The type and the location of OA were not consistent in study participants: most evaluated the knee. Criteria used for assessing OA also varied among studies. A meta-analysis was done to measure pain and function using the Lequesne algofunctional index (LAI) and the Western Ontario MacMaster University Osteoarthritis Index (WOMAC). The LAI is a measurement of pain, walking distance, and activities of daily living, through a series of questions on each area. Versions for both hip and knee pain are available. Scores are given for each question and then added together for a disease severity score [107]. The WOMAC is a self-administered questionnaire of pain, disability, and joint stiffness in knee and hip OA [108].

Collectively, both poor- and high-quality studies showed glucosamine to be superior to placebo for pain and function using the LAI. However, glucosamine was not shown to be more effective than placebo when measured by WOMAC for pain, stiffness, and function. Further, function was shown to improve more with glucosamine than placebo in high-quality studies according to the LAI but when measured by WOMAC glucosamine was not different than placebo.

Two recent studies have contributed more evidence of importance of dosing procedures in determining the efficacy of glucosamine in the treatment of OA [109, 110]. The first of these was the Glucosamine/Chondroitin Arthritis Intervention Trial, which was sponsored by the National Center for Complementary and Alternative Medicine and the National Institute of Arthritis and Musculoskeletal and Skin Diseases [109] . This study evaluated placebo, glucosamine hydrochloride 500 mg three times daily, chondroitin sulfate 400 mg three times daily, combination of glucosamine hydrochloride and chondroitin sulfate, and Celecoxib 200 mg/day in a parallel, blinded, 6-month multicenter study of response in knee OA [109]. Overall, glucosamine hydrochloride + chondroitin sulfate were not significantly better than placebo for reducing knee pain by 20%. However, for patients with moderate-to-severe pain at baseline, the rate of response (Outcome Measures in Arthritis Clinical Trials–Osteoarthritis Research Society criteria) was significantly higher with combined therapy than with placebo (79.2% vs 54.3%, respectively; $p = 0.002$).

An additional study to consider was the Glucosamine Unum In Die (once a day) Efficacy Trial [110, 111]. This 6-month, double-blind, multicenter trial, conducted in Spain and Portugal, compared placebo, glucosamine sulfate 1.5 g once daily, and acetaminophen 3000 mg/day in patients with OA of the knee. The primary efficacy variable was a change in the LAI [107]. Although there was a numerical difference in improvement in the LAI between acetaminophen and placebo, only the improvement in the LAI for glucosamine sulfate versus placebo was significant ($p = 0.032$). Secondary analyses, including the OARSI responder indices, were also significantly favorable for glucosamine sulfate with a p value of 0.004 against placebo.

More recent studies include that of Black et al. [112], which assessed the clinical effectiveness and cost-effectiveness of both glucosamine sulfate, glucosamine HCl, and chondroitin sulfate in modifying the progression of OA of the knee. Electronic databases were searched from 1950 to 2008. There was evidence that glucosamine sulfate shows some clinical effectiveness in the treatment of OA of the knee. Also, Lee et al. [113] assessed the structural efficacies of daily glucosamine sulfate and chondroitin sulfate in patients with knee OA. The authors surveyed randomized controlled studies that examined the effects of long-term (>2 years) daily glucosamine sulfate (two studies [105, 114]) and chondroitin sulfate (four studies [115–117]) on joint space narrowing (JSN) in the knees of patients with OA. Meta-analysis suggested that after 3 years of treatment, glucosamine sulfate produced a small to moderate protective effect on minimum JSN (SMD 0.432, $p < 0.001$).

The same was observed for chondroitin sulfate, which had a small but significant protective effect on minimum JSN in knee of patients with OA after using 2 years (SMD 0.261, $p < 0.001$).

Zhang et al. [118] investigated the effects of glucosamine and chondroitin sulfate on Chinese patients with Kaschin–Beck disease, an interesting articular disorder found in Siberia and northern China. Overall mean change in joint space was significant between the placebo and the drug-treated groups ($p < 0.0001$). Knee joint space of the experimental group narrowed slowly compared with the control group. The authors suggested that glucosamine and chondroitin sulfate might play a protective role in preserving articular cartilage in patients with Kaschin–Beck disease as well as OA. Conversely, another recent study conducted in Norway [119] showed that glucosamine sulfate, when taken in doses of one 0.5 g capsule 3 × per day for 6 months, produced no significant improvement compared with placebo in 125 patients with low back pain or degenerative lumbar OA.

Collectively, these studies and trials suggest that glucosamine is marginally effective in alleviating the pain and clinical symptoms of some types of OA. More specifically, the studies suggest the following: (1) Although it has been proposed [103, 112] that glucosamine sulfate has greater efficacy than glucosamine HCl suggesting a therapeutic role for sulfate [120], the evidence is currently still inconclusive because the most effective studies with glucosamine sulfate used bolus dosing whereas the least effective studies with glucosamine HCl used tablets or capsules; (2) glucosamine given as a daily bolus dose does appear to be more effective than when given in multiple daily doses in capsules or tablets; and (3) the efficacy increases of glucosamine increases with long-term use. These observations are consistent with the pharmacokinetic data.

EVIDENCE THAT ORAL GLUCOSAMINE INCREASES HEXOSAMINE FLUX *IN VIVO*

Ongoing studies at the National Center for Toxicological Research (NCTR) of the U.S. Food and Drug Administration have focused on determining whether glucosamine and/or chondroitin sulfate pose any long-term risk to human health because of their chronic consumption by a significant proportion of the U.S. population. Animal studies involve acute, subchronic, and chronic exposure in diabetic and normal rats that focus on biochemical and mechanistic end points in addition to standard pathological evaluation. Studies are designed to mimic human exposure levels. For example, we have established that oral dosing of lean (Fa/Fa or Fa/fa) Zucker rats with doses of glucosamine HCl ranging from 30 to 600 mg/kg produced peak serum glucosamine concentrations of 0.5–20 μM, which overlap the human exposure range (Figure 20.7). Rats dosed daily for 6 weeks with glucosamine HCl exhibited evidence of increased hexosamine flux associated with induced expression of TGF-β and CTGF in liver, kidney, and articular cartilage and increased hepatic UPD-GlcNAc concentration (see Ali et al. [121] and Ali et al., unpublished observations). Furthermore, similar effects were observed when rats were treated with glucosamine and chondroitin sulfate in combination.

For example, in a recent study, 8-week-old male lean Zucker rats were treated with glucosamine HCl + chondroitin sulfate in combination of 0/0, 30/24, 120/96, 300/240, and 600/480 mg/kg body weight, respectively, via daily oral gavage. After 6 weeks of dosing, expression of TGF-β1 and CTGF mRNA was determined by real-time quantitative polymerase chain reaction in kidney and articular cartilage at 1 and 4 h after the final dose. As shown in Figure 20.8, both TGF-β1 and CTGF mRNA expressions were increased at least twofold in both kidney and cartilage of the rats receiving the highest dose sacrificed at 1 h after dosing. Similar increases were observed in rats sacrificed 4 h after dosing (not shown).

These effects were unexpected because glucosamine is generally used at much greater concentrations (1–20 mM) to stimulate hexosamine flux in cells *in vitro* than the serum glucosamine concentrations 10–20 μM observed in these *in vivo* studies [122]. Although intravenous infusion of glucosamine has been shown in rats to induce insulin resistance and other changes associated with increased hexosamine flux, these effects were achieved with serum glucosamine concentrations of

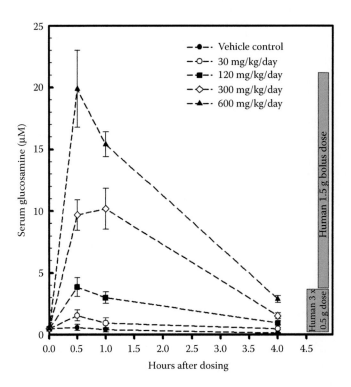

FIGURE 20.7   Serum glucosamine concentrations in tail blood from male lean (Fa/Fa and Fa/fa) 12-week-old Zucker rats treated with glucosamine HCl via oral gavage for 4 weeks. Each point represents mean and SE of eight animals. The shaded boxes on the right depict human plasma glucosamine C_{max} ranges from patients receiving either 0.5 g of glucosamine HCl three times per day or 1.5 g of glucosamine sulfate once per day as reported in references [42] and [40] respectively.

approximately 800 μM [123]. However, Marshall et al. [124] have reported that glucosamine could increase UDP-GlcNAc concentrations in cultured adipocytes with an ED_{50} of 80 μM, suggesting a lower glucosamine threshold dose for some *in vitro* systems. A factor often overlooked in *in vitro* studies of the hexosamine pathway is that flux is dependent on intracellular glutamine and acetyl CoA concentrations as well as fructose 6-phosphate [68, 71]. Fresh culture media generally contain high (3–6 mM) glutamine concentrations and low concentrations of lipid precursors of acetyl CoA. These conditions will tend to minimize the influence of low glucosamine concentrations on hexosamine flux when compared with cells *in vivo*.

The abovementioned studies provide the first evidence that oral doses of glucosamine that produce concentrations in the peripheral circulation that mimic the human exposure range are sufficient to stimulate hexosamine flux and induce hexosamine-dependent growth factor expression. Interestingly, statistically robust responses were only produced by the higher serum concentrations that are equivalent to those of humans receiving 1.5 g bolus doses of glucosamine solution. This suggests that the lower plasma glucosamine concentrations that are associated with consumption of multiple daily doses as capsules will fail to reach threshold levels for stimulation of hexosamine flux in tissues such as cartilage.

Both TGF-β and CTGF are important mediators of chondrocyte maintenance, regeneration, and repair [12, 72, 125–127], and our observations that they are induced only at the higher end of the human exposure range may explain the reported variability of clinical trial data. However, although TGF-β and CTGF are key mediators of chondrocyte proliferation and ECM production, their increased expression may not always lead to successful cartilage healing. In certain cases of

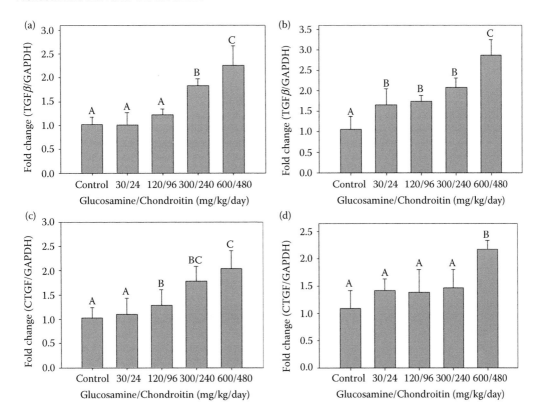

FIGURE 20.8 Upregulation of TGF-β mRNA (a and b) and CTGF mRNA (c and d) in male lean Zucker rats treated via oral gavage with glucosamine HCl (control, 30, 120, 300, and 600 mg/kg/day) in combination with chondroitin sulfate (control, 24, 96, 240, and 480 mg/kg/day) for 6 weeks. Relative mRNA concentrations in kidney (a and c) and articular cartilage (b and d) was determined in samples taken 1 h after the final dose by quantitative real-time polymerase chain reaction standardized against GAPDH (housekeeper gene) expression. Each bar represents the mean and SE of samples from five rats. Bars with different letters are significantly different $p < 0.05$.

OA, TGF-β is expressed in high levels but is inactive because of low expression of TGF-β receptors in the damaged tissue [14, 72, 128]. In such cases, increased TGF-β1 synthesis due to increased hexosamine flux would not provide a therapeutic advantage. Moreover, uncontrolled expression of TGF-β can result in scarring and spur formation in late-stage OA, and experimental injection of TGF-β1 into a normal murine knee joint induced inflammation, synovial hyperplasia, and osteophyte formation as well as prolonged elevation of proteoglycan synthesis and content in the articular cartilage [129]. Studies using a partial-thickness articular cartilage defect model in miniature pigs have shown that the optimal chondrogenic concentration range of TGF-β1 in synovial fluid was from 200 to 1000 ng/mL. At lower concentrations, chondrogenesis did not take place. At higher concentrations and with increasing frequency, adverse side effects such as synovitis, pannus formation, and synovial effusion developed [126]

In addition, prolonged induction of TGF-β and CTGF can stimulate sclerotic or fibrotic damage in other tissues that are susceptible to excessive ECM formation. In all tissues that have the potential to form ECM, a critical balance exists between anabolic-fibrotic factors such as TGF-β1 and catabolic-inflammatory factors such as IL-1β. In disease states, both sets of factors are activated in the attempt to reestablish homeostasis. Hexosamine flux and subsequent UDP-GlcNAc-dependent O-GlcNAcylation of regulatory proteins play a key role in maintaining this balance (Figure 20.9).

In pathological conditions such as chronic hyperglycemia that results from uncontrolled type I or type II diabetes, the most susceptible tissues include the renal glomeruli and the retina [75, 81,

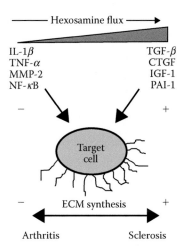

FIGURE 20.9 Influence of hexosamine flux on the balance between sclerosis and arthritis.

130]. In these tissues, chronic hyperglycemia produces pathological profiles that include excessive hexosamine flux and overexpression of TGF-β1 and CTGF, which in turn play a key role in mediating resulting sclerotic damage [81, 82, 131, 132]. Failure to successfully treat these conditions can lead to renal failure and blindness [133]. Although clinical trials have evaluated the effect of bolus glucosamine on insulin resistance, the potential for sclerotic damage was not evaluated [48, 49].

Our observations that oral glucosamine doses in rats, which produce serum glucosamine concentrations equivalent to the human exposure range, can increase TGF-β1 and CTGF expression in the kidney as well as cartilage and raise new concerns about the long-term safety of glucosamine supplements, particularly as new over-the-counter formulations with increased potency become widely available. Such formulations should be used with care and could possibly be contraindicated for diabetics with preexisting sclerotic conditions. Fortunately, our studies have identified an animal model system where these issues can be further investigated, and we are currently evaluating the sclerotic risk of glucosamine using these animal models.

CONCLUSIONS

Recent advances in our understanding of the role UDP-GlcNAc plays in the O-GlcNAcylation of regulatory proteins have provided a potential mechanistic basis for the reported beneficial effects of glucosamine in OA and have potentially elevated the nutraceutical from a simple dietary supplement into an active pharmaceutical agent. Although improvements in formulations that maximize delivery to the peripheral circulation are advantageous for the efficacy of glucosamine in treating OA and possibly other inflammatory conditions, they also increase the potential risk of serious side effects such as sclerotic damage to the kidney, retina, and other susceptible tissues. This may become a serious problem in regions such as North America and Asia, where high potency glucosamine preparations are becoming widely available and consumed by increasing numbers of people in the absence of a physician's oversight.

ACKNOWLEDGMENTS

The opinions expressed in this review are the opinions of authors and should not be concluded as official policy or opinion of the U.S. Food and Drug Administration or any other federal agency. Studies cited in this review that were conducted at the NCTR were supported by an Interagency Agreement (IAG 224-07-007 NCTR/NTP) between the NCTR/USFDA and National Toxicology

Program and the National Institute for Environmental Health Sciences, National Institutes of Health. The authors would like to thank Drs S.M. Lewis, W.T. Allaben, P. Howard, V.H. Frankos, and N. Walker for their critical review of the project; Ms. Florene Lewis, Mr. Delbert Law, and the staff of the Bionetics Corporation for animal husbandry support; and Mr. Alan Warbritton, Ms. Amy Babb, and the staff of the Toxicologic Pathology Associates for assistance in preparation of cartilage and glucosamine analysis. Dr. Ali was supported by funding administered by the Oak Ridge Institute of Science and Education.

REFERENCES

1. Wilder RL, Lafyatis R, Roberts AB, Case JP, Kumkumian GK, Sano H, Sporn MB, Remmers EF. Transforming growth factor-β in rheumatoid arthritis. Ann N Y Acad Sci 1990;593:197–207.
2. Ulrich-Vinther M, Maloney MD, Schwarz EM, Rosier R, O'Keefe RJ. Articular cartilage biology. J Am Acad Orthopaedic Surgn 2003;11:421–430.
3. Bonassar LJ, Frank EH, Murray JC, Paguio CG, Moore VL, Lark MW, Sandy JD, Wu JJ, Eyre DR, Grodzinsky AJ. Changes in cartilage composition and physical properties due to stromelysin degradation. Arthritis Rheum 1995;38:173–183.
4. Standring S. Gray's Anatomy: The Anatomical Basis of Clinical Practice. 40th ed. London: Elsevier; 2008.
5. Huber M, Trattnig S, Lintner F. Anatomy, biochemistry, and physiology of articular cartilage. Invest Radiol 2000;35:573–580.
6. Deal CL, Moskowitz RW. Nutraceuticals as therapeutic agents in osteoarthritis. The role of glucosamine, chondroitin sulfate, and collagen hydrolysate. Rheum Dis Clin North Am 1999;25:379–395.
7. Kim JW, Ahn YH. C/EBP binding activity to site F of the rat GLUT2 glucose transporter gene promoter is attenuated by c-Jun in vitro. Exp Mol Med 2002;34:379–384.
8. Goldring MB. Osteoarthritis and cartilage: the role of cytokines. Curr Rheumatol Rep 2000;2:459–465.
9. Hickery MS, Bayliss MT, Dudhia J, Lewthwaite JC, Edwards JC, Pitsillides AA. Age-related changes in the response of human articular cartilage to IL-1α and transforming growth factor-β (TGF-β): chondrocytes exhibit a diminished sensitivity to TGF-β. J Biol Chem 2003;278:53063–53071.
10. Nishida T, Kawaki H, Baxter RM, Deyoung RA, Takigawa M, Lyons KM. CCN2 (connective tissue growth factor) is essential for extracellular matrix production and integrin signaling in chondrocytes. J Cell Commun Signal 2007;1:45–58.
11. Eguchi T, Kubota S, Kondo S, Kuboki T, Yatani H, Takigawa M. A novel *cis*-element that enhances connective tissue growth factor gene expression in chondrocytic cells. Biochem Biophys Res Commun 2002;295:445–451.
12. Pujol JP, Galera P, Pronost S, Boumediene K, Vivien D, Macro M, Min W, Redini F, Penfornis H, Daireaux M,. Transforming growth factor-β (TGF-β) and articular chondrocytes. Ann Endocrinol (Paris) 1994;55:109–120.
13. Franses RE, McWilliams DF, Mapp PI, Walsh DA. Osteochondral angiogenesis and increased protease inhibitor expression in OA. Osteoarthritis Cartilage 2010;18:563–571.
14. Wang L, Almqvist KF, Veys EM, Verbruggen G. Control of extracellular matrix homeostasis of normal cartilage by a TGFβ autocrine pathway. Validation of flow cytometry as a tool to study chondrocyte metabolism in vitro. Osteoarthritis Cartilage 2002;10:188–198.
15. Bonassar LJ, Jeffries KA, Paguio CG, Grodzinsky AJ. Cartilage degradation and associated changes in biochemical and electromechanical properties. Acta Orthop Scand Suppl 1995;266:38–44.
16. Vincenti MP, Clark IM, Brinckerhoff CE. Using inhibitors of metalloproteinases to treat arthritis. Easier said than done? Arthritis Rheum 1994;37:1115–1126.
17. Flannery CR, Lark MW, Sandy JD. Identification of a stromelysin cleavage site within the interglobular domain of human aggrecan. Evidence for proteolysis at this site *in vivo* in human articular cartilage. J Biol Chem 1992;267:1008–1014.
18. Wu JJ, Lark MW, Chun LE, Eyre DR. Sites of stromelysin cleavage in collagen types II, IX, X, and XI of cartilage. J Biol Chem 1991;266:5625–5628.
19. Chu SC, Yang SF, Lue KH, Hsieh YS, Lee CY, Chou MC, Lu KH. Glucosamine sulfate suppresses the expressions of urokinase plasminogen activator and inhibitor and gelatinases during the early stage of osteoarthritis. Clin Chim Acta 2006;372:167–172.

20. Sadowski T, Steinmeyer J. Effects of tetracyclines on the production of matrix metalloproteinases and plasminogen activators as well as of their natural inhibitors, tissue inhibitor of metalloproteinases-1 and plasminogen activator inhibitor-1. Inflamm Res 2001;50:175–182.

21. Saito S, Katoh M, Masumoto M, Matsumoto S, Masuho Y. Collagen degradation induced by the combination of IL-1α and plasminogen in rabbit articular cartilage explant culture. J Biochem 1997;122:49–54.

22. Okada Y, Shinmei M, Tanaka O, Naka K, Kimura A, Nakanishi I, Bayliss MT, Iwata K, Nagase H. Localization of matrix metalloproteinase 3 (stromelysin) in osteoarthritic cartilage and synovium. Lab Invest 1992;66:680–690.

23. Varghese S. Matrix metalloproteinases and their inhibitors in bone: an overview of regulation and functions. Front Biosci 2006;11:2949–2966.

24. Vetter G. Glucosamine in the therapy of degenerative rheumatism. Dtsch Med J 1965;16:446–449.

25. Vetter G. Topical therapy of arthroses with glucosamines (Dona 200). Munch Med Wochenschr 1969;111:1499–1502.

26. Zerkak D, Dougados M. The use of glucosamine therapy in osteoarthritis. Curr Rheumatol Rep 2004;6:41–45.

27. Curtis CL, Harwood JL, Dent CM, Caterson B. Biological basis for the benefit of nutraceutical supplementation in arthritis. Drug Discov Today 2004;9:165–172.

28. Villacis J, Rice TR, Bucci LR, El-Dahr JM, Wild L, Demerell D, Soteres D, Lehrer SB. Do shrimp-allergic individuals tolerate shrimp-derived glucosamine? Clin Exp Allergy 2006;36:1457–1461.

29. McAlindon T. Why are clinical trials of glucosamine no longer uniformly positive? Rheum Dis Clin North Am 2003;29:789–801.

30. Marshall S, Garvey WT, Traxinger RR. New insights into the metabolic regulation of insulin action and insulin resistance: role of glucose and amino acids. FASEB J 1991;5:3031–3036.

31. Liang Z, Leslie J, Adebowale A, Ashraf M, Eddington ND. Determination of the nutraceutical, glucosamine hydrochloride, in raw materials, dosage forms and plasma using pre-column derivatization with ultraviolet HPLC. J Pharm Biomed Anal 1920;20:807–814.

32. Karamanos NK, Syrokou A, Vanky P, Nurminen M, Hjerpe A. Determination of 24 variously sulfated galactosaminoglycan- and hyaluronan-derived disaccharides by high-performance liquid chromatography. Anal Biochem 1994;221:189–199.

33. National Cancer Institute. Summary of Data for the Chemical Selection of Glucosamine. National Cancer Institute; 2002 :1–27. http://ntp-server.niehs.nih.gov/

34. Abedowale AO, Cox DS, Liang Z, Eddington ND. Analysis of glucosamine and chondroitin sulfate content in marketed products and the Caco-2 permeability of chondroitin sulfate raw materials. J Am Nutraceutical Assoc 2000;3:37–44.

35. Setnikar I, Giacchetti C, Zanolo G. Pharmacokinetics of glucosamine in the dog and in man. Arzneimittelforschung 1986;36:729–735.

36. Setnikar I, Palumbo R, Canali S, Zanolo G. Pharmacokinetics of glucosamine in man. Arzneimittelforschung 1993;43:1109–1113.

37. Setnikar I, Rovati LC. Absorption, distribution, metabolism and excretion of glucosamine sulfate. A review. Arzneimittelforschung 2001;51:699–725.

38. Aghazadeh-Habashi A, Sattari S, Pasutto F, Jamali F. Single dose pharmacokinetics and bioavailability of glucosamine in the rat. J Pharm Pharmaceut Sci 2002;5:181–184.

39. Roda A, Sabatini L, Barbieri A, Guardigli M, Locatelli M, Violante FS, Rovati LC, Persiani S. Development and validation of a sensitive HPLC-ESI-MS/MS method for the direct determination of glucosamine in human plasma. J Chromatogr 2006;844:119–126.

40. Persiani S, Rotini R, Trisolino G, Rovati LC, Locatelli M, Paganini D, Antonioli D, Roda A. Synovial and plasma glucosamine concentrations in osteoarthritic patients following oral crystalline glucosamine sulphate at therapeutic dose. Osteoarthritis Cartilage 2007;15:764–772.

41. Biggee BA, Blinn CM, McAlindon TE, Nuite M, Silbert JE. Low levels of human serum glucosamine after ingestion of glucosamine sulphate relative to capability for peripheral effectiveness. Ann Rheum Dis 2006;65:222–226.

42. Jackson CG, Plaas AH, Sandy JD, Hua C, Kim-Rolands S, Barnhill JG, Harris CL, Clegg DO. The human pharmacokinetics of oral ingestion of glucosamine and chondroitin sulfate taken separately or in combination. Osteoarthritis Cartilage 2010;18:297–302.

43. Hathcock JN, Shao A. Risk assessment for glucosamine and chondroitin sulfate. Regul Toxicol Pharmacol 2007;47:78–83.

44. Anderson JW, Nicolosi RJ, Borzelleca JF. Glucosamine effects in humans: a review of effects on glucose metabolism, side effects, safety considerations and efficacy. Food Chem Toxicol 2005;43:187–201.

45. Echard BW, Talpur NA, Funk KA, Bagchi D, Preuss HG. Effects of oral glucosamine and chondroitin sulfate alone and in combination on the metabolism of SHR and SD rats. Mol Cell Biochem 2001;225:85–91.

46. Sivojelezova A, Koren G, Einarson A. Glucosamine use in pregnancy: an evaluation of pregnancy outcome. J Womens Health (Larchmt) 2007;16:345–348.

47. Muniyappa R, Karne RJ, Hall G, Crandon SK, Bronstein JA, Ver MR, Hortin GL, Quon MJ. Oral glucosamine for 6 weeks at standard doses does not cause or worsen insulin resistance or endothelial dysfunction in lean or obese subjects. Diabetes 2006;55:3142–3150.

48. Biggee BA, Blinn CM, Nuite M, Silbert JE, McAlindon TE. Effects of oral glucosamine sulphate on serum glucose and insulin during an oral glucose tolerance test of subjects with osteoarthritis. Ann Rheum Dis 2007;66:260–262.

49. Pham T, Cornea A, Blick KE, Jenkins A, Scofield RH. Oral glucosamine in doses used to treat osteoarthritis worsens insulin resistance. Am J Med Sci 2007;333:333–339.

50. Bresalier RS, Sandler RS, Quan H, Bolognese JA, Oxenius B, Horgan K, Lines C, et al. Cardiovascular events associated with rofecoxib in a colorectal adenoma chemoprevention trial. N Engl J Med 2005;352:1092–1102.

51. Bosmann HB. Inhibition of protein, glycoprotein, ribonucleic acid and deoxyribonucleic acid synthesis by D-glucosamine and other sugars in mouse leukemic cells L5178Y and selective inhibition in SV-3T3 compared with 3T3 cells. Biochim Biophys Acta 1971;240:74–93.

52. Bekesi JG, Winzler RJ. Inhibitory effects of D-glucosamine on the growth of Walker 256 carcinosarcoma and on protein, RNA, and DNA synthesis. Cancer Res 1970;30:2905–2912.

53. Molnar Z, Bekesi JG. Cytotoxic effects of D-glucosamine on the ultrastructures of normal and neoplastic tissues in vivo. Cancer Res 1972;32:756–765.

54. Hresko RC, Heimberg H, Chi MM, Mueckler M. Glucosamine-induced insulin resistance in 3T3-L1 adipocytes is caused by depletion of intracellular ATP. J Biol Chem 1998;273:20658–20668.

55. Zou L, Yang S, Champattanachai V, Hu S, Chaudry IH, Marchase RB, Chatham JC. Glucosamine improves cardiac function following trauma-hemorrhage by increased protein O-GlcNAcylation and attenuation of NF-κB signaling. Am J Physiol 2009;296:H515–H523.

56. Orth MW, Peters TL, Hawkins JN. Inhibition of articular cartilage degradation by glucosamine-HCl and chondroitin sulphate. Equine Vet J Suppl 2002;34:224–229.

57. Sandy JD, Gamett D, Thompson V, Verscharen C. Chondrocyte-mediated catabolism of aggrecan: aggrecanase-dependent cleavage induced by interleukin-1 or retinoic acid can be inhibited by glucosamine. Biochem J 1998;335:59–66.

58. Varghese S, Theprungsirikul P, Sahani S, Hwang N, Yarema KJ, Elisseeff JH. Glucosamine modulates chondrocyte proliferation, matrix synthesis, and gene expression. Osteoarthritis Cartilage 2007;15:59–68.

59. Bassleer C, Rovati L, Franchimont P. Stimulation of proteoglycan production by glucosamine sulfate in chondrocytes isolated from human osteoarthritic articular cartilage in vitro. Osteoarthritis Cartilage 1998;6:427–434.

60. Uitterlinden EJ, Koevoet JL, Verkoelen CF, Bierma-Zeinstra SM, Jahr H, Weinans H, Verhaar JA, van Osch GJ. Glucosamine increases hyaluronic acid production in human osteoarthritic synovium explants. BMC Musculoskelet Disord 2008;9:120.

61. Chen H, Ing BL, Robinson KA, Feagin AC, Buse MG, Quon MJ. Effects of overexpression of glutamine:fructose-6-phosphate amidotransferase (GFAT) and glucosamine treatment on translocation of GLUT4 in rat adipose cells. Mol Cell Endocrinol 1997;135:67–77.

62. Han DH, Chen MM, Holloszy JO. Glucosamine and glucose induce insulin resistance by different mechanisms in rat skeletal muscle. Am J Physiol 2003;285:E1267–E1272.

63. Bosch RR, Pouwels MJ, Span PN, Olthaar AJ, Tack CJ, Hermus AR, Sweep CG. Hexosamines are unlikely to function as a nutrient-sensor in 3T3-L1 adipocytes: a comparison of UDP-hexosamine levels after increased glucose flux and glucosamine treatment. Endocrine 2004;23:17–24.

64. Huang JB, Clark AJ, Petty HR. The hexosamine biosynthesis pathway negatively regulates IL-2 production by Jurkat T cells. Cell Immunol 2007;245:1–6.

65. Cheng DW, Jiang Y, Shalev A, Kowluru R, Crook ED, Singh LP. An analysis of high glucose and glucosamine-induced gene expression and oxidative stress in renal mesangial cells. Arch Physiol Biochem 2006;112:189–218.

66. Love DC, Hanover JA. The hexosamine signaling pathway: deciphering the "O-GlcNAc code." Sci STKE 2005:2005(312):re13.

67. Teo CF, Wollaston-Hayden EE, Wells L. Hexosamine flux, the O-GlcNAc modification, and the development of insulin resistance in adipocytes. Mol Cell Endocrinol 2010;318:44–53.

68. Slawson C, Copeland RJ, Hart GW. O-GlcNAc signaling: a metabolic link between diabetes and cancer? Trends Biochem Sci 2010;35(10):547–555.

69. Copeland RJ, Bullen JW, Hart GW. Cross-talk between GlcNAcylation and phosphorylation: roles in insulin resistance and glucose toxicity. Am J Physiol 2008;295:E17–E28.

70. Yang X, Ongusaha PP, Miles PD, Havstad JC, Zhang F, So WV, Kudlow JE, et al. Phosphoinositide signalling links O-GlcNAc transferase to insulin resistance. Nature 2008;451:964–969.

71. Hamiel CR, Pinto S, Hau A, Wischmeyer PE. Glutamine enhances heat shock protein 70 expression via increased hexosamine biosynthetic pathway activity. Am J Physiol 2009;297:C1509–C1519.

72. Pujol JP, Chadjichristos C, Legendre F, Bauge C, Beauchef G, Andriamanalijaona R, Galera P, Boumediene K. Interleukin-1 and transforming growth factor-β1 as crucial factors in osteoarthritic cartilage metabolism. Connect Tissue Res 2008;49:293–297.

73. Daniels MC, McClain DA, Crook ED. Transcriptional regulation of transforming growth factor β1 by glucose: investigation into the role of the hexosamine biosynthesis pathway. Am J Med Sci 2000;319:138–142.

74. Kolm-Litty V, Sauer U, Nerlich A, Lehmann R, Schleicher ED. High glucose-induced transforming growth factor β1 production is mediated by the hexosamine pathway in porcine glomerular mesangial cells. J Clin Invest 1998;101:160–169.

75. Buse MG. Hexosamines, insulin resistance, and the complications of diabetes: current status. Am J Physiol 2006;290:E1-E8.

76. Geiser AG, Busam KJ, Kim SJ, Lafyatis R, O'Reilly MA, Webbink R, Roberts AB, Sporn MB. Regulation of the transforming growth factor-β1 and -β3 promoters by transcription factor Sp1. Gene 1993;129:223–228.

77. Weigert C, Sauer U, Brodbeck K, Pfeiffer A, Haring HU, Schleicher ED. AP-1 proteins mediate hyperglycemia-induced activation of the human TGF-β1 promoter in mesangial cells. J Am Soc Nephrol 2000;11:2007–2016.

78. Schleicher ED, Weigert C. Role of the hexosamine biosynthetic pathway in diabetic nephropathy. Kidney Int Suppl 2000;77:S13–S18.

79. Whiteside CI, Dlugosz JA. Mesangial cell protein kinase C isozyme activation in the diabetic milieu. Am J Physiol 2002;282:F975–F980.

80. Blom IE, Goldschmeding R, Leask A. Gene regulation of connective tissue growth factor: new targets for antifibrotic therapy? Matrix Biol 2002;21:473–482.

81. Yamagishi S, Fukami K, Ueda S, Okuda S. Molecular mechanisms of diabetic nephropathy and its therapeutic intervention. Curr Drug Targets 2007;8:952–959.

82. Riser BL, Cortes P. Connective tissue growth factor and its regulation: a new element in diabetic glomerulosclerosis. Ren Fail 2001;23:459–470.

83. Bali JP, Cousse H, Neuzil E. Biochemical basis of the pharmacologic action of chondroitin sulfates on the osteoarticular system. Semin Arthritis Rheum 2001;31:58–68.

84. Nadanaka S, Clement A, Masayama K, Faissner A, Sugahara K. Characteristic hexasaccharide sequences in octasaccharides derived from shark cartilage chondroitin sulfate D with a neurite outgrowth promoting activity. J Biol Chem 1998;273:3296–3307.

85. Volpi N. The pathobiology of osteoarthritis and the rationale for using the chondroitin sulfate for its treatment. Curr Drug Targets Immune Endocr Metabol Disord 2004;4:119–127.

86. Volpi N. Disaccharide mapping of chondroitin sulfate of different origins by high-performance capillary electrophoresis and high-performance liquid chromatography. Carbohydr Polym 2004;55:273–281.

87. Baici A, Horler D, Moser B, Hofer HO, Fehr K, Wagenhauser FJ. Analysis of glycosaminoglycans in human serum after oral administration of chondroitin sulfate. Rheumatol Int 1992;12:81–88.

88. Case JP, Sano H, Lafyatis R, Remmers EF, Kumkumian GK, Wilder RL. Transin/stromelysin expression in the synovium of rats with experimental erosive arthritis. In situ localization and kinetics of expression of the transformation-associated metalloproteinase in euthymic and athymic Lewis rats. J Clin Invest 1989;84:1731–1740.

89. Isnard N, Robert L, Renard G. Effect of sulfated GAGs on the expression and activation of MMP-2 and MMP-9 in corneal and dermal explant cultures. Cell Biol Int 2003;27:779–784.

90. Shikhman AR, Brinson DC, Lotz M. Profile of glycosaminoglycan-degrading glycosidases and glycoside sulfatases secreted by human articular chondrocytes in homeostasis and inflammation. Arthritis Rheum 2000;43:1307–1314.

91. Wood KM, Wusteman FS, Curtis CG. The degradation of intravenously injected chondroitin 4-sulphate in the rat. Biochem J 1973;134:1009–1013.

92. Wood KM, Wusteman FS, Curtis CG. The metabolic fate of chondroitin (35S)sulphate proteoglycan in the rat. Biochem Soc Trans 1975;3:500–502

93. Matsue H, Endo M. Heterogeneity of reducing terminals of urinary chondroitin sulfates. Biochim Biophys Acta 1987;923:470–477.

94. Cho SY, Sim JS, Jeong CS, Chang SY, Choi DW, Toida T, Kim YS. Effects of low molecular weight chondroitin sulfate on type II collagen-induced arthritis in DBA/1J mice. Biol Pharm Bull 2004;27:47–51.

95. Liau YH, Horowitz MI. Desulfation and depolymerization of chondroitin 4-sulfate and its degradation products by rat stomach, liver and small intestine. Proc Soc Exp Biol Med 1974;146:1037–1043.

96. MacNicholl AD, Wusteman FS, Winterburn PJ, Powell GM, Curtis CG. Degradation of [^{3}H]chondroitin 4-sulphate and re-utilization of the [^{3}H]hexosamine component by the isolated perfused rat liver. Biochem J 1980;186:279–286.

97. Wood KM, Curtis CG, Powell GM, Wusteman FS. The metabolic fate of intravenously injected peptide-bound chondroitin sulphate in the rat. Biochem J 1976;158:39–46.

98. Abdel Fattah W, Hammad T. Chondroitin sulfate and glucosamine: a review of their safety profile. J Am Nutraceutical Assoc 2003;3:16–23.

99. Ishidate M Jr, Sofuni T, Yoshikawa K, Hayashi M, Nohmi T, Sawada M, Matsuoka A. Primary mutagenicity screening of food additives currently used in Japan. Food Chem Toxicol 1984;22:623–636.

100. Bassleer CT, Combal JP, Bougaret S, Malaise M. Effects of chondroitin sulfate and interleukin-1β on human articular chondrocytes cultivated in clusters. Osteoarthritis Cartilage 1998;6:196–204.

101. Vangsness CT Jr., Spiker W, Erickson J. A review of evidence-based medicine for glucosamine and chondroitin sulfate use in knee osteoarthritis. Arthroscopy 2009;25:86–94.

102. Vlad SC, LaValley MP, McAlindon TE, Felson DT. Glucosamine for pain in osteoarthritis: why do trial results differ? Arthritis Rheum 2007;56:2267–2277.

103. Bruyere O, Reginster JY. Glucosamine and chondroitin sulfate as therapeutic agents for knee and hip osteoarthritis. Drugs Aging 2007;24:573–580.

104. Towheed TE, Maxwell L, Anastassiades TP, Shea B, Houpt J, Robinson V, Hochberg MC, Wells G. Glucosamine therapy for treating osteoarthritis. Cochrane Database Syst Rev 2005;2:CD002946.

105. Reginster JY, Deroisy R, Rovati LC, Lee RL, Lejeune E, Bruyere O, Giacovelli G, Henrotin Y, Dacre JE, Gossett C. Long-term effects of glucosamine sulphate on osteoarthritis progression: a randomised, placebo-controlled clinical trial. Lancet 2001;357:251–256.

106. Pavelka K, Bruyere O, Rovati LC, Olejarova M, Giacovelli G, Reginster JY. Relief in mild-to-moderate pain is not a confounder in joint space narrowing assessment of full extension knee radiographs in recent osteoarthritis structure-modifying drug trials. Osteoarthritis Cartilage 2003;11:730–737.

107. Lequesne M, Brandt K, Bellamy N, Moskowitz R, Menkes CJ, Pelletier JP, Altman R. Guidelines for testing slow acting drugs in osteoarthritis. J Rheumatol Suppl 1994;41:65–71.

108. Roorda LD, Jones CA, Waltz M, Lankhorst GJ, Bouter LM, van der Eijken JW, Willems WJ, et al. Satisfactory cross cultural equivalence of the Dutch WOMAC in patients with hip osteoarthritis waiting for arthroplasty. Ann Rheum Dis 2004;63:36–42.

109. Clegg DO, Reda DJ, Harris CL, Klein MA, O'Dell JR, Hooper MM, Bradley JD, et al. Glucosamine, chondroitin sulfate, and the two in combination for painful knee osteoarthritis. N Engl J Med 2006;354:795–808.

110. Herrero-Beaumont G, Ivorra JA, Del Carmen Trabado M, Blanco FJ, Benito P, Martin-Mola E, Paulino J, et al. Glucosamine sulfate in the treatment of knee osteoarthritis symptoms: a randomized, double-blind, placebo-controlled study using acetaminophen as a side comparator. Arthritis Rheum 2007;56:555–567.

111. Altman RD, Abramson S, Bruyere O, Clegg D, Herrero-Beaumont G, Maheu E, Moskowitz R, Pavelka K, Reginster JY. Commentary: osteoarthritis of the knee and glucosamine. Osteoarthritis Cartilage 2006;14:963–966.

112. Black C, Clar C, Henderson R, MacEachern C, McNamee P, Quayyum Z, Royle P, Thomas S. The clinical effectiveness of glucosamine and chondroitin supplements in slowing or arresting progression of osteoarthritis of the knee: a systematic review and economic evaluation. Health Technol Assess 2009;13:1–148.

113. Lee YH, Woo JH, Choi SJ, Ji JD, Song GG. Effect of glucosamine or chondroitin sulfate on the osteoarthritis progression: a meta-analysis. Rheumatol Int 2010;30:357–363.

114. Pavelka K, Gatterova J, Olejarova M, Machacek S, Giacovelli G, Rovati LC. Glucosamine sulfate use and delay of progression of knee osteoarthritis: a 3-year, randomized, placebo-controlled, double-blind study. Arch Intern Med 2002;162:2113–2123.

115. Uebelhart D, Malaise M, Marcolongo R, de VF, Piperno M, Mailleux E, Fioravanti A, Matoso L, Vignon E. Intermittent treatment of knee osteoarthritis with oral chondroitin sulfate: a one-year, randomized, double-blind, multicenter study versus placebo. Osteoarthritis Cartilage 2004;12:269–276.

116. Uebelhart D, Thonar EJ, Delmas PD, Chantraine A, Vignon E. Effects of oral chondroitin sulfate on the progression of knee osteoarthritis: a pilot study. Osteoarthritis Cartilage 1998;6(Suppl A):39–46.

117. Michel BA, Stucki G, Frey D, de VF, Vignon E, Bruehlmann P, Uebelhart D. Chondroitins 4 and 6 sulfate in osteoarthritis of the knee: a randomized, controlled trial. Arthritis Rheum 2005;52:779–786.

118. Zhang YX, Dong W, Liu H, Cicuttini F, de Court, Yang JB. Effects of chondroitin sulfate and glucosamine in adult patients with Kaschin–Beck disease. Clin Rheumatol 2010;29:357–362.

119. Wilkens P, Scheel IB, Grundnes O, Hellum C, Storheim K. Effect of glucosamine on pain-related disability in patients with chronic low back pain and degenerative lumbar osteoarthritis: a randomized controlled trial. JAMA 2010;304:45–52.

120. Hoffer LJ, Kaplan LN, Hamadeh MJ, Grigoriu AC, Baron M. Sulfate could mediate the therapeutic effect of glucosamine sulfate. Metabolism 2001;50:767–770.

121. Ali AA, Lewis SM, Badgley HL, Allaben WT, Frankos VH, Leakey JEA. Potential toxicity of glucosamine mediated through transforming growth factor-β (TGF-β) (Abstract). Toxicol Sci 2009;180:(Suppl 1)101.

122. Qu CJ, Jauhiainen M, Auriola S, Helminen HJ, Lammi MJ. Effects of glucosamine sulfate on intracellular UDP-hexosamine and UDP-glucuronic acid levels in bovine primary chondrocytes. Osteoarthritis Cartilage 2007;15:773–779.

123. Virkamaki A, Daniels MC, Hamalainen S, Utriainen T, McClain D, Yki-Jarvinen H. Activation of the hexosamine pathway by glucosamine in vivo induces insulin resistance in multiple insulin sensitive tissues. Endocrinology 1997;138:2501–2507.

124. Marshall S, Nadeau O, Yamasaki K. Dynamic actions of glucose and glucosamine on hexosamine biosynthesis in isolated adipocytes: differential effects on glucosamine 6-phosphate, UDP-N-acetylglucosamine, and ATP levels. J Biol Chem 2004;279:35313–35319.

125. Morales TI, Roberts AB. Transforming growth factor β regulates the metabolism of proteoglycans in bovine cartilage organ cultures. J Biol Chem 1988;263:12828–12831.

126. Hunziker EB, Driesang IM, Morris EA. Chondrogenesis in cartilage repair is induced by members of the transforming growth factor-β superfamily. Clin Orthop Relat Res 2001;391:S171-S181.

127. Nishida T, Kubota S, Kojima S, Kuboki T, Nakao K, Kushibiki T, Tabata Y, Takigawa M. Regeneration of defects in articular cartilage in rat knee joints by CCN2 (connective tissue growth factor). J Bone Miner Res 2004;19:1308–1319.

128. Verdier MP, Seite S, Guntzer K, Pujol JP, Boumediene K. Immunohistochemical analysis of transforming growth factor β isoforms and their receptors in human cartilage from normal and osteoarthritic femoral heads. Rheumatol Int 2005;25:118–124.

129. van Beuningen HM, van der Kraan PM, Arntz OJ, van den Berg WB. Transforming growth factor-β1 stimulates articular chondrocyte proteoglycan synthesis and induces osteophyte formation in the murine knee joint. Lab Invest 1994;71:279–290.

130. Van Geest RJ, Klaassen I, Vogels IM, van Noorden CJ, Schlingemann RO. Differential TGFβ signaling in retinal vascular cells: a role in diabetic retinopathy? Invest Ophthalmol Vis Sci 2010;51:1857–1865.

131. Chen S, Jim B, Ziyadeh FN. Diabetic nephropathy and transforming growth factor-β: transforming our view of glomerulosclerosis and fibrosis build-up. Semin Nephrol 2003;23:532–543.

132. Pohlers D, Brenmoehl J, Loffler I, Muller CK, Leipner C, Schultze-Mosgau S, Stallmach A, Kinne RW, Wolf G. TGF-b and fibrosis in different organs—molecular pathway imprints. Biochim Biophys Acta 2009;1792:746–756.

133. Johnson SL, Tierney EF, Onyemere KU, Tseng CW, Safford MM, Karter AJ, Ferrara A, et al. Who is tested for diabetic kidney disease and who initiates treatment? The Translating Research Into Action For Diabetes (TRIAD) Study. Diabetes Care 2006;29:1733–1738.

21 Safety and Efficacy of a Unique Undenatured Type II Collagen in the Treatment of Arthritis

Siba P. Raychaudhuri, Ramesh C. Gupta,
Hiroyoshi Moriyama, Manashi Bagchi,
Francis C. Lau, and Debasis Bagchi

CONTENTS

INTRODUCTION

Arthritis afflicts as many as one in five Americans, or approximately 20% of the U.S. population [1]. There are more than 100 forms of arthritis, and the two most common and best-known types are osteoarthritis (OA) and rheumatoid arthritis (RA). OA is by far the most prevalent form affecting approximately 60% of all arthritis sufferers. RA is the second most common form of arthritis impinging on 1.3 million adults [1, 2]. OA is a condition in which low-grade inflammation results in pain in the joints, caused by wearing of the cartilage that covers and acts as a cushion inside joints. OA is characterized by articular cartilage degradation with an accompanying periarticular bone response. OA of the knee and hip is a growing health concern because it is the second most common chronic disease leading to Social Security disability payments because of long-term absence from work [3]. It is prevalent in the aging population and affects roughly 12% of elderly (persons 60 years or older) [4]. Patients with OA have pain that typically worsens with weight bearing, including walking and standing. The debilitating pain induced by OA results in decreased movement leading to regional muscle atrophy. Indeed, OA sufferers account for 25% of visits to primary care physicians and half of all nonsteroidal anti-inflammatory drug (NSAID) prescriptions. Consequently, OA imposes a tremendous socioeconomic burden on the U.S. public health system and diminishes the quality of life of millions of people.

The exact causes of OA are not completely understood. It appears that the trigger for OA may be an environmental, a genetic, and/or a biomechanical stressor on the joint. A number of risk factors such as genetics, dietary intake, muscle weakness, obesity, and trauma may initiate various pathogenic pathways leading to OA [5]. Despite considerable medical advances in recent years, treatments of OA are limited. The most common therapies include acetaminophen and NSAIDs targeting pain and inflammation. Unfortunately, many of these agents show limited efficacy and are associated with serious side effects and high toxicities [6]. These side effects include renal and upper gastrointestinal adverse events, increased risk for cardiovascular events, and elevated blood pressure [6, 7]. In addition, recent withdrawal of certain COX-2-selective NSAIDs from the market because of increased risks for heart attack and stroke has prompted many OA sufferers to seek alternative therapies. In fact, there is a growing recognition of the important role of nutraceuticals in the maintenance of bone and joint health [8]. Among these nutraceuticals, a natural collagen extract known as UC-II has gained considerable attention in recent years for its proven safety and efficacy in the treatment of OA.

UC-II is a novel undenatured type II collagen (CII) derived from chicken sternum cartilage. Previous studies have shown that CII is effective in the treatment of RA [9–14]. Subsequent studies in animal [15–21] and human [22, 23] trials have demonstrated UC-II to be effective and safe in treating OA. Recent safety and toxicology studies on UC-II further indicated an overall low toxicity profile. A 90-day subchronic dose-dependent toxicity study showed a broad spectrum of safety for UC-II. This chapter will discuss the safety and efficacy of UC-II in the treatment of arthritis.

UNDENATURED CII IN THE TREATMENT OF RA

Undenatured CII has been researched for its efficacy in the treatment of RA at Harvard University Medical School and other institutions. The first pilot study evaluated the safety and efficacy of CII in 10 patients with recalcitrant RA [13]. In this phase I open-label, dose-escalation, and safety study, 10 RA patients were taken off their immunosuppressive and disease-modifying drugs, supplemented with 0.1 mg of solubilized CII daily for 1 month, and then switched to 0.5 mg for the next 2 months. After the treatment regimen, 6 of the 10 patients experienced a substantial clinical response with a 50% improvement in both swollen and tender joint counts combined with two additional disease measurements improving by 50% and lasting for at least 2 months after the treatment period. A complete response or disease remission with discontinuation of NSAID occurred in one patient previously on methotrexate and continued for 26 months [13]. There were no adverse events reported. The results of this phase I study were promising, which led to a phase II randomized, double-blind, placebo-controlled clinical trial to determine whether clinical efficacy of CII could be demonstrated [13]. Sixty qualified patients with severe and active RA were selected for this phase II trial. The subjects were withdrawn from immunosuppressive drugs if they had been taking them. The subjects were randomized to either a treatment identical to that used in the phase I trial or an indistinguishable placebo to be taken orally for a consecutive 90-day period. Both patients and investigators, except those responsible for medication, were masked as to the identity of the treatment. The demographic, clinical, and laboratory parameters were similar in both treatment and placebo groups [13]. Relative to baseline, there was significant ($p < 0.05$) improvement in the number of swollen joints, the number of tender or painful joints, joint swelling, and tenderness indices, and 15-m walk time at months 1, 2, and 3 in the treatment group as compared with the placebo group. Among the patients receiving CII, the decline in the number of swollen joints, tender joints, and joint swelling and joint tenderness indices was significant (all p values < 0.05). Four of the patients in the treatment group, as compared with none in the placebo group, had complete resolution of disease. Stability or improvement was observed in treatment group while the patients were off immunosuppressives, whereas patients in the placebo group tended to deteriorate. There was no evidence of sensitization to collagen, as measured by antibodies to CII. No side effects or significant changes in laboratory values, including rheumatoid factor and antibodies to CII, were noted [13]. It was concluded that oral administration of small quantities of solubilized native or undenatured CII is safe and can improve the clinical manifestations of active RA.

Another pilot clinical study was conducted to evaluate the efficacy of oral administration of CII in the treatment of juvenile RA (JRA) [9]. Ten juveniles between the ages of 8 and 14 years with active JRA defined by the American College of Rheumatology (ACR) criteria were enrolled in the study. The patients were treated with CII for 3 months, with a daily dose of 0.1 mg of CII for the first month and 0.5 mg thereafter. Clinical efficacy were evaluated monthly by ascertaining parameters including swollen and tender joint count and score, grip strength, 50-ft. walking time, duration of morning stiffness, and patient and physician global scores of disease severity. All patients completed the full course of therapy. Eight patients exhibited reductions in both swollen and tender joint counts after 3 months of CII treatment. The mean changes, relative to baseline, in swollen and tender joint counts for the eight responders at the end of the study were −61% and −54%, respectively. Six patients had greater than 33% reduction in both swollen and tender joint counts. Although the time to onset of response for the patients was variable, one patient achieved almost all of the improvements within the first month. Swollen and tender joint scores relative to baseline decreased in 9 of 10 patients. In addition, mean patient and physician global assessment scores also improved as compared with baseline. One patient had total resolution of arthritis by the end of the treatment and was able to discontinue all medications with no return of symptoms during a 14-month follow-up period. There were no adverse events considered to be treatment related. Therefore, oral supplementation of CII may be a safe and an effective therapy for JRA.

A subsequent NIH-funded multicenter, randomized, double-blind, and placebo-controlled trial confirmed the previous findings that oral administration of CII is both safe and efficacious in the treatment of RA [10]. This research was undertaken to test the safety and efficacy of different dosages of orally administered CII in patients with RA. Patients screened and enrolled in this trial met the ACR classification criteria for RA. Before entering the study, patients were required to discontinue the use of any disease-modifying antirheumatic drugs with variable washout period on the basis of the specific medication. Two hundred seventy-four patients with active RA were enrolled at six different sites and randomized to receive placebo or one of four dosages (20, 100, 500, or 2500 µg/day) of oral CII for 24 weeks. Clinical assessments of efficacy were evaluated at 0 (baseline), 2, 4, 8, 12, 16, 20, and 24 weeks. Individual disease parameters included tender and swollen joint counts and physician and patient global assessments of disease severity. Safety was assessed by comparing the type and incidence of treatment-emergent events as well as blood and urine test results. Adverse events were classified by Coding Symbols for a Thesaurus of Adverse Reaction Terms developed by U.S. Food and Drug Administration [10]. Cumulative response rates (percentage of patients meeting the criteria for response at any time during the study) were analyzed by three composite response indices: the Paulus criteria, the ACR criteria for improvement in RA, and a requirement for greater or equal to 30% reduction in both swollen and tender joint counts. Eighty-three percent of patients completed 24 weeks of treatment, which indicated that CII was well tolerated. Numeric trends in favor of the 20-µg/day treatment group were seen with all three cumulative composite measures. However, a statistically significant increase ($p < 0.05$) in response rate for the 20-µg/day group versus placebo was detected using the Paulus criteria. The safety profile of CII was excellent because the clinical and immunological parameters of CII were indistinguishable from that of placebo. There were no treatment-related adverse events or serious side effects detected with the use of CII.

Research conducted in Berlin, Germany, also indicated the efficacy of CII in the treatment of early RA [24]. Ninety patients with early RA (disease duration less than or equal to 3 years) were treated for 12 weeks with oral bovine CII (BCII) at 1 mg/day ($n = 30$) or 10 mg/day ($n = 30$) or with placebo ($n = 30$) in this double-blind, placebo-controlled, randomized phase II trial. Clinical and laboratory parameters were assessed at 0, 4, 8, and 12 weeks. There was no significant difference between the three groups in terms of response to treatment. However, a higher prevalence of responders in the BCII-treated groups was observed: seven responders in the 10-mg group and six responders in the 1-mg group versus four responders in the placebo group. Furthermore, three patients in the 10-mg and one patient in the 1-mg BCII group but no patient in the placebo group had very good response [24]. These results justify further efforts to identify which patients will have good response to such therapy.

After the initial Berlin trial, a second trial also conducted in Berlin was designed to evaluate the dose range for clinical responsiveness to oral BCII treatment [25]. In this 90-patient double-blind, placebo-controlled, and randomized trial, anti-CII antibody titers were measured before and after the BCII treatment. Sera samples were taken from patients at the beginning, at the end (12 weeks), and at 6 months after the end of the treatment. The results indicated that the titer before treatment did not identify a responder subgroup. BCII treatment reduced CII antibody titers, but only in those patients making a clinical response (responder groups). Administration of a daily dose of 10 mg of BCII reduced the titer in these subsets more effectively than 1 mg/day. The reduction was more pronounced over the 6 months after treatment. The most significant finding from the current trail was that a dose-responsive reduction in titer of anti-undenatured CII antibody was associated with clinical responder status. This observation supported the hypothesis that symptomatic responsiveness to CII treatment may be beneficial to a subset of patients and may be dose dependent. The findings suggested that a titer drop might be useful for identifying those patients who respond to this form of treatment and for determining the optimal dosage required to induce such responsiveness and that the drop might be a valid parameter for detecting the impact of the treatment on the immune system [25].

UC-II VERSUS OTHER CII

Although there are many forms of CII on the market, undenatured or native CII is required for the clinical benefits in the treatment of arthritis [14]. A previous study on bovine CII revealed that the integrity of galactose OH-4 and hydroxylysine side chain primary amino groups play a pivotal role in the activation of T cell [26]. It indicates that the interaction is probably attributed to the formation of hydrogen bonds between the galactosylated epitope and the surface of T cell, which is important in the regulation and activation of T cells that are responsible for attacking CII in the joint cartilage [26].

CII can be obtained from animals such as mice, rats, dogs, pigs, cows, chickens, and even from sharks, fish, and humans; however, the most cost-effective way to extract CII from commercial source is from animals housed and maintained in a pathogen-free environment. In this respect, chickens raised in a controlled environment free of bacteria, viruses, and other microorganisms are the best source of commercial undenatured CII [14]. InterHealth Nutraceuticals uses patented technologies to manufacture high-quality undenatured CII under Good Manufacturing Practice (GMP) guidelines. The final product is verified by ELISA to ensure that it is indeed undenatured. This stable protein extract is marketed under the brand name UC-II, which contains 25% of active undenatured CII. A myriad of research on UC-II has shown that it is both safe and efficacious in the treatment of OA in animal and humans [15–23]. On the basis of these findings, an expert panel of toxicologists concluded that UC-II is safe for human consumption and is generally recognized as safe.

UC-II IN THE TREATMENT OF OA IN ANIMALS

The efficacy of UC-II was evaluated in a placebo-controlled study with 15 osteoarthritic dogs [19]. The animals were randomly divided into three groups. Group 1 received placebo, group 2 received 1 mg/day, and group 3 received 10 mg/day of UC-II orally for 90 days. Lameness and pain were measured on a weekly basis for 120 days (90 days treatment plus 30 days posttreatment). Blood samples were assayed for kidney biomarkers creatinine and blood urea nitrogen (BUN) as well as liver biomarkers alanine aminotransferase and aspartate aminotransferase. Gross observations were noted on a weekly basis for a period of 120 days. Dogs receiving 1 mg or 10 mg of UC-II/day for 90 days showed significant improvement in overall pain and pain during limb manipulation and lameness after physical exertion and with 10 mg of UC-II showed greater improvement. On the other hand, dogs receiving placebo showed no signs of improvement. At either dose of UC-II, no adverse events or significant changes in serum chemistry were noted, which suggested that UC-II was well tolerated without causing any kidney or liver toxicity. In addition, dogs receiving UC-II for 90 days showed increased physical activity level. However, after UC-II withdrawal for a period of 30 days, all dogs experienced a relapse of overall pain, exercise-associated lameness, and pain upon limb manipulation. These results suggest that daily treatment of arthritic dogs with UC-II ameliorates signs and symptoms of arthritis and that UC-II is both safe and well tolerated [19].

A subsequent study compared the effects of UC-II alone and in combination with glucosamine HCl and chondroitin sulfate (G + C) on the treatment of osteoarthritic dogs [18]. In this placebo-controlled study, 20 dogs were randomly divided into four groups ($n = 5$): group 1, placebo; group 2, 10 mg UC-II; group 3, G (2000 mg) + C (1600 mg); and group 4, UC-II (10 mg) + G (2000 mg) + C (1600 mg). The animals were treated daily by oral administration of the assigned treatments for 120 days followed by a 30-day withdrawal period. Dogs were examined monthly for overall pain, pain upon limb manipulation, and exercise-associated lameness (Table 21.1). Serum samples were analyzed for markers of liver function (alanine aminotransferase and bilirubin) and renal function (BUN and creatinine). Body weights were also measured monthly. Dogs on placebo (group 1) did not show any improvement in arthritic conditions. Dogs receiving UC-II alone showed significant reductions in overall pain within 30 days (33%) and pain upon limb manipulation and exercise-associated lameness (66% and 44%, respectively) after 60 days of treatment. Maximum reductions in pain were observed after 120 days of treatment. Overall pain, pain reduction upon limb manipulation and exercise-associated lameness were reduced by 62%, 91%, and 78%, respectively. The overall activity of the dogs in the UC-II supplemented with G + C group (group 4) was significantly better than that in the G + C-supplemented group (group 3). G + C alleviated some pain but in combination

TABLE 21.1
Comparison of the Effects of Various Treatments on Pain Relief in Arthritic Dogs

Duration (days)	Placebo	UC-II	G + C	UC-II + G + C
Overall pain				
0	5.01 ± 0.72	4.79 ± 0.31	4.22 ± 0.30	5.16 ± 0.23
30	4.78 ± 0.75	3.17 ± 0.29*	3.34 ± 0.23	4.06 ± 0.11*
60	4.38 ± 0.73	2.60 ± 0.31*	3.63 ± 0.20	2.81 ± 0.23*
90	5.08 ± 0.83	2.62 ± 0.33*	3.38 ± 0.18	2.50 ± 0.16*
120	4.81 ± 0.87	1.89 ± 0.28*	3.21 ± 0.14	2.16 ± 0.15*
150	5.32 ± 1.03	3.16 ± 0.07*	4.03 ± 0.28	3.62 ± 0.18*
Pain upon limb manipulation				
0	2.57 ± 0.39	2.41 ± 0.19	2.74 ± 0.42	2.70 ± 0.33
30	2.14 ± 0.44	1.68 ± 0.17	2.21 ± 0.37	2.74 ± 0.24
60	2.15 ± 0.24	0.73 ± 0.28*	2.17 ± 0.32	1.98 ± 0.38*
90	2.51 ± 0.36	1.15 ± 0.20*	1.99 ± 0.34	1.69 ± 0.27*
120	2.53 ± 0.34	0.20 ± 0.09	2.01 ± 0.27	1.70 ± 0.29
150	2.52 ± 0.38	1.03 ± 0.26*	2.68 ± 0.39	2.58 ± 0.34
Pain after physical exertion				
0	2.38 ± 0.51	1.71 ± 0.44	2.60 ± 0.41	3.73 ± 0.24
30	2.19 ± 0.56	1.14 ± 0.43	2.01 ± 0.37	2.69 ± 0.37
60	2.03 ± 0.36	0.99 ± 0.06*	1.70 ± 0.38	2.01 ± 0.49*
90	2.00 ± 0.67	1.00 ± 0.43*	1.62 ± 0.39	1.68 ± 0.29*
120	2.47 ± 0.62	0.34 ± 0.32*	1.51 ± 0.36	1.32 ± 0.24*
150	2.70 ± 0.51	0.52 ± 0.21*	2.52 ± 0.39	2.70 ± 0.28

Note: Each value represents mean ± SEM ($n = 5$).

* Statistically significant difference compared with value of day 0 ($p < 0.05$).

with UC-II (group 4) provided significant reductions in overall pain (57%), pain upon limb manipulation (53%), and exercise-associated lameness (53%). After withdrawal of supplements, all dogs in the treatment groups (groups 2–4) experienced a relapse of pain (Table 21.1). No treatment-related adverse events were observed in the animals of this study. No changes in liver or kidney function markers or body weight were noted in the treatment groups as compared with that of the placebo group. Data of this placebo-controlled study demonstrate that daily treatment of arthritic dogs with UC-II alone or in combination with G + C markedly alleviates arthritic-associated pain, and these supplements are safe and well tolerated [18].

Recently, the therapeutic efficacy of UC-II osteoarthritic dogs was confirmed by the ground force plate (GFP) procedure, which objectively measures the peak force and the impulse area [21]. Peak force (N/kg body weight) measures the amount of weight the dog is bearing on a given limb, and impulse area (N·s/kg body weight) measures the amount of force applied by the limb onto the plate. UC-II significantly increased peak force by 18% and impulse area by 44% after 120 days of oral supplementation of 10 mg UC-II/day, suggesting a significant increase in joint comfort and mobility (Figure 21.1). In addition, subjective pain measurements such as pain after limb manipulation and exercise demonstrated a significant increase in joint comfort in these UC-II-supplemented arthritic dogs, which corroborated with the GFP findings. In contrast, dogs on placebo exhibited no significant change in arthritic conditions [21].

The antiarthritic efficacy of UC-II was also investigated in osteoarthritic horses [15]. Osteoarthritic horses were randomly assigned to five groups (five to six horses per group): group 1 horses received placebo; groups 2, 3, and 4 horses received 320, 480, and 640 mg of UC-II daily, respectively; and group 5 horses received a combination of G + C (5.4 + 1.8 g). Treatments for groups 1–5 were given daily for 5 months, whereas treatment for group 5 was administered bid for the first month and once daily thereafter according to product information provided by the supplier (Nutramax). Pain assessment was conducted monthly to evaluate the overall pain and pain after limb manipulation. Evaluation of overall pain was based on a consistent observation of all subjects during a walk and a trot in the same pattern on the same surface. Pain upon limb manipulation was conducted after the walk and trot by placing the affected joint in severe flexion for a period of 60 s. The limb was then placed on to the ground, and the animal was allowed to trot off. The response to the flexion test was noted with the first couple of strides [15]. Overall pain was determined on a 0–10 global

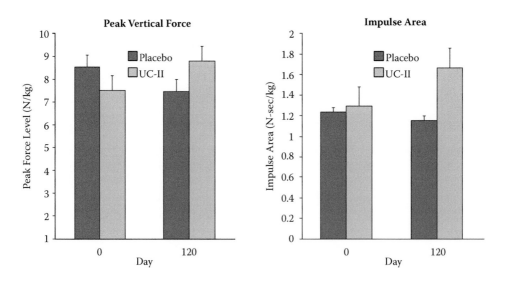

FIGURE 21.1 Quantitative GFP analysis of UC-II efficacy in arthritic dogs. *Significantly different from baseline ($p < 0.05$).

pain assessment scale, whereas pain upon limb manipulation was graded on a 0–4 scale as outlined by the American Association of Equine Practitioners. Body weights and physical wellness of all the horses were evaluated monthly. Blood samples were also collected monthly for the analysis of liver function biomarkers bilirubin, γ-glutamyl transferase, and ALP as well as kidney function biomarkers BUN and creatinine. Horses receiving placebo showed no change in arthritic condition, whereas those receiving 320, 480, or 640 mg UC-II exhibited significant reduction in arthritic pain ($p < 0.05$). UC-II at 480 or 640 mg dose provided equal effects, and therefore 480 mg was considered optimal dose. With this dose, there was an 88% decrease in overall pain and a 78% decrease in pain upon limb manipulation. Although the G + C-treated group showed significant ($p < 0.05$) reduction in pain compared with pretreated values, the efficacy was less than that observed in UC-II. In fact, UC-II at 480 or 640 mg dose was found to be more effective than G + C in the treatment of arthritic horses [15]. Clinical condition (body weight, body temperature, respiration rate, and pulse rate) and liver (bilirubin, γ-glutamyl transferase, and ALP) and kidney (BUN and creatinine) functions remained unchanged, suggesting that these supplements were well tolerated [15].

On the basis of the aforementioned findings of beneficial effects of UC-II on arthritic horses, a recent study was conducted to compare the efficacy of UC-II and G + C. Twenty-eighty arthritic horses were randomized into four groups with seven horses per group. The arthritic horses were supplemented daily for 150 days with placebo (group 1), 480 mg of UC-II (group 2), 5.4 g of G + 1.8 g of C (group 3), or UC-II + G + C at the dosage specified previously (group 4). The efficacy and the tolerability were assessed as described by Gupta et al. [15]. The results are summarized in Table 21.2. UC-II supplementation was found to outperform G + C and UC-II + G + C combinations (Table 21.2). After 150 days of treatment, UC-II significantly reduced overall pain by 90% as compared with 68% and 43% reduction by G + C and UC-II + G + C, respectively. Pain upon limb manipulation was significantly reduced by 78% after 150 days of UC-II supplementation, whereas lesser reductions of 69% and 53% were observed for G + C and UC-II + G + C, respectively (Table 21.2).

TABLE 21.2
Summary of the Effects of Different Supplementations on Pain Relief in Arthritic Horses

Duration (days)	Placebo	UC-II	G + C	UC-II + G + C
Overall pain				
0	5.00 ± 0.30	5.33 ± 0.21	4.40 ± 0.51	4.11 ± 0.11
30	5.00 ± 0.30	3.83 ± 0.17*	3.80 ± 0.58	4.11 ± 0.11
60	5.00 ± 0.30	3.17 ± 0.17*	2.80 ± 0.49*	4.11 ± 0.11
90	4.80 ± 0.33	2.00 ± 0.26*	2.40 ± 0.40*	3.67 ± 0.24
120	5.00 ± 0.39	0.83 ± 0.17*	1.80 ± 0.50*	3.11 ± 0.20*
150	5.00 ± 0.39	0.50 ± 0.34*	1.40 ± 0.40*	2.33 ± 0.33*
Pain upon limb manipulation				
0	2.50 ± 0.11	2.35 ± 0.37	2.60 ± 0.29	2.47 ± 0.11
30	2.45 ± 0.12	1.83 ± 0.19	2.20 ± 0.12	2.47 ± 0.11
60	2.55 ± 0.10	1.73 ± 0.23*	1.80 ± 0.20*	2.33 ± 0.11
90	2.63 ± 0.15	0.60 ± 0.17*	1.50 ± 0.27*	1.97 ± 0.13*
120	2.67 ± 0.14	0.50 ± 0.26*	1.10 ± 0.40*	1.75 ± 0.20*
150	2.50 ± 0.11	0.52 ± 0.18*	0.80 ± 0.34*	1.17 ± 0.27*

Note: Each value represents mean ± SEM ($n = 7$).

* Statistically significant difference compared with value of day 0 ($p < 0.05$).

UC-II HUMAN CLINICAL TRIAL

A pilot human clinical study was conducted in five female patients to test the safety and efficacy of UC-II in the treatment of OA [27]. In this open-label clinical trial, five female subjects (58–78 years) suffering from significant osteoarthritic joint pain who met the ACR criteria were selected to receive a daily dose of 40 mg UC-II (containing 10 mg of active undenatured CII) in the form of enteric capsules for 42 consecutive days. Pain level was evaluated weekly. Significant pain reduction including morning stiffness, stiffness after periods of rest, pain that worsens with use of the affected joint, and loss of joint range of motion and function was observed. The average perceived pain was reduced by 26% [27]. Thus, UC-II may serve as a novel therapeutic tool in people suffering from OA or RA.

A recent phase II human clinical trial was conducted to confirm the safety and efficacy of UC-II in the treatment of OA [23]. This randomized, double-blind clinical study was conducted in two sites in North America on patients with OA of the knee. Fifty-two qualified OA patients were randomized into two groups ($n = 26$). Group 1 received a daily dose of 40 mg of UC-II and group 2 received a daily dose of 1.5 g of glucosamine HCl (G) plus 1.2 g of chondroitin sulfate (C) for 90 days. The efficacy of UC-II as compared with G + C was evaluated at 30-day intervals by three standard OA assessment procedures: the Western Ontario and McMaster Osteoarthritis Index (WOMAC), the Visual Analog Scale (VAS), and the Lequesne functional index. Blood chemistry was examined during patient screening visit and at end of the trial. All subjects were required to record adverse events in a detailed patient diary. Demographic and baseline characteristics of patients indicated that the overall patient profiles with respect to age, sex, height, weight, blood pressure, heart beat, and target knee were similar between both groups. There were no significant interaction terms or between-group differences for treatment compliances. When compliances were compared at each visit, there were no overall between-group differences between the two groups.

In terms of WOMAC scores, the interaction between visit and treatment was statistically significant in the UC-II-treated group for the individual WOMAC components: "pain walking on flat surface," "difficulty walking on flat surface," and "difficulty in performing heavy domestic duties" as compared with the G + C-treated group. There was evidence that UC-II treatment had a significant effect for "ascending stairs" as compared with the G + C treatment. In addition, when groups were compared at each visit, UC-II was significantly better than G + C for "ascending stairs" at 30 and 60 days, "at night while in bed" at 60 days, and "difficulty walking on flat surface" at 90 days. Although there was no significant between-group difference, treatment with UC-II was effective and reduced the WOMAC scores by 33% as compared with 14% in the G + C-treated groups after 90 days. Within-group analysis indicated that UC-II treatment for 90 days significantly ($p < 0.05$) improved WOMAC scores at all treatment time points measured. In contrast, subjects that received G + C did not show any statistical significant change in WOMAC scores at day 90 of treatment (Table 21.3).

With respect to VAS scores, there was evidence that UC-II treatment had a statistically significant effect for "pain during climbing up and down stairs," "night pain," and "resting pain." When groups were compared at each visit, UC-II was significantly better than G + C for "night pain" and "resting pain" at 60 days and "pain during climbing up and down stairs" and "resting pain" at 90 days. Although both the treatments reduced the VAS score, UC-II was found to be more effective with a 40% reduction compared with a 15% decrease in the G + C-treated groups after 90 days of treatment. Within-group analysis indicated that subjects on UC-II showed a significant reduction in total VAS scores at day 60 and day 90 as compared with baseline. However, subjects on G + C showed a significant reduction in total VAS scores only at day 30 and no significant difference was observed at either day 60 or day 90 as compared with baseline (Table 21.3).

The Lequesne functional index was used to determine the effect of different treatments on pain during daily activities. There was evidence that visit had a significant effect in the UC-II-treated group for "pain while up from sitting" and "maximum distance walked" as compared with the G + C-treated group. There was as a strong trend indicating that UC-II was more efficacious than G + C. Specifically, UC-II treatment effectively reduced Lequesne functional index score by 20.2% as

TABLE 21.3
Efficacy of UC-II Compared with Glucosamine plus Chondroitin Combination

	% Relative to Baseline at Day 90	
OA Assessment	UC-II	G + C
WOMAC	66.75 ± 10.67*	85.89 ± 11.82
VAS	59.63 ± 11.42*	84.56 ± 14.93
Lequesne	79.82 ± 9.71*	94.06 ± 9.88

Note: Values are expressed as mean ± SEM.
* Significantly decreased from baseline ($p < 0.05$), indicating an improvement in pain reduction.

compared with 5.9% by G + C treatment. Within-group analysis suggested that subjects on UC-II exhibited a significant reduction in total Lequesne index of severity score from baseline to day 90, whereas no significant difference from baseline was observed for subjects on G + C at any treatment time points evaluated (Table 21.3).

There was no significant difference in the occurrence of adverse events between the two treatment groups, and blood chemistry examination did not show any abnormalities in markers for liver and kidney functions. Therefore, UC-II supplementation may provide relief for OA-related pain, discomfort, and immobility, which enhances daily activities and improves overall quality of life in OA sufferers.

UC-II SAFETY AND TOXICOLOGICAL STUDIES

Safety is of the utmost importance in nutritional supplements. A series of systematic and extensive toxicological studies were conducted on UC-II [28], and the results are summarized in Table 21.4. Acute oral toxicity was performed to assess acute toxicity of UC-II after the up and down procedure. Administration of UC-II at single doses of 175, 550, 1750, or 5000 mg/kg in female rats did not cause any mortality and did not demonstrate any signs of gross toxicity, adverse pharmacologic effects, or abnormal behavior in the treated animals after dosing and during the observation period of 14 days thereafter. No significant changes were observed for all tissues examined. On the basis of these results, the acute oral LD_{50} of UC-II was deemed to be greater than 5000 mg/kg.

Acute dermal toxicity of UC-II was conducted in male and female Sprague–Dawley rats to determine the potential for UC-II to cause toxicity from a single topical application. There were no signs of dermal irritation, gross toxicity, adverse pharmacologic effects, or abnormal behavior. No gross abnormalities were noted for any of the animals during necropsy at the conclusion of the 14-day observation period. The results indicated that the single-dose acute dermal LD_{50} of UC-II is greater than 2000 mg/kg of body weight in both male and female rats. Primary dermal irritation was conducted in male and female New Zealand albino rabbits to evaluate the potential of UC-II to produce irritation after a single topical application. After application of UC-II, all animals appeared active and healthy. There were no signs of gross toxicity, adverse pharmacologic effects, or abnormal behavior. One hour after patch removal, very slight erythema was observed at all three treated sites. The overall incidence and severity of irritation decreased with time. All animals were free of dermal irritation within 24 h posttreatment. Under the conditions of the study, UC-II was classified to be slightly irritating to the skin.

A primary eye irritation test was carried out in New Zealand albino rabbits to determine the potential for UC-II to cause irritation from a single instillation via the ocular route. All animals appeared active and healthy after UC-II instillation. There were no signs of gross toxicity, adverse pharmacologic effects, or abnormal behavior. No corneal opacity or iritis was observed in any treated eye during the study. One hour after UC-II instillation, all treated eyes exhibited conjunctivitis. The overall severity of irritation decreased with time. All animals were free of ocular irritation within 48 h posttreatment. On the basis of these findings, it was concluded that UC-II induces minimal irritation to the eye.

Ames' bacterial reverse mutation assay was used to evaluate whether UC-II can cause mutagenicity. Five strains of *Salmonella typhimurium* (TA98, TA100, TA1535, TA1537, and TA102) were used to evaluate the mutagenic potential of UC-II in the presence and absence of metabolic activation. No toxic effects of UC-II were noted in any of the five tester strains used up to the highest dose group evaluated. No biologically relevant increases in revertant colony numbers of any of the five tester strains were observed after treatment with UC-II at any concentration level in either the presence or the absence of metabolic activation. Therefore, UC-II did not cause gene mutations by base pair changes or frameshifts in the genome of the tester strains used, indicating that UC-II is nonmutagenic.

Cell gene mutation assay in mouse lymphoma cells was also used to evaluate the mutagenic potential of UC-II. No biologically relevant increases in mutants were found after treatment with UC-II (with or without metabolic activation). In addition, UC-II did not induce any clastogenic effect in colony sizing experiment. Under the experimental conditions, UC-II did not induce any mutagenic activities, and UC-II was concluded to be negative for the induction of mutagenicity in the L5178Y murine lymphoma cell line.

A dose-dependent 90-day subchronic toxicity study was conducted in male and female rats to determine the potential of UC-II to produce toxicity. A no-observed-adverse-effect level (NOAEL) was also sought for each sex. Eighty healthy rats (40 males and 40 females) were selected for the test and equally distributed into four groups (10 males and 10 females per dose level). UC-II was administered via intragastric route as 0 mg (group 1, placebo), 40 mg (group 2, low dose), 400 mg (group 3, intermediate dose), or 1000 mg (group 4, high dose) per kg body weight/day dilution in distilled water. The test substance was administered daily for 3 months. Clinical viability was observed for all animals at least twice daily during the study. Individual body weights were recorded, and the average daily body weight gains were calculated for each sex and dose level at each interval and for the overall testing interval. Individual food consumption was measured and was recorded weekly adjusting for spillage. Average daily food consumption was calculated for each sex and each dose level for each week and overall testing interval. Average daily food efficiency was also calculated for each sex and dose level on the basis of body weight gain and food consumption data. Animals were weighed before sacrifice (fasted body weight) for the calculation of organ-to-body weight and organ-to-brain weight ratios. Upon sacrifice, selected organs were immediately dissected and weighed. Blood samples were collected for laboratory tests. Histopathological assessment was performed on selected organs and tissues.

The results from the 90-day subchronic toxicity study did not show any adverse effects in individual body weight or individual organ weight after 90 days of UC-II administration. No significant changes in organ-to-body weight ratios were observed except for the kidney-to-body weight ratio, which was significantly decreased in group 3 males. This finding was not associated with any other clinical findings and did not indicate any corresponding pathologic changes in the high dose animals. Therefore, this change was deemed incidental and of no toxicological interest. There were no test substance-related macroscopic findings. Test substance-related microscopic findings were observed involving the respiratory epithelium of the nasal turbinates in males and females at 1000 mg/kg/day UC-II. Salient microscopic observations included eosinophil infiltrates, goblet cell hypertrophy and hyperplasia, and acute inflammation. Thus, under the conditions of the study, the anatomic pathology NOAEL for UC-II was determined to be 400 mg/kg/day after daily oral gavage to male and female Sprague–Dawley rats for at least 90 days.

Therefore, the wide array of toxicological studies provides unequivocal support for the broad-spectrum safety profile of UC-II (Table 21.4).

CONCLUSIONS

OA is the most prevalent form of arthritis, affecting nearly 21 million people in the United States. This debilitating disease not only imposes a tremendous burden on socioeconomic and health care resources

TABLE 21.4
Summary of UC-II Toxicological Studies

Assay	Result
Acute oral toxicity	$LD_{50} > 5000$ mg/kg
Acute dermal toxicity	$LD_{50} > 2000$ mg/kg
Primary skin irritation	Slightly irritating
Primary eye irritation	Moderately irritating
Ames' bacterial reverse mutation assay	Nonmutagenic
Mouse lymphoma assay	Nonmutagenic
NOAEL	400 mg/kg/day

but also affects the quality of life of millions of Americans. Although there is a vast advancement in medical research, the treatments for OA are limited at best. Current treatment includes physiotherapy/occupational therapy and analgesic/anti-inflammatory drugs. The most common drugs include acetaminophen and NSAIDs. Although they are effective in reducing OA-related pain, these drugs do not reverse the disease. In addition, there are considerable renal and heart side effects associated with the use of these drugs, which were the reasons why some of these drugs were pulled off the market. As a result, people suffering from OA are starting to seek alternative therapeutics or natural nutraceuticals to ease their pain and discomfort. These products are preferred by some consumers because they are well tolerated and considered safe. Currently, glucosamine and chondroitin are the two most commonly used nutraceuticals in the treatment of OA. However, recent randomized controlled trials and meta-analysis of these supplements have shown only small-to-moderate symptomatic efficacy in human OA [29].

Recently, a novel nutraceutical ingredient known as UC-II has received considerable attention in the treatment of OA. UC-II is a branded protein extract of undenatured CII derived from chicken sternum cartilage. Extensive animal and human studies have shown that UC-II is effective in the treatment of OA [15, 18–20, 23, 27]. The latest randomized, double-blind, clinical study further demonstrated that just a small daily dose of 40 mg of UC-II was more than twice as effective as 1500 mg of G + 1200 mg of C in promoting complete joint health. UC-II significantly decreased joint pain, discomfort, and immobility compared with baseline and outperformed the G + C combination using three different OA assessment tools: WOMAC, VAS, and Lequesne functional index [23]. This chapter highlighted the pertinent studies indicating the safety and efficacy of UC-II in the treatment of OA. In this regard, UC-II may present an ideal solution for the treatment and maintenance of joint health for OA sufferers.

REFERENCES

1. Helmick CG, Felson DT, Lawrence RC, Gabriel S, Hirsch R, Kwoh CK, Liang MH, et al. Estimates of the prevalence of arthritis and other rheumatic conditions in the United States. Part I. Arthritis Rheum 2008;58:15–25.
2. Lawrence RC, Felson DT, Helmick CG, Arnold LM, Choi H, Deyo RA, Gabriel S, et al. Estimates of the prevalence of arthritis and other rheumatic conditions in the United States. Part II. Arthritis Rheum 2008;58:26–35.
3. Bitton R. The economic burden of osteoarthritis. Am J Manag Care 2009;15:S230–S235.
4. Felson DT. Developments in the clinical understanding of osteoarthritis. Arthritis Res Ther 2009; 11:203.
5. Felson DT, Lawrence RC, Dieppe PA, Hirsch R, Helmick C, Jordan JM. Osteoarthritis: new insights. Part I: the disease and its risk factors. Ann Intern Med 2000;133:635–646.
6. Sarzi-Puttini P, Cimmino MA, Scarpa R, Caporali R, Parazzini F, Zaninelli A, Atzeni F, Canesi B. Osteoarthritis: an overview of the disease and its treatment strategies. Semin Arthritis Rheum 2005;35:1–10.
7. Berenbaum F. New horizons and perspectives in the treatment of osteoarthritis. Arthritis Res Ther 2008;10(Suppl 2):S1.

8. Goggs R, Vaughan-Thomas A, Clegg PD, Carter SD, Innes JF, Mobasheri A, Shakibaei M, Schwab W, Bondy CA. Nutraceutical therapies for degenerative joint diseases: a critical review. Crit Rev Food Sci Nutr 2005;45:145–164.

9. Barnett ML, Combitchi D, Trentham DE. A pilot trial of oral type II collagen in the treatment of juvenile rheumatoid arthritis. Arthritis Rheum 1996;39:623–628.

10. Barnett ML, Kremer JM, St Clair EW, Clegg DO, Furst D, Weisman M, Fletcher MJ, et al. Treatment of rheumatoid arthritis with oral type II collagen. Results of a multicenter, double-blind, placebo-controlled trial. Arthritis Rheum 1998;41:290–297.

11. Trentham DE. Immunity to type II collagen in rheumatoid arthritis: a current appraisal. Proc Soc Exp Biol Med 1984;176:95–104.

12. Trentham DE. Evidence that type II collagen feeding can induce a durable therapeutic response in some patients with rheumatoid arthritis. Ann N Y Acad Sci 1996;778:306–314.

13. Trentham DE, Dynesius-Trentham RA, Orav EJ, Combitchi D, Lorenzo C, Sewell KL, Hafler DA, Weiner HL. Effects of oral administration of type II collagen on rheumatoid arthritis. Science 1993;261:1727–1730.

14. Trentham DE, Halpner AD, Trentham RA, Bagchi M, Kothari S, Preuss HG, Bagchi D. Use of undenatured type II collagen in the treatment of rheumatoid arthritis. Clin Pract Alternative Med 2001;2:254–259.

15. Gupta RC, Canerdy TD, Skaggs P, Stocker A, Zyrkowski G, Burke R, Wegford K. Therapeutic efficacy of undenatured type-II collagen (UC-II) in comparison to glucosamine and chondroitin in arthritic horses. J Vet Pharmacol Ther 2009; 32:577–584.

16. Bagchi M, Gupta RC, Lindley J, Barnes M, et al. Suppression of arthritic pain in dogs by undenatured type-II collagen (UCII) treatment quantitatively assessed by ground force plate. Abstract presented at the 46th Congress of the European Societies of Toxicology, Dresden, Germany. September 13–16, 2009. Volume 189S: Abstract No. F14, Page S231.

17. Bagchi M, Skaggs P, Gupta RC, Canerdy TD, et al. Therapeutic efficacy of undenatured type II collagen (UC-II) in comparison to glucosamine plus chondroitin in arthritic horses. Abstract presented at Experimental Biology 2008, San Diego, CA. April 5–9, 2008. Abstract No. LB659, Page LB28.

18. D'Altilio M, Peal A, Alvey M, Simms C, Curtsinger A, Gupta RC, Canerdy TD, Good JT, Magchi M, Bagchi D. Therapeutic efficacy and safety of undenatured type II collagen singly or in combination with glucosamine and chondroitin in arthritic dogs. Toxicol Mech Methods 2007;17:189–196.

19. Deparle LA, Gupta RC, Canerdy TD, Goad JT, D'Altilio M, Bagchi M, Bagchi D. Efficacy and safety of glycosylated undenatured type-II collagen (UC-II) in therapy of arthritic dogs. J Vet Pharmacol Ther 2005;28:385–390.

20. Peal A, D'Altilio M, Simms C, Alvey M, Gupta RC, Goad JT, Canerdy TD, Bagchi M, Bagchi D. Therapeutic efficacy and safety of undenatured type-II collagen (UC-II) alone or in combination with (–)-hydroxycitric acid and chromemate in arthritic dogs. J Vet Pharmacol Ther 2007;30:275–278.

21. Gupta RC, Lindley J, Barnes M, Minniear J, et al. Pain reduction measured by ground force plate in arthritic dogs treated with type-II collagen. Abstract presented at Society of Toxicology—48th Annual Meeting and ToxExpo 2009, Baltimore, MD. March 15–19, 2009. Volume 108:No. 1, Abstract No. 769, Page 159.

22. Bagchi M, Lau FC, Bagchi D. Beneficial effects of oral administration of undenatured type II collagen on osteoarthritis: a human clinical trial. Am Col Nutr 2008;27(5):603.

23. Crowley DC, Lau FC, Sharma P, Evans M, Guthrie N, Bagchi M, Bagchi D, Dey DK, Raychaudhuri SP. Safety and efficacy of undenatured type II collagen in the treatment of osteoarthritis of the knee: a clinical trial. Int J Med Sci 2009;6:312–321.

24. Sieper J, Kary S, Sorensen H, Alten R, Eggens U, Huge W, Hiepe F, et al. Oral type II collagen treatment in early rheumatoid arthritis. A double-blind, placebo-controlled, randomized trial. Arthritis Rheum 1996;39:41–51.

25. Gimsa U, Sieper J, Braun J, Mitchison NA. Type II collagen serology: a guide to clinical responsiveness to oral tolerance? Rheumatol Int 1997;16:237–240.

26. Glatigny S, Blaton MA, Marin J, Mistou S, Briand JP, Guichard G, Catherine Fournier C, Chiocchia G. Insights into spatial configuration of a galactosylated epitope required to trigger arthritogenic T-cell receptors specific for the sugar moiety. Arthritis Res Ther 2007;9:R92.

27. Bagchi D, Misner B, Bagchi M, Kothari SC, Downs BW, Fafard RD, Preuss HG. Effects of orally administered undenatured type II collagen against arthritic inflammatory diseases: a mechanistic exploration. Int J Clin Pharm Res 2002;22:101–110.

28. Lau FC, Raychaudhuri SP, Marone PA, Bagchi M, et al. Broad spectrum safety of a novel anti-arthritic supplement: Undenatured type II collagen. Am Col Nutr 2009;28:311.

29. Bruyere O, Reginster JY. Glucosamine and chondroitin sulfate as therapeutic agents for knee and hip osteoarthritis. Drugs Aging 2007;24:573–580.

22 Targeting Inflammatory Pathways by Nutraceuticals for Prevention and Treatment of Arthritis

Bokyung Sung, Gautam Sethi, Kwang Seok Ahn, Manoj K. Pandey, Ajaikumar B. Kunnumakkara, and Bharat B. Aggarwal

CONTENTS

INTRODUCTION

Like most other autoimmune diseases, arthritis is more prevalent in the Western world than in other countries (Devereux, 2006). Although the precise reason for this difference is not understood, lifestyle is known to play a major role. Current treatments for most diseases, including arthritis, tend to be inefficient, have side effects, and tend to be expensive (Aggarwal et al., 2006a). Natural products offer an opportunity that devoid of such disadvantages. Any treatment requires proper understanding of pathogenesis of the disease, such as arthritis. Arthritis is primarily a proinflammatory disease. There are more than 100 different kinds of arthritides. Perhaps three of the most common occurring arthritides in the Western world are gout, osteoarthritis (OA), and rheumatoid arthritis (RA). Gout occurs in response to the presence of crystals of monosodium urate (MSU) in joints, bones, and soft tissues (Becker and Jolly, 2006; Hoskison and Wortmann, 2006; Saag and Choi, 2006). Both acute arthritis and chronic arthropathy (tophaceous gout) are considered part of gout. High serum uric acid or hyperuricemia is the necessary predisposing factor for the development of gout in which a period of hyperuricemia leads to MSU crystal deposition, reaction to which can result in acute and/or chronic inflammation. Although hyperuricemia is a necessary predisposing factor, its presence does not always lead to the development of gout. Indeed, the majority of hyperuricemic patients never develop gout.

Hyperuricemia can be caused by underexcretion or overproduction of uric acid, overconsumption of purine-rich foods that are metabolized to urate, or a combination of both. Phagocytosis of MSU crystals by neutrophils plays a central role in an acute attack of gout (Lee and Terkeltaub, 2006). Macrophage phagocytosis of MSU crystals releases proinflammatory cytokines—interleukin (IL)-1, IL-6, IL-8, and tumor necrosis factor α (TNF-α)—in vitro. Increased levels of IL-6, IL-8, and TNF-α occur in gouty tissues in vivo (Cronstein and Terkeltaub, 2006; Inokuchi et al., 2006). A typical treatment for gout is divided into prompt and safe termination of the acute arthritic attack and chronic prophylaxis to prevent new attacks and decrease hyperuricemia (Terkeltaub, 2003; Lee and Terkeltaub, 2006). The three choices are nonsteroidal anti-inflammatory drugs (NSAIDs), oral or intravenous colchicines, and oral, intravenous, or intra-articular glucocorticoids. All are effective in aborting acute attacks, but they have side effects. Side effects of NSAIDs and corticosteroids are well known. Colchicine causes diarrhea, vomiting, or both in almost all patients. Intravenous colchicine does not have gastrointestinal side effects, but inappropriate use can result in serious systemic reactions, including bone marrow suppression, hepatic necrosis, renal failure, disseminated intravascular coagulation, seizures, and even death. Prophylaxis is usually considered in people with recurrent attacks or other complications related to gout. Effective treatment includes uricosuric agents (e.g., probenecid acid) and xanthine oxidase inhibitor (e.g., allopurinol). However, these treatments are associated with some rare but serious side effects such as hepatotoxicity and Stevens–Johnson syndrome (Terkeltaub, 2003).

OA is the second-most common arthritis affecting worldwide population. OA results from articular cartilage failure induced by a combination of genetic, metabolic, biochemical, and biomechanical factors. The process involves interactive degradation and repair processes of cartilage, bone, and synovium. Chondrocytes are probably the most important cells responsible for the development of the osteoarthritic process (Goldring, 2006). Human and animal studies indicate that chondrocytes exhibit numerous abnormal metabolic features as part of the OA process such as proliferative, synthetic, and degenerative activity (Yasuda, 2006). In most patients, the initiating mechanism is damage to normal articular cartilage by physical forces, which can be either single events of major trauma or repeated microtrauma. Chondrocytes react to this injury by releasing degradative enzymes and elaborating inadequate repair responses. Other factors include genetic predisposition, abnormal mechanical loading, and/or internal derangement. The chondrocytes injury leads to activation of the metalloproteinases—enzymes that are active in the degradation of cartilage and felt to be key elements in the degradation of cartilage and development of OA (Burrage et al., 2006). In addition, cytokines have an important role in the pathogenesis of OA. IL-1β and to a lesser extent IL-6 and TNF-α have been implicated in the development of OA. Conversely, insulin-like growth factor and transforming growth factor are considered to be protective, and low levels of both are seen in the sera and synovial fluids of patients with OA. The goals of management of patients with OA are to control pain and swelling and to minimize disability. There are at present no specific pharmacological therapies that can prevent the progression of joint damage due to OA. Treatment includes use of analgesics such as acetaminophen and opioids, NSAIDs, and intra-articular therapies such as glucocorticoids and hyaluronans. Postinjection flare, characterized by increased pain, swelling, and presence of an inflammatory joint effusion, is a side effect of hyaluronan joint injection in 1.5%–5% of injected knees. Although previous nonrandomized studies showed a beneficial effect of glucosamine and chondroitin in controlling symptoms of OA, a recent large randomized controlled study of combination of glucosamine and chondroitin sulfate showed that the drugs were not significantly more efficacious than placebo for pain relief or functional improvement in patients with OA of the knee (Clegg et al., 2006).

The third most common type of arthritis is RA in which 75% of the sufferers are women, suggesting the importance of hormones. Smoking and stress are thought to contribute to RA. The latter disease is characterized by joint stiffness and swelling, often in a symmetrical pattern on both sides of the body. Fatigue and a low-grade fever also may occur. The synovial membrane in patients with RA is characterized by hyperplasia, increased vascularity, and an infiltrate of inflammatory cells, primarily CD4+ T cells (Choy and Panayi, 2001). Genetic studies have shown a strong link to the major histocompatibility complex class II antigen, and recently it was shown that interaction between distinct environmental risk factors (such as smoking) in genetic contexts (e.g., the presence of HLA-DR shared epitope alleles) can trigger immune reactions (such as autoantibodies to citrullinated peptides) many years before onset of RA, and these immune reactions might contribute to clinical symptoms in a subset of affected patients (Klareskog et al., 2006a–c). Antigen-activated CD4+ T cells stimulate monocytes, macrophages, and synovial fibroblasts to produce the key proinflammatory cytokines—IL-1β, IL-6, and TNF-α, which in turn stimulate the release of matrix metalloproteinases (MMPs) (Choy and Panayi, 2001) (Figure 22.1). Activated CD4+ T cells also stimulate B cells to produce immunoglobulins, including rheumatoid factor. Activated CD4+ T cells express osteoprotegrin ligands that stimulate osteoclastogenesis. TNF-α plays a major role in joint erosion whereas IL-1β is an important contributor of cartilage erosions (manifesting as joint space narrowing). Transcription of many proinflammatory cytokines (IL-1β, IL-6, IL-8, and TNF-α) and adhesion molecules on endothelial cells are coordinated by nuclear factor κB (NF-κB) (Aupperle et al., 2001; Firestein, 2003; Firestein, 2004). NF-κB has been implicated in the pathogenesis of RA (Firestein, 2004).

The goals of management of patients with RA are to control pain and swelling, to delay disease progression, to minimize disability, and to improve quality of life (Emery et al., 1993; Emery, 2006). For pain control and swelling, the treatment includes analgesics such as acetaminophen and opioids, NSAIDs, and intra-articular therapies such as glucocorticoids. In addition, disease-modifying

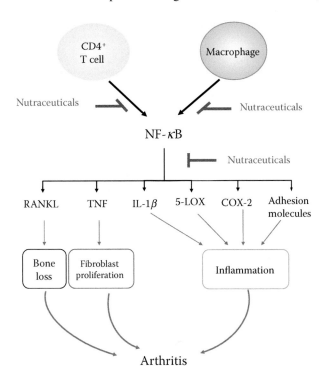

FIGURE 22.1   (See color insert.) Molecular mechanism of development of arthritis and the therapeutic targets of nutraceuticals.

antirheumatic drugs are used to modify the clinical and radiological course of RA. Examples include methotrexate, sulfasalazine, leflunomide, hydroxychloroquine, and newer therapies such as anti-TNF-α therapy (etanercept, infliximab, and adalimumab), anti-CD20 therapy (rituximab), and abatacept. These agents, either as monotherapy or combination, have markedly improved the quality of life of people with RA. However, these agents are associated with side effects, some of them serious (Khanna et al., 2004a, b).

POTENTIAL OF NATURAL AGENTS AGAINST ARTHRITIS

From the previous description, it is clear that agents that can modulate the expression of proinflammatory signals have potential against different type of arthritis. Several plants and plant nutraceuticals have been identified with anti-inflammatory activities (Table 22.1). The molecular targets of these natural agents that are relevant to arthritis are discussed in the next section.

INHIBITORS OF TNF-α EXPRESSION

There are numerous reports that TNF-α plays a major role in different types of arthritis (Darnay and Aggarwal, 1999; Aggarwal, 2000; Feldmann et al., 2004). The monoclonal antibodies against TNF-α (remicade and humira) and soluble TNF-α receptors (enbrel) have been approved for the treatment of arthritis. Macrophages are perhaps the major source of TNF-α (Aggarwal, 2003). Numerous plant-derived nutraceuticals have been identified that can suppress TNF-α expression from macrophages activated by numerous inflammatory stimuli (Table 22.2). These include curcumin, resveratrol, emodin, silymarin, and several others. Thus, these products are likely to be useful for the treatment of this autoimmune disease.

INHIBITORS OF COX-2 EXPRESSION AND ACTIVITY

That COX-2-mediated prostaglandin generation can mediate arthritic symptoms has been established (Sano et al., 1992; Siegle et al., 1998). The therapeutic potential of various "coxibs" and NSAID against arthritis is in part mediated through their ability to suppress prostaglandin E_2 production (Clemett and Goa, 2000). Numerous plant-derived products have been identified that will downregulate the expression of COX-2 and in some cases inhibit the activity of COX-2 (Table 22.3). Therefore, these agents are likely to exhibit activity against arthritis.

INHIBITORS OF 5-LOX EXPRESSION AND ACTIVITY

The conversion of arachidonic acid to leukotrienes (LTs) is catalyzed by the enzyme 5-LOX. LTs are major mediators of inflammation in numerous diseases including arthritis. At present, no 5-LOX inhibitor has been approved for arthritis. Several agents, however, have been identified in plants that can both suppress the expression of this enzyme as well as its activity (Table 22.4). For instance, curcumin can downregulate the expression of 5-LOX (Hong et al., 2004). Curcumin has been shown to suppress the activity of 5-LOX by directly binding to the active site of the enzyme (Huang et al., 1991; Skrzypczak-Jankun et al., 2003). Thus, curcumin and 5-LOX have been cocrystallized together leading to suppression of its activity (Skrzypczak-Jankun et al., 2000).

INHIBITORS OF ADHESION MOLECULES

Cell surface adhesion molecules such as ICAM-1, ELAM-1, and VCAM-1 have been linked with the development of arthritis (Littler et al., 1997). Thus, agents that can suppress the expression of these adhesion molecules or interfere with the adhesion-mediated interaction would have therapeutic potential. There are in fact plant-derived products that can suppress the expression of various adhesion molecules (Table 22.5). Thus, these agents could have therapeutic potential in arthritis.

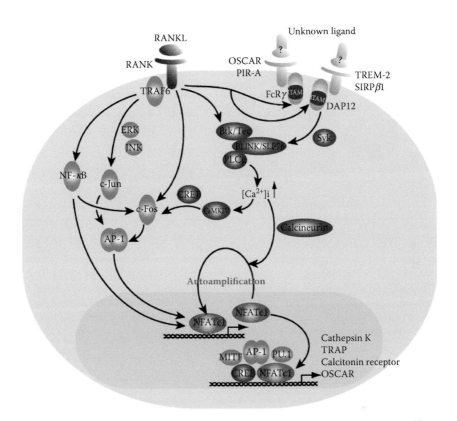

FIGURE 5.1 Signal transduction in osteoclast differentiation. RANKL–RANK binding results in the recruitment of TRAF6, which activates NF-κB and MAPKs. RANKL also stimulates the induction of c-Fos through NF-κB and CaMKIV. NF-κB and c-Fos are important for the robust induction of NFATc1. Several costimulatory receptors associate with the ITAM-harboring adaptors, FcRγ subunit, and DAP12: OSCAR and TREM-2 associate with FcRγ, and SIRPβ1 and PIR-A associate with DAP12. RANK and ITAM signaling cooperate to phosphorylate PLCγ and activate calcium signaling, which is critical for the activation and autoamplification of NFATc1. Tec family tyrosine kinases (Tec and Btk) activated by RANK are important for the formation of the osteoclastogenic signaling complex composed of Tec kinases, B-cell linker (BLNK)/SH2 domain containing leukocyte protein of 76 kDa (SLP76) (activated by ITAM-Syk), and PLCγ, which are essential for the efficient phosphorylation of PLCγ.

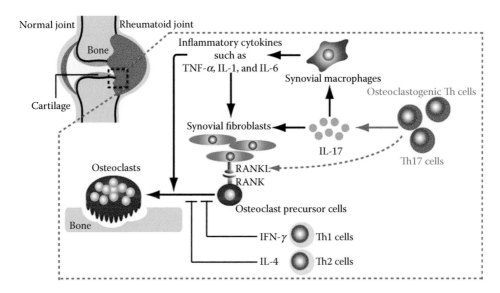

FIGURE 5.2 Regulation of osteoclast differentiation by T cells in RA, Th17 cells have stimulatory effects on osteoclastogenesis and play an important role in the pathogenesis of RA through IL-17, whereas Th1 and Th2 cells have inhibitory effects on osteoclastogenesis through IFN-γ and IL-4, respectively. IL-17 not only induces RANKL on synovial fibroblasts of mesenchymal origin but also activates local inflammation, leading to the upregulation of proinflammatory cytokines, such as TNF-α, IL-1, and IL-6. These cytokines activate osteoclastogenesis by either directly acting on osteoclast precursor cells or inducing RANKL on synovial fibroblasts. Th17 cells also express RANKL on their membrane, which partly contributes to the enhanced osteoclastogenesis.

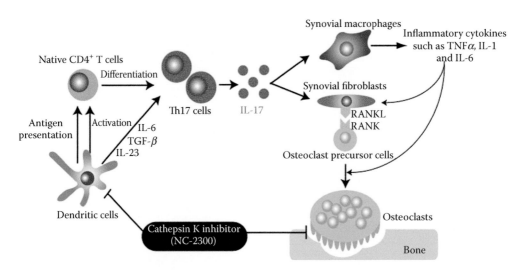

FIGURE 5.3 A cathepsin K inhibitor inhibits both Th17 development and osteoclastogenesis. Cathepsin K is involved in the TLR-9-mediated activation of dendritic cells as well as osteoclastic bone resorption. Cathepsin K inhibition results in the reduced expression of inflammatory cytokines such as IL-6 and IL-23, which are important for the induction of Th17 cells. Therefore, a cathepsin K inhibitor (NC-2300) has dual benefits in the treatment of autoimmune arthritis.

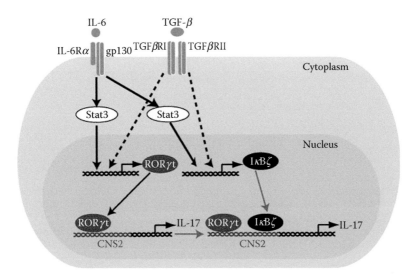

FIGURE 5.4 IκBζ and ROR nuclear receptors synergistically promote Th17 development. IL-6 and TGF-β induce Th17 cell differentiation, in which ROR nuclear receptors, RORγt and RORα, have an indispensable role. The expression of IκBζ is induced by the combination of IL-6 and TGF-β. IκBζ induction is mediated by Stat 3, but not RORγt. IκBζ and ROR nuclear receptor bind directly to the CNS2 region of the *Il17* promoter and cooperatively activate the *Il17* promoter. Notably, recruitment of IκBζ to the CNS2 region was dependent on RORγt, suggesting that the binding of both IκBζ and ROR nuclear receptors to the *Il17* promoter leads to an efficient recruitment of transcriptional coactivators with histone acetylase activity.

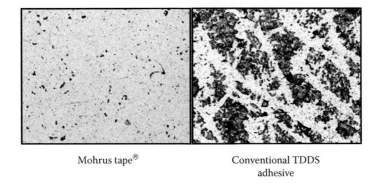

Mohrus tape®   Conventional TDDS
                adhesive

FIGURE 12.1 Optical microscope photograph of the comparison of corneocytes peeling off at patch removal. The corneocytes (stratum corneum) peeling off at patch removal were stained with dye solution (amid black), and stained corneocytes were observed with optical microscopy. (Terahara, unpublished data)

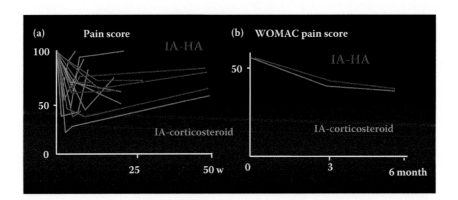

FIGURE 14.1 Effect of intra-articular HA and intra-articular corticosteroid on OA. (a) Pain source. (From Kirwan J. Is there a place for intra-articular hyaluronate in osteoarthritis of the knee? *The Knee* 2001;8:93–101.) (b) WOMAC pain source. (From Leopold SS, Redd BB, Warme WJ, Wehrle PA, Pettis PD, Shott S. Corticosteroid compared with hyaluronic acid injections for the treatment of osteoarthritis of the knee: a prospective, randomized trial. *J Bone Joint Surg. Am.* 2003;85-A:1197–1203.)

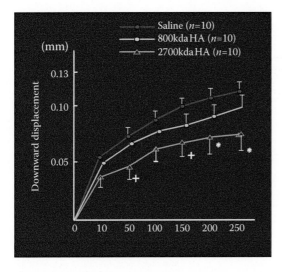

2700-KDa HA maintains a liquid film formation for significantly longer than physiological saline.

⟨Downward Displacement =
Chages in distance between cartilagesarface
& glass plate
⟨MEAN± S.E.⟩
⟨+: $p < 0.10$, *: $p < 0.05$, paired t-test⟩

FIGURE 14.4 Time course of liquid film formation of HA. (From Oka, M., Nakamura, T., and Kitsugi, T., *Nihon Riumachi Kansetsu Geka*, 12, 259–266, 1993.)

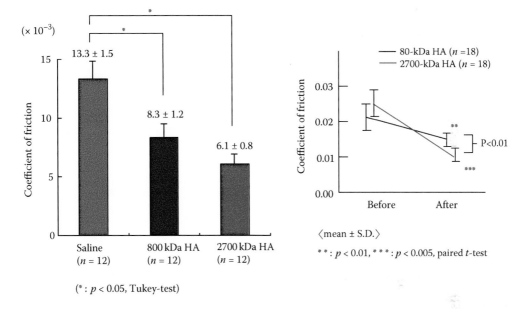

FIGURE 14.5 Boundary-lubricating effect of HA. (From Oka, M., Nakamura, T., Matsusue, Y., Akagi, M., and Horiguchi, M., *Seikei Saigai Geka*, 40, 77–84, 1997.)

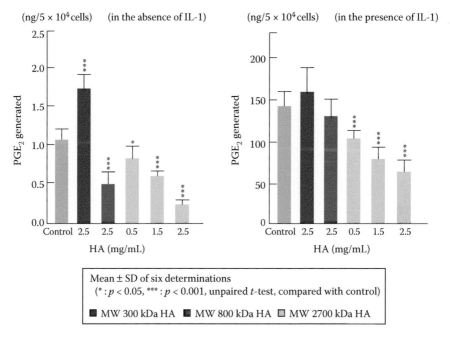

(ng/5 × 10⁴ cells)   (in the absence of IL-1)

(ng/5 × 10⁴ cells)   (in the presence of IL-1)

Mean ± SD of six determinations
($*: p < 0.05$, $***: p < 0.001$, unpaired t-test, compared with control)

■ MW 300 kDa HA   ■ MW 800 kDa HA   □ MW 2700 kDa HA

FIGURE 14.6   Effects of HA on IL-1α-induced PGE$_2$ generation by RA synovial cells. (From Tamoto, K., Nochi, H., and Tokumitsu, Y., *Jpn. J. Rheumatol.*, 5, 227–236, 1994.)

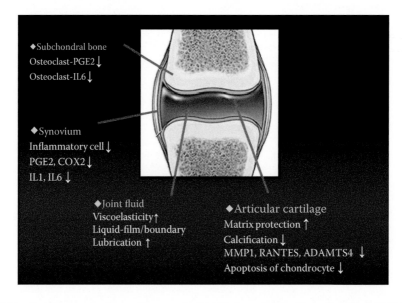

◆Subchondral bone
Osteoclast-PGE2 ↓
Osteoclast-IL6 ↓

◆Synovium
Inflammatory cell ↓
PGE2, COX2 ↓
IL1, IL6 ↓

◆Joint fluid
Viscoelasticity ↑
Liquid-film/boundary
Lubrication ↑

◆Articular cartilage
Matrix protection ↑
Calcification ↓
MMP1, RANTES, ADAMTS4 ↓
Apoptosis of chondrocyte ↓

FIGURE 14.12   Possible mechanisms of intra-articular HA for arthritis. (From Tanaka S, Fujii K, Nishioka K. Possible mechanism of intra-articular hyaluronan injections for arthritis. In "Intra-articular injection of high molecular weight hyaluronan" Medical Tribune, Tokyo, Japan 2003.)

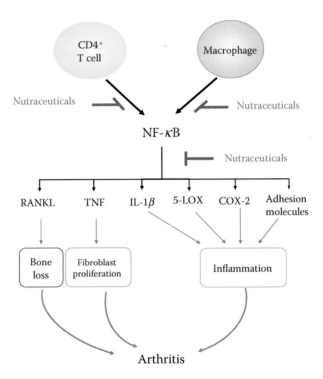

FIGURE 22.1 Molecular mechanism of development of arthritis and the therapeutic targets of nutraceuticals.

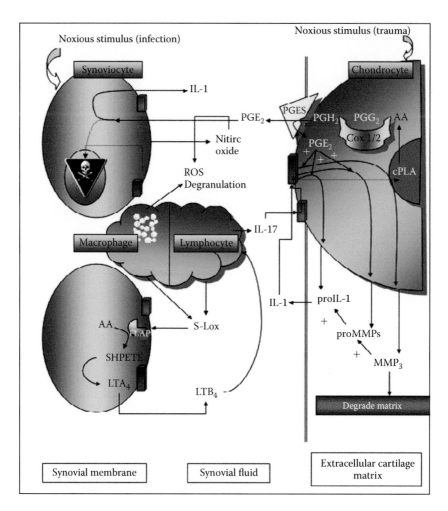

FIGURE 32.2 Cellular response to injury within the joint capsule (Pearson, 2007.) 5HPETE, 5-hydroperoxyeicosatetraenoic acid; 5-Lox, 5-lipoxygenase; AA, arachidonic acid; Cox-1/2, cyclooxygenase-1 and -2; cPLA, cytosolic phospholipase A; FLAP, 5-Lox activating protein; IL-1 and IL-17, interleukin-1 and interleukin-17; LTA$_4$ and LTB$_4$, leukotrienes A$_4$ and B$_4$; MMPs, matrix metalloproteinases; PGE$_2$, PGH$_2$, and PGG$_2$, prostaglandins E$_2$, H$_2$, and G$_2$; PGES, prostaglandin E synthase; proIL-1, pro-interleukin-1; proMMPs, promatrix metalloproteinases; ROS, reactive oxygen species.

TABLE 22.1
A List of Natural Compounds from Plants that Exhibit Anti-inflammatory Potential for Arthritis

Compounds	Source	Botanical Name
Polyphenols		
Blueberry and berry mix	Blueberry, raspberry, strawberry	*Rubus* spp., *Vaccinium* spp., *Vaccinium myrtillus*, *Fragaria ananassa*, *Solanum melongena*
Bakuchiol (drupanol)		*Psoralea corylifolia*
Bisdemethoxycurcumin		*Curcuma zedoaria*
Cannabinol		*Cannabis* spp.
Capsaicinoids (includes capsaicin and its analogs)	Pepper, red chili	*Capsicum* spp., *Euphorbia* spp., *Capsicum annum*
Carnosol	Rosemary	*Rosmarinus officinalis*
Cistifolin	Gravel root	*Eupatorium purpureum*
Curcumin	Turmeric, curry powder	*Curcuma longa*
Catechin and theaflavins (including (–)-epicatechin 3-epicatechin-3-gallate, epigallocatechin gallate)	Green and black teas, berries, spotted knapweed, shea, cocoa	*Centarea maculosa* Lam, *Vitellaria paradoxa*, *Theobroma cacao*, *Polygonum cuspidatum*, *Camellia sinensis*
Ellagic acid	Avocado, red berries, grapes	*Perxea americana* P. mill, *Physalis polygonum*
	Strawberries, raspberries	*Cuspidatum* root, *Fragaria ananassa*
Emodin	Aloe	*Aloe vera*, *Cassia obtusifolia*, *Polygonum emodin*
Ethyl gallate	Grapes, tea, red maple	*Paeonia* spp., *Sophora japonica*, *Vitis vinifera*
Eutigosides B and C		*Eurya emarginata*
Gallic acid	Guava	*Psidium guajava* L., *Erodium glaucophyllum*
Genistein	Soybeans, chickpea, kudzu root	*Pueraria labata radix*, *Cicer arietinum*, *Glycine max*
Gingerol	Ginger	*Zingiber officinale* Roscoe
Morellin	Indica fruit	*Garcinia purpurea*, *Garcinia hanburyi*
Purpurogallin	Black tea	*Piper nigrum*, *Quercus* sp.
Rocaglamides		*Aglaia* spp.
Rosemarinic acid	Rosemary, sage	*R. officinalis*, *Saliva officinalis*
Sanggenon C	Mulberry	*Morus* spp.
Silymarin (including silybin, silibinin, silidian, and silychrist)	Milk thistle, artichokes, wild artichokes	*Cynara scolymus*, *Silybum marianum*
Yakuchinones A and B		*Alpinia oxyphylla*
Terpenes		
Aethiopinone	Mediterranean sage, Lamiaceae	*Salvia aethiopis* L.
Anethol and analogs (Eugenol, bis-eugenol, isoeugenol, anetholdithiolthione)	Broccoli, anise, cloves, cashew	*Brassica oleracea italica*, *Illicum verum*, *Syzygium aromaticum*, *Oscimum sanctum*
Atractylon	Chamomile	*Atractylodes lancea*
Artemisinin ext. (Qinghaosu)		*Artemisia annua*
Avicins (including avicins D and G)		*Acasia victoriae*
Azadirachtin	Neem tree	*Azadirachta indica*
Betulinic acid	Birch tree, almond hulls	*Betula* spp. Quisqualis Fructus, *Coussarea paniculata*
β-Carotene	Carrot, citrus fruits, pumpkin	*Daucus carota sativus*, *Citrus unshiu mar*

continued

TABLE 22.1 (continued)
A List of Natural Compounds from Plants that Exhibit Anti-inflammatory Potential for Arthritis

Compounds	Source	Botanical Name
Celastrol		*Tripterygium wilfordii*
β-Cryptoxanthin	Orange, berries	*Carcica papaya*
Dammarane		*Bruguiera gymnorrhiza*
Ginkgo biloba extract		*Gingko biloba*
Glycyrrhizin	Licorice root	*Glycyrrhiza glabra, Glycyrrhizae radix*
Hypoestoxide		*Hypoestes rosea*
Limonene	Lemon, sweet orange, grapefruit	*Citrus limon, Citrus paradisi, Citrus aurantium*
Lutein	Tomato	*Lycopersicon esculentum*
Lycopene	Tomato	*L. esculentum*
3-Oxo-tirucallic acid	Indian olibanum tree	*Boswellia serrata*
Parthenolide	Feverfew	*Tanacetum parthenium, Michelia champaca*
Petasin and isopetasin	Butterbur	*Petasites hybridus*
Ursolic acid	Basil, salvia, rosemary, berries	*R. officinalis, Ocimum sanctum*
Withanolides		*Withania sominifera*
Alkaloids		
Aquifoline	Berberis	*Mahonia aquifolium*
Berbamine	Berberis	*M. aquifolium*
Conophylline		*Tabernaemontana* spp., *Ervatamia microphylla*
Cucurbitacin	Watermelon, cucumber	*Cucurbita andreana, Trichosanthes kirilowii*
Evodiamine	Goshuyu	*Evodiae fructus, Evodia rutaecarpa*
Higenamine	Lianas	*Aconitum japonicum, Argemone mexicana*
Mahanimbine	Rutaceous	*Murraya koenigii, Clausena dunniana*
Morphine and its analogs		*Rapaver* spp., *Opium poppy*
Piperine	Black pepper	*Garcinia xanthochymu, Piper longum*
Flavonoids		
Apigenin	Plant seeds and vegetables	*Scutellaria* spp., *Cirisium* spp.
2′,8″Biapigenin		*Selaginella tamariscina*
Baicalein and its derivatives (including baicalein, wogonin, and 6-methoxy-baicalein)	Skullcap	*Scutellaria* spp., *Scutellaria lateriflora* L.
Quercetin	Onions, apples, black and green tea	*Allium cepa, C. sinensis*
Cirsimaritin	Basil, sage, rosemary	*O. sanctum, Salvia officinalis*
Eupatilin, 4-demethyleupatilin		*Seriphidium terrae-albae, Artemisia asiatica Nakai*
Flavopiridol		*Dysoxylum binectariferum*
Ginkgetin		*G. biloba*
Hesperidine	Oranges	*C. sinensis* O. Ktze
Kaempferol	Grapefruit	*C. paradisi, Delphinium* spp.
Luteolin	Tea, fruits, and vegetables	*Scutellaria* spp.
Morin	Almond	*P. guajava* L., *Prunus dulcis* (Mill.)
Nobiletin	Citrus fruits	*C. unshiu marc*
Ochnaflavone	Japanese honeysuckle flower	*Lonicera japonica*
Pycnogenol	Citrus fruits	*Citrus retirulata, Pinus maritime*
Persenone A	Tomato, avocado	*L. esculentum, Persea americana* P. Mil
Rhamnetin	Soybeans	*G. max*
Sophoraflavanone G		*Sophora flavescen*

TABLE 22.1 (continued)
A List of Natural Compounds from Plants that Exhibit Anti-inflammatory Potential for Arthritis

Compounds	Source	Botanical Name
Chalcones		
Butein		*Semecarpus anacardium*
Cardamomin	Cardamom	*Alpinia conchigera Griff*
Others		
1′Acetoxychavicol acetate,		*Languas galanga, Alpinia galanga*
1′S-1′-Acetoxyeugenol acetate		
Aesculetin	Lavender	*Santolina oblongifolia*
Ajoene	Garlic	*Allium sativum*
Alkenyl-1,4-benzoquinones (ardisianones A, B, ardisiaquinone A and maesanin)	Marlberry, Myrsinaceae	*Ardisia japonica, Ardisia sieboldii*
Allicin (allyl-thiosulfinate)	Garlic	*A. sativum*
Allixin (phytoalexin)	Garlic	*A. sativum* Linn.
Aucubin (iridoid glycoside)	Algae	*Eucommia* spp., *Veronica* spp., *Globularia* spp.
Bergamottin	Grape	*Citrus paradis*
Calagualine (saponin)		*Polypodium* spp.
Cirsilineol	Holy Basil	*O. sanctum, Lantana montevidensis* Briq
CAPE (caffeic acid phenethyl ester)	Honey bee propolis	*Apis mellifera capensis*
Deguelin		*Mundulea sericea*
Deoxyelephantopin (ESD)		*Elephantopus scaber* Linn.
Diallyl sulfide	Garlic, Chinese leek	*A. sativum*
Diphenyl dimethyl bicarboxylate		*Fructus schizandrae*
Embelin		*Embelin ribes*
2,6-Dihydroxy-1,7-dimethoxyxanthone, 3,4-Dihydroxyxanthone		*Calophyllum membranaceum*
Falcarindiol	Apiacea	*Angelica pubescens f. biserrata*
Flavokavine	Kava kava	*Piper methysticum*
Furocoumarins (imperatorin, isoimperatorin and prantschimgin)		*Cachrys trifida*
F022		*Radix isatidis*
Garcinol and its analog (polyisoprenylated benzophenone)	Indica fruit, African plant	*A. sativum* Linn., *Garcinia huillensis*, *G. purpurea*
Ginkgolide B		*G. biloba*
Harpagoside		*Harpagophytum procumbens*
Honokiol	Magnolia	*Magnolia officinalis*
Humulone		*Humulus lupulus*
7β-Hydroxystigmast-4-en-3-one		*Arbutus unedo*
Hyperforin	St. John's wort	*Hypericum perforatum*
Imperatorin		*C. trifida, Citrus maxima*
Indirubin		*Polygonum tinctorium, Isatis indigotica, Isatis tinctoria*
Indole-3-carbinol	Onions, cabbage	*A. cepa, B. oleracea capita, Brassica*
Isodeoxyelephantopin (ESI)	Asteraceae	*E. scaber* Linn.
Isothymonin	Holy Basil	*O. sanctum*

continued

TABLE 22.1 (continued)
A List of Natural Compounds from Plants that Exhibit Anti-inflammatory Potential for Arthritis

Compounds	Source	Botanical Name
Lanceolitols		*Solanum lanceolatum*
Lapachone (benzo[a]phenazine)	Indian ginseng, lapacha tree	*Tabebuia avellanedae, Tabebuia heptaphylla*
Linoliec acid		*A. pubescens f. biserrata*
α-Lipoic acid	Asparagus, wheat, potato	
Magnonol	Magnolia	*Magnolia obovata* Thunb
5-Methylflavasperone		*Guiera senegalensis*
Neolignans and lignans		*Coptis japonica*
Osthol	Chamomile, Apiaceae	*A. lancea, A. pubescens f. biserrata*
Osthenol		*A. pubescens f. biserrata*
Patridoids I, II, and IIA		*Patrinia saniculaefolia*
Phthalide lactone (Z-ligustilide and senkyunolide A)		*Ligusticum chuanxiong*
Phloroglucinol		*Mallotus japonicus*
Platycodin D and D3		*Platycodon grandiflorum*
Plumbagin (naphthoquinone)		*Plumbago zeylanica*
Pterostilbene		*Pterocarpus marsupium*
Phytylplastoquinone and plastoquinone 7		*Aframomum danielli* K. Schum
Racemosic acid		*Ficus racemosa* L.
Resveratrol and analogs (stilbene)	Grapes, cranberries, etc.	*P. cuspidatum, Veratrum* spp.
Rotenone (benzopyranone)		*Derris* spp.
Saikosaponin		*Bupleurum* spp., *Heteromorpha* spp.
Sedanolide		*Apium graveolens*
Sequiterpene lactones		*T. parthenium*
14,15-Secopregnane derivatives (argelosides K-O (1–5))		*Solenostemma argel*
Sibyllenone		*Ocotea bullata*
Sulphoraphane (glucosinolate)	Broccoli, cauliflower	*B. oleracea italica*
Delta(9)-tetrahydrocanabinoid acid		*Cannabis sativa*
Thymoquinone	Black cumin	*Nigella sativa*
2,4,5-Trimethoxybenzaldehyde		*Daucus carota*
Wedelolactone	false daisy	*Eclipta alba*
Zaluzanin-C and estafiatone		*Ainsliaea*
Zerumbone		*Zingiber zerumbet* Smith

INHIBITORS OF NF-κB ACTIVATION

Whether inflammatory cytokines such as TNF-α, COX-2, 5-LOX, or adhesion molecules, they are all regulated by the transcription factor NF-κB (Aggarwal, 2004). In addition, MMP, also linked with arthritis, is also regulated by NF-κB activation. Moreover, constitutively active NF-κB has been identified in the synovial tissue (Miagkov et al., 1998; Tak and Firestein, 2001). Thus, inhibitors of NF-κB activation are likely to have a potential in the treatment of arthritis. Our laboratory has shown that even some of the currently approved agents against arthritis, such as methotrexate, leflunomide, thalidomide, and celecoxib, suppress NF-κB activation (Manna et al., 2000a; Majumdar and Aggarwal, 2001; Majumdar et al., 2002). Numerous agents from plants have been identified that can suppress NF-κB activation (Table 22.6). Thus, these plant-derived products should be tested for the treatment of arthritis.

TABLE 22.2
A List of Natural Products that Inhibit the Expression of TNF-α

1′-Acetoxychavicol acetate and 1s′-1-acetoxyeugenol acetate (AEA) inhibits lipopolysaccharide (LPS), cytokine, and amyloid Abeta peptide–induced TNF-α expression in THP-1 cell line and antigen–immunoglobulin E antibody-induced TNF-α in RBL-2H3 cells in mice (Matsuda et al., 2003; Grzanna et al., 2004)

Allium sativum inhibits LPS-stimulated TNF-α expression in human placental explants (Makris et al., 2005)

Aloe vera inhibits burn-induced TNF-α expression in rats (Duansak et al., 2003)

Aloe barbadensis inhibits UVB irradiation-induced TNF-α expression in KB cells (Qiu et al., 2000)

Asparagus cochinchinensis inhibits LPS-induced TNF-α expression in primary cultures of mouse astrocytes (Kim et al., 1998a)

Bisdemethoxycurcumin inhibits antigen–immunoglobulin E-induced TNF-α expression in RBL-2H3 cells (Matsuda et al., 2004)

Butein inhibits LPS-induced TNF-α expression in Raw 264.7 cells (Lee et al., 2004)

Cardamomin inhibits LPS-induced TNF-α expression in RAW 264.7 cells (Lee J.H. et al., 2006)

Curcumin inhibits LPS-induced TNF-α expression in Mono Mac 6 cells and in MCL cells (Chan, 1995; Shishodia et al., 2005)

Diphenyl dimethyl bicarboxylate inhibits concanavalin A–induced TNF-α expression in mice (Gao et al., 2005)

Emodin inhibits IL-1-β- and IL-6-induced TNF-α expression in human mesangial cells (Kuo et al., 2001)

Epigallocatechin gallate inhibits bacterial infection-induced TNF-α expression in MH-S cells (Matsunaga et al., 2002)

F022 inhibits LPS-induced TNF-α in murine peritoneal macrophages (Lin et al., 2002)

Ginkgolide B inhibits LPS-induced TNF-α production in mouse peritoneal macrophages and in RAW 264.7 cells (Wadsworth et al., 2001; Nie et al., 2004)

2′-Hydroxychalcone inhibits LPS-induced TNF-α expression in mouse macrophage RAW 264.7 cells (Ban et al., 2004; Abuarqoub et al., 2006)

Hypoestoxide inhibits LPS-induced TNF-α expression in normal human peripheral blood mononuclear cells (Ojo-Amaize et al., 2001)

Inula britannica inhibits LPS-induced TNF-α expression in RAW 264.7 cells (Jin et al., 2006)

Lonicera japonica inhibits trypsin-induced TNF-α expression HMC-1 (Kang et al., 2004)

Neolignans and lignans inhibit LPS-induced TNF-α expression in RAW 264.7 cells (Cho et al., 1998)

Patridoids I, II, and IIA inhibit LPS-induced TNF-α expression in RAW 264.7 cells (Ju et al., 2003)

Phthalide lactone inhibits LPS-induced TNF-α expression in monocytes (Liu et al., 2005)

Phloroglucinol derivatives inhibit LPS-induced TNF-α expression in RAW 264.7 cells (Ishii et al., 2003)

Platycodin D and D3 inhibit LPS- and rIFN-γ-induced TNF-α expression in RAW 264.7 cells (Wang et al., 2004)

Phlebodium decumanum inhibits LPS- and IFN-γ-induced TNF-α expression in peripheral blood mononuclear cells (Punzon et al., 2003)

Phyllanthus amarus inhibits LPS-induced TNF-α expression in RAW 264.7 cells (Kiemer et al., 2003)

Polygala tenuifolia inhibits LPS-induced TNF-α expression in primary cultures of mouse astrocytes (Kim et al., 1998b)

Resveratrol inhibits LPS-induced TNF-α expression in microglia (Bi et al., 2005)

14,15-Secopregnane derivatives argelosides K-O (1–5) inhibit LPS-induced TNF-α expression in RAW 264.7 cells (Perrone et al., 2006)

Silymarin inhibits 12-O-tetradecanoyl phorbol-13 (TPA) and OA-induced TNF-α expression in mouse epidermis (Zi et al., 1997)

Tanacetum microphyllum in LPS-induced TNF-α expression mouse peritoneal macrophages (Abad et al., 2001)

Taraxacum officinale inhibits LPS-induced TNF-α expression in rat astrocytes (H.M. Kim et al., 2000)

Delta(9)-tetrahydrocanabinoid acid inhibits LPS-induced TNF-α expression in U937 macrophages and peripheral blood macrophages (Verhoeckx et al., 2006)

Theobroma cacao inhibits LPS- and IFN-γ-induced TNF-α expression in RAW 264.7 and NR8383 cells (Ramiro et al., 2005)

Uncaria guianensis inhibits LPS-induced TNF-α expression in RAW 264.7 cells (Piscoya et al., 2001)

Yakuchinone A and B inhibit TPA-induced TNF-α expression in mouse skin (Chun et al., 2002)

Zingiber officinale inhibits LPS-, cytokine-, and amyloid Abeta peptide–induced TNF-α expression in THP-1 cells (Grzanna et al., 2004)

Zostera japonica inhibits LPS-induced TNF-α expression in J774A.1 murine macrophages (Hua et al., 2006)

TABLE 22.3
A List of Natural Products that Inhibit Expression and/or Activity of COX-2

Expression

Curcumin suppresses smokeless tobacco-induced COX-2 expression in human oral premalignant and cancer cells (Sharma et al., 2006)

Cardamomin suppresses lipopolysaccharide (LPS)-induced COX-2 expression in RAW 264.7 cells (Lee J.H. et al., 2006)

Eugenol suppresses LPS-induced COX-2 expression in RAW 264.7 cells (Li et al., 2006)

Genistein suppresses PMA-induced COX-2 expression in MCF-7 cells (Lau and Leung, 2006)

Khaya senegalensis bark extract (KSBE) suppressed COX-2 expression in human colorectal cancer (Androulakis et al., 2006)

Ochnaflavone suppresses COX-2 expression in mouse bone marrow-derived mast cells (Son et al., 2006)

Terpene and bioflavonoid suppress LPS-induced COX-2 expression in RAW 264.7 cells (Park et al., 2006)

2′,8″-Biapigenin suppresses LPS-induced COX-2 expression in RAW 264.7 cells (Woo et al., 2006)

Eutigosides B and C suppress COX-2 expression RAW 264.7 cells (Park et al., 2005)

Ginkgetin suppresses COX-2 expression in mouse bone marrow-derived mast cells (Son et al., 2005)

Zaluzanin-C and estafiatone suppress LPS-induced COX-2 expression in RAW 264.7 cells (Shin et al., 2005)

Harpagoside suppresses LPS-induced COX-2 expression in RAW 264.7 and HepG2 cells (Huang et al., 2006)

Petasin and isopetasin suppress COX-2 expression in rat primary microglial cells (Fiebich et al., 2005)

Luteolin, luteolin-7-*O*-glucoside, suppresses LPS-induced COX-2 expression in mouse macrophage RAW264.7 cells (Hu and Kitts, 2004)

Methanolic extract suppresses COX-2 expression in human lung cancer cells (Hung and Chang, 2003)

Ursolic acid suppresses TNF-induced COX-2 expression in leukemic cell line Jurkat (Shishodia et al., 2003)

Evodiamine, rutraecarpin, suppresses TNF-induced and LPS-induced COX-2 expression in KBM-5 (human myeloid leukemia) and RAW 264.7 cells (Moon et al., 1999; Takada et al., 2005b; Choi et al., 2006; Lau and Leung, 2006)

Activity

2,4,5-Trimethoxybenzaldehyde (Momin et al., 2003)

Sedanolide (Momin and Nair, 2002)

Pterostilbene inhibits COX-2 activity *in vivo* (Hougee et al., 2005)

Cirsilineol, cirsimaritin, isothymusin, isothymonin, apigenin, rosmarinic acid (Kelm et al., 2000)

7β-Hydroxystigmast-4-en-3-one (Carcache-Blanco et al., 2006)

Dammarane, triterpenes, inhibits COX-2 activity in HepG2 cells (Homhual et al., 2006)

2,6-Dihydroxy-1,7-dimethoxyxanthone (1) and 3,4-dihydroxyxanthone (Zou et al., 2005)

Lanceolitols inhibits COX-2 activity induced by12-*O*-tetradecanoylphorbol-13-acetate (TPA) in mice (Herrera-Salgado et al., 2005)

Kaempferol (Francis et al., 2004)

(2R,3R)-5′-Methoxyguayarol (Jang et al., 2004)

Racemosic acid (Li et al., 2004)

Cerebrosides (Kang et al., 2001)

Butein (Selvam et al., 2004)

PRECLINICAL AND CLINICAL STUDIES OF NATURAL PRODUCTS AGAINST ARTHRITIS

Numerous agents that are derived from plants have been shown to suppress arthritis in rodent models. These include curcumin, guggulsterone, boswellic acid, withanolides, shogaol, and others. For instance, curcumin has been shown to suppress numerous phases of the development of arthritis. Oral administration of curcumin has been shown to decrease the levels of Gp A72, with concomitant lowering of paw inflammation in arthritic rats (Joe et al., 1997). Neutral matrix MMPs are responsible for the pathological features of RA such as degradation of cartilage, and the messenger RNA upregulation of MMPs was also inhibited by curcumin (Onodera et al., 2000). Curcumin synergistically potentiates

TABLE 22.4
A List of Natural Compounds that Inhibit Activity and/or Expression of 5-Lipoxygenase

Activity

Acetyl-11-keto-β-boswellic acid inhibits LTB4 production in A23187 stimulated rat peritoneal PMNL (Park et al., 2002)

Aesculetin inhibits 5-HETE production in A23187 stimulated mouse peritoneal macrophages (Silvan et al., 1996)

Aethiopinone inhibits LTB4 production in A23187 stimulated human PMNL (Benrezzouk et al., 2001)

Ajoene inhibits 5-HETE production in A23187 stimulated porcine leukocytes (Sendl et al., 1992)

Allicin inhibits 5-HETE production in A23187 stimulated porcine leukocytes (Sendl et al., 1992)

Aquifoline inhibits *in vitro* 5-LOX activity from sunflower seedlings (Bezakova et al., 1996)

Ardisianone A and B inhibit 5-LOX activity from guinea pig peritoneal PMNL (Fukuyama et al., 1993)

Ardisiaquinone A inhibits 5-LOX activity from guinea pig peritoneal PMNL (Fukuyama et al., 1994)

Atractylon inhibits 5-HETE production in porcine leukocytes stimulated by A23187 (Resch et al., 1998)

Berbamine inhibits *in vitro* 5-LOX activity from sunflower seedlings (Bezakova et al., 1996)

Caffeic acid inhibits 5-LOX activity in cultured mastocytoma cells (Koshihara et al., 1983)

Capsaicin inhibits 5-HETE production in human PMNL (Prasad et al., 2004)

Curcumin inhibits LTB4 production in A23187 stimulated rat peritoneal PMNL (Ammon et al., 1993)

4-Demethyleupatilin and eupatilin inhibits 5-LOX activity in cultured mastocytoma cells (Koshihara et al., 1983)

EGCG, EGC, ECG, and theaflavin inhibit 5-, 12-, and 15-HETE production by human 5-LOX from colonic mucosa (Hong et al., 2001)

Eugenol inhibits 5-HETE production in human PMNL (Prasad et al., 2004)

Falcarindiol inhibits 5-HETE production in A23187 stimulated porcine leukocytes (Liu et al., 1998)

[6]-Gingerol inhibits 5-HETE production in RBL-1 cells (Kiuchi et al., 1992)

Hyperforin inhibits LTB4 using A23187 stimulated human PMNL (Albert et al., 2002)

Imperatorin and isoimperatorin inhibit 5-HETE production in porcine leukocytes stimulated by A23187 (Abad et al., 2001)

Linoleic acid inhibits 5-HETE production in porcine leukocytes stimulated by A23187 (Liu et al., 1998)

Magnolol inhibits LTC4 production in RBL-2H3 (Hamasaki et al., 1997)

Maesanin inhibits 5-HETE production in A23187 stimulated porcine leukocytes (Fukuyama et al., 1993)

5-Methylflavasperone inhibits LTB4 and 5-HETE productions A23187 stimulated porcine leukocyte (Bucar et al., 1998)

Osthol and osthenol inhibit 5-HETE production in A23187 stimulated porcine leukocytes (Liu et al., 1998)

3-Oxo-tirucallic acid inhibits 5-HETE production in A23187 stimulated human PMNL (Boden et al., 2001)

Parthenolide inhibits LTB4 production in A23187 stimulated rat peritoneal PMNL (Sumner et al., 1992)

Phytylplastoquinone and plastoquinone 7 inhibit soybean 5-LOX activity using *in vitro* assay system (Odukoya et al., 1999)

Piperine inhibits 5-HETE production in human PMNL (Prasad et al., 2004)

Resveratrol inhibits 5-LOX activity in human PMNL stimulated by A23187 (Kimura et al., 1995)

Rhamnetin inhibits LTB4 and 5-HETE productions in A23187 stimulated porcine leukocyte (Bucar et al., 1998)

Saikosaponin inhibits LTC4 production in A23187 stimulated mouse peritoneal macrophages (Bermejo Benito et al., 1998)

Sanguinarine inhibits 5-HETE and LTB4 production in A23187 stimulated bovine PMNL (Verhoeckx et al., 2006)

Sibyllenone inhibits 5-HETE production in A23187 stimulated porcine leukocytes (Zschocke et al., 2000)

Thymoquinone inhibits 5-HETE production in A23187 stimulated rat peritoneal PMNL (El Gazzar et al., 2006)

Welelolactone inhibits 5-LOX activity in porcine leukocyte stimulated by A23187 (Wagner and Fessler, 1986)

Expression

Curcumin suppresses 5-LOX protein level in LPS-stimulated RAW 264.7 cells (Hong et al., 2004)

TABLE 22.5
A List of Natural Products that Suppress the Expression of Adhesion Molecules

1′-Acetoxychavicol acetate inhibits TNF-α-induced expression of ICAM-1 in human myeloid leukemia (Ichikawa et al., 2005)

Andrographolide inhibits the expression of E-selectin and VCAM-1 in the mouse model of OVA-induced allergic lung inflammation (Xia et al., 2004)

Baicalein inhibits IL-1β- and TNF-α-induced expression of ICAM-1 and ELAM-1 in HUVEC cells (Kimura et al., 1995)

Bergamottin and DHB inhibit TNF-α-induced expression of MAdCAM-1 and ECAMs in murine small vessel endothelial cells (Sasaki et al., 2004)

Carnosol inhibits the expression of E-cadherin in the C57BL/6J/Min/+ (Min/+) mouse (Moran et al., 2005)

Cistifolin inhibits carrageenan-induced expression of β_1, β_2 integrin in rat paw (Habtemariam, 1998)

Curcumin inhibits TNF-α-induced expression of ICAM-1, VCAM-1, and ELAM-1 in HUVEC cells (Kumar et al., 1998)

Emodin inhibits TNF-α-induced expression of ICAM-1, VCAM-1, and ELAM-1 in HUVEC cells (Kumar et al., 1998)

Evodiamine inhibits TNF-α-induced expression of ICAM-1 in Human myeloid leukemia (Takada et al., 2005b)

Honokiol inhibits TNF-α-induced expression of ICAM-1 in Human lung adenocarcinoma (Ahn et al., 2006)

Parthenolide inhibits IL-4-induced expression of VCAM-1 in HUVEC cells (Schnyder et al., 2002)

Sequiterpene lactones inhibit TNF-α-induced expression of ICAM-1 in human T-cell lymphoma (Hehner et al., 1998)

Soy isoflavones inhibit the expression of ICAM-1, VCAM-1, E-selectin, and P-selectin in healthy postmenopausal women (Colacurci et al., 2005)

Withanolides inhibits TNF-α-induced expression of ICAM-1 in human myeloid leukemia (Ichikawa et al., 2006b)

TABLE 22.6
A List of Natural Compounds that Inhibit NF-κB and Their Mechanism(s) of Action

Inhibitors IκBα degradation

- Amentoflavone suppresses TNF-induced IκBα degradation in A549 cells (Banerjee et al., 2002)
- Aucubin suppresses TNF-induced IκBα degradation in RBL-2H3 mast cells (Jeong et al., 2002)
- Beta-lapachone suppresses TNF-induced IκBα degradation in human myeloid U937 cells (Manna et al., 1999a)
- Blackberry extract suppresses lipopolysaccharide (LPS)-induced IκBα degradation in mouse macrophage J774 cells (Pergola et al., 2006)
- Benzyl isothiocyanate suppresses increased protein expression of IκBα in BxPC-3 cells (Srivastava and Singh, 2004)
- Capsaicin suppresses TNF-induced IκBα degradation in human myeloid ML-1a cells (Singh et al., 1996)
- Emodin suppresses TNF-induced IκBα degradation in human umbilical vein endothelial cells (Kumar et al., 1998)
- Ergolide suppresses LPS-induced IκBα degradation in mouse macrophage RAW 264.7 cells (Whan Han et al., 2001)
- Genistein suppresses TNF-induced IκBα degradation in human myeloid U937 cells (Natarajan et al., 1998)
- Glabridin suppresses LPS-induced IκBα degradation in RAW 264.7 cells (Kang et al., 2005)
- Isomallotochromanol and isomallotochromene suppress LPS-induced IκBα degradation in RAW 264.7 cells (Ishii et al., 2003)
- Nobiletin suppresses LPS and interferon-γ-induced IκBα degradation in RAW 264.7 cells (Murakami et al., 2003)
- Platycodon saponins suppresses LPS-induced IκBα degradation in RAW 264.7 cells (Ahn et al., 2005)
- Quercitrin gallate suppresses LPS-induced IκBα degradation in RAW 264.7 cells (Kim B.H. et al., 2005)

Inhibitors of IκBα phosphorylation

- Anethole suppresses TNF-induced IκBα phosphorylation in human myeloid ML-1a cells (Chainy et al., 2000)
- *Artemisia vestita* suppresses LPS-induced IκBα phosphorylation in mouse macrophage RAW 264.7 cells (Sun et al., 2006)
- Baicalein suppresses constitutive IκBα phosphorylation in multiple myeloma U266 cells (Ma et al., 2005)
- Black raspberry suppresses benzo[a]pyrene diol epoxide–induced IκBαphosphorylation in mouse epidermal JB6 Cl 41 cells (Huang et al., 2002)

TABLE 22.6 (continued)
A List of Natural Compounds that Inhibit NF-κB and Their Mechanism(s) of Action

- Calagualine suppresses TNF-induced IκBα phosphorylation in human myeloid U937 cells (Manna et al., 2003)
- [6]-Gingerol suppresses TPA-induced phosphorylation of IκBα in mouse skin (Kim S.O. et al., 2005)
- *Glossogyne tenuifolia* suppresses LPS-induced IκBα phosphorylation in RAW 264.7 cells (Wu et al., 2004)
- Decursin suppresses LPS-induced IκBα phosphorylation in THP-1 cells (Kim J.H. et al., 2006)
- Licorice extracts suppress LPS-induced IκBα phosphorylation in RAW 264.7 cells (Kim J.K. et al., 2006)
- Lupeol suppresses TPA-induced IκBα phosphorylation in skin of CD1 mice (Saleem et al., 2004)
- Oleandrin suppresses TNF-induced IκBα phosphorylation in U937 cells (Manna et al., 2000c)
- Panduratin suppresses LPS-induced IκBα phosphorylation in RAW 264.7 cells (Yun et al., 2003)
- Phytic acid suppresses TNF-induced IκBα phosphorylation in HeLa cells (Ferry et al., 2002)
- Sanguinarine suppresses TNF-induced IκBα phosphorylation in human myeloid ML-1a cells (Chaturvedi et al., 1997)
- Resveratrol suppresses TNF-induced IκBα phosphorylation in U937 cells (Manna et al., 2000b)
- Silymarin suppresses TNF-induced IκBα phosphorylation in U937 cells (Manna et al., 1999b)

Inhibitors of activation/phosphorylation of IκBα kinase (IKK)

- Acetyl-boswellic acid suppresses TNF-induced IκBα kinase activation in myeloid leukemia KBM-5 cells (Takada et al., 2006)
- 1'-Acetoxychavicol acetate suppresses TNF-induced IκBα kinase activation in KBM-5 cells (Ichikawa et al., 2005)
- Anacardic acid suppresses TAK1-mediated IκBα kinase activation in KBM-5 cells (Sung et al., 2008a)
- Asaxanthin suppresses LPS-induced IκBα kinase activation in mouse macrophage RAW 264.7 cells (Lee et al., 2003)
- Berberine suppresses TNF-induced IκBα kinase activation in KBM-5 cells (Pandey et al., 2008)
- Betulinic acid suppresses TNF-induced IκBα kinase activation in epithelial HCT 116 cells (Takada and Aggarwal, 2003)
- Butein suppresses TNF-induced IκBα kinase activation in KBM-5 cells (Pandey et al., 2007a)
- Coronarin D suppresses TNF-induced IκBα kinase activation in KBM-5 cells (Kunnumakkara et al., 2008)
- Deguelin suppresses TNF-induced IκBα kinase activation in KBM-5 cells (Nair et al., 2006)
- 3,4-Dihydroxybenzalacetone suppresses TNF-induced IκBα kinase activation in KBM-5 cells (Sung et al., 2008b)
- Diosgenin suppresses TNF-induced IκBα kinase activation in KBM-5 cells (Shishodia and Aggarwal, 2006)
- Embelin suppresses TNF-induced IκBα kinase activation in KBM-5 cells (Ahn et al., 2007a)
- Escin suppresses TNF-induced IκBα kinase activation in KBM-5 cells (Harikumar et al., 2010a)
- Evodamine suppresses TNF-induced IκBα kinase activation in KBM-5 cells (Takada et al., 2005b)
- Fisetin suppresses TAK1- and RIP-mediated IκBα kinase activation in H1299 cells (Sung et al., 2007)
- Flavopiridol suppresses TNF-induced IκBα kinase activation in KBM-5 cells (Takada and Aggarwal, 2004)
- Gambogic acid suppresses TAK1-mediated IκBα kinase activation in KBM-5 cells (Pandey et al., 2007a)
- Gossypin suppresses TNF-induced IκBα kinase activation in KBM-5 cells (Kunnumakkara et al., 2007)
- Guggulsterone suppresses TNF-induced IκBα kinase activation in nonsmall cell lung adenocarcinoma H1299 cells (Shishodia and Aggarwal, 2004)
- Honokiol suppresses TNF-induced IκBα kinase activation in H1299 (Ahn et al., 2006)
- Indole-3-carbinol suppresses TNF-induced IκBα kinase activation in KBM-5 cells (Takada et al., 2005a)
- Indirubin suppresses TNF-induced IκBα kinase activation in KBM-5 cells (Sethi et al., 2006).
- Isodeoxyelephantopin suppresses TNF-induced IκBα kinase activation in KBM-5 cells (Ichikawa et al., 2006a)
- Kahweol suppresses LPS-induced IκBα kinase activation in RAW 264.7 cells (Kim et al., 2004)
- Morin suppresses TNF-induced IκBα kinase activation in KBM-5 cells (Manna et al., 2007)
- Noscapine suppresses TNF-induced IκBα kinase activation in KBM-5 cells (Sung et al. 2010)
- Ochnaflavone suppresses LPS-induced IκBα kinase activation in RAW 264.7 cells (Suh et al., 2006)
- Pinitol suppresses TAK1-mediated IκBα kinase activation in KBM-5 cells (Sethi et al., 2008b)
- Piceatannol suppresses LPS-induced IκBα kinase alpha and beta phosphorylation in RAW 264.7 cells (Islam et al., 2004)

continued

TABLE 22.6 (continued)
A List of Natural Compounds that Inhibit NF-κB and Their Mechanism(s) of Action

- Rocaglamides suppress PMA-induced IκBα kinase activation in Jurkat T cells (Baumann et al., 2002)
- Sesamin suppresses TAK1-mediated IκBα kinase activation in KBM-5 cells (Harikumar et al. 2010b)
- Simvastatin suppresses TNF-induced IκBα kinase activation in KBM-5 cells (Ahn et al., 2007b)
- Ursolic acid suppresses TNF-induced IκBα kinase activation in Jurkat T cells (Shishodia et al., 2003)
- Withanolides suppresses TNF-induced IκBα kinase activation in KBM-5 cells (Ichikawa et al., 2006b)
- Zerumbone suppresses TNF-induced IκBα kinase activation in H1299 cells (Takada et al., 2005c)
- Celastrol suppresses TAK1-mediated IκBα kinase activation in KBM-5 cells (Sethi et al., 2007)
- γ-Tocotrienol suppresses TAK1- and RIP-mediated IκBα kinase activation in KBM-5 cells (Ahn et al., 2007c)

Inhibitors of p65 expression and/or translocation

- Astragaloside IV inhibits TNF- and LPS-induced nuclear translocation of NF-κB in human umbilical vein endothelial cells (HUVECs) (Zhang et al., 2003)
- Atrovastatin inhibits thrombin-induced nuclear translocation of NF-κB in rat aortic smooth muscle cells (Haloui et al., 2003)
- Carnosol inhibits LPS-induced nuclear translocation of NF-κB in mouse macrophage RAW 264.7 cells (Lo et al., 2002)
- Chiisanoside inhibits LPS-induced p65 expression in RAW 264.7 cells (Won et al., 2005)
- Cyclolinteinone inhibits LPS-induced nuclear translocation of p65 in mouse macrophage J774 cells (D'Acquisto et al., 2000)
- Fluvastatin inhibits the expression of NF-κB in the nuclei of myocardium in experimental autoimmune myocarditis (Azuma et al., 2004)
- Magnolol inhibits TNF-induced nuclear translocation of p65 in human aortic endothelial cells (Chen et al., 2002)
- Oregonin inhibits LPS-induced p65 nuclear translocation in RAW 264.7 cells (Lee et al., 2005)
- Piperine inhibits TNF-induced nuclear translocation in B16F-10 melanoma cells (Pradeep and Kuttan, 2004)
- Pitavastatin inhibits TNF-induced p65 expression in hepatocellular carcinoma (Huh) cells (Wang et al., 2006)
- Inhibitors of p50/p65 binding to DNA
- Andrographolide attenuates TNF-induced NF-κB activation through covalent modification of reduced cysteine 62 of p50 in HEK (A293) cells (Xia et al., 2004)
- Ethyl caffeate impairs the binding of NF-κB to its cis-acting element (Chiang et al., 2005)
- CAPE inhibits binding of p65 to the DNA (Natarajan et al., 1996)
- Eriocalyxin B interferes with the binding of both p65 and p50 to the response element (Leung et al., 2006)
- Luteolin inhibits LPS-stimulated interaction between the p65 subunit of NF-κB and the transcriptional coactivator cyclic-AMP response element binding protein (CREB)-binding protein (CBP) (Kim et al., 2003)
- Picroliv inhibits binding of p65 to the DNA (Anand et al., 2008)
- Plumbagin inhibits binding of p65 to the DNA (Sandur et al., 2006)
- Thymoquinone inhibits binding of p65 to the DNA (Sethi et al., 2008a)
- Xanthohumol inhibits binding of p65 to the DNA (Harikumar et al., 2009)

Inhibitors of IKK activity

- Silibinin directly inhibits IKK activity *in vitro* in human prostate cancer PCA cells (Dhanalakshmi et al., 2002)
- Apigenin suppresses IKK activity *in vitro* in prostate cancer PC-3 cells (Shukla and Gupta, 2004)
- Acetyl-boswellic acid inhibits IKK activity in human monocytes (Syrovets et al., 2005)
- Curcumin inhibits IKK activity in TNF-stimulated U937 cells (Aggarwal et al., 2006b)
- EGCG inhibits IKK activity in TNF-stimulated intestinal epithelial cell IEC-6 (Yang et al., 2001)
- Parthenolide directly binds to and inhibits IKKβ subunit of IKK complex (Kwok et al., 2001)
- Theaflavin inhibits IKK activity in LPS-stimulated mouse macrophage RAW 264.7 cells (Pan et al., 2000)
- Wedelactone inhibits IKK activity in TNF-stimulated BALB c 3T3 cells (Kobori et al., 2004)

the growth-inhibitory and proapoptotic effects of celecoxib in OA synovial adherent cells (Lev-Ari et al., 2006). Funk et al. (2006) determined the *in vivo* efficacy of curcumin in the prevention or treatment of arthritis using streptococcal cell wall–induced arthritis, a model of RA. Curcumin was found to be efficacious in preventing joint inflammation when treatment was started before the onset of joint inflammation. It was not effective against established joint inflammation. However, Jackson et al. (2006) found that the curcumin inhibited neutrophil activation, synoviocyte proliferation, and angiogenesis and strongly inhibited collagenase and stromelysin expression, thus suggesting that curcumin has therapeutic potential for the treatment of crystal-induced arthritis or RA.

Similar to curcumin, 6-shogaol is a component of the ginger rhizome that may contribute to its anti-inflammatory properties. Levy et al. (2006) found that 6-shogaol reduced the chronic inflammatory response in the knees of rats treated with complete Freund's adjuvant. The effect of 6-shogaol was associated with significantly lower concentrations of soluble VCAM-1 in the blood and infiltration of leukocytes, including lymphocytes and monocytes/macrophages, into the synovial cavity of the knee. Fan et al. (2005) examined the effects of an acetone extract of *Boswellia carterii* gum resin on adjuvant-induced arthritis in Lewis rats. The data showed that *B. carterii* extract had significant antiarthritic and anti-inflammation effects and suggest that these effects may be mediated via the suppression of proinflammatory cytokines. Rasool and Varalakshmi (2006) investigated the effect of *Withania somnifera* root powder on paw volume and serum lysosomal enzyme activities in MSU crystal-induced rats. The levels of β-glucuronidase and lactate dehydrogenase were also measured in MSU crystal incubated polymorphonuclear leukocytes (PMNLs). A significant increase in the level of paw volume and serum lysosomal enzymes was observed in MSU crystal-induced rats. The increased β-glucuronidase and lactate dehydrogenase level were observed in untreated MSU crystal incubated PMNLs. On treatment with the *W. somnifera* root powder (500/1000 mg/kg body weight), the previous changes were reverted back to near normal levels. *W. somnifera* also showed potent analgesic and antipyretic effect with the absence of gastric damage at different dose levels in experimental rats. For comparison purpose, NSAID indomethacin was used as a standard. These results provide evidence for the suppressive effect of *W. somnifera* root powder by retarding amplification and propagation of the inflammatory response without causing any gastric damage.

Sharma (1977) compared the anti-inflammatory activity of *Commiphora mukul* (guggul) with those of NSAID (phenylbutazone and ibuprofen) in experimental arthritis induced by mycobacterial adjuvant. Inflammatory syndrome, resembling RA in man, was induced in the right hock joint of albino rabbits by intra-articular injection of the killed mycobacterial adjuvant in liquid paraffin. Development of this arthritic syndrome was studied from a period of 5 months with and without drugs. Anti-inflammatory agents such as phenylbutazone, ibuprofen, and fraction "A" of gum-guggul from *C. mukul* were administered orally at a daily dose of 100, 100, and 500 mg/kg, respectively, for a period of 5 months. All three drugs decreased the thickness of the joint swelling during the course of drug treatment. These results indicate the beneficial role of phenylbutazone, ibuprofen, and fraction "A" of gum-guggul in experimental arthritis.

In another study, Singh et al. (2003) conducted both preclinical and clinical investigations of guggul for reduction of pain, stiffness, and improved function and to determine tolerability in older patients with a diagnosis of OA of the knee. They indicated significant improvement for participants during the trial in both scales and objective measures used for assessment purposes. There were no side effects reported during the trial. Guggul appears to be a relatively safe and effective supplement to reduce symptoms of OA.

Kulkarni et al. (1991) examined the clinical efficacy of a herbomineral formulation containing the roots of *W. somnifera*, the stem of *Boswellia serrata*, the rhizomes of *Curcuma longa*, and a zinc complex (Articulin-F) in a randomized, double-blind, placebo-controlled, crossover study in patients with OA. After a 1-month single-blind run-in period, 42 patients with OA were randomly allocated to receive either a drug treatment or a matching placebo for a period of 3 months. After a 15-day washout period, the patients were transferred to the other treatment for a further period of 3 months. Clinical efficacy was evaluated every fortnight on the basis of severity of pain, morning stiffness, Ritchie articular index, joint score, disability score, and grip strength. Treatment with the herbomineral formulation produced a significant drop in severity of pain and disability score. Radiological assessment, however, did not show any significant changes in both the groups.

RA-11 (ARTREX, MENDAR), a standardized multiplant Ayurvedic drug (*W. somnifera*, *B. serrata*, *Zingiber officinale*, and *C. longa*), is currently used to treat arthritis. Chopra et al. (2004) evaluated the efficacy and safety of RA-11 in patients with symptomatic OA of the knees in a randomized, double-blind, placebo-controlled trial at a single-center, 32-week drug trial. This controlled drug trial demonstrated the potential efficacy and safety of RA-11 in the symptomatic treatment of OA knees more than 32 weeks of therapy.

Avemar, a wheat germ extract, was used as an adjunct therapy in patients with RA who had failed on at least two disease-modifying antirheumatic drugs in an open label trial. The joint score as well as the functional status improved at 1 year. In addition, the patients could reduce the dose of glucocorticoids needed to control symptoms, suggesting good efficacy (Balint et al., 2006). Addition of Suogudan granules along with other traditional Chinese medicine in a 6-week double-blind controlled trial led to significant improvement in joint pain, early morning stiffness, erythrocyte sedimentation rate (ESR), rheumatoid factor (RF), and functional scores as compared with controls in patients with RA (Yu et al., 2005). Cannabis-based medicine spray was better than placebo in reducing pain and disease activity scores in patients with RA. However, majority of patients had minor side effects, and the effect produced by CBM was mild (Blake et al., 2006). Similarly, Meta050 (a mixture of rosemary extract and oleic acid) caused significant pain relief from patient with RA in an 8-week open trial (Lukaczer et al., 2005). Fish oil containing omega-3 fatty acids has been shown to reduce inflammation. In RA, its use reduces joint disease activity. Recent study shows better efficacy when used with olive oil (Berbert et al., 2005). Salicin derived from a willow bark failed to show any efficacy in patients with RA as compared with diclofenac in a 6-week study (Biegert et al., 2004). In a 20-week placebo-controlled study of ethanolic extract of *Tripterygium wilfordii* Hook F, a dose-dependent effect was seen in ACR20 response in patients with RA. Diarrhea was the major side effect seen with *T. wilfordii* Hook F (Tao et al., 2002). Pentacyclic chemotype of *Uncaria tomentosa* showed significant benefit in swollen and tender joint count in a 52-week study with minor side effects (Mur et al., 2002).

Formulations containing curcumin reduce inflammation and disability in patients with RA. RA-1, a polyherbal preparation used by Ayurvedic physicians in India containing extracts of *W. somnifera*, *B. serrata*, *Z. officinale*, and *C. longa*, was tested in a double-blind placebo-controlled study and was found to reduce joint swelling and RF levels. However, because of the high placebo response, no significant difference was seen in the American College of Rheumatology 50% improvement criteria response between the two groups. This trial is one of the best regarding the power of study as well as having well-defined outcome variables (Chopra et al., 2000). A recent systematic review of all randomized controlled trial published on use of these agents in RA revealed that only seven trials met the criteria for inclusion but failed to show a significant benefit because of paucity of good trials (Park and Ernst, 2005). Another systematic review on use of herbal medicines found a moderate usefulness of gamma-linolenic acid in treatment of RA (Soeken et al., 2003).

Extract from *Rosa canina* was tested in a double-blind crossover study in patients with OA. The study drug significantly reduced the disease score (Western Ontario and MacMaster Universities Osteoarthritis Index [WOMAC]) as well as the requirement of analgesics in addition to disability and stiffness, suggesting that it may be an effective treatment for OA (Winther et al., 2005). Hyben vital made from *R. canina* showed a significant improvement in pain and stiffness as compared with placebo in a crossover design study. Patients who received placebo later had a carry over effect of Hyben, suggesting that its efficacy persists even after the drug is discontinued (Rein et al., 2004). Duhuo Jisheng Wan (DJW) is the most widely used Chinese medicine for joint pains. In a double-blind controlled study having 200 patients with OA, it was found comparable with diclofenac sodium, a conventional NSAID. Even the side effect was similar, suggesting that it can be used as an alternative to NSAIDs in management of OA (Teekachunhatean et al., 2004). SK1306X is a mixture of extract of three herbs, namely, *Clematis mandshurica*, *Trichosanthes kirilowii*, and *Prunella vulgaris*. It was found to have efficacy similar to diclofenac but with reduced gastrointestinal toxicity (Lung et al., 2004). In another double-blind controlled study, SK1306X was found to provide better pain relief than placebo (Jung et al., 2001). Guggul, an oleresin from plant *Cammiphora mukkul*, has been used in Ayurveda in Indian traditional medicine system from treatment of various ailments including arthritis. In an open trial, it was found to reduce WOMAC scores and pain in patients with OA (Singh et al., 2003). *B. serrata* extract also contains guggul and was found to significantly reduce knee swelling and pain in patients with OA as compared with placebo (Kimmatkar et al., 2003). Local application of Arnica Montana gel led to significant improvement in pain, stiffness, and function in patients with mild to moderate OA (Knuesel et al., 2002). Ginger has been used traditionally in various Ayurvedic medicines. Concentrated extract from ginger improved pain and WOMAC index as well as requirement of analgesics in patients with OA. It was associated with a modest benefit with minimal toxicity related to gastrointestinal tract (Altman and Marcussen, 2001). However, another study in a crossover design failed to find any benefit of ginger extract. Avocado/soya bean unsaponifiable is better than placebo in relieving pain in patients with OA when used in a dose of 300–600 mg/day. In another placebo-controlled study, avocado/soya bean unsaponifiable administration reduced the need for NSAIDs for pain relief (Ernst, 2003). A compound containing extract from root of *W. somnifera*, stem of *B. serrata*, and rhizome of *C. longa* along with zinc was found to reduce pain and disability in OA patients. Overall, these various preclinical and clinical studies suggest potential natural products for the treatment of arthritis (Kulkarni et al., 1991).

CONCLUSIONS

Overall, from the previous discussion, it is clear that pathogenesis of arthritis is very well defined. Although numerous treatments for various forms of arthritis have been identified, they suffer from various drawbacks, such as lack of efficacy, side effects, and high expense. Usually treatment of arthritis requires treatment of patient for entire life. Thus, less-expensive, less-toxic, and more-efficacious treatments are required. Plant-derived products offer much promise, but they require extensive investigation in various preclinical and clinical settings to prove their usefulness. Because of the lack of intellectual property rights, industry has little motivation to pursue such studies. Hopefully, federal agency will provide the financial backing to support such studies. Thus, natural products serve as great source for the treatment of arthritis.

ACKNOWLEDGMENTS

This research was supported by The Clayton Foundation for Research (to BBA), a program project grant from the National Institutes of Health (NIH CA-124787–01A2), and a grant from the Center for Targeted Therapy of M.D. Anderson Cancer Center. The authors thank Walter Pagel for a careful review of the manuscript.

REFERENCES

Abad MJ, de las Heras B, Silvan AM, et al. Effects of furocoumarins from *Cachrys trifida* on some macrophage functions. J Pharm Pharmacol 2001;53:1163–1168.

Abuarqoub H, Foresti R, Green CJ, Motterlini R. Heme oxygenase-1 mediates the anti-inflammatory actions of 2′-hydroxychalcone in RAW 264.7 murine macrophages. Am J Physiol Cell Physiol 2006;290:C1092–C1099.

Aggarwal BB. Tumour necrosis factors receptor associated signalling molecules and their role in activation of apoptosis, JNK and NF-kappaB. Ann Rheum Dis 2000;59(Suppl 1):i6–i16.

Aggarwal BB. Signalling pathways of the TNF superfamily: a double-edged sword. Nat Rev Immunol 2003;3:745–756.

Aggarwal BB. Nuclear factor-kappaB: the enemy within. Cancer Cell 2004;6:203–208.

Aggarwal BB, Shishodia S, Takada Y, et al. TNF blockade: an inflammatory issue. Ernst Schering Res Found Workshop 2006a;56:S161–S186.

Aggarwal S, Ichikawa H, Takada Y, et al. Curcumin (diferuloylmethane) down-regulates expression of cell proliferation and antiapoptotic and metastatic gene products through suppression of IkappaBalpha kinase and Akt activation. Mol Pharmacol 2006b;69:195–206.

Ahn KS, Noh EJ, Zhao HL, et al. Inhibition of inducible nitric oxide synthase and cyclooxygenase II by *Platycodon grandiflorum* saponins via suppression of nuclear factor-kappaB activation in RAW 264.7 cells. Life Sci 2005;76:2315–2328.

Ahn KS, Sethi G, Aggarwal BB. Embelin, an inhibitor of X chromosome-linked inhibitor-of-apoptosis protein, blocks nuclear factor-kappaB (NF-kappaB) signaling pathway leading to suppression of NF-kappaB-regulated antiapoptotic and metastatic gene products. Mol Pharmacol 2007a;71:209–219.

Ahn KS, Sethi G, Aggarwal BB. Simvastatin potentiates TNF-alpha-induced apoptosis through the down-regulation of NF-kappaB-dependent antiapoptotic gene products: role of IkappaBalpha kinase and TGF-beta-activated kinase-1. J Immunol 2007b;178:2507–2516.

Ahn KS, Sethi G, Krishnan K, Aggarwal BB. Gamma-tocotrienol inhibits nuclear factor-kappaB signaling pathway through inhibition of receptor-interacting protein and TAK1 leading to suppression of antiapoptotic gene products and potentiation of apoptosis. J Biol Chem 2007;282:809–820.

Ahn KS, Sethi G, Shishodia S, et al. Honokiol potentiates apoptosis, suppresses osteoclastogenesis, and inhibits invasion through modulation of nuclear factor-kappaB activation pathway. Mol Cancer Res 2006;4:621–633.

Albert D, Zundorf I, Dingermann T, et al. Hyperforin is a dual inhibitor of cyclooxygenase-1 and 5-lipoxygenase. Biochem Pharmacol 2002;64:1767–1775.

Altman RD, Marcussen KC. Effects of a ginger extract on knee pain in patients with osteoarthritis. Arthritis Rheum 2001;44:2531–2538.

Ammon HP, Safayhi H, Mack T, Sabieraj J. Mechanism of antiinflammatory actions of curcumine and boswellic acids. J Ethnopharmacol 1993;38:113–119.

Anand P, Kunnumakkara AB, Harikumar KB, et al. Modification of cysteine residue in p65 subunit of nuclear factor-kappaB (NF-kappaB) by picroliv suppresses NF-kappaB-regulated gene products and potentiates apoptosis. Cancer Res 2008;68:8861–8870.

Androulakis XM, Muga SJ, Chen F, et al. Chemopreventive effects of *Khaya senegalensis* bark extract on human colorectal cancer. Anticancer Res 2006;26:2397–2405.

Aupperle K, Bennett B, Han Z, et al. NF-kappa B regulation by I kappa B kinase-2 in rheumatoid arthritis synoviocytes. J Immunol 2001;166:2705–2711.

Azuma RW, Suzuki J, Ogawa M, et al. HMG-CoA reductase inhibitor attenuates experimental autoimmune myocarditis through inhibition of T cell activation. Cardiovasc Res 2004;64:412–420.

Balint G, Apathy A, Gaal M, et al. Effect of Avemar—a fermented wheat germ extract—on rheumatoid arthritis. Preliminary data. Clin Exp Rheumatol 2006;24:325–328.

Ban HS, Suzuki K, Lim SS, et al. Inhibition of lipopolysaccharide-induced expression of inducible nitric oxide synthase and tumor necrosis factor-alpha by 2′-hydroxychalcone derivatives in RAW 264.7 cells. Biochem Pharmacol 2004;67:1549–1557.

Banerjee T, Valacchi G, Ziboh VA, van der Vliet A. Inhibition of TNFalpha-induced cyclooxygenase-2 expression by amentoflavone through suppression of NF-kappaB activation in A549 cells. Mol Cell Biochem 2002;238:105–110.

Baumann B, Bohnenstengel F, Siegmund D, et al. Rocaglamide derivatives are potent inhibitors of NF-kappa B activation in T-cells. J Biol Chem 2002;277:44791–44800.

Becker MA, Jolly M. Hyperuricemia and associated diseases. Rheum Dis Clin North Am 2006;32:275–293, v-vi.

Benrezzouk R, Terencio MC, Ferrandiz ML, et al. Inhibition of 5-lipoxygenase activity by the natural anti-inflammatory compound aethiopinone. Inflamm Res 2001;50:96–101.

Berbert AA, Kondo CR, Almendra CL, Matsuo T, Dichi I. Supplementation of fish oil and olive oil in patients with rheumatoid arthritis. Nutrition 2005;21:131–136.

Bermejo Benito P, Abad Martinez MJ, Silvan Sen AM, et al. *In vivo* and *in vitro* antiinflammatory activity of saikosaponins. Life Sci 1998;63:1147–1156.

Bezakova L, Misik V, Malekova L, Svajdlenka E, Kostalova D. Lipoxygenase inhibition and antioxidant properties of bisbenzylisoqunoline alkaloids isolated from *Mahonia aquifolium*. Pharmazie 1996;51:758–761.

Bi XL, Yang JY, Dong YX, et al. Resveratrol inhibits nitric oxide and TNF-alpha production by lipopolysaccharide-activated microglia. Int Immunopharmacol 2005:185–193.

Biegert C, Wagner I, Ludtke R, et al. Efficacy and safety of willow bark extract in the treatment of osteoarthritis and rheumatoid arthritis: results of 2 randomized double-blind controlled trials. J Rheumatol 2004;31:2121–2130.

Blake DR, Robson P, Ho M, Jubb RW, McCabe CS. Preliminary assessment of the efficacy, tolerability and safety of a cannabis-based medicine (Sativex) in the treatment of pain caused by rheumatoid arthritis. Rheumatology (Oxford) 2006;45:50–52.

Boden SE, Schweizer S, Bertsche T, et al. Stimulation of leukotriene synthesis in intact polymorphonuclear cells by the 5-lipoxygenase inhibitor 3-oxo-tirucallic acid. Mol Pharmacol 2001;60:267–273.

Bucar F, Resch M, Bauer R, et al. 5-Methylflavasperone and rhamnetin from *Guiera senegalensis* and their antioxidative and 5-lipoxygenase inhibitory activity. Pharmazie 1998;53:875–878.

Burrage PS, Mix KS, Brinckerhoff CE. Matrix metalloproteinases: role in arthritis. Front Biosci 2006;11:529–543.

Carcache-Blanco EJ, Cuendet M, Park EJ, et al. Potential cancer chemopreventive agents from *Arbutus unedo*. Nat Prod Res 2006;20:327–334.

Chainy GB, Manna SK, Chaturvedi MM, Aggarwal BB. Anethole blocks both early and late cellular responses transduced by tumor necrosis factor: effect on NF-kappaB, AP-1, JNK, MAPKK and apoptosis. Oncogene 2000;19:2943–2950.

Chan MM. Inhibition of tumor necrosis factor by curcumin, a phytochemical. Biochem Pharmacol 1995;49:1551–1556.

Chaturvedi MM, Kumar A, Darnay BG, et al. Sanguinarine (pseudochelerythrine) is a potent inhibitor of NF-kappaB activation, IkappaBalpha phosphorylation, and degradation. J Biol Chem 1997;272:30129–30134.

Chen YH, Lin SJ, Chen JW, Ku HH, Chen YL. Magnolol attenuates VCAM-1 expression *in vitro* in TNF-alpha-treated human aortic endothelial cells and *in vivo* in the aorta of cholesterol-fed rabbits. Br J Pharmacol 2002;135:37–47.

Chiang YM, Lo CP, Chen YP, et al. Ethyl caffeate suppresses NF-kappaB activation and its downstream inflammatory mediators, iNOS, COX-2, and PGE$_2$ *in vitro* or in mouse skin. Br J Pharmacol 2005;146:352–363.

Cho JY, Park J, Yoo ES, et al. Inhibitory effect of lignans from the rhizomes of *Coptis japonica* var. dissecta on tumor necrosis factor-alpha production in lipopolysaccharide-stimulated RAW264.7 cells. Arch Pharm Res 1998;21:12–16.

Choi YH, Shin EM, Kim YS, et al. Anti-inflammatory principles from the fruits of *Evodia rutaecarpa* and their cellular action mechanisms. Arch Pharm Res 2006;29:293–297.

Chopra A, Lavin P, Patwardhan B, Chitre D. Randomized double blind trial of an Ayurvedic plant derived formulation for treatment of rheumatoid arthritis. J Rheumatol 2000;27:1365–1372.

Chopra A, Lavin P, Patwardhan B, Chitre D. A 32-week randomized, placebo-controlled clinical evaluation of RA-11, an Ayurvedic drug, on osteoarthritis of the knees. J Clin Rheumatol 2004;10:236–245.

Choy EH, Panayi GS. Cytokine pathways and joint inflammation in rheumatoid arthritis. N Engl J Med 2001;344:907–916.

Chun KS, Kang JY, Kim OH, Kang H, Surh YJ. Effects of yakuchinone A and yakuchinone B on the phorbol ester-induced expression of COX-2 and iNOS and activation of NF-kappaB in mouse skin. J Environ Pathol Toxicol Oncol 2002;21:131–139.

Clegg DO, Reda DJ, Harris CL, et al. Glucosamine, chondroitin sulfate, and the two in combination for painful knee osteoarthritis. N Engl J Med 2006;354:795–808.

Clemett D, Goa KL. Celecoxib: a review of its use in osteoarthritis, rheumatoid arthritis and acute pain. Drugs 2000;59:957–980.

Colacurci N, Chiantera A, Fornaro F, et al. Effects of soy isoflavones on endothelial function in healthy postmenopausal women. Menopause 2005;12:299–307.

Cronstein BN, Terkeltaub R. The inflammatory process of gout and its treatment. Arthritis Res Ther 2006;8(Suppl 1):S3.

D'Acquisto F, Lanzotti V, Carnuccio R. Cyclolinteinone, a sesterterpene from sponge *Cacospongia linteiformis*, prevents inducible nitric oxide synthase and inducible cyclo-oxygenase protein expression by blocking nuclear factor-kappaB activation in J774 macrophages. Biochem J 2000;346 Pt 3:793–798.

Darnay BG, Aggarwal BB. Signal transduction by tumour necrosis factor and tumour necrosis factor related ligands and their receptors. Ann Rheum Dis 1999;58(Suppl 1):I2–I13.

Devereux G. The increase in the prevalence of asthma and allergy: food for thought. Nat Rev Immunol 2006;6:869–874.

Dhanalakshmi S, Singh RP, Agarwal C, Agarwal R. Silibinin inhibits constitutive and TNFalpha-induced activation of NF-kappaB and sensitizes human prostate carcinoma DU145 cells to TNFalpha-induced apoptosis. Oncogene 2002;21:1759–1767.

Duansak D, Somboonwong J, Patumraj S. Effects of aloe vera on leukocyte adhesion and TNF-alpha and IL-6 levels in burn wounded rats. Clin Hemorheol Microcirc 2003;29:239–246.

El Gazzar M, El Mezayen R, Nicolls MR, Marecki JC, Dreskin SC. Downregulation of leukotriene biosynthesis by thymoquinone attenuates airway inflammation in a mouse model of allergic asthma. Biochim Biophys Acta 2006;1760:1088–1095.

Emery P. Treatment of rheumatoid arthritis. BMJ 2006;332:152–155.

Emery P, Gough A, Salmon M, Devlin J. Medical management of rheumatoid arthritis. BMJ 1993; 307:940.

Ernst E. Avocado–soybean unsaponifiables (ASU) for osteoarthritis—a systematic review. Clin Rheumatol 2003;22:285–288.

Fan AY, Lao L, Zhang RX, et al. Effects of an acetone extract of *Boswellia carterii* Birdw. (Burseraceae) gum resin on adjuvant-induced arthritis in lewis rats. J Ethnopharmacol 2005;101:104–109.

Feldmann M, Brennan FM, Williams RO, Woody JN, Maini RN. The transfer of a laboratory based hypothesis to a clinically useful therapy: the development of anti-TNF therapy of rheumatoid arthritis. Best Pract Res Clin Rheumatol 2004;18:59–80.

Ferry S, Matsuda M, Yoshida H, Hirata M. Inositol hexakisphosphate blocks tumor cell growth by activating apoptotic machinery as well as by inhibiting the Akt/NFkappaB-mediated cell survival pathway. Carcinogenesis 2002;23:2031–2041.

Fiebich BL, Grozdeva M, Hess S, et al. *Petasites hybridus* extracts *in vitro* inhibit COX-2 and PGE$_2$ release by direct interaction with the enzyme and by preventing p42/44 MAP kinase activation in rat primary microglial cells. Planta Med 2005;71:12–19.

Firestein GS. Evolving concepts of rheumatoid arthritis. Nature 2003;423:356–361.

Firestein GS. NF-kappaB: Holy Grail for rheumatoid arthritis? Arthritis Rheum 2004;50:2381–2386.

Francis JA, Rumbeiha W, Nair MG. Constituents in Easter lily flowers with medicinal activity. Life Sci 2004;76:671–683.

Fukuyama Y, Kiriyama Y, Kodama M, et al. Total synthesis of ardisiaquinone A, a potent 5-lipoxygenase inhibitor, isolated from *Ardisia sieboldii*, and degree of 5-lipoxygenase inhibitory activity of its derivatives. Chem Pharm Bull (Tokyo) 1994;42:2211–2213.

Fukuyama Y, Kiriyama Y, Okino J, et al. Naturally occurring 5-lipoxygenase inhibitor. II. Structures and syntheses of ardisianones A and B, and maesanin, alkenyl-1,4-benzoquinones from the rhizome of *Ardisia japonica*. Chem Pharm Bull (Tokyo) 1993;41:561–565.

Funk JL, Oyarzo JN, Frye JB, et al. Turmeric extracts containing curcuminoids prevent experimental rheumatoid arthritis. J Nat Prod 2006;69:351–355.

Gao M, Zhang J, Liu G. Effect of diphenyl dimethyl bicarboxylate on concanavalin A-induced liver injury in mice. Liver Int 2005;25:904–912.

Goldring MB. Update on the biology of the chondrocyte and new approaches to treating cartilage diseases. Best Pract Res Clin Rheumatol 2006;20:1003–1025.

Grzanna R, Phan P, Polotsky A, Lindmark L, Frondoza CG. Ginger extract inhibits beta-amyloid peptide-induced cytokine and chemokine expression in cultured THP-1 monocytes. J Altern Complement Med 2004;10:1009–1013.

Habtemariam S. Cistifolin, an integrin-dependent cell adhesion blocker from the anti-rheumatic herbal drug, gravel root (rhizome of *Eupatorium purpureum*). Planta Med 1998;64:683–685.

Haloui M, Meilhac O, Jandrot-Perrus M, Michel JB. Atorvastatin limits the pro-inflammatory response of rat aortic smooth muscle cells to thrombin. Eur J Pharmacol 2003;474:175–184.

Hamasaki Y, Kobayashi I, Hayasaki R, et al. The Chinese herbal medicine, shinpi-to, inhibits IgE-mediated leukotriene synthesis in rat basophilic leukemia-2H3 cells. J Ethnopharmacol 1997;56:123–131.

Harikumar KB, Kunnumakkara AB, Ahn KS, et al. Modification of the cysteine residues in IkappaBalpha kinase and NF-kappaB (p65) by xanthohumol leads to suppression of NF-kappaB-regulated gene products and potentiation of apoptosis in leukemia cells. Blood 2009;113:2003–2013.

Harikumar KB, Sung B, Pandey MK, et al. Escin, a pentacyclic triterpene, chemosensitizes human tumor cells through inhibition of nuclear factor-kappaB signaling pathway. Mol Pharmacol 2010a;77(5):818–827.

Harikumar KB, Sung B, Tharakan ST, et al. Sesamin manifests chemopreventive effects through the suppression of NF-kappaB-regulated cell survival, proliferation, invasion, and angiogenic gene products. Mol Cancer Res 2010b;8(5):751–761.

Hehner SP, Heinrich M, Bork PM, et al. Sesquiterpene lactones specifically inhibit activation of NF-kappa B by preventing the degradation of I kappa B-alpha and I kappa B-beta. J Biol Chem 1998;273:1288–1297.

Herrera-Salgado Y, Garduno-Ramirez ML, Vazquez L, Rios MY, Alvarez L. Myo-inositol-derived glycolipids with anti-inflammatory activity from Solanum lanceolatum. J Nat Prod 2005;68:1031–1036.

Homhual S, Bunyapraphatsara N, Kondratyuk T, et al. Bioactive dammarane triterpenes from the mangrove plant *Bruguiera gymnorrhiza*. J Nat Prod 2006;69:421–424.

Hong J, Bose M, Ju J, et al. Modulation of arachidonic acid metabolism by curcumin and related beta-diketone derivatives: effects on cytosolic phospholipase A(2), cyclooxygenases and 5-lipoxygenase. Carcinogenesis 2004;25:1671–1679.

Hong J, Smith TJ, Ho CT, August DA, Yang CS. Effects of purified green and black tea polyphenols on cyclooxygenase- and lipoxygenase-dependent metabolism of arachidonic acid in human colon mucosa and colon tumor tissues. Biochem Pharmacol 2001;62:1175–1183.

Hoskison TK, Wortmann RL. Advances in the management of gout and hyperuricaemia. Scand J Rheumatol 2006;35:251–260.

Hougee S, Faber J, Sanders A, et al. Selective COX-2 inhibition by a *Pterocarpus marsupium* extract characterized by pterostilbene, and its activity in healthy human volunteers. Planta Med 2005;71:387–392.

Hu C, Kitts DD. Luteolin and luteolin-7-*O*-glucoside from dandelion flower suppress iNOS and COX-2 in RAW264.7 cells. Mol Cell Biochem 2004;265:107–113.

Hua KF, Hsu HY, Su YC, et al. Study on the antiinflammatory activity of methanol extract from seagrass *Zostera japonica*. J Agric Food Chem 2006;54:306–311.

Huang C, Huang Y, Li J, et al. Inhibition of benzo(a)pyrene diol-epoxide-induced transactivation of activated protein 1 and nuclear factor kappaB by black raspberry extracts. Cancer Res 2002;62:6857–6863.

Huang MT, Lysz T, Ferraro T, et al. Inhibitory effects of curcumin on *in vitro* lipoxygenase and cyclooxygenase activities in mouse epidermis. Cancer Res 1991;51:813–819.

Huang TH, Tran VH, Duke RK, et al. Harpagoside suppresses lipopolysaccharide-induced iNOS and COX-2 expression through inhibition of NF-kappa B activation. J Ethnopharmacol 2006;104:149–155.

Hung WC, Chang HC. Methanolic extract of adlay seed suppresses COX-2 expression of human lung cancer cells via inhibition of gene transcription. J Agric Food Chem 2003;51:7333–7337.

Ichikawa H, Nair MS, Takada Y, et al. Isodeoxyelephantopin, a novel sesquiterpene lactone, potentiates apoptosis, inhibits invasion, and abolishes osteoclastogenesis through suppression of nuclear factor-kappaB (nf-kappaB) activation and nf-kappaB-regulated gene expression. Clin Cancer Res 2006a;12:5910–5918.

Ichikawa H, Takada Y, Murakami A, Aggarwal BB. Identification of a novel blocker of I kappa B alpha kinase that enhances cellular apoptosis and inhibits cellular invasion through suppression of NF-kappa B-regulated gene products. J Immunol 2005;174:7383–7392.

Ichikawa H, Takada Y, Shishodia S, et al. Withanolides potentiate apoptosis, inhibit invasion, and abolish osteoclastogenesis through suppression of nuclear factor-kappaB (NF-kappaB) activation and NF-kappaB-regulated gene expression. Mol Cancer Ther 2006b;5:1434–1445.

Inokuchi T, Moriwaki Y, Tsutsui H, et al. Plasma interleukin (IL)-18 (interferon-gamma-inducing factor) and other inflammatory cytokines in patients with gouty arthritis and monosodium urate monohydrate crystal-induced secretion of IL-18. Cytokine 2006;33:21–27.

Ishii R, Horie M, Saito K, Arisawa M, Kitanaka S. Inhibition of lipopolysaccharide-induced pro-inflammatory cytokine expression via suppression of nuclear factor-kappaB activation by *Mallotus japonicus* phloroglucinol derivatives. Biochim Biophys Acta 2003;1620:108–118.

Islam S, Hassan F, Mu MM, et al. Piceatannol prevents lipopolysaccharide (LPS)-induced nitric oxide (NO) production and nuclear factor (NF)-kappaB activation by inhibiting IkappaB kinase (IKK). Microbiol Immunol 2004;48:729–736.

Jackson JK, Higo T, Hunter WL, Burt HM. The antioxidants curcumin and quercetin inhibit inflammatory processes associated with arthritis. Inflamm Res 2006;55:168–175.

Jang DS, Cuendet M, Su BN, et al. Constituents of the seeds of *Hernandia ovigera* with inhibitory activity against cyclooxygenase-2. Planta Med 2004;70:893–896.

Jeong HJ, Koo HN, Na HJ, et al. Inhibition of TNF-alpha and IL-6 production by Aucubin through blockade of NF-kappaB activation RBL-2H3 mast cells. Cytokine 2002;18:252–259.

Jin HZ, Lee D, Lee JH, et al. New sesquiterpene dimers from *Inula britannica* inhibit NF-kappaB activation and NO and TNF-alpha production in LPS-stimulated RAW264.7 cells. Planta Med 2006;72:40–45.

Joe B, Rao UJ, Lokesh BR. Presence of an acidic glycoprotein in the serum of arthritic rats: modulation by capsaicin and curcumin. Mol Cell Biochem 1997;169:125–134.

Ju HK, Moon TC, Lee E, et al. Inhibitory effects of a new iridoid, patridoid II and its isomers, on nitric oxide and TNF-alpha production in cultured murine macrophages. Planta Med 2003;69:950–953.

Jung YB, Roh KJ, Jung JA, et al. Effect of SKI 306X, a new herbal anti-arthritic agent, in patients with osteoarthritis of the knee: a double-blind placebo controlled study. Am J Chin Med 2001;29:485–491.

Kang JS, Yoon YD, Cho IJ, et al. Glabridin, an isoflavan from licorice root, inhibits inducible nitric-oxide synthase expression and improves survival of mice in experimental model of septic shock. J Pharmacol Exp Ther 2005;312:1187–1194.

Kang OH, Choi YA, Park HJ, et al. Inhibition of trypsin-induced mast cell activation by water fraction of *Lonicera japonica*. Arch Pharm Res 2004;27:1141–1146.

Kang SS, Kim JS, Son KH, Kim HP, Chang HW. Cyclooxygenase-2 inhibitory cerebrosides from phytolaccae radix. Chem Pharm Bull (Tokyo) 2001;49:321–323.

Kelm MA, Nair MG, Strasburg GM, DeWitt DL. Antioxidant and cyclooxygenase inhibitory phenolic compounds from *Ocimum sanctum* Linn. Phytomedicine 2000;7:7–13.

Khanna D, McMahon M, Furst DE. Anti-tumor necrosis factor alpha therapy and heart failure: what have we learned and where do we go from here? Arthritis Rheum 2004a;50:1040–1050.

Khanna D, McMahon M, Furst DE. Safety of tumour necrosis factor-alpha antagonists. Drug Saf 2004b;27:307–324.

Kiemer AK, Hartung T, Huber C, Vollmar AM. Phyllanthus amarus has anti-inflammatory potential by inhibition of iNOS, COX-2, and cytokines via the NF-kappaB pathway. J Hepatol 2003;38:289–297.

Kim BH, Cho SM, Reddy AM, et al. Down-regulatory effect of quercitrin gallate on nuclear factor-kappa B-dependent inducible nitric oxide synthase expression in lipopolysaccharide-stimulated macrophages RAW 264.7. Biochem Pharmacol 2005;69:1577–1583.

Kim H, Lee E, Lim T, Jung J, Lyu Y. Inhibitory effect of *Asparagus cochinchinensis* on tumor necrosis factor-alpha secretion from astrocytes. Int J Immunopharmacol 1998a;20:153–162.

Kim HM, Lee EH, Na HJ, et al. Effect of *Polygala tenuifolia* root extract on the tumor necrosis factor-alpha secretion from mouse astrocytes. J Ethnopharmacol 1998b;61:201–208.

Kim HM, Shin HY, Lim KH, et al. *Taraxacum officinale* inhibits tumor necrosis factor-alpha production from rat astrocytes. Immunopharmacol Immunotoxicol 2000;22:519–530.

Kim JH, Jeong JH, Jeon ST, et al. Decursin inhibits induction of inflammatory mediators by blocking nuclear factor-kappaB activation in macrophages. Mol Pharmacol 2006;69:1783–1790.

Kim JK, Oh SM, Kwon HS, et al. Anti-inflammatory effect of roasted licorice extracts on lipopolysaccharide-induced inflammatory responses in murine macrophages. Biochem Biophys Res Commun 2006;345:1215–1223.

Kim JY, Jung KS, Jeong HG. Suppressive effects of the kahweol and cafestol on cyclooxygenase-2 expression in macrophages. FEBS Lett 2004;569:321–326.

Kim SH, Shin KJ, Kim D, et al. Luteolin inhibits the nuclear factor-kappa B transcriptional activity in Rat-1 fibroblasts. Biochem Pharmacol 2003;66:955–963.

Kim SO, Kundu JK, Shin YK, et al. [6]-Gingerol inhibits COX-2 expression by blocking the activation of p38 MAP kinase and NF-kappaB in phorbol ester-stimulated mouse skin. Oncogene 2005;24:2558–2567.

Kimmatkar N, Thawani V, Hingorani L, Khiyani R. Efficacy and tolerability of *Boswellia serrata* extract in treatment of osteoarthritis of knee—a randomized double blind placebo controlled trial. Phytomedicine 2003;10:3–7.

Kimura Y, Okuda H, Kubo M. Effects of stilbenes isolated from medicinal plants on arachidonate metabolism and degranulation in human polymorphonuclear leukocytes. J Ethnopharmacol 1995;45:131–139.

Kiuchi F, Iwakami S, Shibuya M, Hanaoka F, Sankawa U. Inhibition of prostaglandin and leukotriene biosynthesis by gingerols and diarylheptanoids. Chem Pharm Bull (Tokyo) 1992;40:387–91.

Klareskog L, Padyukov L, Lorentzen J, Alfredsson L. Mechanisms of disease: genetic susceptibility and environmental triggers in the development of rheumatoid arthritis. Nat Clin Pract Rheumatol 2006a;2:425–433.

Klareskog L, Padyukov L, Ronnelid J, Alfredsson L. Genes, environment and immunity in the development of rheumatoid arthritis. Curr Opin Immunol 2006b;18:650–655.

Klareskog L, Stolt P, Lundberg K, et al. A new model for an etiology of rheumatoid arthritis: smoking may trigger HLA-DR (shared epitope)-restricted immune reactions to autoantigens modified by citrullination. Arthritis Rheum 2006c;54:38–46.

Knuesel O, Weber M, Suter A. Arnica montana gel in osteoarthritis of the knee: an open, multicenter clinical trial. Adv Ther 2002;19:209–218.

Kobori M, Yang Z, Gong D, et al. Wedelolactone suppresses LPS-induced caspase-11 expression by directly inhibiting the IKK complex. Cell Death Differ 2004;11:123–130.

Koshihara Y, Neichi T, Murota S, et al. Selective inhibition of 5-lipoxygenase by natural compounds isolated from Chinese plants, Artemisia rubripes Nakai. FEBS Lett 1983;158:41–44.

Kulkarni RR, Patki PS, Jog VP, Gandage SG, Patwardhan B. Treatment of osteoarthritis with a herbomineral formulation: a double-blind, placebo-controlled, cross-over study. J Ethnopharmacol 1991;33:91–95.

Kumar A, Dhawan S, Aggarwal BB. Emodin (3-methyl-1,6,8-trihydroxyanthraquinone) inhibits TNF-induced NF-kappaB activation, IkappaB degradation, and expression of cell surface adhesion proteins in human vascular endothelial cells. Oncogene 1998a;17:913–918.

Kumar A, Dhawan S, Hardegen NJ, Aggarwal BB. Curcumin (Diferuloylmethane) inhibition of tumor necrosis factor (TNF)-mediated adhesion of monocytes to endothelial cells by suppression of cell surface expression of adhesion molecules and of nuclear factor-kappaB activation. Biochem Pharmacol 1998b;55:775–783.

Kunnumakkara AB, Ichikawa H, Anand P, et al. Coronarin D, a labdane diterpene, inhibits both constitutive and inducible nuclear factor-kappa B pathway activation, leading to potentiation of apoptosis, inhibition of invasion, and suppression of osteoclastogenesis. Mol Cancer Ther 2008;7:3306–3317.

Kunnumakkara AB, Nair AS, Ahn KS, et al. Gossypin, a pentahydroxy glucosyl flavone, inhibits the transforming growth factor beta-activated kinase-1-mediated NF-kappaB activation pathway, leading to potentiation of apoptosis, suppression of invasion, and abrogation of osteoclastogenesis. Blood 2007;109:5112–5121.

Kuo YC, Tsai WJ, Meng HC, et al. Immune reponses in human mesangial cells regulated by emodin from *Polygonum hypoleucum* Ohwi. Life Sci 2001;68:1271–1286.

Kwok BH, Koh B, Ndubuisi MI, Elofsson M, Crews CM. The anti-inflammatory natural product parthenolide from the medicinal herb Feverfew directly binds to and inhibits IkappaB kinase. Chem Biol 2001;8:759–766.

Lau TY, Leung LK. Soya isoflavones suppress phorbol 12-myristate 13-acetate-induced COX-2 expression in MCF-7 cells. Br J Nutr 2006;96:169–176.

Lee CJ, Lee SS, Chen SC, Ho FM, Lin WW. Oregonin inhibits lipopolysaccharide-induced iNOS gene transcription and upregulates HO-1 expression in macrophages and microglia. Br J Pharmacol 2005;146:378–388.

Lee JH, Jung HS, Giang PM, et al. Blockade of nuclear factor-kappaB signaling pathway and anti-inflammatory activity of cardamomin, a chalcone analog from *Alpinia conchigera*. J Pharmacol Exp Ther 2006;316:271–278.

Lee SH, Seo GS, Sohn DH. Inhibition of lipopolysaccharide-induced expression of inducible nitric oxide synthase by butein in RAW 264.7 cells. Biochem Biophys Res Commun 2004;323:125–132.

Lee SJ, Bai SK, Lee KS, et al. Astaxanthin inhibits nitric oxide production and inflammatory gene expression by suppressing I(kappa)B kinase-dependent NF-kappaB activation. Mol Cells 2003;16:97–105.

Lee SJ, Terkeltaub RA. New developments in clinically relevant mechanisms and treatment of hyperuricemia. Curr Rheumatol Rep 2006;8:224–230.

Leung CH, Grill SP, Lam W, et al. Eriocalyxin B inhibits nuclear factor-kappaB activation by interfering with the binding of both p65 and p50 to the response element in a noncompetitive manner. Mol Pharmacol 2006;70:1946–1955.

Lev-Ari S, Strier L, Kazanov D, et al. Curcumin synergistically potentiates the growth-inhibitory and pro-apoptotic effects of celecoxib in osteoarthritis synovial adherent cells. Rheumatology (Oxford) 2006;45:171–177.

Levy AS, Simon O, Shelly J, Gardener M. 6-Shogaol reduced chronic inflammatory response in the knees of rats treated with complete Freund's adjuvant. BMC Pharmacol 2006;6:12.

Li RW, Leach DN, Myers SP, et al. A new anti-inflammatory glucoside from *Ficus racemosa* L. Planta Med 2004;70:421–426.

Li W, Tsubouchi R, Qiao S, et al. Inhibitory action of eugenol compounds on the production of nitric oxide in RAW264.7 macrophages. Biomed Res 2006;27:69–74.

Lin, AH, Fang SX, Fang JG, Du G, Liu YH. Studies on anti-endotoxin activity of F022 from *Radix isatidis*. Zhongguo Zhong Yao Za Zhi 2002;27:439–442.

Littler AJ, Buckley CD, Wordsworth P, et al. A distinct profile of six soluble adhesion molecules (ICAM-1, ICAM-3, VCAM-1, E-selectin, L-selectin and P-selectin) in rheumatoid arthritis. Br J Rheumatol 1997;36:164–169.

Liu JH, Zschocke S, Reininger E, Bauer R. Inhibitory effects of *Angelica pubescens f. biserrata* on 5-lipoxygenase and cyclooxygenase. Planta Med 1998;64:525–529.

Liu L, Ning ZQ, Shan S, et al. Phthalide lactones from *Ligusticum chuanxiong* inhibit lipopolysaccharide-induced TNF-alpha production and TNF-alpha-mediated NF-kappaB Activation. Planta Med 2005;71:808–813.

Lo AH, Liang YC, Lin-Shiau SY, Ho CT, Lin JK. Carnosol, an antioxidant in rosemary, suppresses inducible nitric oxide synthase through down-regulating nuclear factor-kappaB in mouse macrophages. Carcinogenesis 2002;23:983–991.

Lukaczer D, Darland G, Tripp M, et al. A pilot trial evaluating Meta050, a proprietary combination of reduced iso-alpha acids, rosemary extract and oleanolic acid in patients with arthritis and fibromyalgia. Phytother Res 2005;19:864–869.

Lung YB, Seong SC, Lee MC, et al. A four-week, randomized, double-blind trial of the efficacy and safety of SKI306X: a herbal anti-arthritic agent versus diclofenac in osteoarthritis of the knee. Am J Chin Med 2004;32:291–301.

Ma Z, Otsuyama K, Liu S, et al. Baicalein, a component of *Scutellaria radix* from Huang-Lian-Jie-Du-Tang (HLJDT), leads to suppression of proliferation and induction of apoptosis in human myeloma cells. Blood 2005;105:3312–3318.

Majumdar S, Aggarwal BB. Methotrexate suppresses NF-kappaB activation through inhibition of IkappaBalpha phosphorylation and degradation. J Immunol 2001;167:2911–2920.

Majumdar S, Lamothe B, Aggarwal BB. Thalidomide suppresses NF-kappa B activation induced by TNF and H_2O_2, but not that activated by ceramide, lipopolysaccharides, or phorbol ester. J Immunol 2002;168:2644–2651.

Makris A, Thornton CE, Xu B, Hennessy A. Garlic increases IL-10 and inhibits TNFalpha and IL-6 production in endotoxin-stimulated human placental explants. Placenta 2005;26:828–834.

Manna SK, Aggarwal RS, Sethi G, Aggarwal BB, Ramesh GT. Morin (3,5,7,2′,4′-Pentahydroxyflavone) abolishes nuclear factor-kappaB activation induced by various carcinogens and inflammatory stimuli, leading to suppression of nuclear factor-kappaB-regulated gene expression and up-regulation of apoptosis. Clin Cancer Res 2007;13:2290–2297.

Manna SK, Bueso-Ramos C, Alvarado F, Aggarwal BB. Calagualine inhibits nuclear transcription factors-kappaB activated by various inflammatory and tumor promoting agents. Cancer Lett 2003;190:171–182.

Manna SK, Gad YP, Mukhopadhyay A, Aggarwal BB. Suppression of tumor necrosis factor-activated nuclear transcription factor-kappaB, activator protein-1, c-Jun N-terminal kinase, and apoptosis by beta-lapachone. Biochem Pharmacol 1999a;57:763–774.

Manna SK, Mukhopadhyay A, Aggarwal BB. Leflunomide suppresses TNF-induced cellular responses: effects on NF-kappa B, activator protein-1, c-Jun N-terminal protein kinase, and apoptosis. J Immunol 2000a;165:5962–5969.

Manna SK, Mukhopadhyay A, Aggarwal BB. Resveratrol suppresses TNF-induced activation of nuclear transcription factors NF-kappa B, activator protein-1, and apoptosis: potential role of reactive oxygen intermediates and lipid peroxidation. J Immunol 2000b;164:6509–6519.

Manna SK, Mukhopadhyay A, Van NT, Aggarwal BB. Silymarin suppresses TNF-induced activation of NF-kappa B, c-Jun N-terminal kinase, and apoptosis. J Immunol 1999b;163:6800–6809.

Manna SK, Sah NK, Newman RA, Cisneros A, Aggarwal BB. Oleandrin suppresses activation of nuclear transcription factor-kappaB, activator protein-1, and c-Jun NH2-terminal kinase. Cancer Res 2000c;60:3838–3847.

Matsuda H, Morikawa T, Managi H, Yoshikawa M. Antiallergic principles from *Alpinia galanga*: structural requirements of phenylpropanoids for inhibition of degranulation and release of TNF-alpha and IL-4 in RBL-2H3 cells. Bioorg Med Chem Lett 2003;13:3197–3202.

Matsuda H, Tewtrakul S, Morikawa T, Nakamura A, Yoshikawa M. Anti-allergic principles from Thai zedoary: structural requirements of curcuminoids for inhibition of degranulation and effect on the release of TNF-alpha and IL-4 in RBL-2H3 cells. Bioorg Med Chem 2004;12:5891–5898.

Matsunaga K, Klein TW, Friedman H, Yamamoto Y. Epigallocatechin gallate, a potential immunomodulatory agent of tea components, diminishes cigarette smoke condensate-induced suppression of anti-Legionella pneumophila activity and cytokine responses of alveolar macrophages. Clin Diagn Lab Immunol 2002;9:864–871.

Miagkov AV, Kovalenko DV, Brown CE, et al. NF-kappaB activation provides the potential link between inflammation and hyperplasia in the arthritic joint. Proc Natl Acad Sci U S A 1998;95:13859–13864.

Momin RA, De Witt DL, Nair MG. Inhibition of cyclooxygenase (COX) enzymes by compounds from *Daucus carota* L. seeds. Phytother Res 2003;17:976–979.

Momin RA, Nair MG. Antioxidant, cyclooxygenase and topoisomerase inhibitory compounds from *Apium graveolens* Linn. seeds. Phytomedicine 2002;9:312–318.

Moon TC, Murakami M, Kudo I, et al. A new class of COX-2 inhibitor, rutaecarpine from *Evodia rutaecarpa*. Inflamm Res 1999;48:621–625.

Moran AE, Carothers AM, Weyant MJ, Redston M, Bertagnolli MM. Carnosol inhibits beta-catenin tyrosine phosphorylation and prevents adenoma formation in the C57BL/6J/Min/+ (Min/+) mouse. Cancer Res 2005;65:1097–1104.

Mur E, Hartig F, Eibl G, Schirmer M. Randomized double blind trial of an extract from the pentacyclic alkaloid-chemotype of *Uncaria tomentosa* for the treatment of rheumatoid arthritis. J Rheumatol 2002;29:678–681.

Murakami A, Matsumoto K, Koshimizu K, Ohigashi H. Effects of selected food factors with chemopreventive properties on combined lipopolysaccharide- and interferon-gamma-induced IkappaB degradation in RAW264.7 macrophages. Cancer Lett 2003;195:17–25.

Nair AS, Shishodia S, Ahn KS, et al. Deguelin, an Akt inhibitor, suppresses IkappaBalpha kinase activation leading to suppression of NF-kappaB-regulated gene expression, potentiation of apoptosis, and inhibition of cellular invasion. J Immunol 2006;177:5612–5622.

Natarajan K, Manna SK, Chaturvedi MM, Aggarwal BB. Protein tyrosine kinase inhibitors block tumor necrosis factor-induced activation of nuclear factor-kappaB, degradation of IkappaBalpha, nuclear translocation of p65, and subsequent gene expression. Arch Biochem Biophys 1998;352:59–70.

Natarajan K, Singh S, Burke TR, Jr., Grunberger D, Aggarwal BB. Caffeic acid phenethyl ester is a potent and specific inhibitor of activation of nuclear transcription factor NF-kappa B. Proc Natl Acad Sci U S A 1996;93:9090–9095.

Nie ZG, Peng SY, Wang WJ. Effects of ginkgolide B on lipopolysaccharide-induced TNFalpha production in mouse peritoneal macrophages and NF-kappaB activation in rat pleural polymorphonuclear leukocytes. Yao Xue Xue Bao 2004;39:415–418.

Odukoya OA, Houghton PJ, Raman A. Lipoxygenase inhibitors in the seeds of Aframomum danielli K. Schum (Zingiberaceae). Phytomedicine 1999;6:251–256.

Ojo-Amaize EA, Kapahi P, Kakkanaiah VN, et al. Hypoestoxide, a novel anti-inflammatory natural diterpene, inhibits the activity of IkappaB kinase. Cell Immunol 2001;209:149–157.

Onodera S, Kaneda K, Mizue Y, et al. Macrophage migration inhibitory factor up-regulates expression of matrix metalloproteinases in synovial fibroblasts of rheumatoid arthritis. J Biol Chem 2000;275:444–450.

Pan MH, Lin-Shiau SY, Ho CT, Lin JH, Lin JK. Suppression of lipopolysaccharide-induced nuclear factor-kappaB activity by theaflavin-3,3′-digallate from black tea and other polyphenols through down-regulation of IkappaB kinase activity in macrophages. Biochem Pharmacol 2000;59:357–367.

Pandey MK, Sandur SK, Sung B, et al. Butein, a tetrahydroxychalcone, inhibits nuclear factor (NF)-kappaB and NF-kappaB-regulated gene expression through direct inhibition of IkappaBalpha kinase beta on cysteine 179 residue. J Biol Chem 2007a;282:17340–17350.

Pandey MK, Sung B, Ahn KS, et al. Gambogic acid, a novel ligand for transferrin receptor, potentiates TNF-induced apoptosis through modulation of the nuclear factor-kappaB signaling pathway. Blood 2007b;110:3517–3525.

Pandey MK, Sung B, Kunnumakkara AB, et al. Berberine modifies cysteine 179 of IkappaBalpha kinase, suppresses nuclear factor-kappaB-regulated antiapoptotic gene products, and potentiates apoptosis. Cancer Res 2008;68:5370–5379.

Park J, Ernst E. Ayurvedic medicine for rheumatoid arthritis: a systematic review. Semin Arthritis Rheum 2005;34:705–713.

Park SY, Lee HJ, Yoon WJ, et al. Inhibitory effects of eutigosides isolated from *Eurya emarginata* on the inflammatory mediators in RAW264.7 cells. Arch Pharm Res 2005;28:1244–1250.

Park YM, Won JH, Yun KJ, et al. Preventive effect of *Ginkgo biloba* extract (GBB) on the lipopolysaccharide-induced expressions of inducible nitric oxide synthase and cyclooxygenase-2 via suppression of nuclear factor-kappaB in RAW 264.7 cells. Biol Pharm Bull 2006;29:985–990.

Park YS, Lee JH, Harwalkar JA, et al. Acetyl-11-keto-beta-boswellic acid (AKBA) is cytotoxic for meningioma cells and inhibits phosphorylation of the extracellular-signal regulated kinase 1 and 2. Adv Exp Med Biol 2002;507:387–393.

Pergola C, Rossi A, Dugo P, Cuzzocrea S, Sautebin L. Inhibition of nitric oxide biosynthesis by anthocyanin fraction of blackberry extract. Nitric Oxide 2006;15:30–39.

Perrone A, Plaza A, Ercolino SF, et al. 14,15-Secopregnane derivatives from the leaves of *Solenostemma argel*. J Nat Prod 2006;69:50–54.

Piscoya J, Rodriguez Z, Bustamante SA, et al. Efficacy and safety of freeze-dried cat's claw in osteoarthritis of the knee: mechanisms of action of the species *Uncaria guianensis*. Inflamm Res 2001;50:442–448.

Pradeep CR, Kuttan G. Piperine is a potent inhibitor of nuclear factor-kappaB (NF-kappaB), c-Fos, CREB, ATF-2 and proinflammatory cytokine gene expression in B16F-10 melanoma cells. Int Immunopharmacol 2004;4:1795–1803.

Prasad NS, Raghavendra R, Lokesh BR, Naidu KA. Spice phenolics inhibit human PMNL 5-lipoxygenase. Prostaglandins Leukot Essent Fatty Acids 2004;70:521–528.

Punzon C, Alcaide A, Fresno M. *In vitro* anti-inflammatory activity of *Phlebodium decumanum*. Modulation of tumor necrosis factor and soluble TNF receptors. Int Immunopharmacol 2003;3:1293–1299.

Qiu Z, Jones K, Wylie M, Jia Q, Orndorff S. Modified *Aloe barbadensis* polysaccharide with immunoregulatory activity. Planta Med 2000;66:152–156.

Ramiro E, Franch A, Castellote C, et al. Flavonoids from *Theobroma cacao* down-regulate inflammatory mediators. J Agric Food Chem 2005;53:8506–8511.

Rasool M, Varalakshmi P. Suppressive effect of *Withania somnifera* root powder on experimental gouty arthritis: an *in vivo* and *in vitro* study. Chem Biol Interact 2006;164:174–180.

Rein E, Kharazmi A, Winther K. A herbal remedy, Hyben Vital (stand. powder of a subspecies of *Rosa canina* fruits), reduces pain and improves general wellbeing in patients with osteoarthritis—a double-blind, placebo-controlled, randomised trial. Phytomedicine 2004;11:383–391.

Resch M, Steigel A, Chen ZL, Bauer R. 5-Lipoxygenase and cyclooxygenase-1 inhibitory active compounds from *Atractylodes lancea*. J Nat Prod 1998;61:347–350.

Saag KG, Choi H. Epidemiology, risk factors, and lifestyle modifications for gout. Arthritis Res Ther 2006;8(Suppl 1):S2.

Saleem M, Afaq F, Adhami VM, Mukhtar H. Lupeol modulates NF-kappaB and PI3K/Akt pathways and inhibits skin cancer in CD-1 mice. Oncogene 2004;23:5203–5214.

Sandur SK, Ichikawa H, Sethi G, Ahn KS, Aggarwal BB. Plumbagin (5-hydroxy-2-methyl-1,4-naphthoquinone) suppresses NF-kappaB activation and NF-kappaB-regulated gene products through modulation of p65 and IkappaBalpha kinase activation, leading to potentiation of apoptosis induced by cytokine and chemotherapeutic agents. J Biol Chem 2006;281:17023–17033.

Sano H, Hla T, Maier JA, et al. *In vivo* cyclooxygenase expression in synovial tissues of patients with rheumatoid arthritis and osteoarthritis and rats with adjuvant and streptococcal cell wall arthritis. J Clin Invest 1992;89:97–108.

Sasaki M, Elrod JW, Jordan P, et al. CYP450 dietary inhibitors attenuate TNF-alpha-stimulated endothelial molecule expression and leukocyte adhesion. Am J Physiol Cell Physiol 2004;286:C931-C939.

Schnyder B, Schnyder-Candrian S, Panski A, et al. Phytochemical inhibition of interleukin-4-activated Stat6 and expression of VCAM-1. Biochem Biophys Res Commun 2002;292:841–847.

Selvam C, Jachak SM, Bhutani KK. Cyclooxygenase inhibitory flavonoids from the stem bark of *Semecarpus anacardium* Linn. Phytother Res 2004;18:582–584.

Sendl A, Elbl G, Steinke B, et al. Comparative pharmacological investigations of *Allium ursinum* and *Allium sativum*. Planta Med 1992;58:1–7.

Sethi G, Ahn KS, Aggarwal BB. Targeting nuclear factor-kappa B activation pathway by thymoquinone: role in suppression of antiapoptotic gene products and enhancement of apoptosis. Mol Cancer Res 2008a;6:1059–1070.

Sethi G, Ahn KS, Pandey MK, Aggarwal BB. Celastrol, a novel triterpene, potentiates TNF-induced apoptosis and suppresses invasion of tumor cells by inhibiting NF-kappaB-regulated gene products and TAK1-mediated NF-kappaB activation. Blood 2007;109:2727–2735.

Sethi G, Ahn KS, Sandur SK, et al. Indirubin enhances tumor necrosis factor-induced apoptosis through modulation of nuclear factor-kappa B signaling pathway. J Biol Chem 2006;281:23425–23435.

Sethi G, Ahn KS, Sung B, Aggarwal BB. Pinitol targets nuclear factor-kappaB activation pathway leading to inhibition of gene products associated with proliferation, apoptosis, invasion, and angiogenesis. Mol Cancer Ther 2008b;7:1604–1614.

Sharma C, Kaur J, Shishodia S, Aggarwal BB, Ralhan S. Curcumin down regulates smokeless tobacco-induced NF-kappaB activation and COX-2 expression in human oral premalignant and cancer cells. Toxicology 2006;228:1–15.

Sharma JN. Comparison of the anti-inflammatory activity of *Commiphora mukul* (an indigenous drug) with those of phenylbutazone and ibuprofen in experimental arthritis induced by mycobacterial adjuvant. Arzneimittelforschung 1977;27:1455–1457.

Shin SG, Kang JK, Lee KR, et al. Suppression of inducible nitric oxide synthase and cyclooxygenase-2 expression in RAW 264.7 macrophages by sesquiterpene lactones. J Toxicol Environ Health A 2005;68:2119–21131.

Shishodia S, Aggarwal BB. Guggulsterone inhibits NF-kappaB and IkappaBalpha kinase activation, suppresses expression of anti-apoptotic gene products, and enhances apoptosis. J Biol Chem 2004;279:47148–47158.

Shishodia S, Aggarwal BB. Diosgenin inhibits osteoclastogenesis, invasion, and proliferation through the down-regulation of Akt, I kappa B kinase activation and NF-kappa B-regulated gene expression. Oncogene 2006;25:1463–1473.

Shishodia S, Amin HM, Lai R, Aggarwal BB. Curcumin (diferuloylmethane) inhibits constitutive NF-kappaB activation, induces G1/S arrest, suppresses proliferation, and induces apoptosis in mantle cell lymphoma. Biochem Pharmacol 2005;70:700–713.

Shishodia S, Majumdar S, Banerjee S, Aggarwal BB. Ursolic acid inhibits nuclear factor-kappaB activation induced by carcinogenic agents through suppression of IkappaBalpha kinase and p65 phosphorylation: correlation with down-regulation of cyclooxygenase 2, matrix metalloproteinase 9, and cyclin D1. Cancer Res 2003;63:4375–4383.

Shukla S, Gupta S. Suppression of constitutive and tumor necrosis factor alpha-induced nuclear factor (NF)-kappaB activation and induction of apoptosis by apigenin in human prostate carcinoma PC-3 cells: correlation with down-regulation of NF-kappaB-responsive genes. Clin Cancer Res 2004;10:3169–3178.

Siegle I, Klein T, Backman JT, et al. Expression of cyclooxygenase 1 and cyclooxygenase 2 in human synovial tissue: differential elevation of cyclooxygenase 2 in inflammatory joint diseases. Arthritis Rheum 1998;41:122–129.

Silvan AM, Abad MJ, Bermejo P, Sollhuber M, Villar A. Antiinflammatory activity of coumarins from *Santolina oblongifolia*. J Nat Prod 1996;59:1183–1185.

Singh BB, Mishra LC, Vinjamury SP, et al. The effectiveness of *Commiphora mukul* for osteoarthritis of the knee: an outcomes study. Altern Ther Health Med 2003;9:74–79.

Singh S, Natarajan K, Aggarwal BB. Capsaicin (8-methyl-*N*-vanillyl-6-nonenamide) is a potent inhibitor of nuclear transcription factor-kappa B activation by diverse agents. J Immunol 1996;157:4412–4420.

Skrzypczak-Jankun E, McCabe NP, Selman SH, Jankun J. Curcumin inhibits lipoxygenase by binding to its central cavity: theoretical and X-ray evidence. Int J Mol Med 2000;6:521–526.

Skrzypczak-Jankun E, Zhou K, McCabe NP, Selman SH, Jankun J. Structure of curcumin in complex with lipoxygenase and its significance in cancer. Int J Mol Med 2003;12:17–24.

Soeken KL, Miller SA, Ernst E. Herbal medicines for the treatment of rheumatoid arthritis: a systematic review. Rheumatology (Oxford) 2003;42:652–659.

Son JK, Son MJ, Lee E, et al. Ginkgetin, a Biflavone from *Ginkgo biloba* leaves, inhibits cyclooxygenases-2 and 5-lipoxygenase in mouse bone marrow-derived mast cells. Biol Pharm Bull 2005;28:2181–2184.

Son MJ, Moon TC, Lee EK, et al. Naturally occurring biflavonoid, ochnaflavone, inhibits cyclooxygenases-2 and 5-lipoxygenase in mouse bone marrow-derived mast cells. Arch Pharm Res 2006;29:282–286.

Srivastava SK, Singh SV. Cell cycle arrest, apoptosis induction and inhibition of nuclear factor kappa B activation in anti-proliferative activity of benzyl isothiocyanate against human pancreatic cancer cells. Carcinogenesis 2004;25:1701–1709.

Suh SJ, Chung TW, Son MJ, et al. The naturally occurring biflavonoid, ochnaflavone, inhibits LPS-induced iNOS expression, which is mediated by ERK1/2 via NF-kappaB regulation, in RAW264.7 cells. Arch Biochem Biophys 2006;447:136–146.

Sumner H, Salan U, Knight DW, Hoult JR. Inhibition of 5-lipoxygenase and cyclo-oxygenase in leukocytes by feverfew. Involvement of sesquiterpene lactones and other components. Biochem Pharmacol 1992;43:2313–2320.

Sun Y, Li YH, Wu XX, et al. Ethanol extract from *Artemisia vestita*, a traditional Tibetan medicine, exerts anti-sepsis action through down-regulating the MAPK and NF-kappaB pathways. Int J Mol Med 2006;17:957–962.

Sung B, Ahn KS, Aggarwal BB. Noscapine, a benzylisoquinoline alkaloid, sensitizes leukemic cells to chemotherapeutic agents and cytokines by modulating the NF-kappaB signaling pathway. Cancer Res 2010;70:3259–3268.

Sung B, Pandey MK, Aggarwal BB. Fisetin, an inhibitor of cyclin-dependent kinase 6, down-regulates nuclear factor-kappaB-regulated cell proliferation, antiapoptotic and metastatic gene products through the suppression of TAK-1 and receptor-interacting protein-regulated IkappaBalpha kinase activation. Mol Pharmacol 2007;71:1703–1714.

Sung B, Pandey MK, Ahn KS, et al. Anacardic acid (6-nonadecyl salicylic acid), an inhibitor of histone acetyltransferase, suppresses expression of nuclear factor-kappaB-regulated gene products involved in cell survival, proliferation, invasion, and inflammation through inhibition of the inhibitory subunit of nuclear factor-kappaBalpha kinase, leading to potentiation of apoptosis. Blood 2008a;111:4880–4891.

Sung B, Pandey MK, Nakajima Y, et al. Identification of a novel blocker of IkappaBalpha kinase activation that enhances apoptosis and inhibits proliferation and invasion by suppressing nuclear factor-kappaB. Mol Cancer Ther 2008b;7:191–201.

Syrovets T, Buchele B, Krauss C, Laumonnier Y, Simmet T. Acetyl-boswellic acids inhibit lipopolysaccharide-mediated TNF-alpha induction in monocytes by direct interaction with IkappaB kinases. J Immunol 2005;174:498–506.

Tak PP, Firestein GS. NF-kappaB: a key role in inflammatory diseases. J Clin Invest 2001;107:7–11.

Takada Y, Aggarwal BB. Betulinic acid suppresses carcinogen-induced NF-kappa B activation through inhi-bition of I kappa B alpha kinase and p65 phosphorylation: abrogation of cyclooxygenase-2 and matrix metalloprotease-9. J Immunol 2003;171:3278–3286.

Takada Y, Aggarwal BB. Flavopiridol inhibits NF-kappaB activation induced by various carcinogens and inflammatory agents through inhibition of IkappaBalpha kinase and p65 phosphorylation: abrogation of cyclin D1, cyclooxygenase-2, and matrix metalloprotease-9. J Biol Chem 2004;279:4750–4759.

Takada Y, Andreeff M, Aggarwal BB. Indole-3-carbinol suppresses NF-kappaB and IkappaBalpha kinase activation, causing inhibition of expression of NF-kappaB-regulated antiapoptotic and metastatic gene products and enhancement of apoptosis in myeloid and leukemia cells. Blood 2005a;106:641–649.

Takada Y, Ichikawa H, Badmaev V, Aggarwal BB. Acetyl-11-keto-beta-boswellic acid potentiates apoptosis, inhibits invasion, and abolishes osteoclastogenesis by suppressing NF-kappa B and NF-kappa B-regulated gene expression. J Immunol 2006;176:3127–3140.

Takada Y, Kobayashi Y, Aggarwal BB. Evodiamine abolishes constitutive and inducible NF-kappaB activa-tion by inhibiting IkappaBalpha kinase activation, thereby suppressing NF-kappaB-regulated antiapop-totic and metastatic gene expression, up-regulating apoptosis, and inhibiting invasion. J Biol Chem 2005b;280:17203–17212.

Takada Y, Murakami A, Aggarwal BB. Zerumbone abolishes NF-kappaB and IkappaBalpha kinase activation leading to suppression of antiapoptotic and metastatic gene expression, upregulation of apoptosis, and downregulation of invasion. Oncogene 2005c;24:6957–6969.

Tao X, Younger J, Fan FZ, Wang B, Lipsky PE. Benefit of an extract of *Tripterygium wilfordii* Hook F in patients with rheumatoid arthritis: a double-blind, placebo-controlled study. Arthritis Rheum 2002;46:1735–1743.

Teekachunhatean S, Kunanusorn P, Rojanasthien N, et al. Chinese herbal recipe versus diclofenac in symp-tomatic treatment of osteoarthritis of the knee: a randomized controlled trial [ISRCTN70292892]. BMC Complement Altern Med 2004;4:19.

Terkeltaub RA. Clinical practice. Gout. N Engl J Med 2003;349:1647–1655.

Verhoeckx KC, Korthout HA, van Meeteren-Kreikamp AP, et al. Unheated *Cannabis sativa* extracts and its major compound THC-acid have potential immuno-modulating properties not mediated by CB1 and CB2 receptor coupled pathways. Int Immunopharmacol 2006;6:656–665.

Wadsworth TL, McDonald TL, Koop DR. Effects of *Ginkgo biloba* extract (EGb 761) and quercetin on lipopolysaccharide-induced signaling pathways involved in the release of tumor necrosis factor-alpha. Biochem Pharmacol 2001;62:963–974.

Wagner H, Fessler B. *In vitro* 5-lipoxygenase inhibition by *Eclipta alba* extracts and the coumestan derivative wedelolactone. Planta Med 1986;52:374–377.

Wang C, Schuller Levis GB, Lee EB, et al. Platycodin D and D3 isolated from the root of *Platycodon grandi-florum* modulate the production of nitric oxide and secretion of TNF-alpha in activated RAW 264.7 cells. Int Immunopharmacol 2004;4:1039–1049.

Wang J, Tokoro T, Higa S, Kitajima I. Anti-inflammatory effect of pitavastatin on NF-kappaB activated by TNF-alpha in hepatocellular carcinoma cells. Biol Pharm Bull 2006;29:634–639.

Whan Han J, Gon Lee B, Kee Kim Y, et al. Ergolide, sesquiterpene lactone from *Inula britannica*, inhibits inducible nitric oxide synthase and cyclo-oxygenase-2 expression in RAW 264.7 macrophages through the inactivation of NF-kappaB. Br J Pharmacol 2001;133:503–512.

Winther K, Apel K, Thamsborg G. A powder made from seeds and shells of a rose-hip subspecies (*Rosa canina*) reduces symptoms of knee and hip osteoarthritis: a randomized, double-blind, placebo-controlled clinical trial. Scand J Rheumatol 2005;34:302–308.

Won JH, Park SY, Nam SG, et al. Inhibition of lipopolysaccharide-induced expression of inducible nitric oxide and cyclooxygenase-2 by chiisanoside via suppression of nuclear factor-kappaB activation in RAW 264.7 macrophage cells. Biol Pharm Bull 2005;28:1919–1924.

Woo ER, Pokharel YR, Yang JW, Lee SY, Kang KW. Inhibition of nuclear factor-kappaB activation by 2′,8″-biapigenin. Biol Pharm Bull 2006;29:976–980.

Wu MJ, Wang L, Ding HY, Weng CY, Yen JH. *Glossogyne tenuifolia* acts to inhibit inflammatory media-tor production in a macrophage cell line by downregulating LPS-induced NF-kappa B. J Biomed Sci 2004;11:186–199.

Xia YF, Ye BQ, Li YD, et al. Andrographolide attenuates inflammation by inhibition of NF-kappa B activation through covalent modification of reduced cysteine 62 of p50. J Immunol 2004;173:4207–4217.

Yang F, Oz HS, Barve S, et al. The green tea polyphenol (–)-epigallocatechin-3-gallate blocks nuclear factor-kappa B activation by inhibiting I kappa B kinase activity in the intestinal epithelial cell line IEC-6. Mol Pharmacol 2001;60:528–533.

Yasuda T. Cartilage destruction by matrix degradation products. Mod Rheumatol 2006;16:197–205.

Yu WY, Shen SW, Yang ZH. A clinical study of Suogudan granule in the treatment of rheumatoid arthritis. Chin J Integr Med 2005;11:255–259.

Yun JM, Kwon H, Hwang JK. *In vitro* anti-inflammatory activity of panduratin A isolated from *Kaempferia pandurata* in RAW264.7 cells. Planta Med 2003;69:1102–1108.

Zhang WJ, Hufnagl P, Binder BR, Wojta J. Antiinflammatory activity of astragaloside IV is mediated by inhibition of NF-kappaB activation and adhesion molecule expression. Thromb Haemost 2003;90:904–914.

Zi, X, Mukhtar H, Agarwal R. Novel cancer chemopreventive effects of a flavonoid antioxidant silymarin: inhibition of mRNA expression of an endogenous tumor promoter TNF alpha. Biochem Biophys Res Commun 1997;239:334–339.

Zou, J, Jin D, Chen W, et al. Selective cyclooxygenase-2 inhibitors from Calophyllum membranaceum. J Nat Prod 2005;68:1514–1518.

Zschocke S, van Staden J, Paulus K, et al. Stereostructure and anti-inflammatory activity of three diastereomers of ocobullenone from Ocotea bullata. Phytochemistry 2000;54:591–595.

23 *Boswellia serrata* for Arthritis Relief
A Journey from Frankincense to Aflapin and 5-Loxin

Alluri Venkata Krishnaraju, Krishanu Sengupta,
Siba P. Raychaudhuri, and Golakoti Trimurtulu

CONTENTS

INTRODUCTION

Inflammation is a complex process triggered in response to noxious stimuli, trauma, or infection. Inflammation is characterized by redness, heat, swelling, and pain, and the response is modulated by inflammatory mediators and inflammatory cells. A number of inflammatory mediators, such as kinins, cytokines, eicosanoids, enzymes, and adhesion molecules, act on specific targets, leading to the local release of other mediators from leukocytes, and they also attract leukocytes to the site of inflammation. Unchecked and improperly phased inflammation can lead to persistent tissue damage, resulting in a wide range of inflammatory disorders including arthritis [1]. Inflammation can be controlled effectively by inhibiting the formation of inflammatory mediators, such as eicosanoids and proinflammatory cytokines. In majority, proinflammatory cytokines such as tumor necrosis factor α (TNF-α) and the various members of interleukin (IL) family, namely, IL-1, IL-6, and IL-8, are responsible to induce inflammatory cascades. Eicosanoids, prostaglandins, and leukotrienes (LTs) are produced primarily from arachidonic acid and are released from the cell membranes [2]. The formation of prostaglandins and LTs from arachidonic acid can be suppressed by inhibiting cyclooxygenase (COX) and lipoxygenase (LOX), respectively. In the enzyme family of COX, inhibition of COX-2 is more desirable. However, recent studies revealed that selective inhibition of COX-2 does reduce inflammation but causes side effects, particularly those leading to cardiovascular complications [3]. On the contrary, 5-LOX inhibition is not known to produce any adverse effects, and it improves bone health and promote fracture healing [4, 5].

Osteoarthritis (OA) is the most prevalent joint disorder characterized by articular cartilage degradation with an accompanying periarticular bone response. It affects various joints, with diverse clinical patterns, but OA of the hip and knee is the major cause of disability in elderly people. It is a growing health concern that has become a major challenge to the health professionals. OA is a slowly developing disorder contributed by complex etiology, including age, genetic, hormonal, and mechanical factors [6]. Pathology of OA involves moderate inflammation of synovial membrane, which may be most pronounced immediately adjacent to the OA lesion, indicating a link between cartilage lesion and synovium inflammation [7]. The inflammatory reaction is further triggered by various mediators released from damaged cartilage, including inflammatory cytokines (mainly IL-1β and IL-6) and arachidonic acid metabolites, for example, prostanoids (PGE$_2$). These stimuli further modulate synovial cells, including macrophages, T cells, and fibroblasts; and produce high levels of inflammatory cytokines, including IL-1β and TNF-α [8].

ALTERNATIVE MEDICINE

Naturally derived or originated compounds play a significant role as drug candidates and as lead structures for the development of synthetic molecules for therapeutic applications [9]. Approximately 50% of the drugs introduced into the market during the last two decades are derived either directly or indirectly from small biogenic molecules. Rational drug discovery approaches failed to yield expected results, and the rate of new drug molecules introduced into the market has shrunken drastically. As such, natural products will continue to play a major role in the future as active substances and model molecules for the discovery and validation of drug targets. A multidisciplinary approach to drug discovery involving the generation of truly novel molecular diversity from natural product sources, combined with total and combinatorial synthetic methodologies, provides the best solution to increase the productivity in drug discovery and development. Screening for new drugs in plants implies the screening of extracts for the presence of novel compounds and an investigation of their biological activities. It is currently estimated that approximately 420,000 plant species exist in nature. For the purpose of lead discovery or for the scientific validation of a traditional medicinal plant or a phytopharmaceutical, active principals in complex matrices need to be identified. Therefore, the interfacing of biological and chemical assessment becomes the critical issue. Drug discovery from plants can be guided by epidemiologic studies facilitated with computer-assisted high-pressure liquid chromatography microfractionation and microplate technology. Epidemiologic studies, for example, have shown that high dietary flavonoid intake may be associated with decreased risk for cardiovascular disease [10].

There are several natural products known to have moderate to potent anti-inflammatory activity. Gum resin of *Boswellia* species, known as Indian frankincense, has been used as an anti-inflammatory agent in traditional Ayurvedic medicine in India. Ancient Ayurvedic texts described its therapeutic use. Clinical studies have shown fair to excellent results in up to 88% of the patients, with no adverse side effects [11, 12].

INDIAN AYURVEDIC MEDICINE

Ayurveda is one of the oldest (more than 5000 years) and complete medical system that originated from the Vedic culture of India to provide healthy life to the mankind. In Sanskrit, *ayus* means "life" and *ved* signifies knowledge or science. It is not simply a health care system but a form of lifestyle to maintain balance between mind, senses, and body. The earliest literature of Ayurveda appeared during the Vedic period in India (3000–2000 BC). Ayurvedic practitioners also identified a number of medicinal preparations and surgical procedures for curing various ailments and diseases. The treatises available on Ayurveda include Astanga Hridayam, Sushruta Samhita, and Charaka Samhita.

BOSWELLIA SERRATA

Boswellia serrata is a medium-sized deciduous tree (Figure 23.1) belonging to Burseraceae family. Its gum exudate is a widely prescribed medicine in alternative systems of medicine including Ayurveda. Burseraceae is a family that consists of 540 species, including shrubs and trees distributed in 17–18 genera, also known as the torchwood family or incense tree family. It is native to tropical regions of Asia, Africa, and America. *B. serrata* is a moderately large branching tree that grows in the hilly regions of India. It grows to a height of approximately 12 ft. (4 m). It is commonly known as Indian Olibanum tree, Luban, Gond, and Gaja-bhaksha (implying its ingestion by elephants). The dried extracts of gum resin (Olibanum or frankincense) is known as sallaki in Ayurveda [13, 14].

The plant parts used are bark and gum resin. Gum resin is also known as frankincense secreted by trees of the genus *Boswellia*. From the very beginning of human civilization, it has been used for various therapeutic applications, in conditions such as pitta, cough, asthma, fevers, urethrorrhea, diaphoresis, convulsions, chronic laryngitis, and jaundice [15]. It has been claimed to decrease the degradation of glycosaminoglycans and thereby helps to prevent the destruction of articular cartilage [16]. It has been used in Europe since the beginning of the 20th century as a component in pharmacopoeia. Frankincense is still used in the region from North Africa to China as a remedy, especially in the traditional Ayurvedic medicine of India. The ethanolic extracts of *Boswellia* gum show various biological activities like anti-inflammatory, antiarthritic, analgesic activities [17], rheumatism, menstrual pain, and wrinkles [18, 19]. During an effort to identify novel biologically active compounds from plant origin and unraveling their mechanisms of action, it was observed that frankincense extracts inhibit LT biosynthesis *in vitro* [20].

CHEMICAL CONSTITUENTS

B. serrata is a host for a wide spectrum of primary and secondary metabolites. The therapeutic value of salai guggal, however, predominantly resides in its gum resin portion. The gum resin

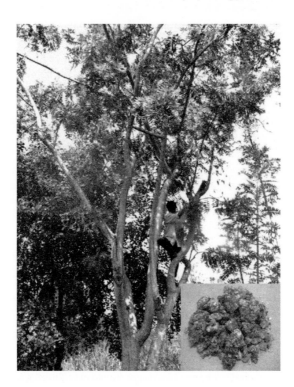

FIGURE 23.1   *Boswellia serrata* tree; inset picture shows dried gum resin.

and its extracts exhibit anti-inflammatory, antiarthritic, antirheumatic, antidiarrheal, antihyperlipidemic, antiasthmatic, anticancer, antimicrobial, and analgesic activities. The oleo-gum resin possesses interesting chemistry, which basically comprises of four groups of phytochemicals. These are the volatile components of essential oil, the nonvolatile neutral components of oil, the acidic components, and the water-soluble pentose and hexose sugar components of gum fraction [21].

The constituents of the essential oil of frankincense were investigated as early as 1840. The components of the essential oil fraction vary depending on the geographic origin of the resin, in addition to climatic and harvest conditions. The volatile oil compounds include (1) α-pinene; (2) α-phellandrene, α-thujene, p-cymene, and δ-limonene; and (3) geraniol, methylchavicol, and cadinene [22]. The prominent among the nonvolatile compounds of the oil is a cembrane-derived diterpene alcohol called (4) serratol [23]. Its concentration in the oil component varies in the range of 5%–10%. The other components of nonvolatile oil include cembrane, isocembrane, incensole, (5) α-amyrine, β-amyrine, (6) lupeol, and lupenoic acid [24, 25].

The anti-inflammatory actions of *B. serrata* gum resin have been attributed primarily to the acidic compounds, which contain predominantly a group of triterpene acids called boswellic acids. The chemical structures of the major constituents of *B. serrata* gum resin extract that include biologically active boswellic acids are depicted in Figure 23.2. These compounds include (7) α-boswellic acid, (8) β-boswellic acid, (9) 3-*O*-acetyl-α-boswellic acid, (10) 3-*O*-acetyl-β-boswellic acid, (11) 11-keto-β-boswellic acid (KBA), and (12) 3-*O*-acetyl-11-keto-β-boswellic acid (AKBA) [26]. The acid functional group in these compounds was taken advantage to selectively enrich these compounds from the gum resin using an aqueous alkali wash during production of commercial grades of *B. serrata* extracts containing 85% total boswellic acids. AKBA is biologically the most active component among its congeners. Other triterpenic acid, 3α-hydroxy-lup-20(29)-en-24-oic acid [25], has been reported as a constituent of gum resin. In addition, 2α,3α-dihydroxy-urs-12-ene-24-oic acid along with urs-12-ene-3α,24-diol was reported from the gum resin extract [27].

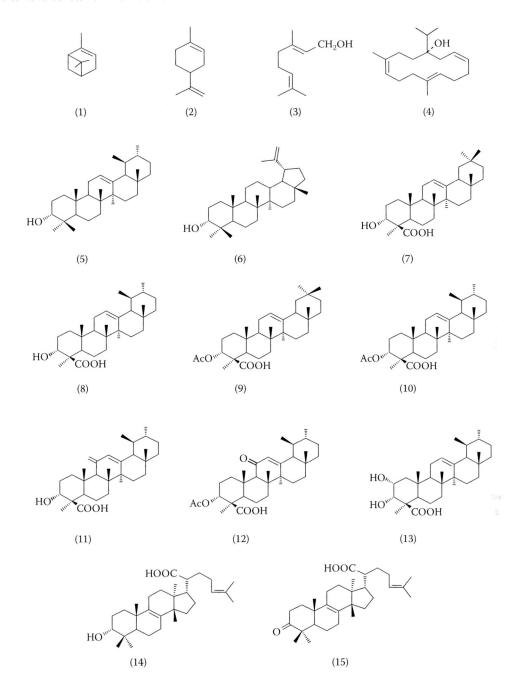

FIGURE 23.2 Chemical structures of the major bioactive compounds in *Boswellia* gum resin extract.

Tetracyclic triterpenoic acids, known as tirucallic acids, have also been reported by Pardhy and Bhattacharya [23, 26]. These compounds include (14) 3α-hydroxy-tirucall-8,24-dien-21-oic acid, (15) 3β-hydroxyl-tirucall-8,24-dien-21-oic acid and 3-keto-tirucall-8,24-dien-21-oic acid, and 3-α-acetoxy tirucall-8,24-dien-21-oic acid [28].

Finally, the water-soluble fraction of the gum resin contains D-galactose, D-arabinose, D-xylose, and D-mannose [21].

MECHANISMS OF ACTION

Boswellic acids, the biologically active ingredients of *B. serrata*, possess anti-inflammatory properties, and AKBA is known to be the most active 5-lipoxygenase inhibitor out of all boswellic acids known so far [29]. It is a potent noncompetitive, nonredox type 5-lipoxygenase inhibitor. In addition, boswellic acids also inhibit leukocyte elastase, which may also contribute to the anti-inflammatory properties of *Boswellia* [30]. AKBA blocks the synthesis of proinflammatory 5-lipoxygenase products, including 5-hydroxyeicosatetraenoic acid (5-HETE) and leukotriene B4 (LTB4), which cause bronchoconstriction, chemotaxis, and increased vascular permeability [31, 32]. In addition to 5-lipoxygenase inhibition, AKBA also exerts its efficacy through inhibiting 5-lipoxygenase activator protein (FLAP) and TNF-α. AKBA including other boswellic acids also inhibits polymorphonuclear leukocyte infiltration, migration, and the classical complement pathway.

PHARMACOLOGICAL ACTIVITIES

ANALGESIC AND PSYCHOPHARMACOLOGICAL EFFECTS

The gum resin of *B. serrata* exhibited marked analgesic activity in addition to mild sedative effect in experimental animals. *B. serrata* extract also produces reduction in the spontaneous motor activity and causes ptosis in rats [33].

ANTI-INFLAMMATORY

The anti-inflammatory actions of boswellic acids evaluated in *in vitro* and in several animal models state that 5-lipoxygenase, the key enzyme in LT biosynthesis, is the key target of their anti-inflammatory activity [20, 34]. LTs have long been recognized as potent mediators of inflammation and allergy. Thus, the concept that suppression of LT formation by boswellic acids as the underlying mechanism of the anti-inflammatory actions of the *Boswellia* extracts appears reasonable. It was first observed that *B. serrata* extracts inhibited the generation of LTB4 in rat neutrophils [20]. Inhibition of LT biosynthesis by isolated boswellic acids (BAs) was later confirmed by other studies. AKBA was identified as the most effective among the other boswellic acids, with IC50 values in the range of 1.5–8.0 μM, depending on the experimental settings (e.g., animal/human, cell type, stimulus, etc.) [29, 34–38]. Although in cell-free systems the direct inhibition of 5-LOX by AKBA was demonstrated independently [36], significantly higher concentrations were required to suppress 5-LOX activity *in vitro* as compared with intact cells. It suggests that potent inhibition of LT formation might be due to interference with cellular events required for activation of the enzyme. Lower concentrations of boswellic acids upregulated 5-LOX activity, whereas higher concentrations of *Boswellia* extracts were needed to inhibit 5-LO product synthesis in stimulated polymorphonuclear leukocytes [35]. Nuclear factor κB (NF-κB) signaling represents a major proinflammatory pathway, and it was found to be suppressed by AKBA in human peripheral monocytes. This blockade caused inhibition of lipopolysaccharide (LPS)-stimulated TNF-α expression, apparently by direct interference with "inhibition of NF-κB kinases" [39]. NF-κB downregulation might also explain altered effector levels observed in a human genome screen using TNF-α-stimulated human microvascular cells [40]. The results of this screen substantiate anti-inflammatory effects of BAs. In addition, in corroboration, a semisynthetic form of AKBA showed the inhibition of P-selectin upregulation and leukocyte–platelet adherence in colitis model of mice [41]. Taken together, boswellic acids exert multidirectional effects on various cell types implicated in inflammation and immunity.

ANTIARTHRITIC ACTIVITIES

Antiarthritic efficacy of mixture of boswellic acids is effective in case of both adjuvant arthritis as well as established arthritis. It also showed antipyretic effect, with no ulcerogenic effect [42]. Boswellic acids and glucosamine exhibited mild anti-inflammatory and moderate antiarthritic activity against mycobacterium-induced arthritis. The combination of boswellic acids and glucos-amine did not showed anti-inflammatory activity but exhibited potent antiarthritic activity [43]. Boswellic acids exhibited dose-dependent efficacy against bovine serum albumin (BSA)–induced arthritis in rabbits. Oral administration of BAs significantly reduced leukocytes population in BSA-injected knee. Local injection of BAs before BSA challenge significantly reduced infiltration of leukocytes in to pleural cavity [44]. These results suggest that *Boswellia* extracts and boswellic acids could be potentially useful as antiarthritic agents.

ANTICOLITIS EFFICACY

Boswellic acids confer protection in experimental murine models of colitis through the inhibition of leukocyte–endothelial cell adhesion. All of the protective responses observed with AKBA supplementation were comparable with that of corticosteroid treatment [41]. On the contrary, the other preclinical efficacy study indicated that BE supplementation resulted in no improvement in murine model of colitis [45]. However, in a randomized placebo-controlled clinical study, *B. serrata* extract has been proven to be clinically effective in collagenous colitis subjects. It was clinically effective against histologically proven colitis. *B. serrata* supplementation for 6 weeks resulted in better remission in clinical symptoms and showed better quality of life scores when compared with placebo [46].

EFFECTS ON LEUKOCYTES MIGRATION

B. serrata exerts marked inhibitory effect on both volume and leukocyte population of pleural exudates induced by carrageenan. This result indicates that *B. serrata* prevents leukocytes migration into the inflammatory exudates [47].

ANTIULCER ACTIVITY

Antiulcerogenic efficacy of *Boswellia* extract was evaluated using various animal models, viz., pyloric ligation, ethanol-HCl, acetylsalicylic acid, indomethacin, and cold restrained stress-induced ulceration in rats. Supplementation of *Boswellia* extract (BE) resulted in a dose-dependent antiulcer efficacy in various experimental models. It showed efficacy in all the tested models with different degrees of inhibition of the ulcer scores toward different ulcerogenic agents [48].

MODULATION OF IMMUNE RESPONSE

Various preparations of *Boswellia* extracts have been subjected to cellular and molecular studies to identify the pharmacological principles and mechanisms of action of the gum resin. First report indicated that *Boswellia* extracts antagonize the host defense system by impairment of leukocyte infiltration and the complement system [30, 49, 50]. Other mechanisms that may contribute to the modulation of the immune response include antiallergic/anaphylactic effects (inhibition of mast cell degranulation and suppression of macrophage nitric oxide production) and alteration of T helper (Th) cell signaling (Th1 cytokine inhibition and Th2 cytokine potentiation) [51–53].

ANTICANCER ACTIVITY

Boswellic acids inhibit glioma cell proliferation in a dose-dependent manner and showed prominent antiedema effect in glioblastoma patients. It was also revealed that boswellic acid–induced apoptosis is protein synthesis dependent and not associated with free radical scavenging activity [54]. Boswellic acids are effective cytotoxic agents, acting through the inhibition of topoisomerase activity. Boswellic acids induce apoptosis in glioma cells in synergy with the cytotoxic cytokine, CD95 ligand [55]. A case study where the subject bearing breast cancer brain metastases was unresponsive to standard therapy was successfully reversed by the chronic supplementation of *B. serrata* extract. The results suggest that boswellic acids can be potential new therapy for breast cancer patients with brain metastases and that BE may be also be useful as an adjuvant to standard therapies [56].

CHOLESTEROL LOWERING AND HYPOLIPIDEMIC ACTIVITIES

B. serrata gum resin extracts are known to play a role in reducing cholesterol. Water-soluble fraction of *B. serrata* extract exhibited significant reduction in total cholesterol and increased high-density lipoprotein in rats fed with atherogenic diet. In addition to its hypolipidemic potential, it can also improve healthy cholesterol level [57].

ANTIATHEROGENIC ACTIVITY

Antiatherosclerotic efficacy of AKBA was evaluated in LPS-induced mice model. Treatment of AKBA resulted in 50% relief from atherosclerotic lesions, and the reduction is statistically significant. AKBA treatment also resulted in significant downregulation of NF-κB-dependent genes [58].

HEPATOPROTECTIVE ACTIVITY

Hexane extract of *B. serrata* was evaluated for hepatoprotective efficacy against carbon tetrachloride, paracetamol, or thioacetamide-induced hepatic injury. *B. serrata* extract significantly reduced the elevated levels of serum marker enzymes and prevented the increase in liver weight in all three models of liver injury [59].

INFLAMMATORY BOWEL DISEASE

B. serrata extract was found to be effective in treating diarrhea in inflammatory bowel syndrome patients without causing constipation. An 8-week, double-blind, placebo-controlled trial of 102 people with Crohn's disease compared the efficacy of standardized *Boswellia* extract against the commercial drug mesalazine [60]. The participants taking *Boswellia* supplement improved at least as good as those taking mesalazine, according to a standard score of Crohn's disease severity. In addition, another human trial also exhibited some indications to suggest that *Boswellia* might offer benefits in ulcerative colitis [12]. The *B. serrata* extract was also found to be effective against diarrhea induced by acetylcholine and barium chloride in rodents [61].

ANTIMICROBIAL ACTIVITY

Essential oil obtained from *B. serrata* exhibited significant antimicrobial activity against *Staphylococcus aureus*, *Escherichia coli*, and *Proteus mirabilis* [62]. *B. serrata* extract exhibited potent antimicrobial activity against *Clostridium perfringens*, *Propionibacterium acnes*, and *Porphyromonas gingivalis* at low concentrations [63].

BIOAVAILABILITY AND METABOLISM

The bioavailability of KBA and AKBA, the most potent among boswellic acids, was evaluated in human subjects under fasting conditions. Both the compounds exhibited poor bioavailability in these pharmacokinetic studies [64]. In a different human study, the bioavailability of the boswellic acids was tested both under fasted and fed conditions. Bioavailability of boswellic acids under fed conditions was found to be five fold better than that observed under fasting conditions [65]. The permeation of KBA and AKBA was examined in human Caco-2 cell line. In addition, the interaction of KBA and AKBA with the organic anion transporter protein 1 B3 (OATP1B3) and the multidrug-resistant proteins P-glycoprotein MRP2 was also evaluated using partly fluorescent-based assays. The permeability studies revealed poor permeability for AKBA, but the KBA showed moderate absorption.

Neither KBA nor AKBA could be identified as substrates of P-glycoprotein. However, both KBA and AKBA modulated the activity of OATP1B3 and MRP2, indicating a possible therapeutic interaction with other anionic drugs [66]. The metabolic stability of KBA and AKBA was investigated in an *in vitro* system using rat liver microsomes and hepatocytes. When rat hepatocytes are incubated with KBA and AKBA, more than 80% of the initial KBA was metabolized after 30 min, whereas 80% of the starting AKBA concentration still remained after 120 min. These *in vitro* findings were correlated with the metabolic profiles of KBA and AKBA obtained in rats *in vivo*. In rat liver microsomes and hepatocytes as well as in human liver microsomes, it was observed that KBA but not AKBA undergoes extensive phase I metabolism. Oxidation to hydroxylated metabolites is the principal metabolic route. During *in vitro* studies, KBA yielded metabolic profiles similar to those obtained *in vivo* in rat plasma and liver, whereas no metabolites of AKBA could be identified *in vivo*. Furthermore, AKBA is not deacetylated to KBA. This study indicates that the AKBA not only exhibits most potent activity but also shows longer biological half-life compared with other boswellic acids. Hence, efficacy of *B. serrata* extract can be improved by increasing its AKBA content or bioavailability of AKBA [67].

TOXICITY STUDIES

The toxicity of *B. serrata* extract was established in two species of animals including rodents and primates. These studies manifested the safety and nontoxic nature of *B. serrata* extracts [68]. The irritation potential of *Boswellia* extract and AKBA was evaluated in *in vitro* cytotoxicity test on human skin-derived cell lines HaCaT, NCTC 2544, and HFFF2. The result indicated that compared with *B. serrata* extract, AKBA showed relatively higher toxicity selectively on lysosomes than that on mitochondria [69]. *B. serrata* hexane extract did not produce any mortality up to the highest concentration (1750 mg/kg) tested [59].

The genotoxic potential of *B. serrata* extract was carried out in Wistar rats using different cytogenetic assay system abnormalities, viz., chromosomal aberrations, sperm morphology, micro nuclei, and comet assays. BE did not show any genotoxicity at any dose level up to the highest concentration (1000 mg/kg) tested, suggesting that *B. serrata* extracts are quite safe for human consumption [70].

CLINICAL STUDIES

Efficacy of *B. serrata* extract was evaluated against different inflammatory aliments in human subjects. The efficacy and the tolerability of BE and their compositions were tested against knee OA in various clinical trials. These studies conferred significant efficacies to BE over placebo. These studies indicated that the onset of efficacy is slower but the efficacy lasts for 1 month after withdrawal [71–73]. The efficacy of nutraceutical preparation containing *B. serrata* extract was tested in a randomized double-blind clinical study against OA. Supplementation of BE for 32 weeks afforded significant ($p < 0.01$) reduction of the Visual Analog Scale and the Western Ontario and MacMaster Universities Osteoarthritis Index pain scores [74]. The efficacy of BE was tested in a double-blind, placebo-controlled clinical study in bronchial asthma subjects. Seventy percent of the patients showed improvement of disease as evident by the disappearance of physical symptoms and signs such as dyspnea, number and frequency of attacks, increase in forced expiratory volume subset 1, forced vital capacity, and peak expiratory flow rate. Only 27% of the patients in the control group showed improvement in disease symptoms. The data showed a definite role of gum resin of *B. serrata* in the treatment of bronchial asthma [12]. In another double-blind controlled clinical study, *B. serrata* extract (900 mg t.i.d.) or sulfasalazine (3 g t.i.d.) were given orally to chronic colitis subjects for 6 weeks. Stool property score, histopathology, and scanning electron microscopy revealed that *B. serrata* might be an effective treatment in controlling chronic colitis with minimal side effects [75]. In another double-blind positive controlled human clinical trial, *B. serrata* was proven to be superior in both efficacy and tolerability over mesalazine in relieving the symptoms of Crohn's disease [76]. *B. serrata* extracts could also be a safe intervention against various cancers including gliomas. A case study where the subject bearing breast cancer brain metastases was not responsive to standard therapy was successfully reversed by chronic supplementation of *B. serrata* extract. The results of this study suggest a potential new area of therapy for breast cancer patients with brain metastases and that *Boswellia* may be useful as an adjuvant to available standard therapies [56, 77]. Many cancer clinical studies of *Boswellia* extracts against various cancers including recurrent glioma (Clinical Trial Registration # NCT00243022) are under progress.

DEVELOPMENT OF AKBA-ENRICHED EXTRACTS

AKBA is the most active constituent of frankincense. 5-Loxin is a novel standardized *B. serrata* extract containing 30% AKBA. It is produced commercially using viable process developed by the researchers at Laila Impex R&D Center (Indian Patent No. 205269). Its efficacy was established at molecular, genetic, and cellular levels using enzymatic and cell-based assays, and its beneficial effects were confirmed by *in vivo* studies [31, 40, 78]. Its safety was proven by a selected battery of preclinical safety studies [79], and its nongenotoxic nature was established using AMES test, mouse lymphoma test, and chromosomal aberration assays [80–82]. Finally, the proof of concept in humans was established by a double-blind placebo-controlled human clinical study [83]. Keeping in perfect consonance with its higher AKBA content, 5-Loxin exhibited significantly better inhibitory activity against 5-lipoxygenase when compared with other commercially available *Boswellia* extracts. In addition, its antibacterial and antiproliferative activities have also been found to be significant compared with the extracts containing lower concentration of AKBA.

IN VITRO EFFICACY STUDIES

The *in vitro* studies revealed superior efficacy of 5-Loxin over regular *Boswellia* extracts containing 3% AKBA. The genetic basis of the anti-inflammatory effects of 5-Loxin was tested in a system of TNF-α-induced gene expression in human microvascular endothelial cells (HMECs). 5-Loxin clearly downregulated 113 genes out of the 522 genes induced by TNF-α in HMECs. These 5-Loxin-sensitive genes are directly related to inflammation, cell adhesion, and proteolysis [40]. The efficacy of 5-Loxin against TNF-α-inducible MMP expression was tested in HMECs. In HMECs, TNF-α caused a dose-dependent induction of MMP3, MMP10, and MMP12. Pretreatment of HMECs with 5-Loxin for 2 days significantly prevented TNF-α-induced expression of MMP3, MMP10, and MMP12. TNF-α significantly induced MMP3 activity, and 5-Loxin treatment significantly inhibited MMP3 activity [78]. 5-Loxin exhibited 42.96% more effectiveness in inhibiting 5-LOX activity in comparison with BE-3. 5-Loxin completely abrogates the overexpression of 5-LOX and FLAP in LPS-induced THP-1 cells. 5-Loxin inhibits the LPS-induced activation of serine/threonine kinases of mitogen-activated protein kinase family. 5-Loxin inhibits IκB phosphorylation and p65 translocation to the nuclear compartment of THP-1 monocytes, thereby blocking LPS-induced NF-κB activation. 5-Loxin and regular BE-3 inhibit the TNF-α production in LPS-induced THP-1 human monocytes in a dose-dependent manner. Interestingly, 5-Loxin exhibited 71.14% ($p < 0.001$) better inhibition of TNF-α production when compared with BE-3 in the inflamed cells [31].

IN VIVO EFFICACY STUDIES

The *in vivo* anti-inflammatory properties of 5-Loxin were tested in rat models of inflammation and experimental arthritis. 5-Loxin exhibited significant and dose-dependent inhibition of carrageenan-induced rat paw edema in albino Wistar rats. It showed 18.23%, 23.65%, and 27.07% inhibition, respectively, at 25, 50, and 100 mg/kg body weight [40]. Antiarthritic efficacy of 5-Loxin was tested against Freund's adjuvant-induced arthritis in Sprague–Dawley (SD) rats. Oral supplementation of 5-Loxin offered a dose-dependent and statistically significant reduction in paw edema and showed 49.3%, 56.7%, and 68% reduction in paw edema at 25, 50, and 100 mg/kg body weight, respectively. The protection shown by 5-Loxin at 50 mg/kg dose was similar to that shown by prednisolone at 10 mg/kg dose level. 5-Loxin showed significantly better inhibition against adjuvant-induced inflammatory response compared with BE-3 [78].

MECHANISM OF ACTION

5-Loxin exerts anti-inflammatory activity by modulation of LT pathway. It is a selective, noncompetitive, nonredox inhibitor of 5-lipoxygenase enzyme. In addition, it also inhibits the activator protein of 5-lipoxygenase enzyme that is FLAP and Cysteinyl LT1 receptor. 5-Loxin inhibits the LPS-induced activation of serine/threonine kinases of mitogen-activated protein kinase family, which are the key players responsible for a variety of cellular responses, including inflammation. 5-Loxin inhibits IkBa phosphorylation and p65 translocation to the nuclear compartment of THP-1 monocytes and thereby blocks LPS-induced NF-κB activation. Collectively, these findings provide molecular basis for the anti-inflammatory properties of 5-Loxin [31]. Figure 23.3 illustrates a schematic diagram showing the molecular targets of 5-Loxin for its anti-inflammatory properties.

TOXICITY STUDIES

A broad-spectrum safety evaluation of 5-Loxin was carried out in a battery of *in vitro* and *in vivo* toxicity studies in microbial strains, cell lines, and animals. These studies indicate no adverse effects for 5-Loxin [79]. Acute oral toxicity tested in SD rats has revealed that the LD50 of 5-Loxin is greater than 5 g/kg body weight, a dose level that is several-fold higher than the recommended daily human dose (100 mg). Acute dermal toxicity tests in SD rats have revealed that its LD50 is greater than 2 g/kg body weight. 5-Loxin is classified as practically nonirritating to skin when topically applied to skin of New Zealand albino rabbits. 5-Loxin is mildly irritating to the eye when instilled in lower eye lids of New Zealand albino rabbits. A dose-dependent 90-day subchronic toxicity study was conducted on male and female SD rats. The animals in the treatment group were supplemented with a feed containing 0.025%, 0.25%, or 2.5% of 5-Loxin corresponding to 0.2, 2, or 20 g of human equivalence dose, respectively, for 90 days. Hematology, serum chemistry, and histopathological evaluations did not show any adverse effects in any of the organs tested. A comprehensive perusal of the safety data indicated that the no observed adverse effect level for male and female SD rats supplemented with 5-Loxin ad libitum is presumed to be at least 20 g/day human equivalence dose. Further, the genotoxic effect of 5-Loxin was evaluated using the Bacterial Reverse Mutation Test (AMES test), and the results show that 5-Loxin is nonmutagenic up to the highest tested concentration of 3000 μg/plate

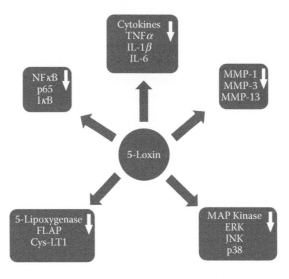

FIGURE 23.3 Molecular basis of anti-inflammatory properties of 5-Loxin.

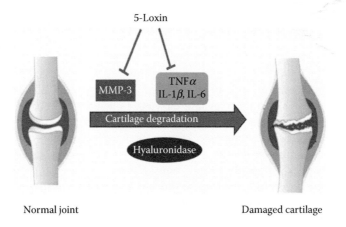

FIGURE 23.4   5-Loxin provides chondroprotection in OA.

[80]. 5-Loxin does not exhibit clastogenic potential to induce micronucleated reticulocytes of mouse peripheral blood in micronucleus assay in BALB/c mice. Also, 5-Loxin does not induce structural chromosome aberration in Chinese Hamster Ovary (CHO) cells with or without metabolic activation. Taken together, these studies confirm that 5-Loxin is nongenotoxic [81, 82].

CLINICAL STUDIES

On the basis of the superior activity shown by 5-Loxin in *in vitro* and *in vivo* studies, its efficacy was evaluated against OA in human subjects in a 90-day, double-blind, placebo-controlled human clinical study (ASRAM, Eluru, AP, India IRB# 06 001; Clinical trial registration number ISRCTN05212803). At both dose levels (100 and 250 mg/day) tested, 5-Loxin conferred clinically and statistically significant improvements in pain, joint stiffness, and physical function scores in OA patients. Interestingly, significant improvement in pain scores was observed in both the treatment groups supplemented with 5-Loxin at as early as 7 days. Figure 23.4 represents possible molecular mechanism of joint protection provided by 5-Loxin in OA.

In corroboration with the improvements in pain scores in the treatment groups, 5-Loxin also reduced the level of the cartilage degrading enzyme MMP3 in synovial fluid, and most importantly, 5-Loxin is safe for human consumption, even in the long term. The safety parameters were virtually unchanged in the treatment groups when compared with those in the placebo group [83]. This clinical study provides important information about the efficacy and safety of 5-Loxin in the treatment of OA and manifests that 5-Loxin can be a promising alternative therapeutic strategy, and it can be used as a nutritional supplement for pain management in OA patients.

Researchers at Laila Impex R&D Center endeavor continuously to develop improved anti-inflammatory products. Recently, we have developed a novel and synergistic composition, namely, Aflapin comprising *B. serrata* extract selectively enriched in AKBA, which possesses superior efficacy as an anti-inflammatory and anti-OA agent and showed better bioavailability than 5-Loxin and other *B. serrata* extracts commercially available in the market. Further validations on preclinical efficacy, clinical efficacy, and safety of Aflapin are under progress.

CONCLUSIONS

Since the early development of modern medicine, biologically active compounds from medicinal plants have played a vital role in providing medicines to combat variety of diseases or disorders. Several hundreds of medicinal plants have been described in Ayurveda, the traditional system of medicine in India, and in Indian folklore medicine for their beneficial effects on human health.

Ayurveda has vast literature in Sanskrit covering various aspects of diseases, therapeutics, and pharmacy. It had evolved through its own theoretical base, which is difficult to comprehend in terms of modern scientific concepts. However, with the advent of modern chemistry and biology and with their synchronized scientific efforts, it has been possible to define the biological activities of significantly large number of medicinal plants and their biologically active compounds in terms of modern scientific concepts.

In Ayurveda and in Indian folklore medicine, *B. serrata* is one of such medicinal plants with a variety of beneficial properties. The family of biologically active compounds in *B. serrata* extract is boswellic acids. The most biologically active member of this family is AKBA. Practically, the AKBA content is only 2%–3% in the highest grade of commercially available extract of *B. serrata*. Thus, the dose requirement to obtain an optimal therapeutic efficacy is very high for the regular extract. In addition, the biological properties of the regular *Boswellia* extract also vary significantly from batch to batch because of varying concentrations of AKBA. Therefore, with an intention to achieve a consistent efficacy at a significantly lower dose, the *Boswellia* extract has been enriched and standardized to contain 30% AKBA, and this is 5-Loxin. The current evidences in favor of anti-inflammatory properties of 5-Loxin are multidirectional. Series of *in vitro*, *in vivo*, and clinical studies reveal that 5-Loxin is able to modify the production and function of multiple number of biologically active molecules involved in inflammation and its related disorders. Interestingly, in corroboration with the hypothesis, the dose requirement of 5-Loxin is several times lower than the *Boswellia* regular extract. In addition, a battery of safety studies in appropriate models revealed that 5-Loxin is systemically and genetically nontoxic. Moreover, 5-Loxin is also safe and well tolerated to human subjects. Taken together, the multiple evidences support that use of 5-Loxin is a promising alternative therapeutic strategy, and it may be used as a dietary supplement against various inflammatory disorders including OA.

In summary, the researchers provided scientific validations in favor of anti-inflammatory properties and therapeutic efficacy of a chemically defined and enriched extract containing a natural compound, isolated from an ancient Indian medicinal plant, widely referred in Ayurveda for various inflammatory disorders in human.

ACKNOWLEDGMENTS

The authors sincerely thank Sri G. Ganga Raju, Chairman, Mr. G. Rama Raju, Director, and Mr. B. Kiran, CEO of Laila Group of Industries, India, for generous support and encouragements.

REFERENCES

1. Nathan C. Points of control in inflammation. Nature 2002;420:846–852.
2. Sharma JN, Mohammed LA. The role of leukotrienes in the pathophysiology of inflammatory disorders: is there a case for revisiting leukotrienes as therapeutic targets? Inflammopharmacology 2006;14:10–16.
3. Segev G, Kaetz RJ. Selective COX-2 inhibitors and risk of cardiovascular events. Hosp Physician 2004;40:39–46.
4. Traianedes K, Dallas MR, Garrett IR, Mundy GR, Bonewald LF. 5-Lipoxygenase metabolites inhibit bone formation in vitro. Endocrinology 1998;139:3178–3184.
5. Cottrell JA, O'Connor JP. Pharmacological inhibition of 5-lipoxygenase accelerates and enhances fracture-healing. J Bone Joint Surg Am 2009;91:2653–2665.
6. Cooper C, McAlindon T, Snow S, Vines K, Young P, Kirwan J, Dieppe P. Mechanical and constitutional risk factors for symptomatic knee osteoarthritis: differences between medial tibiofemoral and patellofemoral disease. J Rheumatol 1994;21:307–313.
7. Ayral X, Pickering EH, Woodworth TG, Mackillop N, Dougados M. Synovitis: a potential predictive factor of structural progression of medial tibiofemoral knee osteoarthritis—results of a 1 year longitudinal arthroscopic study in 422 patients. Osteoarthritis Cartilage 2005;13:361–367.
8. Saha N, Moldovan F, Tardif G, Pelletier JP, Cloutier JM, Martel-pelletier J. Interleukin-1β-converting enzyme/caspase-1 in human osteoarthritic tissues: localization and role in the maturation of IL-1β and IL-18. Arthritis Rheum 1999;42:1577–1587.

9. Vuorela P, Leinonen M, Saikku P, Tammela P, Rauhad JP, Wennberge T, Vuorela H. Natural products in the process of finding new drug candidates. Curr Med Chem 2004;11:1375–1389.

10. Mennen LI, Sapinho D, Arnault N, Bree A, Bertrais S, Galsn P, Hercberg S. Consumption of foods rich in flavonoids is related to a decreased cardiovascular risk in Apparently Healthy French Women. J Nutr 2003;134:923–926.

11. Gerhardt H, Seifert F, Buvari P, Vogelsang H, Repges R. Therapy of active Crohn disease with *Boswellia serrata* extract H15. J Gastroenterol 2001;39:11–17.

12. Gupta I, Gupta V, Parihar A, Gupta S, Ludtke R, Safayhi H, Ammon HP. Effects of *Boswellia serrata* gum resin in patients with bronchial asthma: results of a double-blind, placebo-controlled, 6-week clinical study. Eur J Med Res 1998;3:511–514.

13. Monograph: *Boswellia serrata*. Altern Med Rev 1998;3:306–307.

14. Kulkarni RR, Patki PS, Jog VP, Gandage SG, Patwardhan B. Treatment of osteoarthritis with a herbomineral formulation: a double blind, placebo controlled-cross over study. J Ethanopharmacol 1991;33:91–95.

15. Martinetz D, Lohs K, Janzen J. Weihrauch und Myrrhe: Kulturgeschichtlicheund wirtschaftl. Bedeutung; Botanik, Chemie, Medizin. Z Umwelrchem Okotrox 1990;2:236.

16. Reddy GK, Chandrakasan G, Dhar SC. Studies on metabolism of glycosaminoglycans under the influence of new herbal anti-inflammatory agents. Biochem Pharmacol 1989;38:3527–3534.

17. Mohan Ram HY, Sharma AK, Sukhdev D, Ambasta SP. The wealth of India raw materials, vol. 2-B. Delhi: CSIR; 1988:B.202–B.209.

18. Singh GB, Atal CK. Pharmacology of an extract of salai guggalex-*Boswellia serrata*, a new non-steroidal anti-inflammatory agent. Agents Actions 1986;18:407–412,

19. Reddy GK, Dhar SC, Singh GB. Urinary excretion of connective tissue metabolites under the influence of a new non-steroidal anti-inflammatory agent in adjuvant induced arthritis. Agents Actions 1987;22:99–105.

20. Ammon HPT, Mack T, Singh GB, Safayhi H. Inhibition of leukotrieneB4 formation in rat peritoneal neutrophils by an ethanolic extract of the gum resin exudates of *Boswellia serrata*. Planta Med 1991;57:203–207.

21. Bhargava GG, Negi JJ, Ghua HRD. Studies on the chemical composition of salai gum. Indian Forestry 1978;104:174–181.

22. Wahab SM, Aboutabl EA, El-Zalabani SM, Fouad HA, De Pooter HL, El-Fallaha B. The essential oil of olibanum. Planta Med 1987;53:382–384.

23. Pardhy RS, Bhattacharya SC. Structure of serratol, a new diterpene cembranoid alcohol from *Boswellia serrata* Roxb. Indian J Chem 1978;16B:171–173.

24. Sharma A, Mann AS, Gajbhiye VM, Kharya D. Phytochemical profile of *Boswellia serrata*: an overview. Phcog Rev 2007;1:137–142.

25. Culioli G, Mathe C, Archier P, Vieillescazes C. A lupane triterpene from frankincense (*Boswellia* sp., Burseraceae). Phytochemistry 2003;62:537–541.

26. Pardhy RS, Bhattacharya SC. Boswellic acid, acetyl-boswellic acid and 11-keto-boswellic acid, four pentacyclic triterpenic acids from the resin of *Boswellia serrata* Roxb. Indian J Chem 1978;16B:176–178.

27. Mahajan B, Taneja SC, Sethi VK, Dhar KL. Two triterpenoids from *Boswellia serrata* gum resin. Phytochemistry 1995;39:453–455.

28. Pardhy RS, Bhattacharya SC. Tetracyclic triterpenic acids from the resin of *Boswellia serrata* Roxb. Indian J Chem 1978;16B:174–175.

29. Sailer ER, Subramanian LR, Rall B, Hoernlein H, Ammon P, Safayhi H. Acetyl-11-keto-beta-boswellic acid: structure requirement for binding and 5-lipoxygenase inhibitory activity. Brit J Pharmacol 1996;117:615–618.

30. Kapil A, Moza N. Anticomplementary activity of boswellic acids-an inhibitor of C3-convertase of the classical complement pathway. Int J Immunopharmacol 1992;14:1139–1143.

31. Sengupta K, Golakoti T, Marisetti AK, Tummala T, Ravada SR, Alluri VK, Raychaudhuri SP. Inhibition of TNFα production and blocking of mitogen-activated protein kinase/NFκB activation in lipopolysaccharide-induced THP-1 human monocytes by 3-O-acetyl-11-keto-β-boswellic acid. J Food Lipids 2009;16:325–344.

32. *Boswellia serrata*. Altern Med Rev 2008;13:165–167.

33. Menon MK, Kar A. Analgesic and psychopharmacological activity of gum resin of *Boswellia serrata*. Planta Med 1970;19:51–54.

34. Safayhi H, Mack T, Sabieraj J, Anazodo MI, Subramanian LR, Ammon HP. Boswellic acids: novel, specific, nonredox inhibitors of 5-lipoxygenase. J Pharmacol Exp Ther 1992;261:1143–1146.

35. Safayhi H, Boden SE, Schweizer S, Ammon HP. Concentration-dependent potentiating and inhibitory effects of *Boswellia* extracts on 5-lipoxygenase product formation in stimulated PMNL. Planta Med 2000;66:110–113.
36. Safayhi H, Sailer ER, Ammon HP. Mechanism of 5-lipoxygenase inhibition by acetyl-11 keto-beta-boswellic acid. Mol Pharmacol 1995;47:1212–1216.
37. Werz O, Schneider N, Brungs M. A test system for leukotriene synthesis inhibitors based on the in-vitro differentiation of the human leukemic cell lines HL-60 and Mono Mac 6. Naunyn Schmiedebergs Arch Pharmacol 1997;356:441–445.
38. Werz O, Szellas D, Henseler M, Steinhilber D. Nonredox 5-lipoxygenase inhibitors require glutathione peroxidase for efficient inhibition of 5-lipoxygenase activity. Mol Pharmacol 1998;54:445–451.
39. Syrovets T, Buchele B, Krauss C, Laumonnier Y, Simmet T. Acetyl-boswellic acids inhibit lipopolysaccharide-mediated TNF-alpha induction in monocytes by direct interaction with IkappaB kinases. J Immunol 2005;174:498–506.
40. Roy S, Khanna S, Shah H, Rink C, Phillips C, Preuss H, Subbaraju GV, et al. Human genome screen to identify the genetic basis of the anti-inflammatory effects of *Boswellia* in micro vascular endothelial cells. DNA Cell Biol 2005;24:244–255.
41. Anthoni C, Laukoetter MG, Rijcken E, Vowinkel T, Mennigen R, Müller S, Senninger N, et al. Mechanisms underlying the anti-inflammatory actions of boswellic acid derivatives in experimental colitis. Am J Physiol Gastrointest Liver Physiol 2006;290:G1131–G1137.
42. Singh GB, Atal CK. Assessment of total boswellic acids for anti-inflammatory activity. Indian J Pharmacol 1984;16:51–51.
43. Singh S, Khajuria A, Taneja SC, Khajuria RK, Singh J, Qazi GN. Boswellic acids and glucosamine show synergistic effect in preclinical anti-inflammatory study in rats. Bioorg Med Chem Lett 2007;17:3706–3711.
44. Sharma ML, Bani S, Singh GB. Anti-arthritic activity of boswellic acids in bovine serum albumin (BSA)–induced arthritis. Int J Immunopharmacol 1989;11:647–652.
45. Pawel RK, Anna JM, Nesrin K, Shivanand DJ, Aniko MS, David GB, Barbara NT, Fayez KG. Effects of *Boswellia serrata* in mouse models of chemically induced colitis. Am J Physiol Gastrointest Liver Physiol 2005;288:G798–G808.
46. Ahmed M, Stephan M, Otto E, Jenny M, Bright B, Eberhard K, Elke B, et al. *Boswellia serrata* extract for the treatment of collagenous colitis. A double-blind, randomized, placebo-controlled, multicenter trial. Int J Colorectal Dis 2007;22:1445–1451.
47. Ammon HTP, Mark T, Singh GB, Safayhi H. Inhibition of leukotriene B4 formation in rat peritoneal neutrophils by an ethanolic extract of gum resin exudates of *Boswellia serrata*, Plant Medica 1991;57:203–207.
48. Singh S, Khajuria A, Taneja SC, Khajuria RK, Singh J, Johri RK, Qazi GN. The gastric ulcer protective effect of boswellic acids, a leukotriene inhibitor from Boswellia serrata, in rat. Phytomedicine 2008;15:408–415.
49. Sharma ML, Khajuria A, Kaul A, Singh S, Singh GB, Atal CK. Effect of salai guggal ex-*Boswellia serrata* on cellular and humoral immune responses and leucocyte migration. Agents Actions 1998;24:161–164.
50. Knaus U, Wagner H. Effects of boswellic acid of *Boswellia serrata* and other triterpenic acids on the complement system. Phytomedicine 1996;3:77–81.
51. Pungle P, Banavalikar M, Suthar A, Biyani M, Mengi S. Immunomodulatory activity of boswellic acids of *Boswellia serrata* Roxb. Indian J Exp Biol 2003;41:1460–1462.
52. Pandey RS, Singh BK, Tripathi YB. Extract of gum resins of *Boswellia serrata* L. inhibits lipopolysaccharide induced nitric oxide production in rat macrophages along with hypolipidemic property. Ind J Exp Biol 2005;43:509–516.
53. Chevrier MR, Ryan AE, Lee DY, Zhongze M, Wu-Yan Z, Via CS. *Boswellia carterii* extract inhibits TH1 cytokines and promotes TH2 cytokines in vitro. Clin Diagn Lab Immunol 2005;12:575–580.
54. Boker DK, Winking M. Die Rolle von *Boswellia sauren* in der therapie maligner glione. Deutsches Arzteblatt 1997;94:B958–B960.
55. Glaser T, Winter S, Groscurth P, Safayhi H, Sailer ER, Ammon HPT, Schabet M, Weller M. Boswellic acids and malignant glioma: induction of apoptosis but no modulation of drug sensitivity. Br J Cancer 1999;80:756–765.
56. Flavin DF. A lipoxygenase inhibitor in breast cancer brain metastases. J Neurooncol 2007;82:91–93.
57. Zutsi U, Rao PG, Kaur S. Mechanism of cholesterol lowering effect of salai guggal ex-*Boswellia serrata* Roxb. Indian J Pharmacol 1986;18:182–183.
58. Clarisse C, Ludivine B, Eric B, Corinne C, Daniel SA, Felicitas G. Antiinflammatory and antiatherogenic effects of the NF-κB inhibitor AKBA in LPS-challenged ApoE–/– mice. Thromb Vasc Biol 2008;28:272–277.
59. Jyothi Y, Jagadish VK, Asad M. Effect of hexane extract of *Boswellia serrata* oleo-gum resin on chemically induced liver damage. Pak J Pharm Sci 2007;19:125–129.

60. Gerhardt H, Seifert F, Buvari P, Vogelsang H, Repges R. Therapy of active Crohn disease with *Boswellia serrata* extract H15. Z Gastroenterol 2001;39:11–17.

61. Borrelli F, Capasso F, Capasso R. Effect of *Boswellia serrata* on intestinal motility in rodents: inhibition of diarrhea without constipation. Br J Pharmacol 2006;148:553–560.

62. Kasali AA, Adio AM, Kundayo OE, Oyedeji AO, Adefenwa AOEM, Adeniyi BA. Antimicrobial activity of the essential oil of *Boswellia serrata* Roxb. (fam. Burseraceae) bark. J Essent Oil-Bearing Plants 2002;5:173–175.

63. Weckessera S, Engela K, Simon-Haarhausa B, Wittmerb A, Pelzb K, Schempp CM. Screening of plant extracts for antimicrobial activity against bacteria and yeasts with dermatological relevance. Phytomedicine 2007;14:508–516.

64. Sterk V, Büchele B, Simmet T. Effect of food intake on the bioavailability of boswellic acids from a herbal preparation in healthy volunteers. Planta Med 2004;70:1155–1160.

65. Sharma S, Thawani V, Hingorani L, Shrivastava M, Bhate VR, Khiyani R. Pharmacokinetic study of 11-keto beta-boswellic acid. Phytomedicine 2004;11:1255–1260.

66. Phillip K, Johanna K, Jessica H. Permeation of *Boswellia* extract in the Caco-2 model and possible interactions of its constituents KBA and AKBA with ATP1B3 and MRP2. Eur J Pharm Sci 2009;36:275–284.

67. Kruger P, Daneshfar R, Eckert GP, Klein J, Volmer DA, Bahr U, Müller WE, et al. Metabolism of boswellic acids *in vitro* and *in vivo*. Drug Metab Disp 2008;36:1135–1142.

68. Singh GB, Bani S, Singh S. Toxicity and safety evaluation of boswellic acids. Phytomedicine 1996;3:87–90.

69. Bruno B, Alessandro P, Andrea V, Anna MB. Comparison of the irritation potentials of *Boswellia serrata* gum resin and of acetyl-11-keto-β-boswellic acid by in vitro cytotoxicity tests on human skin-derived cell lines. Toxicolo Lett 2008;177:144–149.

70. Sharma R, Singh S, Singh GD, Khajuria A, Sidiq T, Singh SK, Chashoo G, et al. *In vivo* geno-toxicity evaluation of a plant based antiarthritic and anticancer therapeutic agent boswellic acids in rodents. Phytomedicine 2009;16:1112–1118.

71. Sontakke S, Thawani V, Pimpalkhute S, Kabra P, Babhulkar S, Hingorani L. Open, randomized, controlled clinical trial of Boswellia serrata extract as compared to valdecoxib in osteoarthritis of knee. Ind J Pharmacol 2007;39:27–29.

72. Kimmatkar N, Thawani V, Hingorani L, Khiyani R. Efficacy and tolerability of extract in treatment of osteoarthritis of knee—a randomized double blind placebo controlled trial. Phytomedicine 2003;10:3–7.

73. Farid AB, Tamer E, Adel AS, Samia AH, El-Batoty MF. Boswellia–curcumin preparation for treating knee osteoarthritis: a clinical evaluation. Alt Complementary Ther 2002;8:341–348.

74. Chopra A, Lavin P, Patwardhan B, Chitre D. A 32 week randomized, placebo controlled clinical evaluation of RA-11, an Ayurvedic drug, on osteoarthritis of the knees. J Clin Rheumatol 2004;10(5):236–245.

75. Ahmed M, Stephan M, Otto E, Jenny M, Birgit B, Eberhard K, Elke B, et al. *Boswellia serrata* extract for the treatment of collagenous colitis. A double-blind, randomized, placebo-controlled, multicenter trial. Int J Colorectal Dis 2007;22(12):1445–1451.

76. Herborn G, Rau R, Sander OZ. Therapy of active Crohn disease with *Boswellia serrata* extract H15. Gastroenterol 2001;39:11–17.

77. Winking M, Sarikaya S, Rahmanian A, Jodicke A, Boker DK. Boswellic acids inhibit glioma growth: a new treatment option? J Neurooncol 2000;46:97–103.

78. Roy S, Khanna S, Krishnaraju AV, Subbaraju GV, Yasmin T, Bagchi D, Sen CK. Regulation of vascular responses to inflammation: inducible matrix metalloproteinase-3 expression in human microvascular endothelial cells is sensitive to anti-inflammatory *Boswellia*. Antioxid Redox Signal 2006;3 and 4:653–660.

79. Lalithakumari K, Krishnaraju AV, Sengupta K, Subbaraju GV, Chatterjee A. Safety and toxicological evaluation of a novel, standardized 3-*O*-acetyl-11-keto-β-boswellic acid (AKBA)-enriched *Boswellia serrata* extract (5-Loxin). Toxicol Mech Meth 2006;16:199–226.

80. Indrani BK. Bacterial reverse mutation test with 5-Loxin® Study No. 4477/05. Bangalore, India: Toxicology Department, Advinus Therapeutics Private Limited.

81. Jung-Ti Chang. Micronucleus assay in mice for 5-Loxin. Study No. MN00075. Taipei, Taiwan: Center of Toxicology and Preclinical Sciences, Development Center for Biotechnology; 2008.

82. Jung-Ti Chang. Study number CA00094, In vitro chromosome aberration assay in Chinese hamster ovarian cells for 5-Loxin. Taipei, Taiwan: Center of Toxicology and Preclinical Sciences, Development Center for Biotechnology; 2008.

83. Sengupta K, Krishnaraju AV, Satish AR, Mishra S, Trimurtulu G, Sarma KVS, Dey D, Raychaudhuri SP. Double blind, randomized, placebo controlled study of the efficacy and safety of 5-Loxin for treatment of osteoarthritis of the knee. Arthritis Res Ther 2008;10:R85–R96.

24 Utilization of Marine Products in the Treatment and Prevention of Osteoarthritis

*Tadakazu Tamai, Ayako Honmura, Hisashi Yoshioka,
Tatsuya Konishi, Shisei Kuninaga, Hiroshi Oda,
Akinori Sakamoto, and Tsuyoshi Okada*

CONTENTS

INTRODUCTION

Cartilages used industrially as materials for the production of chondroitin sulfates are derived from pastoral animals such as bovine, porcine, and chicken and aquatic animals such as salmon, shark, stingray, and squid. Of the latter group, the shark is an elasmobranch that has its fin, skull, spine, and bone under the cheeks made from cartilage, and this cartilage is one of the most commonly used materials from sharks that are caught all over the world. In the past several years, the annual catch of sharks in the world has been approximately 700–900 thousand tons, and the main countries that catch sharks are Asian countries such as Indonesia, India, and Taiwan. Countries other than the Asian ones are Spain, the United States, and Mexico. One of the sharks that is used as a material for chondroitin sulfate is a type of a shark called the blue shark (*Prionace glauca*), which inhabit coastal areas and broad oceans of tropic and temperate regions all over the world. The skin is used for the fabrication of leather products, the flesh is transformed into saute and surimi (fish paste used in products such as kamaboko and chikuwa), and the fins become shark-fin soup. The cartilages of the fin that remain after making the shark-fin soup, and other cartilage parts are used as materials for the preparation of chondroitin sulfate for use in foods, cosmetics, and medicines. Other sharks known to be used as a material for chondroitin sulfate are sandbar sharks (*Carcharhinus plumbeus*) and salmon sharks (*Lamna ditropis*), each having a different habitat.

Raw material (shark cartilage) → Extraction → Decoloring and deodorizing → Filtration → Sterilization → Drying
→ Shark cartilage extract

FIGURE 24.1   Manufacturing process to obtain shark cartilage extract.

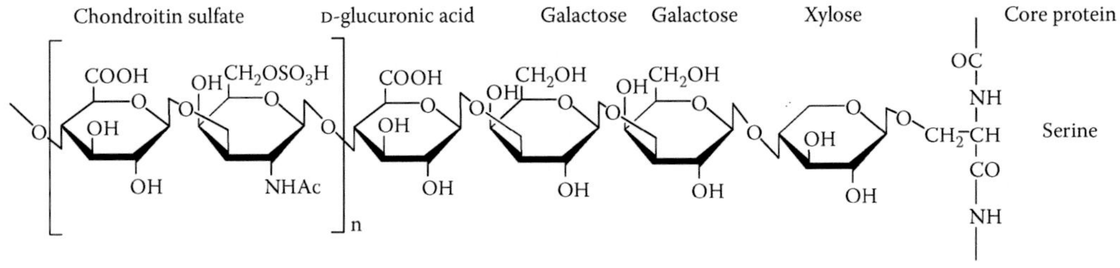

FIGURE 24.2   Structure of chondroitin sulfate peptide.

Each 100 g of dry shark cartilage usually contains several to 20 g of glycosaminoglycans. Other main components are collagen and inorganic materials such as calcium and sodium. Also, it contains many noncollagen proteins and core proteins that bind to the glycosaminoglycans. Other than the disaccharides composing its reducing terminus, chondroitin sulfate in these cartilages usually has trisaccharides composed of two molecules of galactose and xylose. This xylose and the serine in the core protein form the *O*-glycoside bond to result in the proteoglycan. Adding to that structure, the part of amino terminal domain of core proteins of chondroitin sulfate–based proteoglycans forms a noncovalent bond with hyaluronic acid to form a complex with a large molecular weight in the cartilage tissue. Owing to this composition, the macromolecule retains large amounts of water in it to function as a cushion against physical impact.

METHOD FOR PRODUCTION OF SHARK CARTILAGE EXTRACT

Highly purified sodium chondroitin sulfate ester is made by ethanol treating, by membrane treating, or by ion-exchange resin treating the chondroitin sulfate, which is freed by enzymatic treatment or extracted by alkaline solution. In Japan, this sodium chondroitin sulfate ester is on the market exclusively for use as a medicine or food additive according to the Pharmaceutical Affairs Law and the Food Sanitation Law. Also, sodium chondroitin sulfate ester is on the European Pharmacopoeia in Europe, and many countries in Europe, such as Switzerland, Italy, France, and Spain, use it as a medicine. On the other hand, in the 1980s, the Taiyo Fishery Co., Ltd. (presently Maruha Nichiro Foods, Inc., Tokyo, Japan), launched on the Japanese market a shark cartilage extract containing chondroitin sulfate peptide, "SCP," for use in food or as a dietary supplement. Since then, roughly extracted shark cartilages that have gone through simplified purification steps (Figure 24.1) such as decoloring and deodorizing only have been on the health-food market as shark cartilage extracts containing chondroitin sulfate in the form of tablets, capsules, granulated powders, drinks, and so forth. This shark cartilage extract contains chondroitin sulfate bound to a peptide from its core protein (Figure 24.2). Also, small amounts of glycosaminoglycan other than the chondroitin sulfate, collagen peptide, and peptides derived from noncollagen proteins in shark cartilage are contained in a mixed state (Table 24.1). Therefore, the physiological effect that the shark cartilage extract is expected to have is not just the function of chondroitin sulfate to ease joint pain but also the ill-defined beneficial functions of collagen peptide and other noncollagen peptides.

CHONDROITIN SULFATE IN THE SHARK CARTILAGE EXTRACT

Chondroitin sulfate is a linear heteropolymer comprising D-glucuronic acid bound to *N*-acetyl-D-galactosamine by a $\beta1\text{–}3$ bond to form a repeated disaccharide structure. This composing

TABLE 24.1
Analysis Example of Shark Cartilage Extract

Analysis Item	Analysis Result
Mucopolysaccharide	41%
Protein	55%
Fat	0.04%
Residue on ignition	8.7%
pH	6.1

TABLE 24.2
Difference in the Ratio of Composing Disaccharide in Chondroitin Sulfate (Analysis Example)

Unsaturated Disaccharide (%)	ΔDi-0S	ΔDi-6S	ΔDi-4S	ΔDi-diSd	ΔDi-diSb	ΔDi-diSe
Derived from shark	5.2	56.3	30.3	8.3	ND	ND
Derived from salmon	9.9	59.0	29.0	2.0	ND	ND
Derived from squid	13.6	12.4	52.0	ND	ND	22.1
Derived from bovine	4.1	21.0	72.4	0.7	ND	1.1

Note: ΔDi-0S, no sulfate group; ΔDi-4S, chondroitin sulfate A; ΔDi-6S, chondroitin sulfate C; ΔDi-diSb, chondroitin sulfate B; ΔDi-diSd, chondroitin sulfate D; ΔDi-diSe: chondroitin sulfate E; ND, not determined.

disaccharide regularly contains one molecule of *O*-sulfate per disaccharide unit. Chondroitin sulfate with the sulfate group bound to position 4 of the *N*-acetyl-D-galactosamine is called chondroitin sulfate A, and the one with the sulfate group bound to position 6 is called chondroitin sulfate C. Chondroitin sulfate in shark cartilage has these composing disaccharides mixed and repeated to form a macromolecule, but it is thought that these macromolecules contain a relatively high amount of chondroitin sulfate C. Also, chondroitin sulfate of the shark cartilage is known to contain chondroitin sulfate D, which has two molecules of the sulfate group per disaccharide unit, that is, a sulfate group bound to position 2 of the D-glucuronic acid and one bound to position 6 of the *N*-acetyl-D-galactosamine (Table 24.2). Currently, the difference in the physiological effect because of the difference in constituent ratio of the composing disaccharide is being studied, but the effect on joint pain by the different positioning of the sulfate group has yet to be clarified.

As described earlier, there are many types of chondroitin sulfate in the shark cartilage extract, and most of them are bound to the core protein. Although there are differences in the types of chondroitin sulfate and the area of the cartilage from which it is taken, the usual amount of glycosaminoglycan with chondroitin sulfate as its main component is approximately 20%–50% of the shark cartilage extract.

COLLAGEN PEPTIDE IN THE SHARK CARTILAGE EXTRACT

The protein content of the shark cartilage extract is usually approximately 50%, with most being collagen peptide. When the amino acid composition of the shark cartilage extract is compared with that of chicken type II collagen (CII), a high content of characteristic amino acids such as glycine, glutamic acid, proline, and hydroxyproline is seen in both of them (Figure 24.3).

Expected effects of the collagen peptides are improvement of bone density, water retention by the skin, protection of the gastric mucosa, and immunostimulation. Although there are not many examples of this research, in recent years various studies considering the effects of collagen peptides on osteoarthritis and rheumatoid arthritis have begun. In Europe and the United States, clinical trials

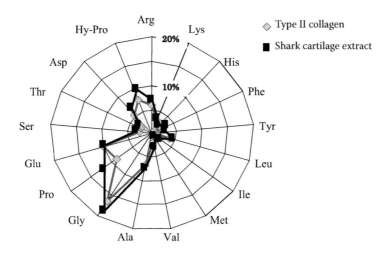

FIGURE 24.3 Comparison of amino acid composition between shark cartilage extract and type II collagen.

focused especially on osteoarthritis patients are in progress, and by administering collagen hydrolysate, improvement of body function and reduction of pain have been reported.

As described earlier, the shark cartilage extract is rich in chondroitin sulfate, which is an important material to alleviate joint pain, and because it also contains large amounts of collagen peptide, this extract is expected to have a synergistic or additive effect on joint pain.

PREVENTIVE EFFECT OF SHARK CARTILAGE EXTRACT IN ARTHRITIS MODEL RATS

The effects of shark cartilage extract for food use (SCP; Maruha Nichiro Foods, Inc.) and purified sodium chondroitin sulfate ester (Japanese Pharmaceutical Codex) manufactured for medical treatment (ChSNa; Maruha Nichiro Foods, Inc.) on CII-induced arthritis (CIA) in rats were evaluated. Dark Agouti/Slc female rats were immunized with bovine-derived CII emulsified in Freund's incomplete adjuvant. SCP or ChSNa at a dose of 5% or 2%, respectively, in the diet, which equaled 2% chondroitin sulfate, was fed to the rats for 14 days before immunization and 15 days afterward. The arthritis index was examined from day 0 to day 15. SCP as well as ChSNa inhibited the progression of the arthritis, as indicated by the drop in the index (Figure 24.4). The reduction in the progression tended to be greater in the SCP group than in the ChSNa one.

The effect of chondroitin sulfate C on CIA in mice was evaluated by Omata et al. [1]. DBA/1J mice were immunized with bovine-derived CII emulsified in Freund's complete adjuvant, followed by a booster injection 21 days later. A dose of 100, 300, or 1000 mg/kg of chondroitin sulfate C was administered orally once a day from 14 days before the initial immunization. The arthritis index and the hind paw edema were examined from day 0 to day 49, after which the mice were killed by ether anesthesia. The arthritis index was reduced by the treatment with chondroitin sulfate C in a dose-dependent manner. Chondroitin sulfate C (1000 mg/kg) significantly inhibited the hind paw edema.

It is well known that taking chondroitin sulfate alone helps to alleviate joint pain. Other than the chondroitin sulfate, the SCP has a high content of collagen peptide, and recent studies show that this collagen peptide would also contribute to improving joint pain. Adam et al. [2] reported that a reduction in pain was confirmed when patients with OA were administered collagen hydrolysate. Deal and Mockowitz [3] and Moskowitz [4] also reported that reduced pain and improvement of body function were seen when patients with OA were administered collagen hydrolysate. The results above show a trend that the SCP works better to inhibit the progression of arthritis compared

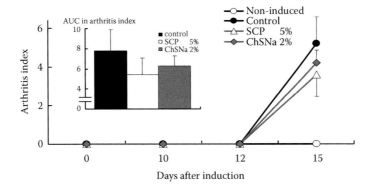

FIGURE 24.4 Effects of dietary and medicinal chondroitin sulfate on CII-induced arthritis rat model. Dark Agouti/Slc rats (9 weeks old) were fed a CRF-1 (Oriental Yeast Co., Ltd.)–based experimental diet containing SCP or ChSNa, both containing 2% chondroitin sulfate. A volume of 0.4 mL of CII (Collagen Research Center) 1.5 mg/10 mM acetic acid, emulsified with an equal volume of Freund's incomplete adjuvant (Difco) by using a high-flex homogenizer (SMT Co.), was injected intradermally into four spots at the base of the tail. Arthritis signs in each paw were evaluated using the scoring system of Mankin et al. Values represent the mean ± SE ($n = 5$).

with the purified sodium chondroitin sulfate ester. This trend suggests that components other than the chondroitin sulfate included in the SCP, especially the collagen peptide, function synergistically or have an additive effect. In fact, products containing chondroitin sulfate alone are a rarity in the health-food market; and chondroitin sulfate is often combined with materials such as glucosamine, collagen peptides, and so forth. Thus, when chondroitin sulfate is used as a measure against joint pain, taking shark cartilage extracts such as SCP, which originally contains chondroitin sulfate and collagen peptides together, is thought to be one of the most effective ways.

COMBINATION OF SHARK CARTILAGE EXTRACT AND OTHER MATERIALS EXPECTED TO HAVE STRONGER EFFECT

The usage of shark cartilage extract is thought to be an effective measure against joint pain because it contains large amounts of chondroitin sulfate and collagen peptide, which give the following physiological effects: chondroitin sulfate (1) protects the existing cartilage from being torn down by inhibiting the action of enzymes that degrade cartilage [5]; (2) helps to prevent the loss of chondrocytes due to aging [6]; (3) stimulates the production of proteoglycans, glycosaminoglycans, and collagen, which are molecules in the cartilage matrix that make new cartilage [7]; (4) increases the production of hyaluronic acid, which makes the joint fluid thicker to have a better cushioning capability [8]; (5) inhibits the negative effects of the interleukin-1β (IL-1β) and blocks the action of tumor necrosis factor α [9], both of which are involved in cartilage destruction; and (6) has a mild anti-inflammatory effect [10].

However, as the anti-inflammatory effect of chondroitin sulfate is relatively mild, it is thought that the effect would be better by combining chondroitin sulfate with another other substance that has a stronger anti-inflammatory effect. Many food materials with anti-inflammatory effects are known, one of which, in particular, is fish oil.

ANTI-INFLAMMATORY EFFECT OF FISH OIL CONTAINING OMEGA-3 FATTY ACIDS

A well-known anti-inflammatory effect of fish oil containing a large amount of docosahexaenoic acid (DHA) and eicosapentaenoic acid (EPA) is the antagonistic activity toward the metabolism of arachidonic acid. That is, it inhibits the production of arachidonic acid–derived mediators of allergic immune reactions, thereby decreasing the intensity of inflammation and allergic reactions. An interesting study was reported by Boileau et al. in 2005 [11] about the effect of a peroxisome proliferator-activated receptor gamma (PPARγ) agonist on an osteoarthritis model. To evaluate the *in vivo* therapeutic effects of pioglitazone, a potent PPARγ agonist, the development of lesions in a canine model of osteoarthritis was observed. The osteoarthritis was surgically induced in dogs by sectioning the anterior cruciate ligament. The dogs were then randomly divided into three treatment groups and then orally administered a placebo, a 15-mg/day pioglitazone, or a 30-mg/day pioglitazone for 8 weeks. After the administration, the severity of the cartilage lesions was scored, and cartilage specimens were then taken for histological evaluation. As a result, pioglitazone reduced the development of cartilage lesions in a dose-dependent manner, with the highest dosage producing a statistically significant change. Thus, new and interesting insights into a therapeutic intervention for osteoarthritis in which PPARγ activation can inhibit major signaling pathways of inflammation have been made.

Yamamoto et al. [12] found that putative metabolites of DHA are strong PPARγ activators. They designed DHA derivatives on the basis of the crystal structure of PPARγ, synthesized them, and evaluated their activities *in vitro* and *in vivo*. The efficacy of 5E-4-hydroxy-DHA as a PPARγ activator was approximately fourfold stronger than that of pioglitazone.

DHA and EPA, the best known of the omega-3 fatty acids, are found in marine plants and fishes. DHA and EPA are actually synthesized by algae, plankton, and seaweed, which are then eaten by certain fishes. Not all fishes are a good source of DHA and EPA. In fact, freshwater fishes have a relatively low DHA and EPA content. Cold water fatty fish caught in the ocean, such as mackerel, anchovies, herring, salmon, sardines, Atlantic sturgeon, and tuna, have the greatest amounts. Eating as little as 1 oz. of fish per day or two fish meals a week can help reduce inflammation. Although it is always better to obtain nutrients from real foods, some people take their omega-3s in the form of a supplement such as fish oil capsules.

IMPROVEMENT OF ARTHRITIS BY COMBINING SHARK CARTILAGE EXTRACT AND FISH OIL

Using the same CIA model rats as mentioned earlier, the efficiency of SCP was evaluated by mixing omega-3 fatty acids in fish hamburger meals at a dose of 0.5 g DHA/kg/day with SCP and feeding rats with it for 8 weeks. As a result, their arthritis tended to be inhibited. The area under the curve for arthritis progression in the SCP + omega-3 group tended to be lower than that of the control group, which was given CRF-1–based diet and fish hamburger supplemented with olive oil instead of fish oil (Figure 24.5). For prevention of arthritis, the combination of chondroitin sulfate and an anti-inflammatory ingredient such as omega-3 polyunsaturated fatty acids (PUFAs) is thought to be optimal.

The usual dose of omega-3 for helping reduce arthritis inflammation is reportedly at least 1000 mg/day and up to 5000 mg/day for more severe cases. Curtis et al. [13] demonstrated that pathologic indicators of degradation and inflammation in human osteoarthritic cartilage were abrogated by exposure to omega-3 fatty acids. To determine whether omega-3 PUFA supplementation (versus treatment with omega-6 PUFA supplement) affects the metabolism of osteoarthritic cartilage or not, they determined the metabolic profile of human osteoarthritic cartilage at the time of harvest and after a 24-h exposure to omega-3 PUFAs or other classes of fatty acids, followed by explant culturing for 4 days in the presence and absence of IL-1β. Measured parameters were the glycosaminoglycan release and the activities of aggrecanase and matrix metalloproteinase. As a result, supplementation with omega-3 PUFA (but not other fatty acids) reduced, in a dose-dependent manner, the endogenous and IL-1β-induced release of proteoglycan metabolites from articular cartilage explants, and it specifically abolished endogenous aggrecanase activity as well as collagenase proteolytic activity [13].

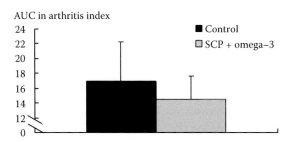

FIGURE 24.5 Effects of dietary chondroitin sulfate in combination with omega-3 on CII-induced arthritis in a rat model. Five percent SCP was mixed with a CRF-1–based diet and fed to rats for 8 weeks before the CII injection and then 16 days after it. Omega-3 in fish hamburger was fed simultaneously to give a dose of 0.5 g/kg as DHA. The amount of CII injected was 0.3 mL/body. Other conditions were the same as described in the legend of Figure 24.4. Values represent the mean ± SE ($n = 6$).

The anti-inflammatory effects of omega-3 PUFA are thought to involve the enhancement of PPARγ action [14]. A PPARγ activator was revealed to be effective against the development of arthritis *in vivo* [11]. In fact, our data suggested that chondroitin sulfate exhibited inhibitory actions against arthritis progression in CIA rats especially in combination with omega-3 PUFA. For prevention of arthritis, the combination of chondroitin sulfate and anti-inflammatory ingredients such as omega-3 PUFA or seaweed [15] might be optimal, but further research should be performed.

CONCLUSIONS

We have cited many studies on materials to countermeasure joint pain. Not only chondroitin sulfate but also shark cartilage extracts including collagen peptide and other components derived from cartilage are effective. Also, the possibility of improving joint pain by combining shark cartilage extracts and fish oil for its anti-inflammatory effect has been described. Research on chondroitin sulfate and other materials to reduce inflammation is underway, and the formulation of new compositions with better effects is expected.

REFERENCES

1. Omata T, Itokazu Y, Inoue N, Segawa Y. Effects of chondroitin sulfate-C on articular cartilage destruction in murine collagen-induced arthritis. Arzneim-Forsch/Drug Res 2000;50(1):148–153.
2. Adam M. Welche wirkung haben gelatinepraparate? Therapiewoche 1991;41:2456–2461.
3. Deal CL, Mockowitz RW. Nutraceuticals as therapeutic agents in osteoarthritis. The role of glucosamine, chondroitin sulfate, and collagen hydrolysate. Rheum Dis Clin North Am 1999;25(2):379–395.
4. Moskowitz RW. Role of collagen hydrolysate in bone and joint disease. Semin Arthritis Rheum 2000;30(2):87–99.
5. Soldani G, Romagnoli J. Experimental and clinical pharmacology of glycosaminoglycans (GAGs). Drugs Exp Clin Res 1991;17(1):81–85.
6. Conrozier T. Death of articular chondrocytes. Mechanisms and protection. Presse Med 1998;27(36)1859–1861.
7. Soldani G, Romagnoli J. Experimental and clinical pharmacology of glycosaminoglycans (GAGs). Drugs Exp Clin Res 1991;17(1):81–85.
8. Nishikawa H, Mori I, Umemoto J. Influences of sulfated glycosaminoglycans on biosynthesis of hyaluronic acid in rabbit knee synovial membranes. Arch Biochem Biophys 1985;240:146–153.
9. Hamon V. Effect of one compound structum on cytokines secretion by human macrophages and PBMC. Pierre Fabre Laboratories—Internal Reports;1997:1–32.
10. Ronca F, Palmieri L, Panicucci P, Ronca G. Anti-inflammatory activity of chondroitin sulfate. Osteoarthritis Cartilage 1998;6(Suppl A):14–21.

11. Boileau C, Martel-Pelletier J, Fahmi H, Mineau F, Boily M, Pelletier JP. The peroxisome proliferator-activated receptor γ agonist pioglitazone reduces the development of cartilage lesions in an experimental dog model of osteoarthritis. Arthritis Rheum 2007;56(7):2288–2298.

12. Yamamoto K, Itoh T, Abe D, Shimizu M, Kanda T, Koyama T, Nishikawa M, et al. Identification of putative metabolites of docosahexaenoic acid as potent PPARgamma agonists and antidiabetic agents. Bioorg Med Chem Lett 2005;15(3):517–522.

13. Curtis CL, Rees SG, Little CB, Flannery CR, Hughes CE, Wilson C, et al. Pathologic indicators of degradation and inflammation in human osteoarthritic cartilage are abrogated by exposure to n-3 fatty acids. Arthritis Rheum 2002;46(6):1544–1553.

14. Keller H, Dreyer C, Medin J, Mahfoudi A, Ozato K, Wahli W. Fatty acids and retinoids control lipid metabolism through activation of peroxisome proliferator-activated receptor-retinoid X receptor heterodimers. Proc Natl Acad Sci USA 1993;90(6):2160–2164.

15. Deutsch L. Evaluation of the effect of Neptune krill oil on chronic inflammation and arthritic symptoms. J Am Coll Nutr 2007;26(1):39–48.

25 Benefits of Fish Oil for Rheumatoid Arthritis
A Review

Christine Dawczynski and Gerhard Jahreis

CONTENTS

CHEMICAL STRUCTURE OF N-3 POLYUNSATURATED FATTY ACIDS

Polyunsaturated fatty acids (PUFA) can be differentiated into two groups according to the position of the double bounds in the fatty acid (FA) chain. Because mammalian cells cannot introduce double bonds at position 3 or 6 from the terminal methyl group, they are unable to produce α-linolenic acid (ALA; C18:3, n-3) and linoleic acid (LA; C18:2, n-6) (Figure 25.1). These FAs are essential for human organisms.

LA and ALA can be converted via elongases and desaturases to long-chain 20- and 22-carbon PUFA (LC-PUFA), such as eicosapentaenoic acid (EPA; C20:5, n-3), docosapentaenoic acid (C22:5, n-3), docosahexaenoic acid (DHA; C22:6, n-3), dihomo-γ-linolenic acid (C20:3, n-6), or arachidonic acid (AA; C20:4, n-6) (Figure 25.2).

ANTI-INFLAMMATORY EFFECTS OF N-3 LC-PUFA

EFFECTS ON EICOSANOID METABOLISM

The n-3 LC-PUFA (EPA and DHA) as well as the n-6 PUFA (AA) present in cell phospholipids can influence structural and metabolic function of cellular membranes. Moreover, both EPA and DHA are involved in numerous physiological processes owing to their effect on membrane fluidity, eicosanoid synthesis, receptor affinity, cell signaling, and gene expression. After its release from cell membranes via phospholipase A2, EPA may compete with AA as a substrate for oxygenation in both the cyclooxygenase (COX) and the 5-lipoxygenase (5-LOX) pathways, resulting in the production of highly metabolically active eicosanoids, including prostaglandins (PGs) and

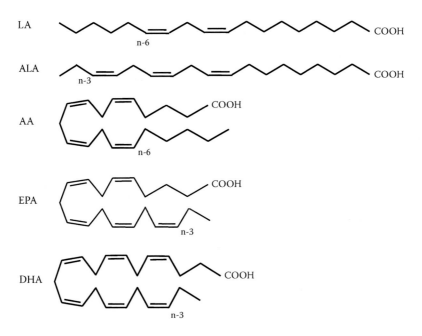

FIGURE 25.1 Chemical structures of important n-6 and n-3 PUFA. AA, arachidonic acid n-6; ALA, α-linolenic acid, n-3; DHA, docosahexaenoic acid, n-3; EPA, eicosapentaenoic acid, n-3; LA, linoleic acid,n-6.

leukotrienes (LTs), respectively (Weber, 1988). COX converts AA to PG metabolites of the two series, whereas LTs of the four series are produced via the LOX pathway (Figure 25.2). LTs not only modulate immune reactivity but also play an important role in the inflammatory process. LT B4, mainly produced in neutrophils, is a strong leukocyte activator responsible for chemotaxis, nondirected migration, aggregation, and lysosomal enzyme release (Ford-Hutchinson et al., 1980; Klickstein et al., 1980; Palmer et al., 1980; Bray et al., 1981; Hoover et al., 1984; Elmgreen et al., 1987). In addition, LTs can significantly affect T- and B-cell activity by modulating the production of certain cytokines, including interleukin-1 (IL-1; Rola-Pleszczynski et al., 1985). Eicosanoids deriving from AA in arthritic joints are associated with numerous undesirable effects (Calder and Zurier, 2001) listed as follows:

PGE_2
- Possesses proinflammatory properties
- Increases
  Vascular permeability
  Vasodilation
  Blood flow
  Local pyrexia
- Potentiates pain caused by other agents
- Promotes the production of matrix metalloproteinases (MMPs)
- Stimulates bone resorption

LT B4
- Increases vascular permeability
- Enhances local blood flow
- Promotes chemotaxis of leukocytes
- Induces release of lysosomal enzymes

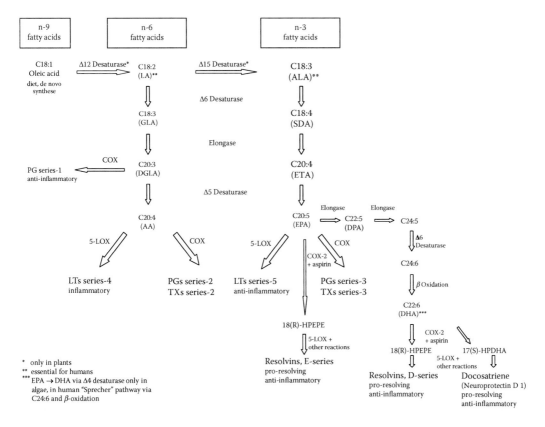

FIGURE 25.2 Pathway of biosynthesis and metabolism of PUFA. 17(S)-HPDHA, 17(S)-hydroperoxydo-cosahexaenoic acid; 18(R)-HPEPE, 18(R)-hydroperoxy-6,8,11,14,17-pentaenoic acid; 5-LOX, 5-lipoxyge-nase/arachidonate 5-lipoxygenase; AA, arachidonic acid; ALA, α-linolenic acid; COX, cyclooxygenase/PG-endoperoxide synthase; DGLA, dihomo-γ-linolenic acid; DHA, docosahexaenoic acid; DPA, docosap-entaenoic acid; EPA, eicosapentaenoic acid; ETA, eicosatetraenoic acid; GLA, γ-linolenic acid; LA, linoleic acid; SDA, stearidonic acid.

- Enhances the generation of reactive oxygen species
- Enhances production of proinflammatory cytokines, tumor necrosis factor α (TNF-α), IL-1, and IL-6

EPA can be oxidized via the COX pathway into PGs, thromboxanes (TXs), and prostacyclins of the three series or into LTs of the five series via the LOX pathway (Figure 25.2; Higgs, 1985; Kelley et al., 1985; Strasser et al., 1985). LT B5 is 10- to 30-fold less potent than LT B4 in assays of leu-kocyte function (Lee et al., 1984; Terano et al., 1984). Hence, EPA acts as an alternative substrate for the enzymes COX and LOX, which leads to the formation of the less proinflammatory PGs and LTs.

Dietary sources of EPA and DHA are marine fish, including shellfish and algae, whereas exog-enous AA is mainly found in animal fat. The intake of AA and its incorporation in cell mem-branes functions as an important regulatory step in the synthesis of both PGs and LTs. An alteration in the composition of dietary FA consisting of supplementing the diet with n-3 LC-PUFA leads to an increase of n-3 LC-PUFA concentrations in individual tissues, whereas AA levels decrease (Volker et al., 2000a; Dawczynski et al. 2009b, c). Thus, intake of PUFA can directly modulate both the synthesis and the action of regulatory eicosanoids and cytokines. A decrease in the ratio of AA to EPA or DHA may decline the production of proinflammatory eicosanoids, cytokines, and cartilage-degrading enzymes providing beneficial effects for patients with inflammatory diseases (Cleland et al., 2003).

Effects on Gene Expression

The effects of dietary fats on human health and disease are most likely mediated by changes in gene expression. Several transcription factors have been shown to respond to FA, including the sterol regulatory element-binding protein 1c, the nuclear factor "kappa-light-chain-enhancer" of activated B cells (NF-κB), the retinoid X receptors, the liver X receptors, the farnesoid X receptor, the hepatocyte nuclear factor 4α, and the peroxisome proliferator-activated receptors (PPARs; Sanderson et al., 2008).

Alteration of gene expression profiles was demonstrated by Bouwens et al. (2009) on analyzing the effects of n-3 LC-PUFA on gene expression profiles in peripheral blood mononuclear cells (PBMCs) in healthy Dutch elderly subjects in a double-blind trial using whole-genome transcriptomics analysis. A total of 111 subjects were randomly allocated to one of three groups: group 1 received 1.8 g EPA + DHA per day ($n = 36$), group 2 consumed 0.4 g EPA + DHA per day ($n = 37$), and group 3 ingested 4.0 g high–oleic acid sunflower oil per day ($n = 38$). Microarray analysis was performed on PBMC RNA in 23 and 25 subjects from groups 1 to 3, respectively. Quantitative real-time polymerase chain reaction was performed in all subjects. A high EPA + DHA intake altered the expression of 1040 genes, whereas high–oleic acid sunflower oil intake changed the expression of only 298 genes. EPA + DHA intake led to a decreased expression of genes involved in inflammatory and atherogenic-related pathways, such as NF-κB signaling, eicosanoid synthesis, scavenger receptor activity, adipogenesis, and hypoxia signaling. The results show that intake of EPA + DHA alters the gene expression profiles to a higher anti-inflammatory and anti-atherogenic status.

PPARs are members of the steroid/retinoid nuclear receptor super family of proteins that mediate ligand-dependent transcriptional activation and repression. These proteins govern genes that regulate metabolic functions, such as lipogenesis, FA oxidation, glucose uptake, inflammation, and cellular differentiation. At present, three isotypes of PPAR (α, β/δ, and γ), each with a specific expression pattern and encoded by different genes, have been characterized. PPARα is expressed in liver, kidney, muscle, heart, and cells from the vascular wall. Although PPARβ/δ is found in a wide range of tissues, its functions are still unclear. PPARγ is mainly expressed in adipose tissue and bone marrow; however, several immune cell types, especially antigen presenting cells, such as macrophages and dendritic cells (Blanquart et al., 2003; Li et al., 2005; Széles et al., 2007; Vanek and Connor, 2007), also express the receptor that plays a role in lipid metabolism and seems to have multiple functions in the immune system (Blanquart et al., 2003; Széles et al., 2007).

PPARs act through dimerization with retinoid X receptor followed by a subsequent regulation of gene expression (Calder, 2003). The transcriptional activity of PPARs is regulated by posttranslational modifications such as phosphorylation and ubiquitination. Phosphorylation of PPARs is controlled by environmental factors that activate different kinase pathways leading to the modulation of their activities. PPARs also control the expression of genes involved in the inflammatory response via negative interference with several inflammatory pathways, such as NF-κB, activator protein 1 (AP-1), CCAAT/enhancer-binding protein β, signal transducers and activator of transcription 1 (STAT-1), and nuclear factor of activated T cells (Blanquart et al., 2003).

For instance, PPARα can repress NF-κB and AP-1 pathways via interaction with the Rel homology domain of the NF-κB p65 subunit and via interaction of the N-terminus DBD (DNA binding domain) containing part of PPARα and the N terminus of *c*-Jun (Delerive et al., 1999a, b). Further, PPARα also induces the expression of I-κB, the major NF-κB inhibitor in smooth muscle cells and hepatocytes resulting in repression of the NF-κB pathway (Delerive et al., 2000). As a result, PPARα can repress the expression of inflammatory mediators induced by extracellular inflammatory stimuli, including the cytokine-induced expression of vascular cell adhesion molecule 1 (VCAM-1; Marx et al., 1999; Pasceri et al., 2000), the thrombin-induced endothelin-1 expression

(Delerive et al., 1999a, b), and the TNF-α-induced intercellular adhesion molecule 1 (ICAM-1) expression in endothelial cells (Pasceri et al., 2000). Moreover, PPARα decreases the secretion of IL-2 and TNF-α in T lymphocytes (Pasceri et al., 2000) as well as repressing the CCAAT/enhancer-binding protein activity, which regulates fibrinogen b and C-reactive protein (CRP) expression in hepatocytes (Gervois et al., 2001; Kleemann et al., 2003).

PPARγ also plays a part in the control of inflammation by repressing the inflammatory pathways (NF-κB and AP-1 signaling) as demonstrated by *in vitro* studies (Delerive et al., 1999a, b, 2001). Further, PPARγ inhibits the expression of inducible nitric oxide synthase (iNOS) via interference with the STAT-1, AP-1, and NF-κB pathways (Li et al., 2000). Finally, PPARγ ligands reduce IL-2 secretion because of an interaction of this nuclear receptor with the nuclear factor of activated T cells in T lymphocytes (Yang et al., 2000).

The anti-inflammatory action of PPARs is due to two mechanisms. First, PPARs interfere with transcription factors, including NF-κB, which are targets for controlling inflammation; and second, they stimulate the breakdown of inflammatory eicosanoids through induction of peroxisomal β-oxidation because LT B4 binding to PPARα results in the activation of PPARα-mediated transcription of enzymes implicated in β-oxidation in the liver. Hence, LT B4 and other FA-derived compounds may induce their own catabolism through stimulation of PPARα via just such a feedback mechanism. The degradation of these compounds results in the termination of the inflammatory process (Chinetti et al., 2000; Delerive et al., 2001).

In summary, PPARs can influence the inflammatory response at several different steps, resulting in a modulation of expression and the production of chemokines, chemokine receptors, adhesion molecules, and eicosanoids.

FAs are natural ligands for PPARs. Relatively high concentrations of around 100 μlmol/L of EPA and DHA are required for PPAR activation; however, they are not selective for PPAR subtypes. Sanderson et al. (2008) showed that PUFA such as DHA and EPA are stronger natural ligands for PPARs than MUFA or SFA.

Eicosanoids can further activate PPARs. Eicosanoid derivates from LOX, for example, LT B4, and 8-S-hydroxytetraenoic acid (8-S-HETE) can activate PPARα, whereas PGs (J2, H1, and H2) and 15-hydroxytetraenoic acid (15-HETE) are selective PPARγ ligands (Blanquart et al., 2003; Li et al., 2005).

PPAR activators were shown to inhibit the activation of inflammatory response genes (such as IL-2, IL-6, IL-8, TNF-α, and MMPs) by negatively interfering with the NF-κB, STAT, and AP-1 signaling pathways (Chinetti et al., 2000).

Effects of n-3 LC-PUFA on the action of the nuclear transcription factor PPARγ are well documented. Li et al. (2005) examined the anti-inflammatory effects of n-3 PUFA via activation of PPARs in human renal tubular cells (human kidney 2 [HK-2] cells). Results illustrate that EPA and DHA, at concentrations of 10 and 100 μmol/L, respectively, effectively decreased LPS-induced NF-κB activation and monocyte chemoattractant protein 1 expression. EPA and DHA also increased both PPARγ messenger RNA and protein activity (two- to threefold) in HK-2 cells. Overexpression of PPARγ further inhibited NF-κB activation compared with the control cells in the presence of EPA and DHA. The data demonstrate that both EPA and DHA downregulate LPS-induced activation of NF-κB via a PPARγ-dependent pathway in HK-2 cells.

Because diets high in n-3 PUFA are known to decrease colon cancer development and suppress colon tumor growth. Allred et al. (2008) evaluated the physiological effects of EPA in human colon cancer cells (HT-29) in association with PPARγ. Incubation of HT-29 cells with EPA at nutritionally relevant concentrations resulted in a stimulation of the PPAR response element reporter assay in a dose-responsive manner. Cotreatment with GW9662 (PPARγ antagonist) significantly inhibited this effect, whereas overexpressing the receptor enhanced it. Further, the authors analyzed whether the functional ligand of PPARγ was EPA or a PG formed from EPA. The results substantiated that EPA is itself a ligand of PPARγ. Moreover, the effect of suppressing HT-29 cell growth by EPA was significantly reversed by the addition of GW, suggesting that physiological actions of EPA result in part from PPARγ activation. The study by Allred et al. identified PPARγ as a molecular mediator of n-3 PUFA actions in colon cancer cells.

Cytochrome P-450 (CYP) 2J2, expressed in vascular endothelial, smooth muscle cells, and cardiomyocytes, metabolizes AA to biologically active epoxyeicosatrienoic acids (EETs). The anti-inflammatory properties of 11,12-EET comprise preventing leukocyte adhesion to endothelial cells by inhibiting the NF-κB pathway. EETs also function as anti-thrombotics via upregulating the tissue plasminogen activator as well as having anti-migratory effects against vascular smooth muscle cells by decreasing the production of reactive oxygen species. Thus, it is thought that CYP 2J2–induced EETs have a protective effect against atherosclerosis and vascular remodeling (Node et al., 1999; Wang et al., 2009). The action of EPA and DHA on expression of CYP 2J2 mRNA by reverse transcriptase polymerase chain reaction in cultured human umbilical vein endothelial cells was investigated by Wang et al. (2009). Interestingly, EPA, but not DHA, increased the expression of CYP 2J2 mRNA in a dose and time-dependent manner. This EPA-induced CYP 2J2 expression was significantly inhibited by pretreatment with a PPARγ antagonist (GW9662). Similarly, only EPA caused a significant increase in cellular levels of 11,12-dihydroxyeicosatrienoic acid, a stable metabolite of 11,12-EET, which was blocked by pretreatment with GW9662. Thus, results depict that EPA increases CYP 2J2 gene expression and EET production via PPARγ in endothelial cells.

It was shown that PPAR activation can inhibit major signaling pathways of inflammation. The effects of EPA and DHA on PPAR activation indicate that n-3 LC-PUFA may represent a class of naturally occurring PPAR ligands with low toxicity and potent anti-inflammatory properties.

There is also an association between PPARγ activation and a reduction in the synthesis of cartilage catabolic factors responsible for articular cartilage degradation. Boileau et al. (2007) determined the *in vivo* effect of a PPARγ agonist, pioglitazone (class thiazolidinedione with hypoglycemic action), on the development of lesions in a canine model of osteoarthritis (OA) in three treatment groups receiving placebo, 15 mg/day, and 30 mg/day oral pioglitazone, respectively, for 8 weeks. After treatment, the severity of cartilage lesions was scored. A reduced development of cartilage lesions and the histologic scores were seen in a dose-dependent manner because of treatment with pioglitazone. In addition, pioglitazone significantly reduced the synthesis of the key OA mediators MMP-1, a disintegrin and metalloproteinase with thrombospondin motifs 5 (ADAMTS-5), and iNOS. At the same time, it inhibited the activation of the signaling pathways for mitogen-activated protein kinases ERK-1/2, p38, and NF-κB. These results indicate the efficacy of pioglitazone in reducing cartilage lesions *in vivo*.

The supplementation of n-3 LC-PUFA may contribute to the prevention of cartilage and bone resorption as FAs are capable of acting as PPARγ agonists (see the section on *Effects of Bone Metabolism and Cartilage Integrity*).

These recent findings indicate a modulatory role for PPARs in the control of inflammatory response and bone remodeling. The ability of n-3 LC-PUFA to interact with PPARs indicates a potential for therapeutic applications for the treatment of inflammation-related diseases, such as rheumatoid arthritis (RA) and atherosclerosis.

EFFECTS ON PRODUCTION OF CYTOKINES

Various cells of synovial origin and in the immune system are involved in the etiopathogenic process of RA leading to disease development and progression. Furthermore, numerous functionally active cytokines are expressed in the synovial tissue. TNF-α and IL-1, produced in monocytes and macrophages, are important mediators of inflammation and tissue damage in active RA. In addition, IL-6 is involved in the induction of the acute phase protein response, differentiation of hematopoietic precursor cells, and proliferation of synovial fibroblasts (Sundrarjun et al., 2004). An increase in concentrations of IL-1 and TNF-α affect synovial tissue and cartilage metabolism, a feature characteristic in autoimmune inflammatory disease such as RA (Dayer et al., 1986).

A reduction in production of proinflammatory mediators including cytokines (e.g., TNF-α, IL-1) belongs to the well-described anti-inflammatory effects of n-3 LC-PUFA. The promoter region of TNF-α gene contains several potential regulatory elements including κB. Binding of the transcription factor, NF-κB, to the κB site resulted in the maximal LPS-induced TNF-α expression in human monocytic cells (Shakhov et al., 1990; Ziegler-Heitbrock et al., 1993; Trede et al., 1995; Yao et al., 1997; Udalova et al., 1998). The inactive NF-κB heterotrimer found in the cytosol of resting inflammatory cells has an inhibitory subunit I-κB. Upon stimulation, a signaling cascade activates the I-κB kinase protein complex, which in turn phosphorylates I-κB, causing its dissociation from the rest of the inactive NF-κB trimer (Karin and Ben-Nerjah, 2000; Karin and Delhase, 2000). Phosphorylation and subsequent ubiquitination of I-κB lead to its degradation. The remaining NF-κB heterodimer rapidly translocates to the nucleus, binds to target DNA elements, and activates the transcription of target genes, for example, TNF-α (Baeuerle and Baltimore, 1988; Baldwin, 1996; Sha, 1998). Inappropriate activation of NF-κB is associated with a wide range of human ailments including inflammatory diseases, atherosclerosis, and cancer (Chen et al., 1999; Grossmann et al., 1999; Calder, 2003; Zhao et al., 2004).

Zhao et al. (2004) investigated the effects of EPA on LPS-induced expression of TNF-α and activation of NF-κB in human monocytic THP-1 cells. TNF-α production and expression induced by LPS were significantly decreased because of preincubation with EPA. LPS-induced NF-κB activation, translocation of the p65 subunit to the nucleus, phosphorylation, and degradation of I-κB-α were partially prevented by EPA. According to the authors, suppression of TNF-α expression by EPA is partly attributed to its inhibitory effect on NF-κB activation. EPA appears to inhibit NF-κB activation by preventing the phosphorylation of I-κB-α. In addition to its effect on TNF-α expression, the transcription factor of NF-κB is involved in the induction of numerous inflammatory genes, including COX-2, ICAM-1, VCAM-1, E-selectin, IL-1β, IL-6, nitric oxide synthase, acute phase proteins, and MMPs in response to inflammatory stimuli (Christman et al., 1998; Chen et al., 1999; Calder, 2003).

The inhibitory effects of EPA and DHA on the production of the inflammatory mediators IL-1β, TNF-α, IL-6, and IL-8 are well documented in cell culture studies with monocytes, macrophages, or venous endothelial cells (Calder, 2003, 2006a, b). In healthy human volunteers, diet supplementation with fish oil providing more than 2.4 g/day EPA plus DHA resulted in a decreased production of TNF-α, IL-1, and IL-6 by mononuclear cells (Endres et al., 1989; Meydani et al., 1991; Gallai et al., 1993; Caughey et al., 1996; Kelley et al., 1999; Calder, 2003).

The recent study by Weaver et al. (2009) examined the effect of reducing dietary n-6/n-3 PUFA ratio on expression of inflammatory pathway genes in mononuclear cells. Healthy humans were placed on a controlled diet for 1 week, then given fish oil and borage oil containing 775 mg EPA per day and 831 mg GLA per day, respectively, for an additional 4 weeks. The study period was followed by a 2-week washout phase during which the volunteers resumed their normal diets. The *ex vivo* LT B4 production from stimulated neutrophils measured at the start and end of the supplementation period and after the 2-week washout had decreased by 31%. In addition, a significant reduction in expression of the proinflammatory cytokines IL-1β, IL-10, and IL-23 was observed as well as a strong trend toward a decreased expression of IL-5 and IL-17. No changes were seen for TNF-α ($p = 0.11$) and IL-6 ($p = 0.27$). However, levels of IL-1β showed a significant and continual decrease from week 5 to week 7, whereas expression of the other cytokines showed a tendency toward an increase to baseline week 1 values during the washout phase. Further, the expression of phosphoinositide 3-kinases α (PI3Kα) and PI3Kγ plus the quantity of PI3Kα protein in mononuclear cells had declined after supplementation. PI3K plays an important role in eicosanoid formation, cell growth, survival, and inflammation by using downstream effectors including NF-κB.

In patients with RA, dietary supplementation with 27 mg EPA + 18 mg DHA/kg body weight (low), 54 mg EPA + 36 mg DHA/kg body weight (high), or olive oil as placebo more than 24 weeks led to a decrease of IL-1 production in macrophages by 54.7% in the high-dose group ($p = 0.0005$), by 40.6% in the low-dose group $(p = 0.06)$, and by 38.5% in the olive oil group, respectively (NS; Kremer et al., 1990).

A significant decrease of serum IL-1β concentration was also determined in the follow-up intervention study with RA patients by Kremer et al. (1995) with dietary fish oil supplementation (130 mg n-3 LC-PUFA/kg body weight/day; 26 weeks). However, an inhibitory effect of supplementation with dietary fish oils on the serum concentrations of IL-2, IL-6, IL-8, or TNF-α could not be demonstrated. Similar results were found by Espersen et al. (1992) in a comparable study.

A significant reduction of TNF-α in stimulated PBMCs was found by Adam et al. (2003) only in the second period of the crossover due the consumption of 30 mg n-3 LC-PUFA/kg body weight more than 12 weeks, although the decrease in IL-1β concentration was not significant.

Sundrarjun et al. (2004) determined the effects of a diet low in n-6 PUFA + n-3 LC-PUFA (3.36 g n-3 LC-PUFA per day) in comparison with a diet low in n-6 PUFA + placebo supplement and a control group without special diet or intervention more than 12 weeks. The patients consumed food containing less than 12.5 g/day of n-6 FA from cooking oils. In the fish oil group, a significant reduction of the soluble TNF receptor p55 was observed. In addition, a significant drop in serum IL-6 and TNF-α concentrations was seen in all groups; the percentage change in TNF-α from baseline in the fish oil group was greater (difference = 40.7%) than that in the control group (NS), whereas there was no significant difference between the fish oil and the placebo group.

Thus, in most studies, a reduced production of inflammatory cytokines was observed in healthy volunteers or patients with RA owing to supplementation with n-3 LC-PUFA. The data reveal that n-3 LC-PUFA may exert clinically beneficial effects via their capacity to regulate the expression of genes for both signal transduction and proinflammatory cytokines.

Worthy of note is, however, that several other studies failed to show any effect of dietary n-3 LC-PUFA on the production of inflammatory cytokines in humans. One possible explanation for the discrepancy lies in the occurrence of polymorphism in genes affecting cytokine production, as illustrated by the TNF genotypes (Grimble et al., 2002).

EFFECTS ON THE PRODUCTION OF "PRORESOLVING" MEDIATORS (RESOLVINS, PROTECTINS, AND MARESINS)

Endogenous "proresolving" mediators control the process of resolution of acute inflammation. These factors switch off leukocyte trafficking to the inflamed site and reverse vasodilatation and vascular permeability, thus allowing tissues to return to a state of homeostasis (Gilroy et al., 2004).

A number of recent studies have identified a novel group of mediators from n-3 LC-PUFA. These oxygenated derivatives are capable of potent anti-inflammatory, immunoregulatory, and proresolving actions. The trivial name *resolvin* (resolution phase interaction products) has been introduced for these bioactive compounds (Serhan et al., 2004). E-series resolvins are formed from EPA by COX-2 in the presence of aspirin (ASA) and DHA-derived mediators termed D-series resolvins, docosatrienes, and neuroprotectins, also produced by COX-2 in the presence of ASA (Figure 25.2). These mediators are synthesized during the spontaneous resolution phase of acute inflammation when specific cell–cell interactions occur.

Organic synthesis was achieved revealing the complete stereochemical assignment of RvE1 as 5S,12R,18R-trihydroxy-6Z,8E,10E,14Z,16E-EPA. RvE1 possesses unique counter-regulatory actions including inhibition of *in vitro* transendothelial migration of polymorphonuclear neutrophils (PMNs), inhibition of leukocyte infiltration, dendritic cell migration, and inhibition of proinflammatory gene expression, including IL-12 p40, TNF-α, and iNOS in murine models (Arita et al., 2005). Thus, RvE1 counter-regulates leukocyte-mediated tissue injury and proinflammatory gene expression. The key histological event in tissue resolution is the loss of inflammatory PMNs, which are one of the main cellular targets of the anti-inflammatory actions of RvE1.

Arita et al. (2007) examined the mechanisms responsible for these effects. The receptor BLT1 is a high-affinity LT B_4 receptor responsible for its chemotactic actions (Yokomizo et al., 1997). The results from Arita et al. (2007) indicate that RvE1 binds to BLT1 as a partial agonist, potentially serving as a local damper of BLT1 signals on leukocytes along with other receptors (e.g., ChemR23-mediated counter-regulatory actions) to mediate the resolution of inflammation. Further, RvE1 attenuates LT B_4-dependent proinflammatory signals such as mobilization of intracellular calcium and NF-κB activation via interaction with BLT1. The authors concluded that acting as a proresolving ligand, RvE1 probably blocks proinflammatory signals mediated by LT B4.

Hasturk et al. (2006) evaluated the regulatory actions of RvE1 in neutrophil tissue destruction and resolution of inflammation in patients with localized aggressive periodontitis (LAP), a well-understood example of leukocyte-mediated bone loss and inflammation. The pathogenic features in LAP are similar to those observed in other inflammatory diseases such as arthritis. The actions of an ASA-triggered lipoxin (LX) analog and RvE1 were compared in the study. Interestingly, neutrophils from LAP did not react with anti-inflammatory molecules of the LX series, whereas LAP neutrophils responded to RvE1. Further, RvE1 was found specifically bound to human neutrophils at a site that is functionally distinct from the LX receptor. Moreover, in a rabbit model, topical application of RvE1 for periodontitis conferred dramatic protection against inflammation-induced tissue and bone loss. These findings show that RvE1 effectively stops inflammation-induced bone loss *in vivo* in experimental periodontitis.

On the basis of the findings from Hasturk et al. (2006), the direct action of RvE1 on osteoclast (OC) development and bone resorption were analyzed in primary OC cultures derived from mouse bone marrow by Herrera et al. (2008). The presence of RvE1 caused a marked decrease of OC growth and resorption pit formation. In addition, OC differentiation was inhibited by RvE1 as demonstrated by a decreased number of multinuclear OC, a delay in the time course of OC development, and a reduction of receptor activator for NF-κB ligand-induced nuclear translocation of the NF-κB p50 subunit. Hence, RvE1 inhibits OC growth and bone resorption by interfering with OC differentiation.

Acetylation of COX-2 by aspirin enabled the biosynthesis of *R*-containing precursors of endogenous anti-inflammatory mediators. Human COX-2 converted DHA to 13-hydroxy-DHA that switched with ASA to 17*R*-HDHA, in turn proving a major route in hypoxic endothelial cells. Human neutrophils transformed COX-2-ASA-derived 17*R*-hydroxy-DHA into two sets of novel di- and trihydroxy products. These novel compounds inhibited (IC50 ~ 50 pM) microglial cell cytokine expression and *in vivo* dermal inflammation and peritonitis at monogram doses (Serhan et al., 2002).

Schwab et al. (2006, 2007) examined the effects of protectin D1 (PD1, DHA-derived mediator) and RvE1 in a model of murine peritonitis. The authors report that RvE1 and PD1 in nanogram quantities promote phagocyte removal during acute inflammation by regulating leukocyte infiltration, increasing macrophage ingestion of apoptotic PMNs *in vivo* and *in vitro*, and enhancing the appearance of phagocytes carrying engulfed zymosan in lymph nodes and spleen. These results demonstrate that RvE1 and PD1 are potent agonists for resolution of inflamed tissues.

A third group of lipid-derived mediators, the maresins identified by Serhan et al. (2009), control both the magnitude and duration of inflammation because of their potent anti-inflammatory and proresolving effects comparable with those of RvE1. Maresins are produced by macrophages (MPhis) from DHA during the resolution of mouse peritonitis. Characterization of physical and biological properties of the products demonstrated a novel 14-lipoxygenase pathway, generating bioactive 7,14-dihydroxydocosa-4Z,8,10,12,16Z,19Z-hexaenoic acid, named *MPhi mediator in resolving inflammation* (maresin), which are involved in enhancing resolution.

Defective resolution mechanism(s) could play an important role in chronic inflammatory diseases, for example, RA. Specialized proresolving mediators, including resolvins, protectins, and maresins, are biosynthesized from n-3 LC-PUFA. The previous data suggest that resolvins endogenously formed from n-3 LC-PUFA enhance the proresolution status in addition to blocking proinflammatory signals. These mediators could provide a targeted approach toward the treatment of chronic inflammatory diseases such as RA, and cardiovascular (CV) disease by virtue of their beneficial effects on bone remodeling, bone sparing, and proresolving activity.

Summary: Anti-inflammatory Effects of n-3 LC-PUFA (modified according to Calder, 2006a)

- Decreased incorporation of AA in cell membrane phospholipids
  - Decreased induction of COX-2, 5-LOX, and 5-LOX-activating protein (pivotal enzymes in the temporal generation of proinflammatory mediators)
  - Decreased generation of AA-derived eicosanoids (many with inflammatory actions)
- Increased content of EPA and DHA in cell membrane phospholipids
  - Increased generation of EPA-derived eicosanoids (many with less inflammatory actions than those produced from AA)
  - Increased generation of EPA and DHA-derived resolvins (with anti-inflammatory and proresolving actions)
- Activation of PPARs, altered activity of other transcription factors (differential effects of n-3 LC-PUFA vs AA and their derived eicosanoids)
  - Blocking of inflammatory pathways (e.g., NF-κB: interaction with the p65 subunit)
  - Decreased phosphorylation of I-κB (inhibitory unit)
  - AP-1: interaction with c-Jun
  - Decreased generation or expression of inflammatory cytokines (TNF-α, IL-1β, IL-6, IL-8) and inflammatory mediators (VCAM-1, ICAM-1, endothelin-1)
- Decreased leukocyte chemotaxis
- Decreased generation of reactive oxygen species

n-3 LC-PUFA inhibit production of proinflammatory chemical mediators because of their influence on various steps of the inflammatory pathways that includes eicosanoid production, inhibition of enzymes and/or antagonism of receptors, and the production of proresolving mediators. Today, therapy with selective COX inhibitors and anti-TNF-α medications is widely used to control the inflammatory process in RA. Thus, dietary intake of n-3 LC-PUFA can support anti-inflammatory therapy in RA patients.

EFFECTS ON BONE METABOLISM AND CARTILAGE INTEGRITY

RA is a chronic autoimmune disease characterized by joint inflammation involving the synovial tissue and the destruction of cartilage and bone.

Both LC-PUFA and the lipid mediator derivatives have been assigned critical roles in the regulation of a variety of biological processes including bone metabolism. Dietary FAs are implicated in a variety of different mechanisms that affect bone metabolism: the effect on calcium balance and on osteoblastogenesis plus osteoblast activity, the change of membrane function, a decrease in inflammatory cytokines such as IL-1, IL-6, and TNF-α, and the modulation of PPARγ (Maggio et al., 2009).

AA is the precursor for a range of proinflammatory eicosanoids that are bioactive in both soft and mineralized tissue. In bone, the AA-derived proinflammatory lipid mediator PGE$_2$ has an integral role in the regulation of both osteoblast and OC formation and function (Poulsen et al., 2007). The OC differentiation factor (ODF; also known as osteoprotegerin ligand and receptor activator of NK-κB ligand or TNF-related activation-induced cytokine) and osteoprotegerin represent newly identified factors that participate in bone cell differentiation (Watkins et al., 2001). ODF, induced by many osteotrophic hormones and cytokines (e.g., parathyroid hormone, glucocorticoids, TNF-α, IL-1, IL-6, IL-11), appears to be a common mediator of OC formation. Osteoprotegerin, a decoy receptor for ODF, functions reciprocally with ODF to regulate the induction of mature osteoclastic cells. The ODF–osteoprotegerin ratio may be a regulatory mechanism controlling bone resorption. Evidence also suggests that the stimulatory effect of PGE$_2$ on osteoclastogenesis may be mediated by the inhibition of osteoprotegerin expression in bone cells. PGE_2 downregulated osteoprotegerin mRNA level in human bone marrow stromal cells (Bränström et al., 1998) and decreased osteoprotegerin expression in mouse calvarial osteoblasts that supported an increase in osteoclastogenesis (Murakami et al., 1998; Watkins et al., 2001).

Dietary n-3 LC-PUFA, especially EPA, modulates prostanoid synthesis from AA (e.g., PGE_2) via competitive inhibition of AA oxygenation by COX. Hence, n-3 LC-PUFA can influence bone metabolism because of their ability to reduce an overproduction of PGE_2.

Watkins et al. (2000) determined the effects of dietary PUFA on *ex vivo* bone PGE_2 production and the bone formation rate in weaning male Sprague–Dawley rats. The rats were fed a diet containing 70 g/kg of added fat for 42 days. The dietary lipid treatments were formulated with safflower oil and menhaden oil to provide the following ratios of n-6/n-3 PUFA: 23.8 (SMI), 9.8 (SMII), 2.6 (SMIII), and 1.2 (SMIV). *Ex vivo* PGE_2 production in liver homogenates and bone organ cultures were significantly lower in rats fed a lower dietary ratio of n-6/n-3 PUFA than in those fed with a higher ratio. Regression analysis revealed a significant positive correlation between bone PGE_2 and the ratio of AA/EPA but significant negative correlations between bone formation rate and the ratio of AA/EPA or the PGE_2 in bone. Activity of serum alkaline phosphatase isoenzymes, including the bone-specific isoenzyme, was higher in rats fed a diet high in n-3 or with a low ratio of n-6/n-3 PUFA. These results demonstrate the positive action of n-3 PUFA on bone formation via modulation of bone PGE_2 production and activity of serum bone-specific isoenzyme in growing rats.

Hankenson et al. (2000) studied the n-3 and n-6 PUFA modulation of *in vitro* model ligament healing in pig knee medial collateral ligament fibroblasts. The cells were exposed to bovine serum albumin (control), EPA, or AA. Improved healing of *in vitro* wounds was achieved after incubation (72 h) by AA and EPA. In addition, EPA raised the collagen biosynthesis and the overall percentage of collagen produced, whereas AA decreased collagen production together with total protein levels. Although the level of PGE_2 was increased because of exposition with AA and reduced owing to exposition with EPA, a linear correlation ($r^2 = 0.57$) between IL-6 levels and collagen production was observed. Thus, n-3 PUFA (EPA) improved the healing characteristics of medial collateral ligament cells and may provide a noninvasive treatment method to improve ligament healing.

The loss of proteoglycan (aggrecan) from cartilage via aggrecanases and collagenases is an early event leading to degradation and joint tissue destruction in degenerative joint diseases. Three members of the ADAMTS family of proteinases, ADAMTS-1, ADAMTS-4, and ADAMTS-5, have been identified. Aggrecanases that cleave the Glu373–Ala374 bond of the aggrecan core protein play a key role in the early stages of cartilage destruction in both RA and OA. Later events involve the breakdown and release of collagen, mediated by members of the MMPs family of enzymes (specifically MMPs 1, 8, 13, and 14). MMPs, which are also found in arthritic joints, cleave aggrecans at a distinct site (i.e., Asn341-Phe342; Cawston, 1998; Nagase and Kashiwagi, 2003). Significant proteolysis of type II collagen may represent the point of irreversible cartilage damage. Curtis et al. (2002b) analyzed the effects of n-3 PUFA (ALA and EPA), supplementation (vs n-6 PUFA; LA and AA), and other FA supplements (C16:0 and C18:1) on the metabolism of OA cartilage. The metabolic profile of human OA cartilage harvested from patients who had undergone knee replacement surgery was determined at the time of harvest and after a 24-h exposure to the FA classes, followed by explant culture for 4 days in the presence or absence of IL-1. The supplementation with n-3 PUFA, but not n-6 PUFA, reduced the endogenous and IL-1-induced release of proteoglycan metabolites from articular cartilage explants in a dose-dependent manner and specifically abolished endogenous aggrecanase and collagenase proteolytic activity. Similarly, expressions of mRNA for ADAMTS-4 (aggrecanase), MMP-13 (collagenase), and MMP-3 (stromelysin) but not tissue inhibitors of metalloproteinases-1, -2, or -3 were also specifically diminished because of n-3 PUFA supplementation. In addition, n-3 PUFA supplementation reduced the expression of mRNA for mediators of inflammation (COX-2, 5-LOX, 5-LOX-activating protein, TNF-α, IL-1α, and IL-1β) without affecting the normal tissue homeostasis. These findings provide evidence that n-3 LC-PUFA supplementation may protect against cartilage degradation because of their influence on the pathologic indicators.

Curtis et al. (2004) could reproduce these results in a small study with 31 OA patients before knee replacement surgery. All patients received two capsules per day containing either 1000 mg cod liver oil or placebo oil (with the same amount of vitamins A and D) for 10–12 weeks. Six patients dropped out of the study leaving 14 on cod liver oil and 11 on placebo. A preliminary report stated that in 86% of patients given cod liver oil, greatly reduced levels of aggrecanase were found in cartilage and joint tissue taken at surgery compared with 26% of those on placebo. There was a similar reduction in collagenase activity in 73% of patients on cod liver oil but only in 18% of those on placebo. Furthermore, gene expression for aggrecanases was reduced in 93% of cod liver oil patients, and the levels of the inflammatory mediators (IL-1 and TNF) were also found to be reduced.

Curtis et al. (2000) had also shown that incorporation of n-3 PUFA (but not other PUFA or SFA) into articular cartilage chondrocyte membranes results in a dose-dependent reduction in the expression and activity of proteoglycan-degrading enzymes (aggrecanases) and the expression of inflammation-inducible cytokines (IL-1α and TNF-α) and COX-2 (not the constitutively expressed COX-1).

Weiss et al. (2005) investigated the association between n-6/n-3 PUFA ratio and bone mineral density (BMD) in 1532 community-dwelling men and women aged 45–90 years. The dietary data were obtained through self-administered food-frequency questionnaires; the medical history and current medication were also documented. The results of the age and multiple-adjusted linear regression analyses showed a significant inverse association between the ratio of dietary LA/ALA and BMD in the hips in 642 men, 564 women not using hormone therapy, and 326 women using hormone therapy (independent of age, body mass index, and lifestyle factors), respectively. Further, an increasing ratio of n-6/n-3 PUFA was also significantly and independently associated with lower BMD in the hips in all women and in the spine in women not using hormone therapy. These findings indicated that a higher ratio of n-6/n-3 PUFA is associated with lower BMD in the hips in both sexes and the relative amounts of dietary PUFA may play a vital role in preserving skeletal integrity in older age.

Högström et al. (2007) conducted a cohort study on 78 healthy young men (mean baseline age = 16.7 years). BMD (g/cm^2) of total body, hip, and spine was measured at baseline and at 22 and 24 years of age. In addition, FA concentrations were measured in the phospholipid fraction in serum at 22 years of age. The authors found a positive correlation between concentrations of n-3 PUFA and total BMD ($r = 0.27$, $p = 0.02$) or BMD at the spine ($r = 0.25$, $p = 0.02$) at 22 years of age. This association was especially relevant for DHA concentrations and total BMD ($r = 0.32$, $p = 0.004$) or BMD at the spine ($r = 0.30$, $p = 0.008$) at 22 years of age. Also, a negative association was found between higher ratios of n-6/n-3 PUFA and spinal BMD accrual between ages 16 and 22 years. In this cohort of healthy young men, the concentrations of n-3 PUFA, particularly DHA, were positively associated with peak BMD in the total body and spine and with bone accrual in the spine. Study limitations included the fact that the cohort was not randomly selected from the general population but rather consisted of volunteers from high schools and sports clubs. Information on dietary patterns that may have been useful to further strengthen the relation between FA and BMD was unavailable. Finally, although the authors reported a relationship between changes in BMD and both palmitoleic acid and AA, they do not provide a plausible explanation for these findings.

A correlation between increased dietary consumption of n-3 and some n-6 LC-PUFA on limiting postmenopausal bone loss in ovariectomized (OVX) rats was conducted by Poulsen et al. (2007). Rats were either fed a control diet or one supplemented with 0.5 g/kg body weight/day of GLA, EPA, DHA ethyl esters, or a mixture of all three FAs for 16 weeks. It was shown that GLA, DHA, and possibly EPA are bioactive in bone *in vivo*, albeit with different mechanism of action and with divergent effects. Under study conditions, DHA was the most effective at maintaining bone mineral content post-OVX. GLA exacerbated post-OVX bone mineral loss, possibly as a result of parathyroid hormone–induced bone catabolism. Further, the ratio of n-3 to n-6 LC-PUFA in the diet and bone marrow was the same in both EPA-supplemented and DHA-supplemented animals; however, a beneficial effect of supplementation on bone mass was observed only in DHA-fed animals. Hence, this result suggests that the overall ratio of n-3 to n-6 LC-PUFA is perhaps not as important as the type of LC-PUFA in the diet for optimizing bone mass.

Animal *in vitro* and *in vivo* studies have shown that a higher dietary intake of n-3 LC-PUFA is associated with a decrease of PGE_2 overproduction, the inflammatory mediators (IL-1 and TNF-α), and the activity of proteolytic enzymes (aggrecanases and collagenases). In addition, there is a positive association between dietary n-3 LC-PUFA intake and BMD. These effects suggest a benefit for n-3 PUFA on skeletal health. But at this point in time, there is no definitive conclusion regarding the value of n-3 LC-PUFA supplementation in clinical practice.

EFFECTS OF FISH OIL–DERIVED N-3 LC-PUFA ON THERAPY OF RA (HUMAN INTERVENTION TRIALS)

Epidemiological studies support the hypothesis that consumption of fish prevents the development of RA, as seen in the population of Eskimos and habitants of the Faroe Islands, who show a reduced incidence of RA associated with a diet rich in marine organisms, for example, fish and whale meat with a high n-3 LC-PUFA content (Horrobin, 1987; Recht et al., 1990). Moreover, improvements in the clinical and immunological parameters of RA via n-3 LC-PUFA consumption have been shown in more than 20 intervention studies dating back to the first reported publication in 1985 (Kremer et al., 1985; Table 25.1).

RA patients taking dietary supplements of n-3 LC-PUFA exhibit an improvement in clinical parameters of disease activity from baseline, including the disease activity score DAS 28 (Das Gupta et al., 2009; Dawczynski et al., 2009c), visual analog scale for pain evaluation by patients or physicians (Tulleken et al., 1990; Kremer et al., 1995; Berbert et al., 2005; Das Gupta et al., 2009; Dawczynski et al., 2009b), grip strength (Cleland et al., 1988; Berbert et al., 2005), duration of morning stiffness (van der Tempel et al., 1990; Nielsen et al., 1992; Kremer et al., 1995; Berbert et al., 2005), and number of tender or swollen joints (Cleland et al., 1988; Kremer et al., 1990; Tulleken et al., 1990; van der Tempel et al., 1990; Nielsen et al., 1992; Kremer et al., 1995; Table 25.1).

The inflammatory mediators LT B4, IL-1β, IL-6, and TNF-α are characteristically elevated in patients with RA. The improvement of disease activity because of increased consumption of n-3 LC-PUFA is associated with significant decreases in levels of serum IL-1β (Kremer et al., 1990, 1995), IL-6 (Sundrarjun et al., 2004), TNF-α (Sundrarjun et al., 2004), LT B4 (Cleland et al., 1988; Kremer et al., 1990; van der Tempel et al., 1990; Adam et al., 2003), and PG metabolites (Adam et al., 2003; Table 25.1).

In addition to the effects on clinical parameters, supplementation with n-3 LC-PUFA caused a reduction in patient's nonsteroidal anti-inflammatory drugs (NSAIDs) requirement without deterioration in the clinical and laboratory parameters of RA activity (Sköldstam et al., 1992; Lau et al., 1993; Geusens et al., 1994; Adam et al., 2003; Galarraga et al., 2008; Table 25.1). However, patients showed an accentuated improvement on ingesting supplements containing both fish and olive oil. According to Berbert et al. (2005), this development may relate to the ability of olive oil to decrease the expression of ICAM-1 and to increase the incorporation of n-3 PUFA into cell membranes. They also suggest that eicosatrienoic acid (20:3n-9) synthesized from oleic acid under reduced n-6 PUFA levels inhibits the synthesis of LT B4, thereby altering the balance of eicosanoids toward a less inflammatory mixture. A similar premise has been proposed by James et al. (2003).

In contrast, Geusens et al. (1994) found no improvement for the combination of n-3 LC-PUFA and olive oil, although when the latter was used as placebo, a low improvement of disease activity was observed in some studies (Cleland et al., 1988; Kremer et al., 1990; Dawczynski et al., 2009c; Table 25.1).

TABLE 25.1

Intervention Studies with Fish Oil in RA Patients (Human Intervention Trials)

Author	Design/Duration of Treatment Periods	RA Patients/Dropout (n)	Dosage and Intervention (n-3 LC-PUFA/Placebo)	Effect on NSAID Consumption	Effect on Disease Activity Parameters
Intervention studies with fish oil in RA patients					
Das Gupta et al. (2009)	Placebo-controlled parallel-designed study with two groups/12 weeks	100/19	Intervention: 75 mg indomethacin + 3 g n-3 PUFA per day (capsules) Placebo: 75 mg indomethacin capsule per day	Stable dose of prescribed NSAIDs during study. No differences in consumption between groups were described	Fish oil group: significant decrease of DAS28, swollen and tender joint count, duration of morning stiffness, VAS pain, patients global pain, ESR Placebo: significant decrease of DAS28, swollen and tender joint count, duration of morning stiffness, VAS pain, patients global pain, ESR, and CRP Better improvement in the intervention group (in comparison with placebo): DAS28 and swollen and tender joint count physical functioning, physical role, bodily pain, general health, vitality, social functioning, and duration of morning stiffness (but these changes were not significant in the intervention group)
Dawczynski et al. (2009a)	Double-blind, placebo-controlled crossover study/12 weeks (8-week washout)	45/6	Intervention: 2.4 g n-3 PUFA per day (1.1 g ALA + 0.7 g EPA + 0.1 g DPA+ 0.4 g DHA) in dairy products Placebo: common dairy products	Stable dose of prescribed NSAIDs during study. No differences in consumption between groups were described.	Fish oil group: improvement of HDL, lipoprotein A, and TAG. No effects on disease activity Placebo: improvement of HDL and lipoprotein a Dairy products: significant decrease of hydroxylpyridinium crosslink excretion and diastolic blood pressure

Reference	Study design	Patients/dropouts	Intervention	NSAID	Results
Dawczynski et al. (2009b, c)	Double-blind, placebo-controlled parallel-designed study with four groups/12 weeks	54 RA patients + 6 patients with psoriasis arthritis/7 dropouts	Four groups: (A) 3 g n-3 LC-PUFA per day; (B) 3 g GLA per day; (C) 1.6 g n-3 LC-PUFA + 1.8 g GLA per day; (D) 3 g olive oil Capsules	Stable dose of prescribed NSAIDs during study. No differences in consumption between groups were described	(A) Significant increase of n-3 LC-PUFA in PL, CE, EM, significant decrease of AA in EM and AA/EPA ratio in PL and EM (B) Significant increase of GLA, DGLA in CE, and EM (C) Low increase of n-3 LC-PUFA, GLA in PL, CE, and EM (D) No effect on n-3 LC-PUFA, GLA, DGLA in PL, CE, and EM (A, B, D) Significant decrease of DAS28 (A) Significant decrease of VAS pain (trend in group B)
Galarraga et al. (2008)	Dual-center, double-blind placebo-controlled randomized study/9 months	97 RA patients/17 dropouts of 49 patients in the fish oil group and 22 dropouts of 48 patients in the placebo group	Intervention: 10 g cod liver oil per day (containing 2.2 g of n-3 LC-PUFA) Placebo: air-filled identical capsules	At 12 weeks of the study, patients were instructed to gradually reduce, and if possible, stop their NSAID intake 19 (59%) of 32 patients in the fish oil group and 5 (19%) of 26 patients in the placebo group were able to reduce their daily NSAID requirement by more than a third at 9 months ($p = 0.003$) The reduction of NSAID intake had no worsening effects on disease activity	No differences between the groups with respect to HAQ, early morning stiffness, DAS-28-CRP, CRP, and grip strength Fish oil group: significant decrease of VAS for pain (-6.7 ± 3.05 mm) compared with the placebo group (1.9 ± 2.40 mm)

continued

TABLE 25.1 (continued)
Intervention Studies with Fish Oil in RA Patients (Human Intervention Trials)

Author	Design/Duration of Treatment Periods	RA Patients/ Dropout (n)	Dosage and Intervention (n-3 LC-PUFA/Placebo)	Effect on NSAID Consumption	Effect on Disease Activity Parameters
Berbert et al. (2005)	Parallel randomized design with three groups/24 weeks	55/12	Placebo (G1): soy oil Intervention 1 (G2): 3 g n-3 PUFA per day (fish oil) Intervention 2 (G3): 3 g n-3 PUFA per day (Fish oil) + 9.6 mL of olive oil	Stable dose of prescribed NSAIDs during study. No differences in consumption between groups were described	Significant improvement in the intervention groups (G2, G3) in relation to G1 regarding joint pain intensity, right and left handgrip strength after 12 and 24 weeks, duration of morning stiffness, onset of fatigue, Ritchie's articular index for pain joints after 24 weeks, ability to bend down to pick up clothing from the floor, and getting in and out of a car after 24 weeks G3, but not G2, in relation to G1 showed additional improvements with respect to duration of morning stiffness after 12 weeks, patient global assessment after 12 and 24 weeks, ability to turn faucets on and off after 24 weeks, rheumatoid factor after 24 weeks G3 showed a significant improvement in patient global assessment in relation to G2 after 12 weeks
Remans et al. (2004)	Double-blind placebo-controlled, parallel group study/4 months	66/11	Intervention: formula drink (1.4 g EPA + 0.21 g DHA + 0.5 g GLA + micronutrients) Placebo: formula drink without supplements	Stable dose of prescribed NSAIDs during study. No differences in consumption between groups were described	Both groups: no significant change from baseline in the clinical parameters (tender and swollen joint count, VAS pain, disease activity, grip strength, functionality score, and morning stiffness) Intervention: significant increase in PL concentrations of vitamin E, EPA, DHA, DPA, and decrease of AA Significant intergroup differences for PUFA and vitamin E

Reference	Study design/duration		Intervention/Placebo	Results
Kremer et al. (1995)	Double-blind, placebo-controlled, prospective study/26 or 30 weeks	66/10	Intervention: 130 mg n-3 LC-PUFA/kg body weight/day Placebo: corn oil capsules Diclofenac (75 mg/twice a day) Placebo diclofenac was substituted at week 18 or 22 (fish oil supplements were continued for 8 weeks (to week 26 or 30)) No further differences in consumption of NSAID between groups were described	Fish oil group: significant decrease in the number of tender joints, duration of morning stiffness, physician's and patient's evaluation of global arthritis activity, physician's evaluation of pain (the decrease in the number of tender joints remained significant 8 weeks after discontinuing diclofenac in patients taking fish oil and the decrease in the number of tender joints at this time was significant compared with the placebo group) Fish oil group: significant decrease of IL-1β (weeks 18, 22) Placebo group: no improvement in clinical parameters from baseline
Lau et al. (1993)	Double-blind, randomized study, parallel design with two groups/12 months + 3 months placebo treatment for all patients	64/–	Intervention: 10 MaxEPA capsules per day (171 mg EPA + 114 mg DHA/capsule = 2.85 g n-3 LC-PUFA per day) Placebo: air-filled capsules	No influence on clinical and laboratory variables of RA (articular index, grip strength, duration of morning stiffness, VAS pain, ESR, hemoglobin level, leukocyte and platelet count, hematocrit, mean corpuscular volume and mean corpuscular hemoglobin, IgM RF titer, and CRP NSAID requirement at entry visit = 100% Patients were instructed to slowly reduce their NSAID dosage after the first 6 weeks of the study providing there was no worsening of their symptoms Intervention: NSAID intake was decreased to 71.1% at 3 months compared with 89.7% in placebo, continued during the study (maximum at month 12; mean requirement for NSAIDs was reduced to 40.6% of the original dose compared with 84.1% in the placebo group; effect persisted to month 15)

continued

TABLE 25.1 (continued)
Intervention Studies with Fish Oil in RA Patients (Human Intervention Trials)

Author	Design/Duration of Treatment Periods	RA Patients/ Dropout (n)	Dosage and Intervention (n-3 LC-PUFA/Placebo)	Effect on NSAID Consumption	Effect on Disease Activity Parameters
Nielsen et al. (1992)	Multicenter, randomized, placebo-controlled, double-blind study/12 weeks	57/6	Intervention: 6 n-3 LC-PUFA capsules (2.0 g EPA + 1.2 g DHA g/day) Placebo: six capsules with fat composition equivalent to the average Danish diet	Stable dose of prescribed NSAIDs during study. No differences in consumption between groups were described	Intervention: significant improvement of morning stiffness and joint tenderness
Sköldstam et al. (1992)	Randomized, controlled, double-blind study/6 months	46/3	Intervention: capsules with 10 g fish oil per day (37% n-3 PUFA, including 18% EPA, 12% DHA = 3.0 g n-3 LC-PUFA per day) Placebo: a mixture of maize, olive, and peppermint oil with <2% ALA + <0.5% n-3 LC-PUFA	Decrease in NSAID consumption in treatment group at 3 and 6 months	Fish oil group: increase of n-3 PUFA in serum phosphatidylcholine, significant improvement in status of global arthritic activity at 3 months in physician's assessment Placebo: significant increase of global arthritic activity at 6 months No change was found in patient assessment of pain, duration of morning stiffness, functional capacity, and biochemical markers of inflammation
van der Tempel et al. (1990)	Randomized, double-blind, placebo-controlled crossover/12-week treatment periods (+12-week run-in period without FA supplementation)	16/–	Intervention: capsules with 12 g fish oil per day (2.04 g EPA + 1.32 g DHA per day) Placebo: fractionated coconut oil flavored with fish oil	Stable dose of prescribed NSAIDs during study. No differences in consumption between groups were described	Fish oil group: significant improvement of joint swelling index (2 ± 1 vs 8 ± 3 points) and duration of early morning stiffness (15 ± 5 vs 50 ± 13 min) in comparison to placebo; increase of EPA, DHA in CE, neutrophil membrane phospholipid fractions (mainly at the expense of n-6 PUFA); mean neutrophil LT B4 production in vitro significantly reduced; LT B5 production increase (not detected during control or placebo periods)

Study	Study design/duration	n	Co-treatment	Results
Tulleken et al. (1990)	Randomized, placebo-controlled study in parallel design with two groups/3 months	28/1	Intervention: 6 g fish oil per day (2.04 g EPA + 1.32 g DHA per day), 12.9 mg α-tocopherol per day, $n = 13$; Placebo: α-tocopherol-enriched coconut oil supplements flavored with fish oil (10.3 mg α-tocopherol per day), $n = 14$	NSAID consumption during the study and type of NSAID not reported	Fish oil group (compared with the control treatment): significant decrease of joint pain index (from 27 (3–103) to 6 (0–4)), Ritchie articular index (from 18 (3–49) to 6 (0–49)), and joint swelling index (from 7 (0–26) to 4 (1–16)). Control group: some clinical improvement (clinical improvement greater in the fish oil group). No influence on laboratory indices (complete blood cell count, ESR, plasma CRP, and IgM rheumatoid factor) of disease activity in both groups
Kremer et al. (1990)	Prospective, double-blind, randomized study/24 weeks	51/15	Intervention 1: 27 mg EPA + 18 mg DHA/kg body weight, low dose, $n = 20/18$; Intervention 2: 54 mg EPA + 36 mg DHA/kg body weight, high dose, $n = 17/15$; Placebo: olive oil capsules containing 6.8 g of oleic acid, $n = 14/3$	Stable dose of prescribed NSAIDs during study. No differences in consumption between groups were described	Fish oil group 1: significant decrease in number of tender joints at week 24 (−1.9 (−3.7 to 0.0)). Fish oil group 2: significant decrease in number of tender joints (at week 18 (−2.6 (−5.1 to 0.0)) and week 24 (−1.7 (−3.1, −0.2)). Fish oil group 1: significant decrease in number of swollen joints at week 12 (−2.7 (−4.4 to 1.0)), week 18 (−3.6 (−5.6 to 1.5)), week 24 (−4.1 (−6.9 to −1.8)), and week 36 (−4.1 (−6.9 to −1.8)). Fish oil group 2: significant decrease in number of swollen joints at week 12 (−2.9 (−4.0, −1.8)), week 18 (−2.3 (−3.9, −0.7)), and week 24 (−2.8 (−5.0, −0.7)). Fish oil groups: significant decrease of neutrophil LTB4 production (group 1 by 19%, group 2 by 20%), macrophage IL-1 production (group 1 by 40.6%, group 2 by 54.7%); increase of IL-2 (by 32.8% in group 1, by 16% in group 2; NS)

continued

TABLE 25.1 (continued)
Intervention Studies with Fish Oil in RA Patients (Human Intervention Trials)

Author	Design/Duration of Treatment Periods	RA Patients/ Dropout (n)	Dosage and Intervention (n-3 LC-PUFA/Placebo)	Effect on NSAID Consumption	Effect on Disease Activity Parameters
					Placebo: decrease of macrophage IL-1 production by 38.5% (NS)
					All groups: no significant changes in hemoglobin levels, ESR, and rheumatoid factor titer
					A total of 5 of 45 clinical measures were significantly changed from baseline in the olive oil group, 8 of 45 in the low-dose fish oil (1), and 21 of 45 in the high-dose fish oil (2) during the study
Cleland et al. (1988)	Double-blind, placebo-controlled non-crossover study/12 weeks followed by a 4-week washout	60/–	Intervention: 18 g fish oil per day in gelatin capsules (3.2 g EPA + 2.0 g DHA per day). Placebo: olive oil	Stable dose of prescribed NSAIDs during study. No differences in consumption between groups were described	Fish oil group: improvement in tender joint score, grip strength; reduction in production of LT B4 by isolated neutrophils stimulated *in vitro* by 30% (unchanged in the olive oil). Both groups: improvement of mean duration of morning stiffness, analog pain score (only significant in the olive oil group)

Intervention studies with fish oil in RA patients with reduced n-6 PUFA intake

Author	Design/Duration of Treatment Periods	RA Patients/ Dropout (n)	Dosage and Intervention (n-3 LC-PUFA/Placebo)	Effect on NSAID Consumption	Effect on Disease Activity Parameters
Sundrarjun et al. (2004)	Parallel randomized design with three groups/24 weeks, divided into (a) 6-week dietary advice period, (b) 12-week treatment, and (c) 6-week follow-up	60/25	Intervention (G1): diet low in n-6 FA + n-3 LC-PUFA (4 Omacor capsules with 470 mg EPA + 370 mg DHA = 3.36 g n-3 LC-PUFA per day), $n = 23$. Placebo (G2): diet low in n-6 FA + placebo supplement, $n = 23$	Stable dose of prescribed NSAIDs during study. No differences in consumption between groups were described	Fish oil group (G1) week 18: significant reductions in CRP, soluble TNF receptor p55, significant increase of serum EPA, and DHA compared with baseline; week 24: significant reductions in serum IL-6, TNF-α in all groups (G1–G3); percentage change in TNF-α from baseline in the fish oil group (G1) was greater than that in G3 (difference was NS). No significant difference between the fish oil and placebo group

Reference	n	Design	Intervention	Results	
			Control (G3): no special diet/intervention, n = 14. Patients were asked to use cooking oils containing less than 12.5 g/day of n-6 FA		No significant differences in the clinical variables (swollen joint count, tender joint count, ESR, VAS, Patient Global Assessment, and modified HAQ) between or within the three groups
Adam et al. (2003)	68/8	Double-blind, placebo-controlled crossover study with two groups (normal WD and AID)/3-month treatment (2-month washout)	WD group: normal western diet. AID group: anti-inflammatory diet—AA intake <90 mg/day. Patients in both groups were allocated to receive placebo or fish oil capsules (30 mg/kg body weight in crossover)	Decrease in NSAID consumption in treatment group (AID). AID (fish oil treatment): reduction of the NSAID dose (significant during fish oil in months 6–8). AID/WD (fish oil): significant reduction of corticosteroid doses	AID (not in WD): significant decrease in numbers of tender and swollen joints (placebo treatment). AID (compared with WD): significant reduction in the numbers of tender (28% vs 11%) and swollen (34% vs 22%) joints in the fish oil group. AID fish oil group: increase of EPA in EM, significant decrease of LT B4, 11-dehydro-TX B2, PG metabolites, and CRP. Both AID and WD on MTX ($n = 28$): significant decrease in CRP with fish oil treatment (not seen in patients with or without other DMARDs). AID versus WD (placebo treatment): reduction in the numbers of tender or swollen joints, patients' and physicians' global assessments of disability indicated improvement (NS), and patients' assessment of pain (significant); fish oil treatment reduced disease activity in both groups; overall improvement for joint parameters averaged 14% with AID, 17% with fish oil on WD, and 31% with fish oil and AID

continued

TABLE 25.1 (continued)
Intervention Studies with Fish Oil in RA Patients (Human Intervention Trials)

Author	Design/Duration of Treatment Periods	RA Patients/ Dropout (*n*)	Dosage and Intervention (n-3 LC-PUFA/Placebo)	Effect on NSAID Consumption	Effect on Disease Activity Parameters
					AID patients on fish oil (during months 5–8): the improvement was 37% (*P* < 0.001) for tender and swollen joints, the patients' (−31%) and physicians' (−40%) global assessments of disease activity, and the patients' assessments of pain (−40%) improved significantly more in the AID than in the WD group
					Fish oil treatment: 38% of the AID patients had at least 20% improvement according to ACR criteria, over baseline values of the corresponding period (*p* < 0.01), whereas only 24% of patients on WD fulfilled these criteria. 11-dehydro-TX B2, PGM lowered to a greater extent in AID than in WD patients
					Placebo treatment: increase of 11-dehydro-TX B2, urinary PGM (WD), and decrease of PGs in AID patients
					AID (fish oil treatment): significant decrease in LT B4 (WD: significant difference was only found on intake of fish oil during months 6–8 of the observation period); TNF-α decreased significantly in both WD/AID (this effect was not seen in patients on fish oil between months 1 and 3)
					At baseline: TNF-α and IL-1β were significantly higher in WD than in AID when fish oil was ingested between months 6 and 8

Study	Design/duration	N	Intervention	Medication/diet notes	Results
Volker et al. (2000b)	Placebo-controlled, double-blind, randomized study/15 weeks	50/–	Background diet: <10 g n-6-PUFA per day. Intervention: 3–6 fish oil capsules (60% n-3 PUFA) per day (40 mg n-3 LC-PUFA/kg body weight). Placebo: olive/corn oil capsules	Stable dose of prescribed NSAIDs during study. No differences in consumption between groups were described	Intervention: significant improvement of nine clinical variables compared with the placebo group (e.g., duration of morning stiffness, pain score, number of swollen joints, patients' and physicians' global assessment of disease activity, overall health assessment); five subjects (intervention) and three subjects (placebo) met the American College of Rheumatology 20% improvement criteria. Fish oil treatment: significant increase in EPA in PL and monocyte lipids
Geusens et al. (1994)	Double-blind, randomized study, parallel design with three groups/12 months	90/30	Intervention A: capsules with 2.6 g n-3 LC-PUFA per day. Intervention B: capsules with 1.3 g n-3 LC-PUFA per day + 3 g olive per day. Placebo: 6 g olive oil per day. Intake of animal fat was <100 g/day in all groups	Decrease in NSAID consumption in treatment group. Group A: 47% of patients were able to decrease these medications versus 15% in the placebo group. Group B: 29% of patients could decrease these medications (not significantly different from the other treatment groups)	Fish oil group (A): significant improvement in the patient's global evaluation and the physician's assessment of pain in comparison with placebo group (this difference was already observable after 3 months of supplementation and was sustained, tending to further increase, throughout the 12-month treatment period). Fish oil group (A): a significantly greater proportions of patients reported global improvement and were found to have a reduction in their pain score as assessed by the physician (compared with the placebo group, not seen in group B)

continued

TABLE 25.1 (continued)
Intervention Studies with Fish Oil in RA Patients (Human Intervention Trials)

Author	Design/Duration of Treatment Periods	RA Patients/ Dropout (n)	Dosage and Intervention (n-3 LC-PUFA/Placebo)	Effect on NSAID Consumption	Effect on Disease Activity Parameters
Intervention studies with fish oil in RA patients with respect to SFA intake					
Magaro et al. (1988)	Prospective, double-blind, randomized study/1 month	12/–	Intervention: diet high in PUFA (PUFA:SFA [P:S] ratio 5.0, supplemented with 1.6 g EPA + 1.1 g DHA per day) Placebo: diet high in SFA (P:S ratio 1.33)	Stable dose of prescribed NSAIDs during study. No differences in consumption between groups were described	Fish oil group: significant decrease in Ritchie's index (10.6 ± 3.48 vs 17.2 ± 3.38) and morning stiffness (22 ± 8.45 vs 33 ± 7.34 min); significant increase in grip strength (136 ± 12.88 vs 116 ± 13.26 mmHg); significant difference between the two groups at the end of the study: Ritchie's index (10.6 ± 3.48 vs 21.4 ± 3.2), morning stiffness (22 ± 8.45 vs 36 ± 10.17 min), and grip strength (136 ± 12.88 vs 104 ± 21.58 mmHg) Placebo: no statistical difference in clinical parameters; a nonsignificant alteration in neutrophil chemiluminescence (2.66 ± 0.38 vs 3.25 ± 0.58 cpm/PMN; p = NS) Fish oil group: significant reduction of neutrophil chemiluminescence (2.04 ± 0.3 vs 3.67 ± 0.87 cpm/PMN) Both groups: no significant changes in ESR, hemoglobin concentration, TAG, or cholesterol dietary levels

Kremer et al. (1985)	Prospective, double-blind, controlled study/12 weeks + follow-up	52/15	Intervention: diet high in PUFA and low in SFA + supplementation of 1.8 g EPA per day in capsules, $n = 17$ Placebo: diet lower in PUFA to SFA ratio + a placebo supplement (paraffin wax capsules)	Stable dose of prescribed NSAIDs during study. No differences in consumption between groups were described	Fish oil group: significant decrease of morning stiffness, number of tender joints Follow-up evaluation (1 and 2 months after stopping the diet): significant deterioration in the fish oil group in patient and physician global evaluation of disease activity, pain assessment, and number of tender joints Improvement in the placebo group: morning stiffness and number of tender joints

Abbreviations: AID, anti-inflammatory diet; CE; cholesterol esters; DGLA, dihomo-γ-linolenic acid; DPA, docosapentaenoic acid; EM, erythrocyte membranes; HAQ, Health Assessment Questionnaire; PL, plasma lipids; VAS, visual analog scale; WD, Western diet.

Recent studies report an increase in the beneficial effects of EPA + DHA, due to reducing the dietary intake of AA from animal fat (Geusens et al., 1994; Volker et al., 2000a, b; Adam et al., 2003; Sundrarjun et al., 2004; Table 25.1). Because of the simultaneous decrease of AA intake in the intervention studies by Sundrarjun et al. (2004) and Adam et al. (2003), the inflammation parameters CRP, IL-1, TNF-α, LT B4, PG metabolites, and TX B2 were significantly decreased in the fish oil treatment groups. Adam et al. (2003) found an average overall improvement for joint parameters of 14% because of the anti-inflammatory diet (Table 25.1) without fish oil intake, an improvement by 17% for the western diet with fish oil intake, and the improvement increased to 31% (28% for tender joints, 34% for swollen joints) with fish oil and anti-inflammatory diet. In conclusion, a diet low in AA ameliorates clinical signs of inflammation in patients with RA and augments the beneficial effect of fish oil supplementation suggesting a synergism between low AA intake and fish oil supplementation.

In previous studies, effective daily n-3 LC-PUFA dosages lay between 2.2 g/day (Galarraga et al., 2008) and 9 g/day (Kremer et al., 1995) for duration between 12 weeks and 12 months (Table 25.1). The main finding from the existing human intervention studies suggests that daily fish oil supplementation at dosages of around 3 g n-3 LC-PUFA per day for approximately 12 weeks is sufficient to effectuate a clinical benefit in patients with RA (Table 25.1). Berbert et al. (2005) demonstrated a greater benefit at 24 weeks rather than at 12 weeks. Studies with lower dosages did not show superior clinical benefit or anti-inflammatory effects of the daily supplementation with n-3 LC-PUFA in RA patients (Kremer et al., 1985; Geusens et al., 1994 [Group B]; Remans et al., 2004; Dawczynski et al., 2009a; Table 25.1).

The systematic validation of results regarding the efficacy of fish oil treatment in RA was achieved by means of meta-analyses. Seven published studies and three additional trials were included in the meta-analysis by Fortin et al. (1995). Data showed a significant reduction in tender joint count (rate difference = –2.9, 95% confidence interval [CI] = –3.8 to –2.1, $p = 0.001$) and duration of morning stiffness (rate difference = –25.9, 95% CI = –44.3 to –7.5, $p < 0.01$) associated with a 3-month supplementation with dietary fish oil compared with heterogeneous dietary control oils. For outcome variables including swollen joint count, grip strength, and patient and physician global assessment, erythrocyte sedimentation rate (ESR) did not achieve significance ($p > 0.10$).

A second meta-analysis by Goldberg and Katz (2007) included 17 randomized controlled trials assessing the pain-relieving effects of n-3 PUFA in patients with RA or joint pain secondary to inflammatory bowel disease and dysmenorrhea. The supplementation with n-3 PUFA for 3–4 months reduced patient reported joint pain intensity (standardized mean difference [SMD] = –0.26, 95% CI = –0.49 to –0.03, $p = 0.03$), minutes of morning stiffness (SMD = –0.43, 95% CI = –0.72 to –0.15, $p = 0.003$), number of painful and/or tender joints (SMD = –0.29, 95% CI = –0.48 to –0.10, $p = 0.003$), and NSAID consumption (SMD = –0.40, 95% CI = –0.72 to –0.08, $p = 0.01$). Significant effects were not detected for physician-assessed pain (SMD = –0.14, 95% CI = –0.49 to 0.22, $p = 0.45$) or for the Ritchie articular index (SMD = 0.15, 95% CI = –0.19 to 0.49, $p = 0.40$) at 3–4 months. The results suggest that n-3 PUFA are an attractive adjunctive treatment for joint pain associated with RA, inflammatory bowel disease, and dysmenorrhea.

These two meta-analyses are in accordance regarding the lack of a significant effect of n-3 LC-PUFA on swollen joint count, ESR, and patient's global assessment. Significant beneficial effects of n-3 LC-PUFA supplementation relate rather to number of tender joints, duration of morning stiffness, and requirement for NSAID treatment. The NSAID-sparing effect of n-3 LC-PUFA is beneficial for patients with RA because of the dose-dependent gastrointestinal and CV side effects correlated with the long-term use of NSAIDs. This is an important aspect that needs to be considered because RA is known to be associated with increased CV mortality (DeMaria, 2002).

In summary, fish oil supplements principally influence subjective signs of inflammation like joint tenderness, grip strength, fatigue, pain scale intensity, and the need for pain-relieving drugs. Biochemical indicators of inflammation, for example, CRP or ESR, were not significantly influenced in most intervention studies (Table 25.1).

On the basis of the totality of the data, a recommendation for the daily intake of dietary supplements containing a minimum of 3 g n-3 LC-PUFA for a minimum period of 12 weeks can be recommended for RA patients with an aim at reducing the NSAID dose and improving pain outcomes. The dietary supplement should not, however, replace the standard medical therapeutic regimen.

LIMITATIONS OF HUMAN INTERVENTION STUDIES WITH N-3 PUFA IN RA PATIENTS

Several factors may influence the outcome of intervention studies with RA patients. For instance, patient management is a complex task because of the variety of treatment drugs administered, alone or in combination, either to suppress symptoms or to modify disease activity. Intervention studies are designed to evaluate the add-on therapeutic effect of n-3 LC-PUFA supplementation in RA patients with persistent disease activity despite antiphlogistic and antirheumatic medication. Because study subjects are allowed to continue full treatment either with disease-modifying antirheumatic drugs (DMARD) or NSAID treatment regimens, observing and assessing the effects because of PUFA is not quite so straight forward for a number or reasons. For example, the considerable number of side effects in extensively treated patients may lead to a disruption of the therapy. In addition, the continued use of NSAIDs may have an effect on the metabolism of n-3 LC-PUFA (e.g., inhibition of COX due to NSAIDs).

Additional limiting factors that include n-3 LC-PUFA dosage, duration of the treatment period, background diet (AA intake and n-6/n-3 ratio in the diet), and type of placebo used (olive oil also has anti-inflammatory effects) have a significant influence on the observed effects. Finally, the genotype of the study subjects can also affect treatment outcome.

Long-term compliance of n-3 LC-PUFA intake is also an important issue because of the disagreeable side effects associated with fish oil intake, for example, gastrointestinal symptoms, nausea, flatulence, diarrhea, fishy taste or odor, and fishy regurgitation (MacLean et al., 2004). Appropriate markers of long-term compliance to n-3 LC-PUFA-rich fish oil supplements are denoted by concentrations of EPA and DHA in erythrocyte lipids (Sun et al., 2007), which may also serve as a guide to assess the success of therapeutic and preventive strategies aimed to increase the intake of dietary n-3 PUFA. Finally, gas chromatographic analysis of FA distribution in plasma, erythrocyte lipids, or other tissues can be a clear indicator of noncompliance to experimental conditions.

The rate of dropout from long-term studies before completion is relatively high (Table 25.1). A variety of reasons quoted for withdrawing include the inconvenience of scheduling and keeping study appointments, especially by patients in the placebo group, gastrointestinal side effects because of the high dosage of fish oil, changes in medication because of a new diagnosis (e.g., cancer), and a modification of DMARDs because of increased clinical disease manifestations. Other reasons that were cited comprised an increase in oral corticosteroid dose and the need for intra-articular steroid injection.

EFFECT OF FISH OIL ON INFLAMMATION PARAMETERS DEPEND ON GENOTYPE

Inflammation as part of the immune response induces the exaggerated production of proinflammatory cytokines in RA, for example, IL-1, IL-6, and TNF-α. Several but not all intervention studies have reported inhibitory effects of n-3 LC-PUFA on production of TNF-α. The influence of genotype might explain the inconsistency associated with the release of inflammatory cytokines in response to fish oil treatment. There is accumulating evidence implicating single nucleotide polymorphisms (SNP) in genes controlling proinflammatory cytokine production in influencing the individual level of cytokine production (Grimble, 2001).

Grimble et al. (2002) analyzed the relationship between TNF-α and lymphotoxin α genotypes and the ability of dietary fish oil (6 g n-3 LC-PUFA per day for 12 weeks) to suppress TNF-α production by PBMCs. The polymorphisms in the TNF-α (TNF*1 and TNF*2) and lymphotoxin α (TNFB*1 and TNFB*2) genes were determined in 111 healthy young men. A significant decrease of the TNF-α production after the n-3 LC-PUFA intake was observed in patients with the highest TNF-α baseline values. The extent of the cytokine production depended on its genotype. Medium and high inherent TNF-α production was associated with homozygosity for the LTα +252 (TNFB)2 allele, and individuals with medium or low levels of TNF-α production were more likely to experience the anti-inflammatory effects of fish oil if they were heterozygous for the LTα +252 (TNFB) alleles). Without consideration of these relations (baseline levels of TNF-α, genotypes), there was no overall effect of n-3 LC-PUFA supplementation on TNF-α production. These results indicate that only individuals with specific genotypes (TNF-α –308 and lymphotoxin α +252 SNPs) and inherent TNF-α production before supplementation will benefit from fish oil intervention. Paradoxically, fish oil caused enhanced TNF-α production in some subjects, particularly those in the tertile with the lowest TNF-α production before supplementation. Markovica et al. (2004) also described an association between carrying the genotypes and the increase of inflammatory stress because the ability of fish oil to reduce lipid levels or to behave in a anti-inflammatory manner in healthy men was influenced by BMI as well as the possession of the lymphotoxin α +252 SNPs.

EFFECTS OF N-3 LC-PUFA ON THE RISK FOR CORONARY HEART DISEASES

Patients with RA suffer from excessive CV morbidity and mortality when compared with age and sex-matched individuals. The increased incidence of CV events in RA patients is independent of traditional CV risk factors. This suggests that additional mechanisms are responsible for CV disease in RA (del Rincon et al., 2001).

The meta-analysis by Avina-Zubieta et al. (2008) determined the magnitude of risk of CV mortality in RA patients in comparison with the general population. The inclusion criteria for the observational studies (24 studies, comprising 111,758 patients with 22,927 CV events) were as follows: (1) prespecified RA definition; (2) clearly defined CV disease (CVD) outcome, including ischemic heart disease and cerebrovascular accidents; and (3) reported standardized mortality ratios (SMRs) and 95% CI. Overall, there was a 50% increased risk of CVD death in patients with RA (meta-SMR = 1.50, 95% CI = 1.39–1.61). In addition, the mortality risk for ischemic heart disease and cerebrovascular accident was increased by 59% and 52%, respectively (meta-SMR = 1.59, 95% CI = 1.46–1.73 and meta-SMR = 1.52, 95% CI = 1.40–1.67). Subgroup analyses showed that inception cohort studies (n = 4, comprising 2175 RA cases) were the only group that did not show a significantly increased risk for CVD (meta-SMR = 1.19, 95% CI = 0.86–1.68). The authors identified an increase in CVD mortality of 50% in RA patients compared with the general population.

The meta-analysis by Meune et al. (2009) included all cohort studies that had analyzed the association between overall increase in CV mortality and RA from January 1960 to November 2008. All cohort studies reporting CV mortality risk were included (17 studies, corresponding to a total of 91,916 patients). The overall pooled SMR was 1.6 (95% CI = 1.5–1.8, I^2 = 93%, p(heterogeneity [het]) < 0.0001). Mid-cohort year ranged from 1945 to 1995 (<1980, seven studies; 1980–1990, five studies; >1990, five studies). Meta-regression analyses revealed neither a trend in SMR over time (p = 0.784) nor any correlation with disease duration at the time of inclusion (p = 0.513). The results demonstrate that RA is associated with a 60% increase in risk of CV death compared with the general population. Despite changes in RA course over the past decades, SMR for CV death has not changed.

Numerous studies and reviews underline the beneficial effects of n-3 LC-PUFA in the prevention and management of CVD (Holub and Holub, 2004; Hjerkinn et al., 2005; Breslow, 2006). Evidence from clinical trials indicates that n-3 LC-PUFA decrease the risk of coronary heart disease by reducing myocardial susceptibility to lethal arrhythmias (Marchioli et al., 2002; Leaf et al., 2003; Geelen et al., 2005). Both EPA and DHA lower nonfatal and CV events by enhancing plaque stability (Thies et al., 2003), by decreasing the endothelial activation (Hjerkinn et al., 2005), and by acting anti-atherosclerotically via improving the vascular patency (Harris, 2007). An accumulation of EPA and DHA in platelets is associated with decreased platelet adhesiveness and aggregation and an overall reduction of thrombogenicity (Holub, 2002) because n-3 LC-PUFA replaced AA, the TX A2 precursor in blood platelet membrane phospholipids. In addition, EPA acts in an inhibitory manner on the COX-dependent formation of TX A2 from AA (Holub, 2002). Further, n-3 LC-PUFA improve blood lipids by lowering very low density lipoprotein (VLDL) cholesterol and triacylg-lycerides (TAG), which are important risk factors for atherosclerosis (Holub and Holub, 2004; De Roos et al., 2008; Milte et al., 2008). The TAG-lowering mechanism of n-3 LC-PUFA relates to their favorable effects on reducing hepatic production and secretion of VLDL and VLDL apolipoprotein B particles, along with favorable effects on plasma lipolytic activity through lipoprotein lipase-mediated clearance as well as stimulation of β-oxidation of other FA in the liver (Jacobson, 2008). The lipid-modulatory effects of high intakes of the fish oil FAs (EPA and DHA) are well established and likely to contribute to cardioprotective benefits.

The meta-analysis of Hartweg et al. (2007) determined the effects of n-3 LC-PUFA on lipopro-teins and other CV risk markers in patients with type II diabetes. The authors included 23 trials, involving 1075 subjects with mean treatment duration of 8.9 weeks. Compared with placebo, n-3 LC-PUFA had a statistically significant effect on the following four outcomes: (1) reduction of TAG (18 trials, 969 subjects) by 25% (mean = 0.45 mmol/L, 95% CI = −0.58 to −0.32, $p < 0.00001$); (2) VLDL cholesterol (7 trials, 238 subjects) by 36% (mean = 0.07 mmol/L, 95% CI = −0.13 to 0.00, $p = 0.04$); and (3) VLDL triacylglycerol (6 trials, 178 subjects) by 39.7% (mean = 0.44 mmol/L, 95% CI = −0.83 to −0.05, $p = 0.03$) but slightly increasing low-density lipoprotein (LDL) (16 trials, 565 subjects) by 5.7% (mean = 0.11 mmol/L, 95% CI = 0.00 to 0.22, $p = 0.05$). There were no significant effects on total cholesterol (TC), apolipoproteins, or lipid subfractions. The hypotriacylglyceridemic properties are related to both the dose of n-3 LC-PUFA used and the baseline TAG concentra-tions of the population. In patients with TAG concentrations >5.7 mmol/L, 4 g n-3 LC-PUFA has been shown to reduce TAG by 45%, VLDL by 42%, and non–high-density lipoprotein by 10.2% (Jacobson, 2008). Further, existing large-scale clinical trials such as the GISSI-Prevenzione Study and JELIS using low doses of n-3 FA (1–2 g) showed a clinical benefit in reducing coronary heart diseases without substantial changes in concentrations of TAG or other lipids (Jacobson, 2008).

The effects of n-3 LC-PUFA-supplementation on circulating lipid concentrations could be influ-enced by genetic variations. Madden et al. (2008) examine how SNPs in the CD36 gene modify the effects of fish oil on fasting plasma TAG, LDL, and HDL cholesterol concentrations in 111 healthy, middle-aged, Caucasian men. Subjects consumed habitual diets while taking 6 g MaxEPA daily for 12 weeks. TAG decreased from 1.48 to 0.11 mmol/L, and HDL rose from 1.27 to 0.04 mmol/L, respectively, irrespective of genotype. Significant falls in TAG only occurred in individuals with the GG variant of the 25444, 30294, –31118, or –33137 SNPs. These TAG-lowering effects could be due to stimulation of CD36 activity in extrahepatic tissue in individuals with the GG variants of these SNPs.

Caslake et al. (2008) determined the effect of moderate EPA and DHA intakes (< 2 g/day) on the lipid profile in 312 adults aged 20–70 years, who were prospectively recruited according to age, sex, and *APOE* genotype. Participants consumed control oil, 0.7 g EPA + DHA per day (0.7FO), and 1.8 g EPA + DHA per day (1.8FO) capsules in random order, each for an 8-week intervention period, separated by 12-week washout periods.

In the group as a whole, 8% and 11% lower plasma TAG concentrations were evident after 0.7FO and 1.8FO, respectively ($p < 0.001$): significant sex × treatment ($p = 0.038$) and sex × geno-type × treatment ($p = 0.032$) interactions were observed, and the greatest TAG-lowering responses (reductions of 15% and 23% after 0.7FO and 1.8FO, respectively) were evident in *APOE4* men. Furthermore, lower VLDL cholesterol ($p = 0.026$) and higher LDL cholesterol ($p = 0.010$), HDL cholesterol ($p < 0.001$), and HDL2 ($p < 0.001$) concentrations were evident after fish oil intervention. These results are indicative of a greater TAG-lowering action of n-3 LC-PUFA in men than that in women and the involvement of the APOE4 genotype.

Georgiadis et al. (2006) described differences in the lipid profile of patients with early RA (n = 58) in comparison with healthy volunteers (n = 63). The RA patients exhibited higher serum levels of total cholesterol, LDL cholesterol, and TAG, whereas their serum HDL cholesterol levels were significantly lower compared with controls. As a consequence, the atherogenic ratio of TC/HDL as well as that of LDL/HDL was significantly higher in patients with early RA compared with controls. After treatment with methotrexate (MTX), the first-choice DMARD in RA and prednisone, a significant reduction of the atherogenic ratios was observed, a phenomenon primarily due to the increase of serum HDL levels. These changes inversely correlated with laboratory changes, especially CRP and ESR. These results indicate that immunointervention to control disease activity may reduce the risk of the atherosclerotic process and CV events in patients with RA. Similar results were also found by Westlake et al. (2010). These literature data suggest that MTX use is associated with a reduced risk of CVD events in patients with RA (Westlake et al., 2010).

The literature data show an increased risk for CVD and CV death in RA patients in comparison with healthy controls. There is evidence to suggest that because of their influence on the risk factors, medication like MTX and a diet rich in n-3 LC-PUFA can decrease this risk for CVD. The supplementation of n-3 LC-PUFA could contribute toward a reduction in CV mortality, which should be considered as an important issue in RA therapy.

REFERENCES

Adam O, Beringer C, Kless T, Lemmen C, Adam A, Wiseman M, Adam P, Klimmek R, Forth W. Anti-inflammatory effects of a low arachidonic acid diet and fish oil in patients with rheumatoid arthritis. Rheumatol Int 2003;23:27–36.

Allred CD, Talbert DR, Southard RC, Wang X, Kilgore MW. PPARg1 as a molecular target of eicosapentaenoic acid in human colon cancer (HT-29) cells. J Nutr 2008;138:250–256.

Arita M, Ohira T, Sun YP, Elangovan S, Chiang N, Serhan CN. Resolvin E1 selectively interacts with leukotriene B4 receptor BLT1 and ChemR23 to regulate inflammation. J Immunol 2007;178:3912–3917.

Arita M, Yoshida M, Hong S, Tjonahen E, Glickman JN, Petasis NA, Blumberg RS, Serhan CN. Resolvin E1, an endogenous lipid mediator derived from omega-3 eicosapentaenoic acid, protects against 2,4,6-trinitrobenzene sulfonic acid-induced colitis. PNAS 2005;102:7671–7676.

Avina-Zubieta JA, Choi HK, Sadatsafavi M, Etminaan M, Esdaile JM, Lacaille D. Risk of cardiovascular mortality in patients with rheumatoid arthritis: a meta-analysis of observational studies. Arthritis Rheum 2008;59:690–1697.

Baeuerle PA, Baltimore D. Activation of DNA-binding activity in an apparently cytoplasmic precursor of the NF-kappaB transcription factor. Cell 1988;53:211–217.

Baldwin AB Jr. The NF-κB and IκB proteins: new discoveries and insights. Annu Rev Immunol 1996;14:649–681.

Berbert AA, Kondo CR, Almendra CL, Matsuo T, Dichi I. Supplementation of fish oil and olive oil in patients with rheumatoid arthritis. Nutrition 2005;21:131–136.

Blanquart C, Barbier O, Fruchart JC, Staels B, Glineur C. Peroxisome proliferator-activated receptors: regulation of transcriptional activities and roles in inflammation. J Steroid Biochem Mol Biol 2003;85:267–273.

Boileau C, Martel-Pelletier J, Fahmi H, Mineau F, Boily M, Pelletier J-P. The peroxisome proliferator-activated receptor γ agonist pioglitazone reduces the development of cartilage lesions in an experimental dog model of osteoarthritis. Arthritis Rheum 2007;56:2288–2298.

Bouwens M, van de Rest O, Dellschaft N, Bromhaar MG, de Groot L, Geleijnse JM, Müller M, Afman L A. Fish-oil supplementation induces antiinflammatory gene expression profiles in human blood mononuclear cells. Am J Clin Nutr 2009;90:415–424.

Brändström H, Jonsson KB, Ohlsson C, Vidal O, Ljunghall S, Ljunggren O. Regulation of osteoprotegerin mRNA levels by prostaglandin E_2 in human bone marrow stroma cells. Biochem Biophys Res Commun 1998;247:338–341.

Bray MA, Ford-Hutchinson AW, Smith MJH. Leukotriene B4: an inflammatory mediator *in vivo*. Prostaglandins 1981;22:213–222.

Breslow JL. N-3 fatty acids and cardiovascular disease. Am J Clin Nutr 2006;83:1477–1482.

Calder PC, Zurier RB. Polyunsaturated fatty acids and rheumatoid arthritis. Curr Opin Clin Nutr Metab Care 2001;4:115–121.

Calder PC. Dietary modification of inflammation with lipids. Proc Nutr Soc 2002;61:345–358.

Calder PC. n-3 polyunsaturated fatty acids and inflammation: from molecular biology to the clinic. Lipids 2003;38:343–352.

Calder PC. n-3 polyunsaturated fatty acids, inflammation, and inflammatory diseases. Am J Clin Nutr 2006a;83:1505–1519.

Calder PC. Polyunsaturated fatty acids and inflammation. Prostaglandins Leukot Essent Fatty Acids 2006b;75:197–202.

Caslake MJ, Miles EA, Kofler BM, Lietz G, Curtis P, Armah CK, Kimber AC, et al. Effect of sex and genotype on cardiovascular biomarker response to fish oils: the FINGEN Study. Am J Clin Nutr 2008; 88:618–629.

Caughey GE, Mantzioris E, Gibson RA, Cleland LG, James MJ. The effect on human tumor necrosis factor a and interleukin 1b production of diets enriched in n-3 fatty acids from vegetable oil or fish oil. Am J Clin Nutr 1996;63:116–122.

Cawston T. MMPs and TIMPs: properties and implications for the rheumatic diseases. Mol Med Today 1998;4:130–137.

Chen F, Castranova V, Shi X, Demers LM. New insights into the role of nuclear factor-κB, a ubiquitous transcription factor in the initiation of diseases. Clin Chem 1999;45:7–17.

Chinetti G, Fruchart JC, Staels B. Peroxisome proliferator-activated receptors (PPARs): nuclear receptors at the crossroads between lipid metabolism and inflammation. Inflamm Res 2000;49:497–505.

Christman JW, Lancaster LH, Blackwell TS. Nuclear factor-κB: a pivotal role in systemic inflammatory response syndrome and new target for therapy. Int Care Med 1998;24:1131–1138.

Cleland GL, French KJ, Betts HW, Murphy AG, Elliott JM. Clinical and biochemical effects of dietary fish oil supplements in rheumatoid arthritis. J Rheumatol 1988;15:1471–1475.

Cleland GL, James JM, Proudman MS. The role of fish oil in the treatment of rheumatoid arthritis. Drugs 2003;63:845–853.

Curtis LC, Hughes EC, Flannery RC, Little BC, Harwood LJ, Caterson B. Modulate catabolic factors involved in articular cartilage degradation. J Biol Chem 2000;275:721–724.

Curtis LC, Rees GS, Cramp J, Flannery RC, Hughes EC, Little BC, Williams WR, Dent MC, Harwood LJ, Caterson B. Effects of n-3 fatty acids on cartilage metabolism. Proc Nutr Soc 2002a;61,381–389.

Curtis LC, Rees S, Evans R, Dent MC, Caterson B, Harwood LJ. The effects of n-3 polyunsaturated fatty acids on cartilage metabolism in patients with osteoarthritis: the results of a pilot clinical trail. Proc Eur Fed Sci Technol Lipids 2004:216.

Curtis LC, Rees GS, Little BC, Flannery RC, Hughes EC, Wilson C, Dent MC, Otterness GI, Harwood LJ, Caterson B. Pathologic indicators of degradation and inflammation in human osteoarthritic cartilage are abrogated by exposure to n-3 fatty acids. Arthritis Rheum 2002b;46:1544–1553.

Das Gupta BA, Hossain M, Islam H, Dey RS, Khan LA. Role of omega-3 fatty acid supplementation with indomethacin in suppression of disease activity in rheumatoid arthritis. Bangladesh Med Res Counc Bull 2009;35:63–68.

Dawczynski C, Schubert R, Hein G, Müller A, Eidner T, Vogelsang H, Basu S, Jahreis G. Long-term moderate intervention with n-3 long-chain PUFA-supplemented dairy products: effects on pathophysiological biomarkers in patients with rheumatoid arthritis. Br J Nutr 2009a;101:1517–1526.

Dawczynski C, Hackermeier U, Viehweger M, Stange R, Springer M, Jahreis G. Einbau von langkettigen mehrfach ungesättigten n-3 Fettsäuren (n-3 LC-PUFA) und gamma-Linolensäure (GLA) in Plasmalipide, Cholesterolester und Erythrozytenmembranen bei Patienten mit rheumatoider Arthritis. Z Rheumatol 2009b;68:1–104.

Dawczynski C, Hackermeier U, Viehweger M, Stange R, Springer M, Jahreis G. Incorporation of n-3 LC-PUFA and GLA in plasma lipids, cholesterol esters, and erythrocyte membranes and their influence on disease activity of rheumatoid arthritis. 7th Euro Fed Lipid Congress "Lipids, Fats and Oils: From Knowledge to Application" 2009c, Graz, Austria.

Dayer MJ, de Rochemonteix B, Bums B, Demczuk S, Dinarello AC. Human recombinant interleukin-1 stimulates collagenase and prostaglandin E, production by human synovial cells. J Clin Invest 1986; 77:645–648.

De Roos B, Geelen A, Ross K, Rucklidge G, Reid M, Duncan G, Caslake M, Horgan G, Brouwer AI. Identification of potential serum biomarkers of inflammation and lipid modulation that are altered by fish oil supplementation in healthy volunteers. Proteomics 2008;8:1965–1974.

del Rincon DI, Williams K, Stern PM, Freeman LG, Escalante A. High incidence of cardiovascular events in a rheumatoid arthritis cohort not explained by traditional cardiac risk factors. Arthritis Rheum 2001;44:2737–2745.

Delerive P, De Bosscher K, Besnard S, Vanden Berghe W, Peters MJ, Gonzalez JF, Fruchart CJ, Tedgui A, Haegeman G, Staels B. Peroxisome proliferator-activated receptor alpha negatively regulates the vascular inflammatory gene response by negative cross-talk with transcription factors NF-kappaB and AP-1. J Biol Chem 1999a;274:32048–32054.

Delerive P, Fruchart CJ, Staels B. Peroxisome proliferator-activated receptors in inflammation control. J Endocrinol 2001;169:453–459.

Delerive P, Gervois P, Fruchart CJ, Staels B. Induction of IkappaBalpha expression as a mechanism contributing to the anti-inflammatory activities of peroxisome proliferator-activated receptor alpha activators. J Biol Chem 2000;275:36703–36707.

Delerive P, Martin F, Chinetti G, Trottein F, Fruchart CJ, Najib J, Duriez P, Staels B. PPAR activators inhibit thrombin-induced endothelin-1 production in human vascular endothelial cells by inhibiting the AP-1 signalling pathways. Circ Res 1999b;85:394–402.

DeMaria NA. Relative risk of cardiovascular events in patients with rheumatoid arthritis. Am J Cardiol 2002;89:33–38.

Elmgreen J, Nielsen HO, Ahnfelt-Ronne I. Enhanced capacity for release of leucotriene B4 by neutrophils in rheumatoid arthritis. Ann Rheum Dis 1987;46:501–505.

Endres S, Ghorbani R, Kelley EV, Georgilis K, Lonnemann G, van der Meer MJW, Cannon GJ, et al. The effect of dietary supplementation with n-3 polyunsaturated fatty acids on the synthesis of interleukin-1 and tumor necrosis factor by mononuclear cells. N Engl J Med 1989;320:265–271.

Espersen TG, Grunnet N, Lervang HH, Nielsen LG, Thomsen SB, Faarvang LK, Dyerberg J, Ernst E. Decreased interleukin-1 beta levels in plasma from rheumatoid arthritis patients after dietary supplementation with n-3 polyunsaturated fatty acids. Clin Rheumatol 1992;11:393–395.

Ford-Hutchinson WA, Bray AM, Doig VM, Shipley EM, Smith JMH. Leukotriene B, a chemokinetic and aggregating substance released from polymorphonuclear leukocytes. Nature 1980;286:264–265.

Fortin RP, Lew AR, Liang HM, Wright AE, Beckett AL, Chalmers CT, Sperling IR. Validation of a meta-analysis: the effects of fish oil in rheumatoid arthritis. J Clin Epidemiol 1995;48:1379–1390.

Galarraga B, Ho M, Youssef MH, Hill A, McMahon H, Hall C, Ogston S, Nuki G, Belch JJF. Cod liver oil (n-3 fatty acids) as a non-steroidal anti-inflammatory drug sparing agent in rheumatoid arthritis. Rheumatology 2008;47:665–669.

Gallai V, Sarchielli P, Trequattrini A, Franceschini M, Floridi A, Firenze C, Alberti A, Di Benedetto D, Stragliotto E. Cytokine secretion and eicosanoid production in the peripheral blood mononuclear cells of MS patients undergoing dietary supplementation with n-3 polyunsaturated fatty acids. J Neuroimmunol 1993;56:143–153.

Geelen A, Brouwer A, Schouten GE, Maan CA, Katan BM, Zock LP. Effects of n-3 fatty acids from fish on premature ventricular complexes and heart rate in humans. Am J Clin Nutr 2005;81:416–420.

Georgiadis NA, Papavasiliou CE, Lourida SE, Alamanos Y, Kostara C, Tselepis DA, Drosos AA. Atherogenic lipid profile is a feature characteristic of patients with early rheumatoid arthritis: effect of early treatment—a prospective, controlled study. Arthritis Res Ther 2006;8:R82.

Gervois P, Vu-Dac N, Kleemann R, Kockx M, Dubois G, Laine B, Kosykh V, Fruchart CJ, Kooistra T, Staels B. Negative regulation of human fibrinogen gene expression by peroxisome proliferator-activated receptor alpha agonists via inhibition of CCAAT box/enhancer-binding protein beta. J Biol Chem 2001;276:33471–33477.

Geusens P, Wouters C, Nijs J, Jiang Y, Dequeker J. Long-term effect of omega-3 fatty acid supplementation in active rheumatoid arthritis. A 12-month, double-blind, controlled study. Arthritis Rheum 1994;37:824–829.

Gilroy WD, Lawrence T, Perretti M, Rossi GA. Inflammatory resolution: new opportunities for drug discovery. Nat Rev Drug Discov 2004;3:401–416.

Goldberg JR, Katz J. A meta-analysis of the analgesic effects of omega-3 polyunsaturated fatty acid supplementation for inflammatory joint pain. Pain 2007;129:210–223.

Grimble FR, Howell MW, O'Reilly G, Turner JS, Markovic O, Hirrell S, East MJ, Calder CP. The ability of fish oil to suppress tumor necrosis factor alpha production by peripheral blood mononuclear cells in healthy men is associated with polymorphisms in genes that influence tumor necrosis factor alpha production. Am J Clin Nutr 2002;76:454–459.

Grimble FR. Nutritional modulation of immune function. Proc Nutr Soc 2001;60:389–397.

Grossmann M, Nakamura Y, Grumont R, Gerondakis S. New insights into the roles of ReL/NF-kappaB transcription factors in immune function, hemopoiesis and human disease. Int J Biochem Cell Biol 1999;10:1209–1219.

Hankenson DK, Watkins AB, Schoenlein AI, Allen GKD, Turek JJ. Omega-3 fatty acids enhance ligament fibroblast collagen formation in association with changes in interleukin-6 production. Proc Soc Exp Biol Med 2000;223:88–95.

Harris SW. Omega-3 fatty acids and cardiovascular disease: a case for omega-3 index as a new risk factor. Pharmacol Res 2007;55:217–223.

Hartweg J, Farmer JA, Perera R, Holman RR, Neil AH. Meta-analysis of the effects of n-3 polyunsaturated fatty acids on lipoproteins and other emerging lipid cardiovascular risk markers in patients with type 2 diabetes. Diabetologia 2007;50:1593–1602.

Hasturk H, Kantarci A, Ohira T, Arita M, Ebrahimi N, Chiang N, Petasis AN, Levy DB, Serhan NC, Van Dyke ET. RvE1 protects from local inflammation and osteoclast-mediated bone destruction in periodontitis FASEB J 2006;20:401–403.

Herrera SB, Ohira T, Gao L, Omori K, Yang R, Zhu M, Muscara NM, Serhan NC, Van Dyke ET, Gyurko R. An endogenous regulator of inflammation, resolvin E1, modulates osteoclast differentiation and bone resorption. Br J Pharmacol 2008;155:1214–1223.

Higgs AG. The effects of dietary intake of essential fatty acids on prostaglandin and leukotriene synthesis. Proc Nutr Soc 1985;44:181–187.

Hjerkinn ME, Seljeflot I, Ellingsen I, Bergstad P, Hjermann I, Sandvik L, Arnesen H. Influence of long-term intervention with dietary counseling, long chain n-3 fatty acid supplements, or both on circulation markers of endothelial activation in men with long-standing hyperlipidemia. Am J Clin Nutr 2005; 81:583–589.

Högström M, Nordström P, Nordström A. n-3 fatty acids are positively associated with peak bone mineral density and bone accrual in healthy men: the NO_2 Study. Am J Clin Nutr 2007;85:803–807.

Holub JB. Clinical Nutrition: 4. Omega-3 fatty acids in cardiovascular care. CMAJ 2002;166:608–615.

Holub JD, Holub JB. Omega-3 fatty acids from fish oils and cardiovascular disease. Mol Cell Biochem 2004;263:217–225.

Hoover LR, Karnovsky JM, Austen FK, Corey JE, Lewis AR. Leukotriene B4 action on endothelium mediates augmented neutrophil/endothelial adhesion. Proc Natl Acad Sci U S A 1984;81:2191–2193.

Horrobin FD. Low prevalence of coronary heart disease, psoriasis, asthma and rheumatoid arthritis in Eskimos: are they caused by high dietary intake of eicosapentaenoic acid, a genetic variation of essential fatty acid metabolism, or a combination of both? Med Hypotheses 1987;22:421–428.

Jacobson AT. Role of n-3 fatty acids in the treatment of hypertriglyceridemia and cardiovascular disease. Am J Clin Nutr 2008;87:1981–1990.

James JM, Proudman MS, Cleland GL. Dietary n-3 fats as adjunctive therapy in a prototypic inflammatory disease: issues and obstacles for use in rheumatoid arthritis. Prostaglandins Leukot Essent Fatty Acids 2003;68:399–405.

Karin M, Ben-Neriah Y. Phosphorylation meets ubiquination: the control of NF-κB activity. Annu Rev Immunol 2000;18:621–663.

Karin M, Delhase M. The IκB Kinase (IkK) and NF-κB: key elements of proinflammatory signalling. Semin Immunol 2000;12:85–98.

Kelley SD, Taylor CP, Nelson JG, Schmidt CP, Ferretti A, Erickson LK, Yu R, Chandra KR, Mackey EB. Docosahexaenoic acid ingestion inhibits natural killer cell activity and production of inflammatory mediators in young healthy men. Lipids 1999;34:317–324.

Kelley EV, Ferretti A, Izui S, Strom BT. A fish oil diet rich in eicosapentaenoic acid reduces cyclooxygenase metabolites, and suppresses lupus in mrl-lpr mice. J Immunol 1985;3:1914–1919.

Kleemann R, Gervois PP, Verschuren L, Staels B, Princen MH, Kooistra T. Fibrates down-regulate IL-1-stimulated C-reactive protein gene expression in hepatocytes by reducing nuclear p50-NFκB-C/EBP-b complex formation. Blood 2003;101:545–551.

Klickstein BL, Shapleigh C, Goetzl JE. Lipooxygenation of arachidonic acid as a source of polymorphonuclear leukocyte chemotactic factors in synovial fluid and tissue in rheumatoid arthritis and spondyloarthritis. J Clin Invest 1980;66:1166–1170.

Kremer MJ, Bigauoette J, Michalek VA, Timchalk AM, Lininger L, Rynes IR, Huyck C, Zieminski J, Bartholomew EL. Effects of manipulation of dietary fatty acids on clinical manifestations of rheumatoid arthritis. Lancet 1985;1:184–187.

Kremer MJ, Jubiz W, Michalek A, Rynes IR, Bartholomew EL, Bigaouette J, Timchalk M, Beeler D, Lininger L. Fish-oil fatty acid supplementation in active rheumatoid arthritis. A double-blinded, controlled, crossover study. Ann Intern Med 1987;106:497–503.

Kremer MJ, Lawrence AD, Jubiz W, DiGiacomo R, Rynes R, Bartholomew LE, Sherman M. Dietary fish oil and olive oil supplementation in patients with rheumatoid arthritis. Clinical and immunologic effects. Arthritis Rheum 1990;33:810–820.

Kremer JM, Lawrence DA, Petrillo GF, Litts LL, Mullaly PM, Rynes RI, Stocker RP, et al. Effects of high-dose fish oil on rheumatoid arthritis after stopping nonsteroidal antiinflammatory drugs. Clinical and immune correlates. Arthritis Rheum 1995;38:1107–1114.

Lau SC, Morley DK, Belch JJ. Effects of fish oil supplementation on non-steroidal anti-inflammatory drug requirement in patients with mild rheumatoid arthritis—a double-blind placebo controlled study. Br J Rheumatol 1993;32:982–989.

Leaf A, Kang XJ, Xiao FY, Billman EG. Clinical prevention of sudden cardiac death by n-3 polyunsaturated fatty acids and mechanism of prevention of arrhythmias by n-3 fish oils. Circulation 2003;107:2646–2652.

Lee HT, Mencia-Huerta MJ, Shih C, Corey JE, Lewis AR, Austen FK. Characterization and biologic properties of 5,12-dihydroxy derivatives of eicosapentaenoic acid, including leukotriene B5 and the double lipoxygenase product. J Biol Chem 1984;4:2383–2389.

Li H, Ruan ZX, Powis HS, Fernando R, Mon YW, Wheeler CD, Moorhead FJ, Varghese Z. EPA and DHA reduce LPS-induced inflammation responses in HK-2 cells: evidence for a PPAR-c–dependent mechanism. Kidney Int 2005;67:867–874.

Li M, Pascual G, Glass KC. Peroxisome proliferator-activated receptor gamma-dependent repression of the inducible nitric oxide synthase gene. Mol Cell Biol 2000;20:4699–4707.

MacLean HC, Mojica AW, Morton CS, Pencharz J, Hasenfeld RG, Tu W, Newberry SJ, et al. Effects of omega-3 fatty acids on lipids and glycemic control in Type II diabetes and the metabolic syndrome and on inflammatory bowel disease, rheumatoid arthritis, renal disease, systemic lupus erythematosus, and osteoporosis. Summary, Evidence Report/Technology Assessment No. 89. (Prepared by the Southern California/RAND Evidence-based Practice Center, Los Angeles, CA.) AHRQ Publication No. 04-E012-1. Rockville, MD: Agency for Healthcare Research and Quality; March 2004.

Madden J, Carrero JJ, Brunner A, Dastur N, Shearman PC, Calder CP, Grimble FR. Polymorphisms in the CD36 gene modulate the ability of fish oil supplements to lower fasting plasma triacylglycerol and raise HDL cholesterol concentrations in healthy middle-aged men. Prostaglandins Leukot Essent Fatty Acids 2008;78:327–335.

Magaro M, Altomonte L, Zoli A, Mirone L, De Sole P, Di Mario G, Lippa S, Oradei A. Influence of diet with different lipid composition on neutrophil chemiluminescence and disease activity in patients with rheumatoid arthritis. Ann Rheum Dis 1988;47:793–796.

Maggio M, Artoni A, Lauretani F, Borghi L, Nouvenne A, Valenti G, Ceda PG. The impact of omega-3 fatty acids on osteoporosis. Curr Pharm Des 2009;15:4157–4164.

Marchioli R, Barzi F, Bomba E, Chieffo C, Di Gregorio D, Di Mascio R, Franzosi GM, et al. Early protection against sudden death by n-3 polyunsaturated fatty acids after myocardial infarction—time course analysis of the results of the Gruppo Italiano per lo Studio della Sopravvivenza nell`Infarto Myocardio (GISSI)-Prevenzione. Circulation 2002;105:1897–1903.

Markovica O, O'Reillya G, Fussellb MH, Turnerb JS, Calder CP, Howell HW, Grimble FR. Role of single nucleotide polymorphisms of proinflammatory cytokine genes in the relationship between serum lipids and inflammatory parameters, and the lipid-lowering effect of fish oil in healthy males. Clin Nutr 2004;23:1084–1095.

Marx N, Sukhova KG, Collins T, Libby P, Plutzky J. PPARalpha activators inhibit cytokine-induced vascular cell adhesion molecule-1 expression in human endothelial cells. Circulation 1999;24:3125–3131.

Meune C, Touze E, Trinquart L, Allanore Y. Trends in cardiovascular mortality in patients with rheumatoid arthritis over 50 years: a systematic review and meta-analysis of cohort studies. Rheumatology 2009;48:1309–1313.

Meydani NS, Endres S, Woods MM, Goldin RB, Soo C, Morrill-Labrode A, Dinarello C, Gorbach LS. Oral (n-3) fatty acid supplementation suppresses cytokine production and lymphocyte proliferation: comparison between young and older women. J Nutr 1991;121:547–555.

Milte MC, Coates MA, Buckley DJ, Hill MA, Howe RP. Dose-dependent effects of docosahexaenoic acid-rich fish oil on erythrocyte docosahexaenoic acid and blood lipid levels. Br J Nutr 2008;99:1083–1088.

Murakami T, Yamamoto M, Ono K, Nishikawa M, Nagata N, Motoyoshi K, Akatsu T. Transforming growth factor-beta1 increases mRNA levels of osteoclastogenesis inhibitory factor in osteoblastic/stromal cells and inhibits the survival of murine osteoclast-like cells. Biochem Biophys Res Commun 1998;252:747–752.

Nagase H, Kashiwagi M. Aggrecanases and cartilage matrix degradation. Arthritis Res Ther 2003;52:94–103.

Nielsen LG, Faarvang LK, Thomsen SB, Teglbjaerg LK, Jensen TL, Hansen MT, Lervang HH, Schmidt BE, Dyerberg J, Ernst E. The effects of dietary supplementation with n-3 polyunsaturated fatty acids in patients with rheumatoid arthritis: a randomized, double blind trial. Eur J Clin Invest 1992;22:687–691.

Node K, Huo Y, Ruan X, Yang B, Spiecker M, Ley K, Zeldin CD, Liao KJ. Anti-inflammatory properties of cytochrome P450 epoxygenase-derived eicosanoids. Science 1999;285:1276–1279.

Palmer MR J, Stepney JR, Higgs AG, Eakins EK. Chemokinetic activity of arachidonic acid lipoxygenase products on leukocytes of different species. Prostaglandins 1980;2:411–418.

Pasceri V, Wu DH, Willerson TJ, Yeh TE. Modulation of vascular inflammation *in vitro* and *in vivo* by peroxisome proliferator-activated receptor-gamma activators. Circulation 2000;101:235–238.

Poulsen CR, Firth CE, Rogers WC, Moughan JP, Kruger CM. Specific effects of a-linolenic, eicosapentaenoic, and docosahexaenoic ethyl esters on bone post-ovariectomy in rats. Calcif Tissue Int 2007;81:459–471.

Recht L, Helin P, Rasmussen OJ, Jacobsen J, Lithman T, Schersten B. Hand handicap and rheumatoid arthritis in a fish-eating society (the Faroe Islands). J Internal Med 1990;227:49–55.

Remans HP, Sont KJ, Wagenaar WL, Wouters-Wesseling W, Zuijderduin MW, Jongma A, Breedveld CF, Van Laar MJ. Nutrient supplementation with polyunsaturated fatty acids and micronutrients in rheumatoid arthritis: clinical and biochemical effects. Eur J Clin Nutr 2004;58:839–845.

Rola-Pleszczynski M, Lemaire I. Leukotrienes augment interleukin-1 production by human monocytes. J Immunol 1985;135:3958–3961.

Sanderson LM, de Groot PJ, Hooiveld GJ, Koppan A, Kalkhoven E, Müller, M, Kersten S. Effect of synthetic dietary triglycerides: a novel research paradigm for nutrigenomics. PLoS One 2008;3:e1681.

Schwab JM, Serhan CN. Lipoxins and new lipid mediators in the resolution of inflammation. Curr Opin Pharmacol 2006;6:414–420.

Schwab MJ, Chiang N, Arita M, Serhan NC. Resolvin E1 and protectin D1 activate inflammation-resolution programmes. Nature 2007;447:869–875.

Serhan NC, Gotlinger K, Hong S, Arita M. Resolvins, docosatrienes, and neuroprotectins, novel omega-3-derived mediators, and their aspirin-triggered endogenous epimers: an overview of their protective roles in catabasis. Prostaglandins Other Lipid Mediat 2004;73:155–172.

Serhan NC, Hong S, Gronert K, Colgan PS, Devchand RP, Mirick G, Moussignac R-L. Resolvins: a family of bioactive products of omega-3 fatty acid transformation circuits initiated by aspirin treatment that counter proinflammation signals. J Exp Med 2002;196:1025–1037.

Serhan NC, Yang R, Martinod K, Kasuga K, Pillai SP, Porter FT, Oh FS, Spite M. Maresins: novel macrophage mediators with potent antiinflammatory and proresolving actions. J Exp Med 2009;206:15–23.

Sha CW. Regulation of immune responses by NF-κB/Rel transcription factors. J Exp Med 1998;187:143–146.

Shakhov NA, Collart AM, Vassalli P, Nedospasov AS, Jongeneel VC. KappaB-type enhancers are involved in lipopolysaccharide mediated transcriptional activation of the tumor necrosis factor alpha gene in primary macrophages. J Exp Med 1990;171:35–47.

Sköldstam L, Börjesson O, Kjällman A, Seiving B, Akesson B. Effect of six months of fish oil supplementation in stable rheumatoid arthritis. A double-blind, controlled study. Scand J Rheumatol 1992;21:178–185.

Strasser T, Fisher S, Weber CP. Leukotriene B5 is formed in human neutrophils after dietary supplementation with eicosapentaenoic acid. Proc Natl Acad Sci U S A 1985;82:1540–1543.

Sun Q, Ma J, Campos H, Hankinson ES, Hu BF. Comparison between plasma and erythrocyte fatty acid content as biomarkers of fatty acid intake in US woman. Am J Clin Nutr 2007;86:74–81.

Sundrarjun T, Komindr S, Archararit N, Dahlan W, Puchaiwatananon O, Angthararak S, Udomsuppayakul U, Chuncharunee S. Effects of n-3 fatty acids on serum interleukin-6, tumour necrosis factor-alpha and soluble tumour necrosis factor receptor p55 in active rheumatoid arthritis. J Int Med Res 2004;32:443–454.

Széles L, Töröcsik D, Nagy L. PPARγ in immunity and inflammation: cell types and diseases. Biochim Biophys Acta 2007;1771:1014–1030.

Terano T, Salmon AJ, Moncado S. Biosynthesis and biological activity of leukotriene B5. Prostaglandins 1984;27:217–232.

Thies F, Garry MJ, Yaqoob P, Rerkasem K, Williams J, Shearman PC, Gallagher JP, Calder CP, Grimble FR. Association of n-3 polyunsaturated fatty acids with stability of atherosclerotic plaques: a randomised controlled trial. Lancet 2003;361:477–485.

Trede SN, Tsytsykova VA, Chatila T, Goldfeld EA, Geha SR. Transcriptional activation of the human TNF-alpha promoter by superantigen in human monocytic cells: role of NF-kappaB. J Immunol 1995;155:902–908.

Tulleken EJ, Limburg CP, Muskiet AF, van Rijswijk HM. Vitamin E status during dietary fish oil supplementation in rheumatoid arthritis. Arthritis Rheum 1990;33:1416–1419.

Udalova AI, Knight CJ, Vidal V, Nedospasov AS, Kwiatkowski D. Complex NF-κB interactions at the distal tumor necrosis factor promoter region in human monocytes. J Biol Chem 1998;273:21178–21186.

van der Tempel H, Tulleken EJ, Limburg CP, Muskiet AF, van Rijswijk HM. Effects of fish oil supplementation in rheumatoid arthritis. Ann Rheum Dis 1990;49:76–80.

Volker HD, Fitzgerald EP B, Garg LM. The eicosapentaenoic to docosahexaenoic acid ratio of diets affects the pathogenesis of arthritis in LEW/SSN rats. J Nutr 2000a;130:559–565.

Volker D, Fitzgerald P, Major G, Garg M. Efficacy of fish oil concentrate in the treatment of rheumatoid arthritis. J Rheumatol 2000b;27:2343–2346.

Wang D, Hirase T, Nitto T, Soma M, Node K. Eicosapentaenoic acid increases cytochrome P-450 2J2 gene expression and epoxyeicosatrienoic acid production via peroxisome proliferator-activated receptor γ in endothelial cells. J Cardiol 2009;54:368–374.

Watkins AB, Li Y, Allen GKD, Hoffmann EW, Seifert FM. Dietary ratio of (n-6)/(n-3) polyunsaturated fatty acids alters the fatty acid composition of bone compartments and biomarkers of bone formation in rats. J Nutr 2000;130:2274–2284.

Watkins AB, Li Y, Seifert FM. Lipids as modulators of bone remodelling. Curr Opin Clin Nutr Metab Care 2001;4:105–110.

Weaver LK, Ivester P, Seeds M, Case DL, Arm PJ, Chilton HF. Effect of dietary fatty acids on inflammatory gene expression in healthy humans. J Biol Chem 2009;284:15400–15407.

Weber PC. Membrane phospholipid modification by dietary omega-3 fatty acids: effects on eicosanoid formation and cell function. In: Karnovsky ML, ed. Biological Membranes: Aberrations in Membrane Structure and Function. New York: Alan R. Liss; 1988.

Weiss AL, Barrett-Connor E, von Mühlen D. Ratio of n-6 to n-3 fatty acids and bone mineral density in older adults: the Rancho Bernardo Study. Am J Clin Nutr 2005;81:934–938.

Westlake LS, Colebatch NA, Baird J, Kiely P, Quinn M, Choy E, Ostor JA, Edwards JC. The effect of methotrexate on cardiovascular disease in patients with rheumatoid arthritis: a systematic literature review. Rheumatology 2010:295–307.

Yang YX, Wang HL, Chen T, Hodge RD, Resau HJ, DaSilva L, Farrar LW. Activation of human T lymphocytes is inhibited by peroxisome proliferator-activated receptor gamma (PPARgamma) agonists. PPARgamma co-association with transcription factor NFAT. J Biol Chem 2000;275:4541–4544.

Yao J, Mackman N, Edgington ST, Fan TS. Lipopolysaccharide induction of tumor necrosis factor-α promoter in human monocytic cells. J Biol Chem 1997;272:177795–177801.

Yokomizo T, Izumi T, Chang K, Takuwa T, Shimizu T. A G-protein-coupled receptor for leukotriene B4 that mediates chemotaxis. Nature 1997;387:620–624.

Zhao Y, Joshi-Barve S, Barve S, Chen HL. Eicosapentaenoic acid prevents LPS-induced TNF-α expression by preventing NF-κB activation. J Am Coll Nutr 2004;23:71–78.

Ziegler-Heitbrock WH, Sternsdorf T, Liese J, Belohradsky B, Weber C, Wedel A, Schreck R, Bauerle P, Strobel M. Pyrrolidine dithiocarbamate inhibits NF-kappaB mobilization and TNF production in human monocytes. J Immunol 1993;151:6986–6993.

26 Potential Health Benefits of n-3 and -6 Fatty Acids in Selected Plant Seed Oils in Rheumatoid Arthritis

Hiroyuki Takeuchi, Hiroyoshi Moriyama,
Debasis Bagchi, and Siba P. Raychaudhuri

CONTENTS

INTRODUCTION

Arthritis is a broad term used to describe encompassing more than 100 chronic and debilitating diseases of the joints, bones, and muscles [1, 2]. The two most common types are rheumatoid arthritis (RA) and osteoarthritis (OA). RA is a chronic inflammatory disease that is characterized by the attack of killer T cells on type II joint collagen, resulting in damage to cartilage with manifestations of joint swelling, pain, and inflammation and further into the deformity and destruction of joints and bones [3–6]. RA is known as an "autoimmune" arthritis, whereas OA is recognized as an age-related "wear-and-tear" arthritis [2]. More specifically, OA is a degenerative disease in which the joint cartilage deteriorates; as a consequence, pain, stiffness, and loss of movement become notable [7, 8]. In addition, inflammatory response has a common mediator in both types of arthritis; for example, T cells in RA and OA synovial membrane produce predominantly TH1 cytokines [9].

According to the Pharmaceutical Society of Japan, the RA population represents approximately 0.8% or 0.8 million people, the majority of which is found in women aged between 20 and 40 years, whereas an increase in the population ages older than 65 years has been apparent in Japan [10]. Existing and available treatments of RA, for example, include nonsteroidal anti-inflammatory drugs (NSAIDs) [11], steroid, and selective cyclooxygenase-2 (COX-2) inhibitors [12], which are designed to retard the disease progression and further joint deterioration. Thus, patients who are undergoing on such treatments potentially develop dependency on the medications and encounter side effects.

A survey conducted in Japan on the use of the "so-called health foods" (SCHF) as commonly defined primarily for dietary supplements [13] revealed that approximately 60% of definite patients with RA under the treatment of RA specialists had ever used SCHF in Japan [14]. Similarly, another research indicated that people who are suffering from chronic pain in RA and those who were not satisfied with present treatment tended to seek alternate therapeutics such as herbal supplementation, that is, 60%–90% of people with arthritis use complementary and alternative medicines [15]. In fact, the aforementioned are common to mitigate inflammation and pain involved in RA symptoms, while supplementation of SCHF such as glucosamine, chondroitin, shark cartilage, and undenatured type II collagen as an innovative ingredient [16] has been widely used for the alleviation of moderate inflammation and pain associated with another type of arthritis, OA, in Japan. However, in recent years, the anti-inflammatory effects of n-3 fatty acids (FAs) from fish oils have been demonstrated in studies using animal models and of humans, revealing potential benefits of improving RA symptoms [17].

The present chapter provides potential benefits of n-3 and/or n-6 FAs, for example, α-linolenic acid (ALA; 18:3) derived from various plant seed oils as a precursor of eicosapentanoic acid (EPA; 20:5), which has demonstrated to alleviate inflammation associated with RA. Selected plant seed oils containing FAs are briefly reviewed, whereas certain FAs possess suppressions of inflammation occurred in RA. Also, those plant seed oils with high contents of n-3 and/or n-6 FAs, such as flaxseed, borage, blackcurrant, and evening primrose seeds, which are commonly used and also prevalent in daily diets or from dietary supplement, are discussed in light of potential health benefits in patients with RA.

PLANT SEED OILS

HISTORY OF PLANT SEED OILS

In ancient times, the cold press technology, which was not well developed to produce plant seed oils as now, can be obtained easily and affluently in the marketplace; as a result, the oil was highly valued. Therefore, much of the oil was not used as edible oil in the daily diets but rather as for fuel, medicines, and cosmetics. However, in Greece, olive which is rich in oil had a long historical use as initiated from the Iron Age because oil was easily obtained from olive by using simple pressing, and olive had already been actively cultivated in Greece. In addition to olive, sesame was considered as an oldest crop grown, in which the seeds were used for producing oil. Furthermore, sesame was cultivated in diverse regions in the world, including ancient India, Egypt, Greece, and Rome, and even today sesame seeds are prevalent and grown throughout the world.

PRODUCTION METHODOLOGY

In general, most of the oils and fats derived from seeds of edible plants are separated from the plant body first by means of mechanical force. In addition, the residue after the separation is extracted with hexane. Then, the crude oil obtained requires further refining. After the removal of impurities such as phospholipids and nonesterified FAs, absorbent is added to the crude oil to decolorize. In addition, steam distillation is performed to eliminate undesired odor from the oil. The refined oil resin collected thus has slightly yellowish color with transparency, and it is tasteless and odorless. The oil is finally distributed as the edible oil in the market.

COMPOSITIONS OF PLANT OILS

Presently, oils such as palm oil, soybean oil, sunflower oil, and rapeseed oil are used as the main plant oils with rich sources of FAs. The composition of FAs therefore significantly varies by the origins of vegetables and plant seeds, thereby resulting in the difference not only in the FA composition but also in the physiological character. Table 26.1 shows the typical compositions of FAs contained in plant seed oils, including saturated FAs, monounsaturated FAs, and polyunsaturated FAs (PUFAs). The different types of FAs play a vital role in the body metabolism related to essential physiological activities.

FAs AND METABOLISM

CLASSIFICATIONS OF FAs

FA structurally is a compound with the carboxyl group at the end of chained hydrocarbon, and it mainly exists as the composing chemical of triacylglycerols. In nature, a wide variety of FAs are

TABLE 26.1
FA Composition of Plant Seed Oils (% Total FA)

	Palm Oil	Soybean Oil	Sunflower Oil	Rapeseed Oil
SFA				
12:0[a]	0.5	–	–	0.1
14:0	1.1	0.1	–	0.1
15:0	0.1	–	–	–
16:0	44.0	10.6	6.0	4.3
18:0	4.4	4.3	4.3	2.0
20:0	0.4	0.4	0.2	0.6
22:0	0.1	0.4	0.2	0.3
24:0	0.1	0.1	–	0.2
MUFA				
16:1	0.2	0.1	0.1	0.2
18:1	39.2	23.5	28.4	62.7
20:1	0.1	0.2	0.1	1.2
24:1	–	–	–	0.2
PUFA				
18:2 (n-6)	9.7	53.5	60.1	19.9
18:3 (n-3)	0.2	6.6	0.4	8.1

Source: Data obtained from Michio Yamaguchi, ed., Nihon Shokuhin Bunseki Hyou (Japan Food Analysis Table), 2nd ed., pp. 402–403, Ishiyaku, Tokyo, Japan, 2006 [in Japanese]. These data are from Standard Tables of Food Composition in Japan fifth Revised and Enlarged Edition, Fatty Acid Section reported by the Subdivision on Resources, the Council for Science and Technology, the Ministry of Education, Culture, Sports, Science And Technology, Japan.

Abbreviations: 12:0, lauric acid; 14:0, myristic acid; 15:0, pentadecylic acid; 16:0, palmitic acid; 16:1, palmitoleic acid; 18:0, stearic acid; 18:1, oleic acid; 18:2 (n-6), LA; 18:3 (n-3), ALA; 20:0, arachidic acid; 20:1, eicosanoic acid; 22:0, behenic acid; 24:0, lignoceric acid; 24:1, tetracosenoic acid; MUFA, monounsaturated FA; PUFA, polyunsaturated FA; SFA, saturated FA.

[a] Number of carbon atoms : number of double bonds.

found in different structures, depending on the number of carbon atoms and double bonds as well as the positions of the double bonds. The major dietary FAs can be divided into three series on the basis of the metabolic pathways in mammals: (1) the saturated and monounsaturated series, (2) the ALA series, and (3) the linoleic acid (LA) series. Typical food sources of ALA (n-3 series) and LA series (n-6 series) are summarized in Table 26.2.

In mammals, both PUFAs that are physiologically important cannot be synthesized because of the absence of desaturases required for the productions of the PUFAs. Those FAs that cannot be synthesized in the body are called essential FAs (EFAs), and the biosynthetic pathways of n-6 and n-3 FAs and their structures are shown in Figure 26.1.

TABLE 26.2
PUFAs and the Food Sources

FA	Examples of Food Sources
n-3 PUFA	
ALA	Flaxseed oil (linseed oil), soybean oil, and canola oil
EPA	Fish oils
DHA	Fish oils
n-6 PUFA	
LA	Safflower, corn, soybean, cottonseed, and sunflower oils
GLA	Evening primrose seed, borage seed, and black currant seed oils
AA	Meat, poultry, and eggs

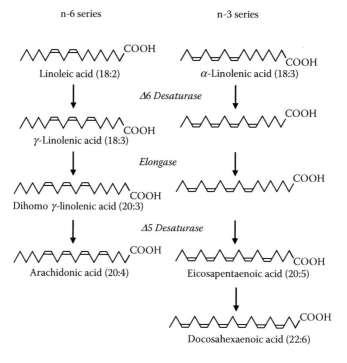

FIGURE 26.1 Metabolic pathways of n-6 and n-3 series FAs. The pathways involve desaturation and elongation.

Ingested FAs

FAs orally taken in the form of triacylglycerol, which is partially hydrolyzed by lipases at the small intestine, are absorbed into the gut. It is resynthesized to triacylglycerol at the wall of the small intestine again, and then chylomicron is formed and flowed into the blood and finally distributed inside the body. FA undergoes β-oxidation for the adenosine 5'-triphosphate production and is ultimately decomposed to carbon dioxide [18].

A part of the FAs are taken into lipid complexes such as phospholipids and become components of the cellular membrane. The cellular membrane plays an important role in transmitting signal information from outside of the cell through receptors. For example, proteins exist unevenly on the membrane with the presence of 30–40 phospholipid molecules for each protein. Such proteins may act as receptors, form ion channels, or have various functions such as surface enzymatic activities [19].

FAs and Eicosanoids

It is also known that that FAs act as precursors of various hormone-like substances. Physiological functions of such substances called eicosanoids produced are considered to be different depending on families of FAs. Furthermore, because FAs can be ligands of the nuclear receptors, it has been elaborated that the FAs also regulate the gene expressions. Thus, FA not only is used as energy or fuel in the human body but also *per se* regulates important biological functions through physical, chemical, and biochemical mechanisms. In fact, accumulated experimental data from different studies on molecular and cellular understandings on roles if the certain PUFAs in the human body have arisen remarkable increase in the scientific attention and public interest in n-3 FAs for their multifaceted health benefits related to cancer, inflammatory bowel disease, psoriasis, and RA [20].

PUFA-DERIVED EICOSANOIDS IN RA

Different Eicosanoids

However, much of the attention was directed to n-3 FAs from fish oils to assess the impact of FAs on the immune system in connection to suppression of inflammation [19–21], whereas eicosanoids derived from certain FA metabolites as mediators of inflammation and immune cell function play a vital role. The eicosanoids represent four families, including prostaglandins (PGs), prostacyclins, thromboxanes (TXAs), and leukotrienes (LTs). Different eicosanoids are derived from n-3 or n-6 EFAs. Briefly, the eicosanoid is synthesized from the cellular stimulation *via* arachidonic acid (AA), which is the most abundant eicosanoid precursor and has crucial influence on inflammation/immune-mediated diseases such as asthma and RA in humans [20].

The initial activating compound is LA and then into γ-linolenic acid (GLA) and dihomo-GLA (DGLA) in the n-6 FA series, while ALA is metabolized into EPA in the n-3 FA series (Figure 26.1). However, the eicosanoids produced *in vivo* are mostly derived from AA and are proinflammatory. Thus, the biosynthesis involving such eicosanoids is often called as the AA cascade. This biosynthesis more likely occurred in the Western diet rich in n-6 FAs, which contain high contents of LA [22, 23]. Moreover, n-6 EFAs (e.g., AA) are generally known to play proinflammatory roles, whereas n-3 EFAs (e.g., EPA) exhibit less proinflammatory or anti-inflammatory activities [22]. Balanced intake of EFAs of n-6 and n-3 series FAs from diets or dietary supplements seems to affect the body's eicosanoid-regulated physiological functions, such as mitigating inflammation associated with RA [22, 23].

RA-linked Eicosanoids

It has been reported that genetic, environmental, and infectious factors are also important in triggering complex mechanistic actions of RA [24–27]. Most likely, such factor(s) might activate macrophage, B cells, T cells, and monocytes as well as inflammatory and other immune-related cells at the sites of synovial membranes. Briefly, during the course of proinflammatory events, B cells within the synovium produce rheumatoid factor as an autoantibody to denatured immunoglobulin G. Rheumatoid factor binds to the autologous immunoglobulin G, forming immune complexes inducing the migration and activation of neutrophils. Neutrophilic activation is a characteristic occurrence in RA because high amounts of neutrophils are found in the synovial fluid of patients with RA [28]. The activated neutrophils release eicosanoids such as PGE_2 and LTB_4 derived from AA, proteolytic enzymes including metalloproteases, and reactive oxygen species, which are potent effectors of cartilage destruction. In parallel, the activated macrophages release interleukin1β (IL-1β) and tumor necrosis factor α (TNF-α), which are primary proinflammatory mediators, stimulating the synovial membrane, leading to tissue inflammation and eventually resulting in cartilage destruction. Moreover, IL-1β, TNF-α, and other mediators promote the proliferation of synovial cells by forming pannus, which is the granulation tissue at synovial membranes, propagating the joint destruction. Thus, IL-1β, TNF-α, and other inflammation-related cytokines along with PGE_2 and LTB_4 as the metabolites of AA (PUFA) play crucial roles in RA [17, 23, 27, 29, 30].

PUFA AND EICOSANOIDS

Because of the functional differences between AA-derived PGs and LTs and LA-derived eicosanoids (Figure 26.2), their effects on the inflammation of the synovial membrane associated with RA vary according to series of the PUFAs ingested in the diet or taken from the supplement. When cells are exposed to dissimilar physiological and pathological stimuli, AA is liberated from membrane phospholipids by phospholipase A_2 and is converted to PGH_2 by prostaglandin H synthase (COX-1 or COX-2) and peroxidase. PGH_2 is the common substrate for a number of different synthases that

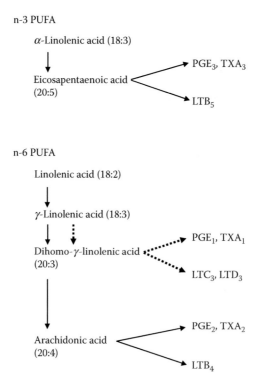

FIGURE 26.2 Metabolic pathways of n-3 and n-6 PUFAs in the formations of proinflammatory and antiinflammatory eicosanoids. Dashed lines show pathways to the anti-inflammation.

produce the major prostanoids or series 2 PGs, including PGD_2, PGE_2, PGF_2, prostacyclin (PGI_2), and TXA_2. In the other biosynthetic pathway, AA is converted by 5′-lipoxygenase (5-LOX) into series 4 LTs, such as LTA_4, LTB_4, LTC_4, LTD_4, and LTE_4. On the other hand, EPA can act as a substrate for both COX and 5-LOX, generating series 3 PGs/TXAs or series 5 LTs, respectively [22, 29].

In Figure 26.2, AA-derived eicosanoids such as PGE_2 and LTB_4 promote such inflammation and ultimately to cartilage destruction; however, it seems that AA, a bioactive FA, exerts a downregulating effect at high concentrations [30]. On the other hand, EPA-derived PG and LT is synthesized in the cell, but they have weak physiological activities. Therefore, inflammation associated with RA is potentially regulated with a decrease in the amounts and activities of inflammatory mediators by lowering the concentration of AA in the cell membrane and concomitantly by increasing the concentrations of EPA [29]. Administered n-3 FA is converted to EPA, which does not only increase the concentrations of EPA in the cell membrane phospholipids but also potentially inhibit a metabolic pathway from LA to AA. It is noteworthy that this pathway exhibits the same enzymatic actions that convert ALA to EPA, involving Δ6 desaturase, elongase, and Δ5 desaturase (Figure 26.1).

PUFAs AND INFLAMMATORY DISEASES: RA

Little attention has been paid to n-3 derived from plant seed oils such as flaxseed oil (FXO); however fish oils enriched with n-3 PUFA such as EPA and decosahexaenoic acid (DHA; 22:6) have been previously shown to have health benefits in patients with RA [19–21]. Studies of PUFAs derived from fish oils and also plant seed oils on the therapy of RA were extensively conducted since 1980s, in which results were reported and reviewed in light of assessing efficacies and also elucidating the suppressive mechanism of inflammatory action in *ex vivo* and *in vivo* using animal models, and evaluating human clinical trials [17, 23, 29–32].

α-LINOLENIC ACID

Flaxseed (linseed) oil (FXO), for example, contains approximately 60% of ALA (Table 26.3), whereas other known oils such as rapeseed oil (canola oil) and soybean oil only contain approximately 10% of ALA [34]. Part of the ingested ALA, if not all, from the diet is converted into EPA then further into DHA *via* the process of desaturation and chain elongation in the body (Figure 26.1).

ALA was found to have a wide range of health benefits, such as helping in maintaining appropriate neural function, and also it became apparent that n-3 FA is EFA along with another independent EFA, that is, n-6 FA including LA. For example, n-3 PUFAs such as EPA and DHA are essential for normal cell growth, playing an important role in the prevention and treatment of coronary artery disease, hypertension, cancer, and other inflammatory and autoimmune disorders which include

TABLE 26.3
Typical Composition of n-6 and n-3 FAs in Selected Plant Seed Oils (Typical %)

Predominant Fatty Acids	FXO	BSO	BCO	EPO
18:2[a] (n-6)		38	47	72
18:3 (n-6)		23	17	9
18:3 (n-3)	60			

Note: 18:2 (n-6), LA; 18:3 (n-6), GLA; 18:3 (n-3) ALA.

Abbreviations: BCO, blackcurrant seed oil; BSO, borage seed oil; EPO, evening primrose seed oil; FXO, flaxseed oil.

[a] Number of carbon atoms : number of double bonds.

RA [20]. To obtain maximum effects on such chronic diseases, the ratio of n-6/n-3 FA is remarkably important [33, 34].

In a previous review, the inhibitory mechanism of inflammation by n-3 FAs at the molecular and cellular levels has gradually become more evident, and such FAs seem to accumulate in membranes, playing either structural function or role as substrate and interacting with the membrane proteins [35]. Also, it discussed the effects of free FAs into phospholipids [35].

The scientific evidence potentially interprets anti-inflammatory effects of the selected FAs acting as a competitive substance or substrate of AA resident in membranes to suppress the formation of proinflammatory eicosanoids such as PGE_2 and LTB_4 [22, 29]. More recently, it has been shown that EPA and DHA produce novel anti-inflammatory lipids such as resolvins and protectins to possess anti-inflammatory effects as proposed by investigations using animal models [36, 37]. Furthermore, it has been shown that EPA and DHA inhibit activation of the transcription factor nuclear factor κB and the release of cytokines such as IL-1β and TNF-α as key regulators of inflammation [38, 39]. In addition, investigation demonstrated that EPA could suppress the proliferation of fibroblast like synoviocytes *in vitro* [40].

A study tested patients with RA to take supplements containing 3–6 g of n-3 FAs daily for more than 12 weeks while continuing to receive the standard therapeutic medical regimen. Ingestion of 3 g or more of n-3 FAs (EPA/DHA) potentially affected reductions in the release of LTB_4 from activated neutrophils and also of IL-1 from monocytes, while those eicosanoids were proinflammatory molecules in RA. Furthermore, it revealed that it could possibly reduce the NSAID dose under the supervision of a physician after taking n-3 FAs supplements for 3–4 months [41].

The other review provided a meta-analysis examining the pain alleviating effects of n-3 FAs and EPA/DHA in patients with RA [32]. In the study, 17 studies were included in the meta-analysis, of which 16 studies were conducted against patients with RA. In a study reported in the review, FXO was used as the source of n-3 PUFA, in which human study was conducted in a double-blind, placebo-controlled and randomized manner [42]. Details are discussed in the next section.

Although human clinical trials using n-3 FA (ALA) of botanical origins have not been positive, the mechanism in which n-3 PUFA such as EPA behaves is hypothesized in that intake of fish oils rich in EPA/DHA inhibits the formation of COX and LOX products derived AA [43, 44], thus providing a modest anti-inflammatory action in patients with RA [45, 46].

Flaxseed Oil

Seeds of flax (*Linum usitatissimum* L.) is a good source of oil with high content of ALA. FXO is obtained in liquid and softgel capsule forms. When the oil is stored, it requires special packaging because it is easily vulnerable to heat, light, and oxygen like any other edible oils. Consequently, products containing FXO must be produced and distributed with care considering the above adversary factors. Also, it should be free of heavy metals such as lead and mercury to assure maximum health benefits.

Generally, the dosage of FXO recommended for adult is one to two tablespoonfuls daily or as a supplement one to two capsules a day. Flaxseed in liquid form contains approximately 7 g of ALA/15 mL [47]. It is however presumed that there are possible interactions with medications because flaxseed possibly slows down the absorption of orally taken medicines when concomitantly taken. Potential interactions may include blood thinning, blood sugar lowering, and cholesterol-lowering medications, cyclosporine, etretinate, and topical steroids although effects vary in some extents [47].

It contains approximately 60% n-3 FAs in the form of ALA [34], which is almost double that contained in fish oil. However, it seems that ALA in plant seed oil unlike EPA in fish oils, which is not readily bioavailable in the body when ingested, is converted less efficiently to the form of effective n-3 FAs [42]. Although both ALA and EPA belong to n-3 series FA, the extent of health benefits thus such as for hyperlipidemia, hypertension, and RA considerably differ. For example, EPA is specially known to reduce inflammation involved in arthritis diseases, RA in particular [22]. Such discrepancy in efficacies using PUFAs in the same n-3 series but from the different sources is still remained to be elucidated.

The previous review also stated that the FXO study [42] showed no improvements in RA symptoms after 3 months of ALA supplementation. But in the same review, higher dosages of n-3 PUFA from fish oils could decrease the levels of triglyceride in the blood with daily intake of 2–4 g, and a minimum of 3 g/day was required to reduce RA symptoms such as morning stiffness in patients with RA [48]. It immediately suggested that dosage might be one of the factors affecting any results in human studies.

Further, to evaluate the study of FXO in humans [42], the experimental design was examined for its validity. In the study, the treatment group received 30 g of FXO (32% ALA), or approximately 9. 5 g of ALA/day for 3 months was administered to the treatment group (11 patients) compared with the placebo group (11 patients) who received 30 g of safflower oil (33% LA). The study used patient's and investigator's five-scale global assessments, functional classification [49], Kaarela's joint score index [50], and subjective visual analog scale for pain [51] and the measurement of the laboratory values such as erythrocyte sedimentation rate, C-reactive protein, and hemoglobin [52]. The result of the study did not show any improvements in the above assessments. In addition, the investigation was considered as one of the early studies using FXO for ALA to gauge efficacy of botanical n-3 series FA in patients with RA and also was an initial attempt to examine the potential conversion of ALA to EPA and also to observe the effect of AA reduction by ALA in the human body, which was later hypothesized by other studies [22, 33]. Also, the study argued that the conversion might require zinc, which possibly regulates desaturase enzyme activities in the conversion from ALA to EPA [42]; zinc was reported to play a pivotal role in the involvement of FA metabolism and membranes [53].

An *in vitro* study was conducted to observe the effects of an FXO-based diet on the production of TNF-α and IL-1β. In the study, FXO containing approximately 56% of ALA and 18% LA was administered to healthy male volunteers ($n = 15$) in their diet and the control group ($n = 15$) ingested sunflower. The results of the study demonstrated that the concentrations of mononuclear cell FAs such as ALA and EPA were enhanced 3.0-fold and 2.3-fold, respectively, while TNF-α, IL-1β, thromboxane B_2 (TXB_2), and PGD_2 productions decreased by approximately 30% after 4 weeks [54]. The result of the study was likely to support evidence that part of the ingested ALA in FXO could be converted into EPA.

Nevertheless, the clinical study suggested that ALA from FXO was not effective [42]. When the health benefit of n-3 series FAs is to test patients, for example, in RA, it is now important to consider the background of elaborated dietary habits of the patients undergoing clinical trials [41]. Further, *in vitro* and *in vivo* studies need to enhance the detailed understanding on the biochemical pathway of ALA to EPA, which is still unclear, particularly the enzymes involved in desaturation and elongation in the presence of other series of PUFA in FXO in the body. It is obviously meaningful to design dexterous human clinical trials using ALA from other plant seed oils, if not FXO, to determine whether obtaining anti-inflammatory effects of ALA as comparable with those of EPA and DHA from fish oils is possible.

γ-LINOLENIC ACID

Oils containing rich GLA are limited to special plant seeds such as borage, blackcurrant, and evening primrose. Recently, culturing microorganisms has been used to produce GLA [55–57].

In the human body, ingested LA may be converted into GLA, DGLA, and AA on the basis of the biosynthetic pathway (Figure 26.1). Eicosanoids such as PGs and other bioactive compounds are generated from AA in the cell membrane, which regulate various important physiological activities. For example, DGLA and LA change AA metabolism by neutrophils, which play a key role in the synovitis, although such neutrophils are counted more than 5×10^4 per mm^3 in the synovial fluids of patients with RA [28]. In addition, proinflammatory eicosanoid, LTB_4, produced by neutrophils was suppressed by both DGLA and LA, whereas DGLA and LA demonstrated 85% and 60% inhibitions, respectively [58]. The same study also confirmed increase in the 15-LOX metabolites, which directly inhibited LTB_4 synthesis by neutrophils [58].

Furthermore, GLA is metabolized into DGLA as the immediate precursor of PGE_1, an eicosanoid with anti-inflammatory and immunoregulatory activities [59]. Also, DGLA has been shown to modulate immune response by enacting directly on T cells in a PG-independent manner [60, 61]. Similarly, the concentration level of DGLA in the cellular membrane is a factor that affects the production of AA, the primary source of proinflammatory eicosanoids, and also the formation of PGE_1 and TXA_1 *via* COX as well as (15OH)DGLA and LTC_3 *via* LOX as anti-inflammatory eicosanoids, which are dependent on the activity of Δ^5 desaturase [31, 62, 63].

As shown in Figure 26.2, when GLA was ingested, series 1 PGs and TXAs as well as series 3 were produced after being converted to DGLA. Because PGE_1, a DGLA-derived eicosanoid, suppressed IL-1β, DGLA was thus found to possess inhibitory effect [22]. Moreover, addition of GLA *in vitro* inhibited the release of IL-1β from human monocytes that were stimulated with lipopolysaccharide. Consequently, in the study, GLA reduced autoinduction, an amplification of IL-1β, while maintaining the initial IL-1β response to lipopolysaccharide intact [64].

Borage Seed Oil

Borage (*Boragao officinalis* L.) is a herb that originated in Syria and is now widely cultivated for culinary and medicinal uses throughout Europe, North Africa, and North America. Specifically, oil derived from the seeds is rich in GLA. The profiles of representative FAs are palmitic acid, stearic acid, oleic acid, and LA.

An *in vitro* study showed that TNF-α might play a role as a central mediator of inflammatory and joint destructive processes in RA, where GLA in the borage seed oil (BSO) increased PGE levels that further enhanced cyclic AMP levels that in turn suppressed TNF-α synthesis [65].

A pilot study reported seven patients with active RA who received 11 g/day of GLA for 12 weeks [66]. In the study, increased proportions of the GLA metabolite, DGLA, were detected in circulating mononuclear cells. Also, significant reduction in PGE_2, LTB_4, and LTC_4 produced by stimulated monocytes was observed after 12 weeks of GLA administration. Majority of the enrolled patients showed clinical improvement [66].

Efficacy and side effects of GLA were assessed in 27 patients with RA completed, of which 19 received GLA and 13 patients received cotton seed oil as placebo [67]. The clinical study showed that treatment with 1.4 g/day of GLA in the form of BSO compared with the patients in the placebo group received cotton seed oil for 6 months. The result of the study demonstrated that GLA group showed a significant difference in reductions in clinical parameters and symptoms of RA ($p < 0.05$), whereas patients in the placebo group showed no change or any aggravation. Specifically, GLA reduced the tender joint score by 45%, the swollen joint count by 28%, and the swollen joint score by 41% as compared with the placebo group. Side effects of GLA intake were negligible [67].

In another study, 56 patients ingested either 2.8 g/day of GLA derived from BSO or sunflower seed oil as placebo. As similar to the above study, patients treated with BSO at the end of 6 months indicated significant improvement compared with the placebo in parameters such as tender joint count, swollen joint count, and pain expressed in a visual analog scales. Among the patients completed in the first 6 months of the study, side effects were belching (three patients in the GLA group and two patients in the placebo group) and diarrhea (four patients in the GLA group and one patient in the placebo group) [68].

The effects of BSO supplementation were evaluated against patients with RA (functional class I–III) who fulfilled the American College of Rheumatology (ARC) criteria for RA. Such patients, who consisted of 22 women and 6 men, were randomized to receive either 6 g/day of the active BSO containing a total of 1320 mg GLA in 12 capsules, whereas the placebo group received the same number of capsules containing peanut oil with no GLA [69]. Supplementing 6 g/day of

BSO resulted in improvements in the symptoms of RA. Furthermore, supplementation might poten-tially help reduce NSAID dose, thereby minimizing the serious gastrointestinal and renal side effects with the drug. Side effects in the study were reported in three patients in the placebo group, such as one or more symptoms of an upper respiratory tract infection, shingles, nausea, and diz-ziness, while five patients in the BSO group had side effects, including mild diarrhea and nausea, which did not necessitated any medication [69].

Blackcurrant Seed Oil

Blackcurrant (*Ribes nigrum* L.) is native to central and northern Europe and northern Asia. Oil derived from blackcurrant seed is rich in GLA (Table 26.3). The other FAs contained in the oil are ALA, LA, and stearidonic acid (SDA), which is an 18-carbon n-3 PUFA with four double bonds. High content of GLA in addition to substantial contents of ALA and SDA in blackcurrant seed oil (BCO) provides health benefit in the treatment of inflammatory disease [70].

In the study, BCO (3 g/day) was administered to both healthy volunteers and patients with RA for 6 weeks, whereas sunflower oil was given at the same dosage in the control group. The study exhib-ited no altered secretion of IL-1, and IL-6 occurred in stimulated monocytes from the sunflower oil treatment group, whereas some reduction of the cytokines was noted in the BCO group [70].

The mechanistic action of BCO is attributable to the presence of GLA (n-3 series), ALA (n-6 series), and SDA. GLA participates in the synthesis of PGE_1, and ALA is a precursor in the biosyn-thesis of EPA, which is a precursor of 3 series PGEs, 3 series TXAs, and 5 series LTDs. Thereby, it could be hypothesized that well-balanced and sufficient concentrations of both n-3 series and n-6 series FAs might synergistically increase the treatment of RA [71].

Another study examined whether dietary supplementation of BCO could improve response of healthy elderly subjects and determined whether the altered immune response was mediated by a change in the factors associated with T-cell activation. In the study, BCO was compared with soy bean oil as placebo [72]. The clinical trial was conducted in a randomized, double-blind, placebo-controlled manner for 2 months to examine effects of BCO on the immune responses of 40 healthy subjects 65 years or older. The finding concluded that BCO had a moderate immune-enhancing effect attributable to its ability to reduce PGE_2 production [72]. There was also evidence that BCO suppressed inflammation in an animal model study using rats. In the animal study, BCO that also contained ALA or other series 3 PUFAs, which presumably converted to EPA to exhibit anti-in-flammatory effects, enhanced anti-inflammatory effect of GLA as compared with the findings of other studies [73, 74].

The result of a study revealed that BCO might have some effects on RA *in vitro*, evaluating the inflammatory mediators of volunteers and also of arthritis patients. Volunteers randomly received capsules containing safflower oil or 525 mg/day GLA in the form of BCO capsules for 6 weeks followed immediately by a 6-week washout period. There were remarkable decreases in proinflam-matory cytokines such as IL-1β, IL-6, and PGE_2 in patients with intake of BCO for 6 weeks, but not for the safflower oil. Furthermore, healthy volunteer group also showed statistically significant decreases in all measured cytokines with the exception of IL-1β [75].

In a clinical trial conducted for 6 months, 34 patients participated, of which 20 patients took BCO in capsule and 14 patients received soybean oil as placebo. The daily dose of BCO was 10.5 g containing 2 g GLA. The results of the study suggested that the treated group showed significant improvements in joint tenderness count and tenderness score compared with the placebo group. Side effects were observed in the placebo group ($n = 2$), whereas none was found in the treatment group [76].

Overall RA studies using BCO demonstrated promising results in regulating RA inflammation, whereas BCO contains fair amounts of ALA (12%) compared with evening primrose seed oil (EPO) or BSO [31]. The composition of n-3 series and n-6 series FAs in BCO might be an efficacious ratio in the treatment of patients with RA as revealed that ALA to EPA conversion was potentiated [73, 74].

Evening Primrose Seed Oil

Evening primrose (*Oenothera biennis* L.) is a wildflower grown throughout the United States. The oil obtained from the seeds is rich in GLA. The oil also contains LA. Hexane as solvent is used to extract the oil, which is prepared as medicine; for example, it has been reported that EPO helps with symptoms of premenstrual syndrome [77].

EPO has been shown to reduce chronic inflammation in laboratory animals [78]. The GLA in EPO is believed to reduce RA potentially by two mechanisms. First, it is metabolized to the anti-inflammatory series 1 PGs (Figure 26.2). Second, it may competitively suppress the synthesis of the proinflammatory series 2 PGs and series 4 LTs that are involved in RA (Figures 26.2 and 26.3).

In a study conducted in 1983, 432 mg/day of GLA in the form of EPO was supplied to 20 patients with RA for treatment [79]. However, its validity was equivocal whether the study was appropriately performed to provide a high dose of GLA for a longer period of time [71]. Another human clinical study was designed in such a way that administering 540 mg GLA/day in the form of EPO for 12 months in a double-blind manner [80]. Although there was a significant improvement in the patients' self-assessment, the result was questioned because it was not reflected in any of the conventional measurements of disease activity [71]. In addition, the study showed side effects in the treatment group such as nausea and diarrhea ($n = 4$), and none was found in the placebo group.

Additional double-blind, placebo-controlled study was performed in 40 patients with RA [81]. In the trial, 19 patients received 6 g/day of EPO, which is equivalent to 540 mg/day of GLA compared with a group of 21 patients who received 6 g/day of olive oil as the placebo. The results revealed that the group that ingested EPO might have showed mild improvement in RA, whereas many benefits were observed in the group of patients with olive oil [81]. However, the study again might be misleading to conclude whether EPO was efficacious because olive oil was used as the placebo. It has been known that olive oil itself had beneficial effects in RA [82]; therefore, olive oil should not be used as a placebo in any of the investigations using PUFAs, particularly in studies to examine inflammatory effects. Similarly, there was another case that failed to show the effect of EPO on RA because olive oil was used as the placebo [83]. Furthermore, a letter stated that the period of the study was too short to draw any conclusions on the effects of EPO in RA [84].

An investigation using EPO was demonstrated to be efficacious in RA as described in GLA [68]. In this study, no patients withdrew from GLA treatment because of adverse reactions, where BSO and EPO were used as the sources of GLA. Few studies demonstrated the beneficial effects of EPO in RA as described earlier; however, experimental designs such as the uses of appropriate

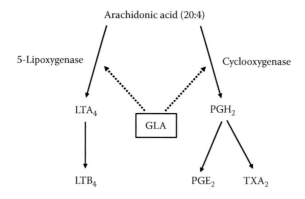

FIGURE 26.3 GLA in the suppression of AA metabolic pathways to proinflammatory eicosanoids. The suppression involves the formation of DGLA, which is metabolized from GLA, competing with AA for access to the COX and lipoxygenase. Dashed lines indicate pathways affecting the formation of eicosanoids involved in the inflammation.

placebo, the dosage, and also the study period made the results of the studies less conclusive and thus evidence ultimately became weak [85].

PERSPECTIVES

Most of the RA studies using n-3 and/or n-6 FAs are derived from fish oils and/or plant seed oils as used for an alternative suppression of inflammation associated with RA. However, it is difficult to ingest high amounts of n-3 and n-6 FAs from the daily diets, particularly in a well-balanced ratio of n-6/n-3 FAs for RA. In a recent report, such importance of the ratio was emphasized in the prevention and possible treatment of cardiovascular disease and other chronic diseases, which include coronary artery disease, hypertension, diabetes, arthritis, osteoporosis, other inflammatory and autoimmune disorders, cancer, and mental health [33]. For example, a ratio of 2–3:1 (n-6/n-3 FAs) seems to be effective in controlling inflammation in patient with RA.

In the Western diet, n-6 PUFAs are predominant compared with the amounts of n-3 PUFAs from plant seed oils or fish oils, possibly causing high risks of the occurrence of cardiovascular and other lifestyle-related diseases. After World War II in Japan, lifestyle change or the so-called "western-ization" rapidly took place, for example, the Japanese diets becoming animal based, while decreasing the incorporation of Japanese traditional food sources such as fish, seaweeds, and soybeans to name few into daily diets. As a result, upsurge of lifestyle-related diseases including obesity has become prevalent and is now a social health concern in Japan [13].

Coupling the aging population's ever growing demands for establishing the preventive and thera-peutic interventions of OA has been leading to another social challenge in Japan. A study estimated the annual occurrence of knee OA at approximately 900,000, representing 87% of the patients older than 50 years in Japan [86]. It can be said that Japan is a largest population with OA in the world along with the United States.

Under a phenomenon of "shrinking and graying" taking place in Japan, a well-recognized age-related disorder, OA, has obviously become very prominent in Japan; in fact, the Ministry of Health, Labor, and Welfare estimated 30 million patients with OA [87]. As previously described, OA is characterized as an age-related "wear-and-tear" arthritis [2]. In addition, obesity [88–90], as a major risk factor, plays a vital role in increasing the population of OA.

Current pharmacological strategies for effective intervention in processes of the both arthri-tis diseases and also for promotion of cartilage remodeling primarily address immune suppres-sion and anti-inflammatory approaches. Most recently, fish oil n-3 PUFAs were supplemented to weight-bearing dogs with OA to evaluate its effects on arthritis [91]. In the study, supplementation of 3.5% fish oil n-3 FAs as the test-food group improved by conducting orthopedic evaluation and force-plate analyses of the most severely affected limb of each dog compared with the control-food group. Another dog study was conducted to assess the effect of food rich with fish oil n-3 FAs and with a low n-6/n-3 ratio on dogs with OA [92]. Results similarly showed that ingestion of the food rich in low ratio of n-6/n-3 FAs was suggestive to improve the arthritic condition in tested dogs with OA.

Thus, in the future, it is anticipated that human clinical trials are designed using plant seed oils or fish oils rich in n-3 PUFAs and/or in well-balanced n-6/n-3 PUFA ratio as in dietary supplements for health benefits of patients with not only RA but also OA. Supplement such as undenatured type II collagen [93] has been already available in Japan, in the United States, and in other countries, which is effective against patients with OA as well as RA, although the mechanistic action is not yet fully clarified, but only speculated [93].

CONCLUSIONS

Immunoregulatory and anti-inflammatory properties of n-3 and n-6 FAs have been extensively stud-ied for the potential prevention and therapy of chronic diseases in the past few decades, particularly in RA, because inhibition of TNF-α and IL-1β as well as inhibition of enzymes such as COX and 5-LOX required for the production of eicosanoids. Because the selected plant seed oils in this chapter are rich in EFAs and also are readily available as dietary supplement, if not taken from the diets, it is highly recommended to take daily in the manner that n-6/n-3 FAs are low enough. It is beneficial to have dietary supplement containing n-3 and/or n-6 FAs because dosage can be managed easily and regulated in accordance of amounts of estimated FAs in the daily diets. Prolong use of medication such as NSAIDs is not favored for potential side effects for patients with RA, whereas the selected oils as described are known to be safe on the basis of historical and cultural eating experience. Furthermore, supplementation of n-3 and/or n-6 FAs in proper ratio ensures quality of life of patients with RA. However, it is not escapable that further safety studies on PUFAs for prolong administration are required for patients with RA because side effects such as stool softening, belching, and diarrhea have been noted in the plant seed oils. Lastly, additional well-designed and rigorous human clinical trials are awaited to conclude real health benefits of n-3 and/or n-6 derived from plant seed oils in patients with RA.

REFERENCES

1. Trentham DE, Halpner A, Trentham RA, Bagchi M, Kothari S, Preuss HG, Bagchi A. Treatment of rheumatoid arthritis using undenatured type II collagen. The original internist. March 2002;12–15.
2. Trentham DE, Halpner AD, Trentham RA, Bagchi M, Kothari S, Preuss HG, Bagchi D. Use of undenatured type II collagen in the treatment of rheumatoid arthritis. Clin Prac Alter Med 2001;2:254–259.
3. Trentham DE, Dynesius-Trentham RA, Orav EJ, Combitchi D, Lorenzo C, Sewell KL, Hafler DA, Weiner HL. Effects of oral administration of type II collagen on rheumatoid arthritis. Science 1993;261:1727–1730.
4. Barnett ML, Combitchi D, Trentham DE. A pilot trial of oral type II collagen in the treatment of juvenile rheumatoid arthritis. Arthritis Rheum 1996;39:623–628.
5. Barnett ML, Kremer J, St. Clair EW, Clegg DO, Furst D, Weisman M, Fletcher MJ, et al. Treatment of rheumatoid arthritis with oral type II collagen. Results of a multicenter, double-blind, placebo-controlled trial. Arthritis Rheum 1998;41:290–297.
6. Nagler-Anderson C, Bober LA, Robinson ME, Siskind GW, Thoebecker GJ. Suppression of type II collagen-induced arthritis by intragastric administration of soluble type II collagen. Proc Natl Acad Sci U S A 1986;83:7443–7446.
7. Peat G, McCarney R, Croft P. Knee pain and osteoarthritis in older adults: a review of community burden and current use of primary health care. Ann Rheum Dis 2001;60:91–97.
8. Bellamy N, Carr A, Dougados M, Shea B, Wells G. Towards a definition of 'difference' in osteoarthritis. J Rheumatol 2001;28:427–430.
9. Sakkas LI, Johanson NA, Scanzello CR, Burkholder J, Mitra A, Salgame, P, Katsetos CD, Platsoucas CD. Interleukin-12 is expressed by infiltrating macrophages and synovial lining cells in rheumatoid arthritis and osteoarthritis. Cell Immunol 1998;188:105–110.
10. Yakugaku yougo kaisetu (Explanation an Pharmaceutical Terms), The Pharmaceutical Society of Japan. [Internet on RA] http://www.pharm.or.jp/dictionary/. Accessed February 22, 2010 [in Japanese].
11. Langford RM. Pain management today-what have we learned? Clin Rheumatol 2006;25:2–8.
12. Andersohn F, Suissa S, Garbe E. Use of first-and second-generation nonsteroidal anti-inflammatory drugs and risk of acute myocardial infarction. Circulation 2006;113:1950–1957.
13. Ohama H, Ikeda H, Moriyama H. Health foods and foods with health claims in Japan. Toxicology 2006;221:95–111.
14. Ikuyama S, Imamura-Takase E, Tokunaga S, Oribe M, Nishimura J. Sixty percent of patients with rheumatoid arthritis in Japan have used dietary supplements or health foods. Mod Rheumatol 2009;19:253–259.
15. Rao JK, Mihaliak K, Kroenke K, Brandley J, Tierney W, Weinberg M. Use of complementary therapies for arthritis among patients of rheumatologists. Ann Intern Med 1999;131:409–416.
16. Crowley DC, Lau FC, Sharma P, Evans M, Guthrie N, Bagchi M, Bagchi D, Dey DK, Raychaudhuri SP. Safety and efficacy of undenatured type II collagen in the treatment of osteoarthritis of the knee: a clinical trial. Int J Med Sci 2009;6:312–322.
17. Fritsche K. Fatty acids as modulators of the immune response. Annu Rev Nutr 2006;26:45–73.
18. Bach AC, Babayan VK. Medium-chain triglycerides: an update. Am J Clin Nutr 1982;36:950–962.
19. Alexander JW. Immunonutrition; the role of ω-3 fatty acids. Nutrition 1998;14:627–633.

20. Simopoulos AP. Omega-3 fatty acids in inflammation an autoimmune diseases. J Am Coll Nutr 2002;21:495–505.
21. Dawczynski C, Schubert R, Hein G. Long-term moderated with *n*-3 long-chain PUFA-supplemented dairy products: effects on pathophysiological biomarkers in patients with rheumatoid arthritis. Br J Nutr 2009;101:1517–1526.
22. James MJ, Gibson RA, Cleland LG. Dietary polyunsaturated fatty acids and inflammatory mediator production. Am J Clin Nutr 2000;71:343S-348S.
23. Chilton FH, Rudel LL, Parks JS, Arm JP, Seeds MC. Mechanisms by which botanical lipids affect inflammatory disorders. Am J Clin Nutr 2008;87:498S-503S.
24. Decker JL, Malone DG, Haraoui B, Wahl SM, Schrieber L, Klippel JH, Steinnverg AS, Wilder RL. NIH conference. Rheumatoid arthritis: evolving concepts of pathogenesis and treatment. Ann Intern Med 1984;101:810–824.
25. Firestein GS. The immunopathogenesis of rheumatoid arthritis. Curr Opin Rheumatol 1991;3:398–406.
26. Wordsworth BP, Bell JL. The immunogenetics of rheumatoid arthritis. Springer Semin Immunopathol 1992;14:59–78.
27. Smith JB, Haynes MK. Rheumatoid arthritis-a molecular understanding. Ann Inter Med 2002;136: 908–922.
28. Harris DE. Rheumatoid arthritis: pathophysiology and implications of therapy. N Engl J Med 1990;322: 1277–1289.
29. Calder PC. n-3 polyunsaturated fatty acids, inflammation, and inflammatory diseases. Am J Clin Nutr 2006;83:1505S-1509S.
30. Rothman D, DeLuca P, Zurier R. Botanical lipids: effects on inflammation, immune responses, and rheumatoid arthritis. Semin Arthritis Rheum 1995;25:87–96.
31. Barre DE. Potential of evening primrose, borage, blackcurrant, and fungal oils in human health. Ann Nutr Metab 2001;45:47–57.
32. Goldberg RJ, Katz JM. A meta-analysis of the analgesic effects of mega-3 polysaturated fatty acid supplementation for inflammatory joint pain. Pain 2007;129:210–223.
33. Simopoulos AP. The importance of the omega-6/omega-3 fatty acid ratio in cardiovascular disease and other chronic diseases. Exp Biol Med 2008;233:674–688.
34. Leonard EC. Dietary fatty acids: effect of the n-6/n-3 balance on human nutrition and disease. Lipid Technol 1999;11,110–114.
35. Jenski LJ. Omega-3 fatty acids and the expression of membrane proteins: emphasis on molecules of immunologic importance. Curr Org Chem 2000;4:1185–1200.
36. Arita M, Yoshida M, Hong S, Tjonahen E, Glickman JN, Petasis NA, Blumberg RA, Serhan CN. Revolvin E_1, an endogenous lipid mediator derived from omega-3 eicosapentaenoic acid, protects against 2,4,6-trinitrobenzene sulfonic acid-induced colitis. Proc Natl Acad Sci U S A 2005;102:7671–7676.
37. Hudert CA, Weylandt KH, Lu Y, Wang J, Hong S, Dignass A, Serhan CN, Kang JX. Transgenic mice rich in endogenous omega-3 fatty acids are protected from colitis. Proc Natl Acad Sci U S A 2006;103,11276–11281.
38. Novak TE, Babcock TA, Jho DH, Helton WS, Espat NJ. NF-kappa B inhibition by omega-3 fatty acids modulates LPS-stimulated macrophage TNF-alpha transcription. Am J Physiol Lung Cell Mol Physiol 2003;284: L84-L89.
39. Zhao Y, Joshi-Barve S, Barve S, Chen LH. Eicosapnetanoenoic acid prevents LPS-induced TNF-alpha expression by preventing NF-kappaB activation. J Am Coll Nutr 2004;23:71–78.
40. Hamaguchi M, Kawahito Omoto A, Hamaguchi M, Kawahito Y, Omoto A, Tsubouchi Y, Kohno M, Seno T, Kadoya M, et al. Eicosapentaenoic acid suppresses the proliferation of synoviocytes from rheumatoid arthritis. J Clin Biochem Nutr 2008;43:126–128.
41. Kremer JM. N-3 fatty acid supplements in rheumatoid arthritis. Am J Clin Nutr 2000;71:349S-351S.
42. Nordström DC, Honkanen VE, Nasu Y, Antila E, Friman C, Konttinen YT. Alpha-linolenic acid in the treatment of rheumatoid arthritis: a double-blind placebo-controlled and randomized study: flaxseed vs. safflower seed. Rheumatol Int 1995;14:231–234.
43. Needleman P, Raz A, Minkes MS, Ferrendelli JA, Sprecher H. Triene prostaglandins: prostacyclin and thromboxane biosynthesis and unique biological properties. Proc Natl Acad Sci U S A 1979;76:944–948.
44. Lee TH, Hoover RL, Williams JD, Sperling RI, Revalese III, J, Spur BW, Robinson DR, Corey EJ, Lewis RA, Austen KF. Effect of dietary enrichment with eicosapentanaenoic and docosahexaenoic acids on in vitro neutrophil and monocyte leukotriene generation and neutrophil function. N Engl J Med 1986;312:1217–1224.

45. Kremer JM, Jubiz W, Michalek A, Rynes RI, Bartholomew LD, Bigouette J, Timchalk M, Belleer D, Lininger L. Fish-oil fatty acid supplementation in rheumatoid arthritis. Ann Intern Med 1987;106:497–504.

46. Cleland LG, French JK, Betts WH, Murphy GA, Elliot J. Clinical and biochemical effects of dietary fish oil supplements in rheumatoid arthritis. J Rheumatol 1988;15:1471–1475.

47. Flaxseed oil. [Internet on flaxseed] University of Maryland Medical Center, http://www.umm.edu/altmed/articles/flaxseed-oil-000304.htm. Accessed January 11, 2010.

48. Covington MB. Omega-3 fatty acids. Am Fam Physician 2004;70:133–140.

49. Hochberg MC, Chang RW, Dwosh I, Lindsey S, Pincus T, Wolfe F. The American College of Rheumatology 1991 revised criteria for the classification of global functional status in rheumatoid arthritis. Arthritis Rheum 1992;35:498–502.

50. Kaarela K. Prognostic factors and diagnostic criteria in early rheumatoid arthritis [thesis]. Scand J Rheumatol 1985;57:1–54.

51. Huskisson EC. Measurement of pain. Lancet 1974;11:1127–1131.

52. Meike H, Deicher H. Correlation of inflammatory RA disease activity with laboratory parameters. Scand J Rheumatol 1985;14:22–24.

53. Cunnane SC. Role of zinc in lipid fatty acid metabolism and in membranes. Prog Nutr Sci 1988;12:151–188.

54. Caughey GE, Mantzioris E, Gibson RA, Cleland LG, Maes MJ. The effect on human tumor necrosis factor α and interleukin 1β production of diets enriched in n-3 fatty acids from vegetable oil or fish oil. Am J Nutr 1996;63:116–122.

55. Conti E, Stredansky M, Stredanska S, Zanetti F. gamma-Linolenic acid production by solid-state fermentation of Mucorales strains on cereals. Bioresour Technol 2001;76:283–286.

56. Jang HD, Lin YY, Yang SS. Effect of culture media and conditions on polysaturated fatty acids production by *Mortierella alpina*. Bioresour Technol 2005;96:1633–1644.

57. Jang HD, Yang SS. Polysaturated fatty acids production with a solid-state column reactor. Bioresour Technol 2008;99:6181–6189.

58. Baker DG, Krakauer KA, Tate G, Laposata M, Zurier RB. Suppression of human synovial proliferation by dihomogammalinoleic acid. Arthritis Rheum 1989;32:1273–1281.

59. Iverson L, Fogh K, Bojesen G. Linoleic acid and dihomogammalinolenic acid inhibit leukotriene formation and stimulate the formation of their 15-lipoxygnease products by human neutrophils in vitro. Evidence of formation of anti-inflammatory compounds. Agents Actions 1991;33:286–291.

60. Santoli D, Zurier RB. Prostaglandin E, precursor fatty acids inhibit human IL-2 production by a prostglanding E-independent mechanism. J Immunol 1989;143:1303–1309.

61. Santoli D, Phillips PD, Colt TL, Zurier RB. Suppression of interleukin 2-dependent human T cell growth by prostaglandin (PGE) and their precursor fatty acids. Evidence for a PGE-independent mechanism of the inhibition by the fatty acids. J Clin Invest 1990;85:424–432.

62. Kirtland SJ. Prostaglandin E_1: a review. Prostaglandins Leukot Essent Fatty Acids 1988;32:165–174.

63. Belch J. Eicosanoids and rheumatology: inflammatory and vascular aspects. Prostaglandins Leukot Essent Fatty Acids 1989;36(4):219–234.

64. Furse RK, Rossetti RG, Zurier RB. Gammalinolenic acid, an unsaturated fatty acid with anti-inflammatory properties, blocks amplification of IL-1β production by human monocytes. J Immunol 2001;167:490–496.

65. Kast RE. Borage oil reduction of rheumatoid arthritis activity may mediated by increased cAMP that suppresses tumor necrosis factor-alpha. Int Immunopharmcol 2001;1:2197–2199.

66. Pullman-Mooar S, Laposata M, Lem D, Holman RT, Levanthal LJ, Bemarco D, Zurier RB. Alteration of the cellular fatty acid profile and production of eicosanoids in human monocytes by gamma-linolenic acid. Arthritis Rheum 1990;33:1526–1533.

67. Levanthanl LJ, Boye EG, Zurier RB. Treatment of rheumatoid arthritis with gammalinolenic acid. Ann Inter Med 1993;119:867–873.

68. Zurier RB, Rossetti RG, Jacobson EW. Gammma-linolenic acid treatment of rheumatoid arthritis: a randomized, placebo-controlled trial. Arthritis Rheum 1996;39:1808–1817.

69. Kumar P, Strang A, Ho M, Maple C, Radederstoff D, Morley K, Belch J. The effects of borage oil supplementation on non-steroidal anti-inflammatory drug requirements in patients with rheumatoid arthritis. J Complement Integr Med 2008;5:1–9.

70. Byars ML, Watson J, McGill PE. Black currant seed oil as a source of polyunsaturated fatty acids in the treatment of inflammatory disease. Biochem Soc Trans 1992;20:139S.

71. Rothman D, DeLuca P, Zurier RB. Botanical lipids: effects on inflammation, immune responses, and rheumatoid arthritis. Semin Arthritis Rheum 1995;26:87–96.

72. Wu D, Meydani SM, Leka LS, Nightingale Z, Handelman J, Blumberg JB, Meydani SM. Effect of dietary supplementation with black currant seed oil in the immune response of heath elderly subjects. Am J Clin Nutr 1999;70:536–543.

73. Tate GA, Zurier RB. Suppression of monosodium urate crystal-induced inflammation by black currant seed oil. Agents Actions 1994;43:35–38.

74. Tate GA, Mandell BF, Karmali RA, Laposata M, Baker DG, Schumatcher HR Jr, Zurier RB. Suppression of monosodium urate crystal-induced acute inflammation by diets enriched with gamma-linolenic acid and eicosapentaenoic acid. Arthritis Rheum 1988;31:1543–1551.

75. Watson J, Byars ML, Mc Gill P, Kelman AW. Cytokine and prostaglandin production by monocytes of volunteers and arthritis patients treated with dietary supplements of blackcurrant seed oil. Br J Rheumatol 1993;32:1055–1058.

76. Levanthal LJ, Boyce EG, Zurier RB. Treatment rheumatoid arthritis with blackcurrant seed oil. Br J Rheumatol 1994;33:847–852.

77. Horrobin DF. The role of essential fatty acids metabolism and prostaglandins in the premenstrual syndrome. J Reprod Med 1983;28:465–468.

78. Kunkel SL, Ogawa H, Ward PA, Zurier RB. Suppression of chronic inflammation by evening primrose oil. Prog Lipid Res 1982;20:885–888.

79. Hansen TM, Lerche A, Kassis V, Lorenz I, Sondergaard J. Treatment of rheumatoid arthritis with prostaglandin E_1 precursors cis-linoleic acid and γ-linolenic acid. Scand J Rheumatol 1983;12:85–88.

80. Belch JJF, Ansell D, Madhok R, O'Dowd A, Sturrock RD. Effects of altering dietary essential fatty acids on requirements for non-steroidal anti-inflammatory drugs in patients with rheumatoid arthritis: a double blind placebo controlled study. Ann Rheum Dis 1988;47:96–104.

81. Brzeski M, Madhok R, Capell HA. Evening primrose oil in patients with rheumatoid arthritis and side effects of non-steroidal inflammatory drugs. Br J Rheumatol 1991;30:370–372.

82. Darlington LG, Ramsey NW. Olive oil for rheumatoid patients? Br J Rheumatol 1987;26:215.

83. Jäntti J, Seppälä E, Vapaataalo H, Isomäki H. Evening primrose oil and olive oil in treatment of rheumatoid arthritis. Clin Rheumatol 1989;8:238–244.

84. Horrobin DF. Effects of evening primrose oil in the rheumatoid arthritis. Ann Rheum Dis 1989;48:965–966.

85. Belch JJ, Hill A. Evening primrose oil and borage oil in rheumatologic conditions. Am J Clin Nutr 2000;71:352S-356S.

86. Kawamura H, Sugioka Y, Hirota Y, Kurosawa M, Ogata K, Shiina M, Fujii K. Epidemiology of osteoarthritis of the knee investigation of incidence and the results of a case study [in Japanese]. Orthoped Traumatol 1995;44:12–15.

87. Setaiin no kenkoujyoutai (Health conditions of the members of householders), the Ministry of Health, Labour, and Welfare (MHLW). [Internet:MHLW]http://www.mhlw.go.jp/toukei/saikin/hw/k-tyosa/k-tyosa04/3–1.html. Accessed January 11, 2010 [in Japanese].

88. Felson DT, Anderson JJ, Naimark A, Walker AM, Meenan RF. Obesity and knee osteoarthritis. The Framingham Study. Ann Intern Med 1988;109:18–24.

89. Oliveria SA, Felson DT, Cirillo PA, Reed JI, Walker AM. Body weight, body mass index, and incident symptomatic osteoarthritis of the hand, hip, and knee. Epidemiology 1999;10:161–166.

90. Yoshimura N, Nishioka S, Kinoshita H, Hori N, Nishioka T, Ryujin M, Mantani Y, Miyake M, Coggon D, Cooper C. Risk factors for knee osteoarthritis in Japanese women: heavy weight, previous joint injuries, and occupational activities. J Rheumatol 2004;31:157–162.

91. Roush JK, Cross AR, Renberg WC, Dodd CE, Sixby KA, Fritsch DA, Allen TA, et al. Evaluation for the effects of dietary supplementation with fish oil omega-3 fatty acids on weight bearing in dogs with osteoarthritis. J Am Vet Med Assoc 2010;236:67–73.

92. Roush JK, Dodd CE, Fritsch DA, Allen TA, Jewell DE, Schoenherr WD, Richardson DC, Leventhal PS, Hahn KA. Multicenter veterinary practice assessment of the effects of omega-3 fatty acid on osteoarthritis in dogs. J Am Vet Med Assoc 2010;236:59–66.

93. Bagchi D, Misner B, Bagchi M, Kothari SC, Downs BW, Fafard RD, Preuss HG. Effects of orally administered undenatured type II collagen against arthritic inflammatory disease: a mechanistic exploration. Int J Clin Pharmacol Res 2002;XXII:101–110.

27 Antiarthritic Potential of Bromelain from *Ananas comosus* and Its Combination

Dilip Ghosh

CONTENTS

INTRODUCTION

Arthritis is often referred to as a single disease, but in reality it is an umbrella term for more than 100 medical conditions that affect the musculoskeletal system, specifically joints where two or more bones meet. Arthritis is the major cause of disability that creates global chronic economic pain, at a cost to the economy of more than several trillion dollars each year in medical care and indirect costs such as loss of earnings and lost production. This can result in joint weakness, instability, and deformities that can interfere with the most basic daily tasks such as walking, driving a car, and preparing food.

Rheumatoid arthritis (RA) is a chronic form of this disease, for which multiple pharmacotherapies are generally applied. Because once acquired the disease generally requires lifelong treatment, it is not surprising that 33%–75% of RA patients believe food plays an important role in their symptom severity and 20%–50% will have tried dietary manipulation in an attempt to relieve their suffering (Stamp et al., 2005). Osteoarthritis (OA) is the most common type of this disease and one of the leading causes of chronic disability. Recent estimates suggest that symptomatic knee OA occurs in 13% of persons 60 years and older, and the prevalence is expected to increase further as the population ages.

COMPLEMENTARY AND ALTERNATIVE MEDICINE IN ARTHRITIS MANAGEMENT

There are various complementary and alternative medicine (CAM) products for OA and RA that have been advocated. CAM for the treatment of RA is becoming more prevalent worldwide

(Pullar et al., 1982; Kaboli et al., 2001; Kim and Seo, 2003; Sleath et al., 2005; Kikuchi et al., 2009). Continuous pain is characteristic of OA patients, and the rate of CAM usage for the treatment OA is estimated to be high. Gray (1985) was the first person to advocate the use of CAM for the treatment of OA for the elderly patients having multiple diseases. Further, as the aging of society progresses, more attention is being focused on the effectiveness of CAM products in OA and RA (Kikuchi et al., 2009). In the United Kingdom, Pullar et al. (1982) investigated the significance of CAM for the treatment of RA from the patients' expenditure point of view, and they found that CAM ranging from cheap copper rings to expensive acupuncture treatments were used and accounted for 30% of the treatment and care for rheumatic diseases. In the United States, RA patients frequently use CAM, and in Japan, usage rate of CAM by RA patients was estimated as 35%. Usage rates in Canada and Australia were reported to be 34%–60%, and usage rates were found to vary among countries rather than among ethnic groups (see review by Kikuchi et al., 2009). CAM users were found to be predominantly women, patients of a high academic background, and dissatisfied with ordinary medication. The variation in usage rates among countries seems to be the result of differences in social welfare and medical systems.

ANANAS COMOSUS AND BROMELAIN: PART OF CAM TREATMENTS

Botanicals such as *Ananas comosus* (pineapple) and their extracts (bromelain) have been used clinically as anti-inflammatory agents in RA, soft tissue injuries, colonic inflammation, chronic pain, and asthma (Taussigand Batkin, 1988; Maurer, 2001; Hale et al., 2005; Secor et al., 2005). Bromelain is an aqueous extract of pineapple that contains a complex mixture of thiol proteases and nonprotease components (Chobotova et al., 2010). Proteases constitute the major components of bromelain and include stem bromelain (80%), fruit bromelain (10%), and ananain (5%). Among nonprotease components are phosphatases, glucosidases, peroxidases, cellulases, glycoproteins, and carbohydrates (Maurer, 2001). Assays for the individual protease components of bromelain have recently been established, thus raising the possibility of standardizing bromelain preparations (Hale et al., 2005).

MECHANISM OF ACTION

The major mechanism of action of bromelain appears to be proteolytic in nature, although an immunomodulatory and hormone-like activity acting via intracellular signaling pathways is also suggested. Although poorly understood, the pleiotropic effects of bromelain are considered to be due to the complex mixture of closely related cysteine proteinases, proteinase inhibitors, phosphatases, glucosidases, peroxidases, and other undefined compounds (Kalra et al., 2008). Immune cells are a vital part of the body defense against infections, but when inappropriately or excessively activated, they can induce a state of uncontrolled systemic or local inflammation. Such hyperactivation of inflammatory cells often leads to chronic progressive diseases like glomerulonephritis, RA, multiple sclerosis, or inflammatory bowel disease (Manhart et al., 2002). In these diseases, the ability to modulate T-cell activation has important implications because they are thought to attribute and perpetuate inflammatory processes (Oleg et al., 1999).

IN VITRO STUDIES

In vitro incubation with a mixture of bromelain, trypsin, and antioxidant rutoside called Phlogenzym (PHL) showed that accessory molecules such as CD4, CD44, and B7–1, which are involved in T-cell co-stimulation, were cleaved by PHL, which is consistent with an increased T-cell activation threshold (Hale and Haynes, 1992; Targoin et al., 1999; Hale et al., 2002). On the other hand, the inhibitory action of bromelain on T cells is not simply caused by a degradative action on cell surface molecules because bromelain blocked signaling by receptor-independent agonists (Secor et al., 2009). Recently, Engwerda et al. (2001) showed that bromelain simultaneously enhanced and inhibited T-cell responses *in vitro* and *in vivo* via a stimulatory action on accessory cells and a direct inhibitory action on T cells. *In vitro* studies have shown that bromelain can inhibit PMA-induced T-cell production of the Th2 cytokine interleukin-4 and to a lesser degree the Th1 cytokines interleukin-2 and interferon-α via modulation of the extracellular regulated kinase-2 intracellular signaling pathway (Mynott et al., 1999). Bromelain has also been shown to reduce cell surface receptors such as the hyaluronan receptor CD44, which is associated with leukocyte migration and induction of proinflammatory mediators (Engwerda et al., 2001). Another recent study (Secor et al., 2005) demonstrated the effect of bromelain on CD4[+] T-cell activation, specifically the expression of CD25 *in vitro*. Bromelain treatment of anti-CD3-stimulated CD4[+] T cells reduced CD25 expression in a dose- and time-dependent manner, and this reduction was dependent on the proteolytic action of bromelain as the addition of E64 (a cysteine protease inhibitor) abrogated this response. The concentration of CD25 was increased in supernatants of bromelain-treated activated CD4[+] T cells as compared with control cells, suggesting that bromelain proteolytically cleaved cell surface CD25. This novel mechanism of action identifies how bromelain may exert its therapeutic benefits in inflammatory conditions (Secor et al., 2009).

In Vivo Animal Studies

Evidences from animal studies as well as a number of human studies have demonstrated anti-inflammatory and analgesic properties of orally administered bromelain (Maurer, 2001). Experimental trials showed that proteases like bromelain or a mixture of bromelain, trypsin, and antioxidant rutoside called PHL affect T-cell reactivity. PHL administration led to an increased T-cell activation threshold in an animal model of T-cell-mediated autoimmune disease. Also, bromelain has been shown to significantly reduce CD4[+] T lymphocytes, which are primary effectors in animal models of inflammation (Manhart et al., 2002). Bromelain, a cysteine protease, has been shown to have anti-inflammatory effects in other animal disease models such as EAE and inflammatory bowel disease (Oleg et al., 1999; Hale et al., 2005; Fitzhugh et al., 2008).

Clinical Evidence

Bromelain can be absorbed in human intestines without degradation and without losing its biological activity (Castell et al., 1997). It is well tolerated in high doses (up to 3 g/day) for prolonged periods of therapy, even up to several years when taken orally (Taussig and Batkin, 1988; Castell et al., 1997; Brien et al., 2004). Bromelain has been used either alone or in a multienzyme preparation, most commonly combined with trypsin and rutin, in multiple clinical trials in both humans and animals. The overall beneficial effects were suggested or proven in a variety of inflammatory diseases and models of inflammation, such as experimental allergic rheumatologic diseases in mice and humans (Wittenborg et al., 2000; Akhtar et al., 2004) and also in OA of the knee and hip (Klein et al., 2006).

Early evidence came from Cohen and Goldman (1964), who administered bromelain (60–160 mg/day) to patients with moderate or severe arthritis with residual joint swelling after long-term steroid therapy. Nearly three-quarters of the patients reported either complete or near total reduction of swelling after the treatment, with a corresponding reduction in pain and soreness. Another small, blinded, multicenter study conducted in Germany reported a positive outcome compared with placebo for patients with arthritis (Vogler, 1988). A double-blinded 3-week trial of 73 patients suffering OA of knee joint using the oral enzyme preparation PHL (which contains bromelain, trypsin, and rutin) with a nonsteroidal anti-inflammatory drug (NSAID) (diclofenac; Klein and Kullich, 2000) demonstrated the effectiveness of PHL as diclofenac in significantly reducing pain indices (by approximately 80% after 3 weeks of treatment), and this decrease was sustained for

4 weeks posttreatment. Tilwe et al. (2001) also compared PHL with diclofenac in 50 patients with arthritis of the knee joint and likewise found reductions in pain, tenderness, and swelling in both groups after 3 and 4 weeks posttreatment.

Several relatively recent randomized clinical trials (RCT) have been conducted with mixed outcomes. In an RCT study, Brien et al. (2006) used single fixed dose of bromelain 800 mg/day for 12 weeks in patients with moderate-to-severe OA of the knee ($n = 47$) along with placebo. Both treatment groups showed clinically relevant improvement in the Western Ontario and MacMaster Universities Osteoarthritis Index disability subscale only. This study suggests that bromelain is not efficacious as an adjunctive treatment of moderate to severe OA.

In another multicenter, double-blind, randomized, parallel group design study (Kerkhoffs et al., 2004) with the triple combination, the PHL (rutoside, bromelain, and trypsin) with double combinations, the single substances, and the placebo also suggested that the PHL was not found to be superior to the three two-drug combinations, the three single substances, or the placebo for treatment of patients with acute unilateral sprain of the lateral ankle joint.

A double-blind prospective randomized study with similar combination of oral enzyme–rutoside, containing rutoside and the enzymes bromelain and trypsin, was completed with comparison of diclofenac in OA patients (Akhtar et al., 2004). The result indicates that oral enzyme–rutoside can be considered as an effective and safe alternative to NSAIDs, such as diclofenac, in the treatment of painful episodes of OA of the knee. The potential limitation of this study in the fact is the lack of placebo control.

COMMENTARY

Recently, bromelain, an extract from pineapple stem (*A. comosus*), has been used clinically for a wide variety of maladies including edema, thrombophlebitis, sinusitis, inflammation, RA, and OA and as adjuvant in cancer treatment (Yuan et al., 2006).

A number of clinical trials have assessed the use of bromelain in joint inflammation, and these have been briefly reviewed in this article. Majority of the studies are either open studies or equivalence studies designed to assess the comparative effectiveness against standard NSAID treatment. Their findings suggest that bromelain may be beneficial in the treatment of OA and as effective as a standard NSAID treatment. In addition, safety reports reveal no serious adverse reactions, and tolerability appears good. Although minor adverse events have been reported, these are mainly confined to mild gastrointestinal symptoms. However, there are a number of methodological concerns surrounding these studies. Firstly, the period of treatment in these arthritic studies is much shorter (average 3–4 weeks) than that used in clinical practice (3–4 months). Therefore, the safety and efficacy of longer-term treatment is still unknown. In addition, comparison of efficacy between trials is problematic because the dosage varies. Finally, in all but one (open) study, bromelain was used in conjunction with other additional proteolytic enzymes of variable doses, leaving doubts about the specific efficacy of bromelain alone.

Despite some promising studies on bromelain as part of an enzyme complex, there are currently no well-controlled human studies on the effects of bromelain alone. These limitations support the need for a long-term RCT trial using both bromelain alone and in combination form.

REFERENCES

Akhtar NM, Naseer R, Farooqi AZ, Aziz W, Nazir M. Oralenzyme combination versus diclofenac in the treatment of osteoarthritis of the knee—a double-blind prospective randomized study. Clin Rheumatol 2004;23:410–415.

Brien S, Lewith G, Walker A, Hicks SM, Middleton D. Bromelain as a treatment for osteoarthritis: a review of clinical studies. Evid Based Complement Altern Med 2004;1:251–257.

Brien S, Lewith G, Walker A, Middleton D, Prescott P, Bundy R. Bromelain as an adjunctive treatment for moderate-to-severe osteoarthritis of the knee: a randomized placebo-controlled pilot study. QJM 2006;99:841–850.

Castell JV, Friedrich G, Kuhn CS, Poppe GE. Intestinal absorption of undegraded proteins in men: presence of bromelain in plasma after oral intake. Am J Physiol 1997;273:G139-G146.

Chobotova K, Vernallis AB, Majid FAA. Bromelain's activity and potential as an anti-cancer agent: current evidence and perspectives. Cancer Lett 2010;290:148–156.

Cohen A, Goldman J. Bromelian therapy in rheumatoid arthritis. Pa Med J 1964;27–30.

Engwerda CR, Andrew D, Ladhams A, Mynott TL. Bromelain modulates T cell and B cell immune responses in vitro and in vivo. Cell Immunol 2001;210:66–75.

Fitzhugh DJ, Mark SS, Dewhirst W, Hale LP. Bromelain treatment decreases neutrophil migration to sites of inflammation. Clin Immunol 2008;128:66–74.

Gray D. The treatment strategies of arthritis sufferers. Soc Sci Med 1985;21:507–515.

Hale LP, Greer PK, Sempowski GD. Bromelain treatment alters leukocyte expression of cell surface molecules involved in cellular adhesion and activation. Clin Immunol 2002;104:183–190.

Hale LP, Greer PK, Trinh CT, Gottfried MR. Treatment with oral bromelain decreases colonic inflammation in the IL-10 deficient murine model of inflammatory bowel disease. Clin Immunol 2005;5:783–793.

Hale LP, Haynes BF. Bromelain treatment of human T cells removes CD44, CD45RA, E2/MIC2, CD6, CD7, CD8, and Leu 8/LAM1 surface molecules and markedly enhances CD2-mediated T cell activation. J Immunol 1992;149:3809–3816.

Kaboli PJ, Doebbeling BN, Saag KG, Rosenthal GE. Use of complementary and alternative medicine by older patients with arthritis: a population-based study. Arthritis Rheum 2001;45:398–403.

Kalra N, Bhui K, Roy P, Srivastava S, George J, Prasad S, Shukla Y. Regulation of p53, nuclear factor κB and cyclooxygenase-2 expression by bromelain through targeting mitogen-activated protein kinase pathway in mouse skin. Toxicol Appl Pharmacol 2008;226:30–37.

Kerkhoffs GMMJ, Struijs PAA, de Wit C, Rahlfs VW, Zwipp H, van Dijk CN. A double blind, randomised, parallel group study on the efficacy and safety of treating acute lateral ankle sprain with oral hydrolytic enzymes. Br J Sports Med 2004;38:431–435.

Kikuchi M, Matsuura K, Matsumoto Y, Inagaki T, Ueda R. Bibliographical investigation of complementary alternative medicines for osteoarthritis and rheumatoid arthritis. Geriatr Gerontol Int 2009;9:29–40.

Kim HA, Seo YI. Use of complementary and alternative medicine by arthritis patients in a university hospital clinic serving rheumatology patients in Korea. Rheumatol Int 2003;23:277–281.

Klein G, Kullich W. Short term treatment of painful osteoarthritis of the knee with oral enzymes: a randomised, double-blind study versus diclofenac. Clin Drug Invest 2000;19:15–23.

Klein G, Kullich W, Schnitker J, Schwann H. Efficacy and tolerance of an oral enzyme combination in painful osteoarthritis of the hip. A double-blind, randomised study comparing oral enzymes with nonsteroidal anti-inflammatory drugs. Clin Exp Rheumatol 2006;24:25–30.

Manhart N, Akomeah R, Bergmeister H, Spittler A, Ploner M, Rotha E. Administration of proteolytic enzymes bromelain and trypsin diminish the number of CD4+ cells and the interferon-c response in Peyer's patches and spleen in endotoxemic balb/c mice. Cell Immunol 2002;215:113–119.

Maurer HR. Bromelain: biochemistry, pharmacology and medical use. Cell Mol Life Sci 2001;58:1231–1245.

Mynott TL, Ladhams A, Scarmato P, Engwerda CR. Bromelain, from pineapple stems, proteolytically blocks activation of extracellular regulated kinase-2 in T cells. J Immunol 1999;163:2568–2575.

Oleg S, Lehmann MT, Lehmann PV. Prevention of murine EAE by oral hydrolytic enzyme treatment. J Autoimmun 1999;12:191–198.

Pullar T, Pullar T, Capell HA, Millar A, Brooks RG. Alternative medicine: cost and subjective benefit in rheumatoid arthritis. Br Med J 1982;285:1629–1631.

Secor Jr ER, Carson WF, Cloutier MM, Guernsey LA, Schramm CM, Wu CA. Bromelain exerts anti-inflammatory effects in an ovalbumin-induced murine model of allergic airway disease. Cell Immunol 2005;237:68–75.

Secor ER Jr., Singh A, Guernsey LA, McNamara JT, Zhan L, Maulik M, Thrall RS. Bromelain treatment reduces CD25 expression on activated CD4+ T cells in vitro. Int Immunopharmacol 2009;9:340–346.

Sleath B, Callahan L, DeVellis RF, Sloane PD. Patients' perceptions of primary care physicians' participatory decision-making style and communication about complementary and alternative medicine for arthritis. J Altern Complement Med 2005;11:449–453.

Stamp LK, James MJ, Cleland LG. Diet and Rheumatoid Arthritis: A Review of the Literature. Semin Arthritis Rheum 2005;35:77–94.

Targoni OS, Tary-Lehmann M, Lehmann PV. Prevention of murine EAE by oral hydrolytic enzyme treatment. J Autoimmun 1999;12:191–198.

Taussig SJ, Batkin S. Bromelain, the enzyme complex of pineapple (*Ananas comosus*) and its clinical application. An update. J Ethnopharmacol 1988;22:191–203.

Tilwe GH, Beria S, Turakhia NH, Daftary GV, Schiess W. Efficacy and tolerability of oral enzyme therapy as compared to diclofenac in active osteoarthrosis of knee joint: an open randomized controlled clinical trial. J Assoc Physicians India 2001;49:617–621.

Vogler W. Enzymtherapie beim Weichteilrheumatismus. Natur-Ganzheits-Med 1988;1:27.

Wittenborg A, Bock PR, Hanisch J, Saller R, Schneider B. Comparative epidemiological study in patients with rheumatic diseases illustrated in a example of a treatment with nonsteroidal anti-inflammatory drugs versus an oral enzyme combination preparation. Arzneimittel-Forschung 2000;50:728–738.

Yuan G, Wahlqvist ML, He G, Yang M, Li D. Natural products and anti-inflammatory activity. Asia Pac J Clin Nutr 2006;15:143–152.

28 Anti-Inflammatory Properties of *Zingiber officinale* var. Rubra (Red Ginger Extract)

Hiroshi Shimoda

CONTENTS

INTRODUCTION

Rheumatism and knee osteoarthritis are degenerative disorders with aging. With the progression of rheumatism, patients suffer severe pain and joint deformities. Steroids, cyclooxygenase-2 (COX-2)-selective nonsteroidal anti-inflammatory drugs, SH compounds, and immunosuppressants are prescribed to treat rheumatism. Osteoarthritis is characterized as a disease with the deterioration of joint cartilage resulting in pain and dyskinesis. After disease progression, the joint cavity narrows and osteophytes are formed in the affected joint. These morphological changes cause severe pain and mobility limitations. Nonsteroidal anti-inflammatory drugs are commonly prescribed for pain relief, whereas nutritional supplements (e.g., chondroitin sulfate [1], glucosamine [2], and hyaluronic acid [3]) are used for prevention and palliative care of osteoarthritis.

Ginger (*Zingiber officinale* Roscoe) is commonly prescribed in over-the-counter drugs for stomachic, antinausea, and analgesic purposes. In studies of the anti-inflammatory and analgesic effects of ginger, highly purified ginger extracts were reported to improve knee pain and the osteoarthritis composite index in patients with osteoarthritis [4]. [6]-Gingerol (2), a principal vanilloid in ginger oil [5], with inhibitory activity against COX-2 expression [6] and nitric oxide (NO) production [7], has been considered to be a major anti-inflammatory ingredient [8]. Red ginger (*Z. officinale* var. Rubra) is a variant of the *Z. officinale* species cultivated in Indonesia and Malaysia. The surface is reddish-purple and so it is called "Jahe Merah," which means "red ginger" in Indonesia [9]. The rhizome contains gingerols and shogaols as oily ingredients, and its skin contains anthocyanidins and tannins [10]. Red ginger has been used as a spice for cooking and prescribed in traditional medicine for rheumatism, osteoporosis, asthma, and cough. In this paper, we describe the anti-inflammatory effects of red ginger and its inhibitory properties [11].

PROFILE OF RED GINGER EXTRACT AND ITS CONSTITUENTS

We used 40% ethanolic extract prepared from defatted dried red ginger for the experiments described below. The yield of red ginger extract (RGE) was 7.4% and the contents of principal gingerol derivatives (Figure 28.1) determined by HPLC were [4]-gingerol (1), 0.10%; [6]-gingerol

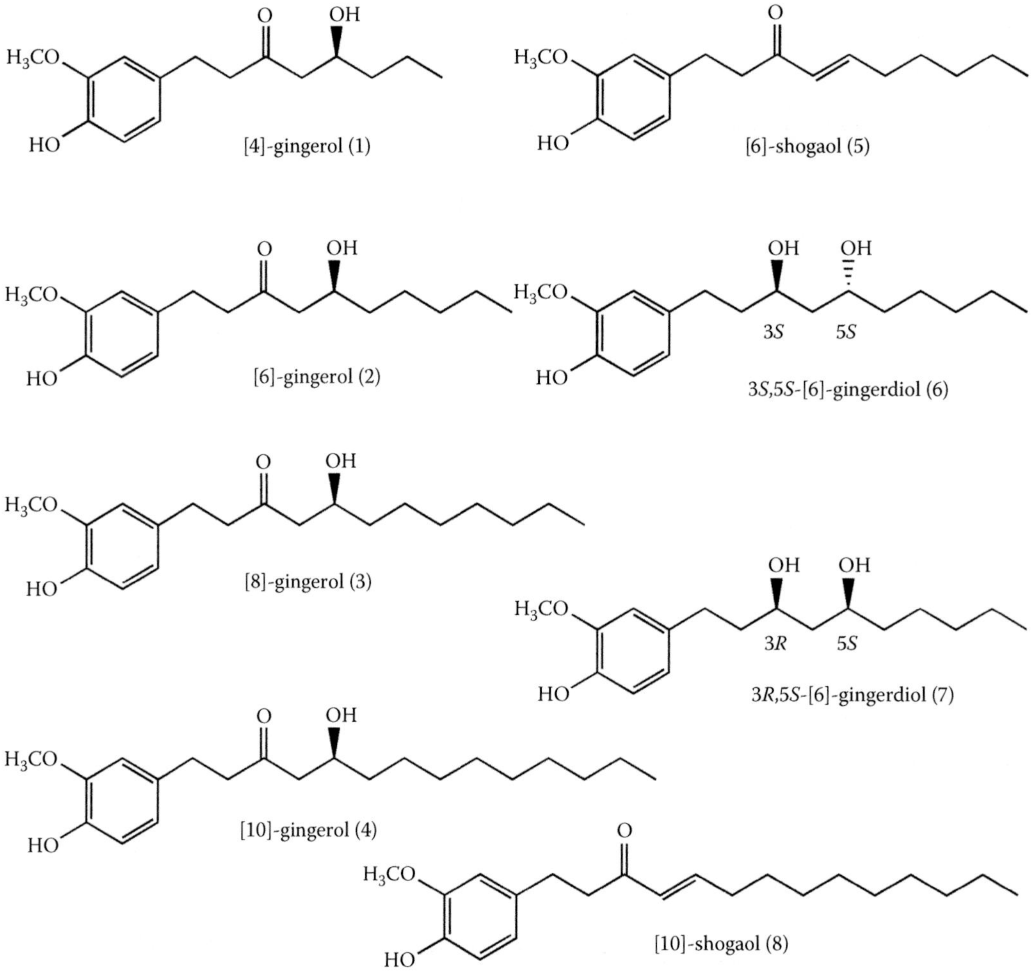

FIGURE 28.1 Structures of compounds isolated from red ginger.

(2), 2.7%; [6]-shogaol (5), 1.7%; and [10]-gingerol (4), 0.16%. The contents of the other gingerol derivatives (3, 6, 7, and 8) were less than 0.1%. The amount of colorimetric products reacting to vanillin/HCl reagent was 1.9% (procyanidine B2 equivalent). To separate a red dye fraction (RDF) containing proanthocyanidins, the extract from red ginger by acidified MeOH extraction was subjected to silica gel column chromatography with $CHCl_3/MeOH/H_2O$ (7:3:1, lower phase) → $CHCl_3/MeOH/H_2O$ (65:35:10, lower phase)→MeOH to provide a light brown fraction. The fraction was further eluted by ODS with $H_2O/MeOH/CF_3COOH$ (90:10:0.1)→$MeOH/CF_3COOH$ (100:0.1) to afford RDF including crude proanthocyanidins.

ANTI-INFLAMMATORY EFFECTS IN ANIMAL MODELS

We evaluated the anti-inflammatory effects of RGE on acute and chronic inflammation models. In an acetic acid–induced mouse writhing model [12], single oral treatment with RGE (10–100 mg/kg) suppressed the number of writhings and dye leakage in a dose-dependent manner (Figure 28.2). RGE was found to exhibit analgesic and anti-inflammatory effects against acute inflammation after oral treatment.

Subsequently, we examined the effect of RGE on chronic inflammation using a rat adjuvant arthritis model. The arthritis was induced in the right hind paw in SD rats by subcutaneous injection

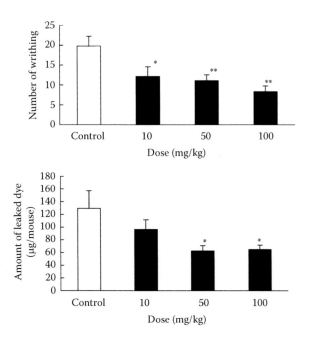

FIGURE 28.2   Effect of RGE on acetic acid–induced writhing and inflammation in mice. RGE was given orally to fasted mice and pontamine sky blue solution was injected (200 mg/kg) intravenously 55 min later. Then, acetic acid (100 mg/kg) was given intraperitoneally 5 min after the injection. The writhing frequency was counted for 15 min beginning at 5 min after the acetic acid injection. The mice were sacrificed and the leaked dye in the abdominal cavity was washed with saline. The absorbance of collected dye solution was measurement at 590 nm. Each column represents the mean with the SE of 12 animals. Asterisks denote significant differences from the control at $*p < 0.05$ and $**p < 0.01$, respectively.

of Freund's complete adjuvant containing inactivated *Mycobacterium butyricum*. RGE was given daily after immunization and edema was determined by measuring the hind paw volume. As shown in Figure 28.3, continuous oral treatment with RGE (10 mg/kg/day) for 13 days significantly suppressed hind paw edema. The suppressive effect was weaker than indomethacin, but it was considered to be potent for a naturally occurring extract. X-ray images of the hind paw treated with the adjuvant were shown in Figure 28.4. Severe joint destruction was observed in the controls, whereas joint destruction in rats treated with RGE and indomethacin was less severe. The joint specimens were observed under a microscope. In the control (Figure 28.5a), papillary growth of villus in the articular cavity and medium-level bone destruction were observed. Invasion of osteoclasts to the surface of the bone was also observed. On the other hand, the articular cavity in the tissue treated with RGE (10 mg/kg) was quite clear and no bone destruction was observed (Figure 28.5b). From the above observation, RGE was suggested to suppress edema and cartilage destruction in an animal chronic inflammation model. Levy et al. [13] reported that daily oral administration of [6]-shogaol (5, 6.2 mg/kg) suppressed adjuvant arthritis in rats. [6]-Shogaol (5) content in RGE was 1.7%, therefore, 10 mg/kg of RGE equates to 0.17 mg/kg [6]-shogaol (5). The content of [6]-shogaol (5) in RGE was not considered sufficient to exhibit a suppressive effect in an adjuvant arthritis model. Therefore, the participation of constituents in RGE other than [6]-shogaol (5) was suggested to be involved in the anti-chronic inflammatory effect of RGE.

In further research with regard to the anti-inflammatory effect of RGE on chronic inflammation, we evaluated the effect on collagen-induced arthritis in mice [14]. RGE was given to mice already suffering from arthritis in the ankles. As shown in Figure 28.6, RGE (10 mg/kg) significantly suppressed edema in the ankles by continuous administration. RGE was found to suppress chronic

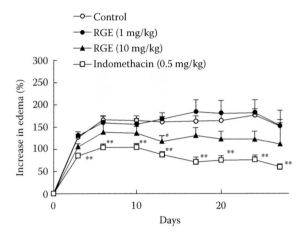

FIGURE 28.3 Effect of RGE on adjuvant arthritis in rats. Adjuvant arthritis in rat feet was induced by a subcutaneous injection of a mixture of Freund's incomplete adjuvant (0.1 mL) and *M. butyricum* (1 mg) into the hind paw. RGE was given daily after adjuvant injection and the increase in edema in the hind paw was measured. Each point represents the mean with the SE of seven animals. Asterisks denote significant differences from the control at $*p < 0.05$ and $**p < 0.01$, respectively.

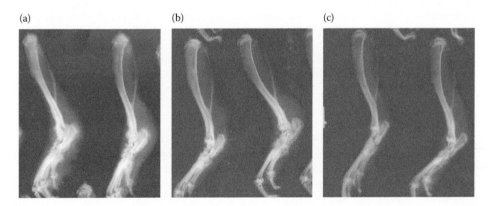

FIGURE 28.4 X-ray images of the rat hind paw. (a) control; (b) RGE (10 mg/kg); (c) indomethacin (0.5 mg/kg).

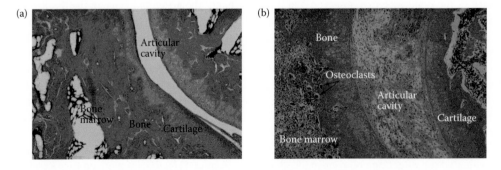

FIGURE 28.5 Microscopic illustration of joint tissues of rats treated with adjuvant H&E staining, ×10; (a) control; (b) RGE (10 mg/kg).

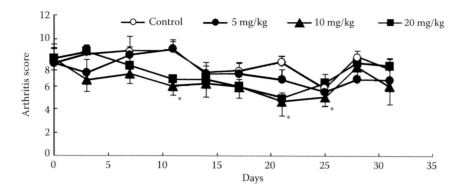

FIGURE 28.6   Effect of RGE on collagen-induced arthritis in mice. An equal volume of bovine type II collagen and Freund's complete adjuvant (100 μL) was intradermally injected into the base of the tail in mice (male DBA/1J, 5 weeks). Booster immunization was performed similarly 3 weeks later. Mice were divided into four groups to adjust the mean severity levels to equality. RGE was given orally once a day at different concentrations (5, 10, and 20 mg/kg). The intensity of inflammation was determined every 3 or 4 days for 31 days. The intensity of inflammation was determined according to Banerjee et al., with an arthritis score in five levels on the basis of average total scores of four legs (16 at the maximum). Each point represents the mean value with the SE of seven mice. Asterisks denote a significant difference from the control at *$p < 0.05$.

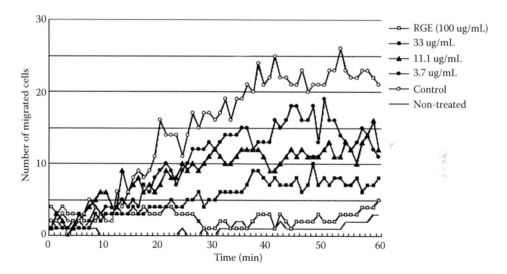

FIGURE 28.7   Effect of RGE on the migration of human monocytes induced by MCP-1. A crude monocyte fraction was obtained from human peripheral blood by dextran solution and Lymphorep. The fraction was suspended in a medium containing microbeads with CD13 and CD19 followed by application to an LD column (Miltenyi Biotec). A nonabsorbed fraction (monocyte fraction) was used for the experiment. Monocytes (2×10^6 cells/mL) were treated with RGE for 1 h at 37°C and migration of monocytes was induced by MCP-1 (10 nM) in a TAXIScan.

inflammation which was induced by collagen. From these in vivo examinations, RGE was found to possess potent analgesic and anti-inflammatory effects.

ANTI-INFLAMMATORY MECHANISM

To investigate the anti-inflammatory mechanism of RGE, we evaluated the effect on macrophages. Macrophages infiltrate inflamed sites and release inflammatory cytokines such as prostaglandins

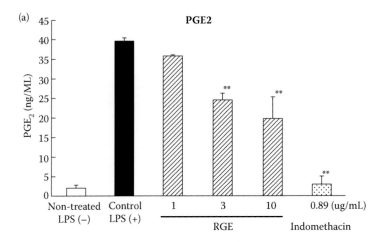

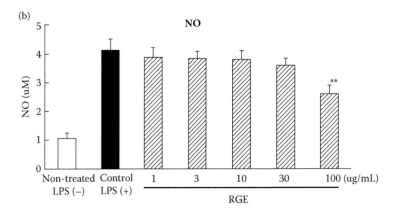

FIGURE 28.8 Effect of RGE on PGE_2 and NO production from RAW264 induced by LPS. RAW264 cells (2×10^5 cells) in 200 μL medium were precultured for 24 h. The medium was replaced with FCS-free medium and each test sample solution and LPS (20 μg/mL) were added. The cells were cultured for 20 h and the supernatant was collected. Each column represents the mean with the SE of four to six experiments. Asterisks denote significant differences from the control at $**p < 0.01$.

(PG) and NO. The effect of RGE on macrophage migration was examined in a chemotactic chamber (TAXIScan, Effecter Cell Institute, Japan). Human monocytes prepared from peripheral blood were used and the migration was induced by macrophage chemoattractant protein (MCP-1). As illustrated in Figure 28.7, RGE demonstrated a concentration-dependent suppression of the migration of monocytes. RGE appeared to inhibit macrophage migration to inflammatory sites in arthritis.

Ginger extract has been reported to inhibit macrophage activation induced by lipopolysaccharide (LPS) [15]. Therefore, we investigated the effect of RGE on LPS-induced PGE_2 and NO production from RAW264 cells. The cells are macrophage-like cells and have been frequently used to evaluate the effect of samples on the release of cytokines and inflammatory mediators induced by inflammatory stimulation [16]. RGE (1–10 μg/mL) suppressed PGE_2 production in a concentration dependent-manner (Figure 28.8a). The IC_{50} value was 10 μg/mL. The suppressive effect of ginger constituents on PGE_2 production have been reported for Chinese white ginger and Japanese yellow ginger [17, 18]. Inhibition of PGE_2 production is thought to be the principal mechanism of the anti-inflammatory action of ginger. In our experiment, we confirmed that red ginger also suppressed LPS-induced PGE_2 production from RAW264 cells. Inhibition of COX-2 activity was reported to be involved in the mechanism of ginger suppression of PGE_2 production [19]. Among the constituents of ginger, [8]-paradol, [8]-shogaol, and [8]-gingerol (3) have been

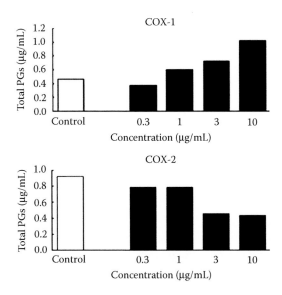

FIGURE 28.9 Effect of RGE on COX-1 and COX-2 activity. Each column represents the mean of two experiments.

reported to be potent COX-2 inhibitors [20]. However, these compounds inhibit COX-1 activity [21], meaning selectivity is lacking in the action. We identified [8]-gingerol (3) in RGE, but the content was less than 0.1% and its involvement in the suppression of PGE2 production was suggested to be slight. On the other hand, Kiuchi et al. [22]. reported that [6]-gingerol (2), [8]-gingerol (3), [10]-gingerol (4), and [6]-shogaol (5) inhibited prostaglandin synthase prepared from rabbit kidney medulla with IC_{50} values of 4.6, 5.0, 2.5, and 1.6 µM, respectively. Flynn et al. [23] also reported that gingerol-related compounds were inhibitors of COX. The contents of [6]-gingerol (2) and [6]-shogaol (5) in RGE were 2.7% and 1.7%, respectively. Considering these reports, we examined the COX-inhibitory activity of RGE. As shown in Figure 28.9, RGE inhibited COX-2 activity at 3 and 10 µg/mL. Hence, major compounds in RGE are suggested to be involved in the inhibitory activity of RGE on PGE_2 synthesis. However, RGE did not inhibit COX-1 activity at the same concentrations. Further investigation is required to clarify this interesting observation.

Excessive NO production by inducible NO synthase is closely related to rat adjuvant arthritis [24]. Inhibitors of NO synthase were reported to potently suppress adjuvant arthritis [25]; therefore, we examined the effect of RGE on NO production from LPS-stimulated RAW264 cells. As for LPS-stimulated NO production from RAW264 cells, a high concentration of RGE (100 µg/mL) significantly suppressed it (Figure 28.8b). Imanishi et al. [26] reported that an extract prepared from common ginger (*Z. officinale* Roscoe) suppressed NO production in RAW264.7 cells at 100 µg/mL. Our data, obtained from red ginger (*Z. officinale* var. Rubra), were similar to their results. Regarding the suppressive effect of ginger constituents on NO production, only [6]-gingerol (2) [7] and its metabolite, [6]-dihydroparadol [27], reportedly suppressed NO production with IC_{50} values of 7.2 and 2.1 µg/mL in LPS-stimulated macrophage cell lines. Therefore, we evaluated the effect of the other constituents in RGE, including RDF. Table 28.1 shows the suppressive effects of the compounds on NO production. Inhibitory effects of [4]-, [6]-, [8]-, and [10]-gingerols (1, 2, 3, 4) and [10]-shogaol (8) were weak or ineffective. On the other hand, [6]-shogaol, 3S,5S-[6]-gingerdiol (6), and 3R,5S-[6]-gingerdiol (7) suppressed NO production with more than 70% inhibition at 100 µg/mL. [6]-Shogaol was the most potent suppressor among gingerols and shogaols. This result is similar to a report by Koh et al. [28]. We investigated RDF containing proanthocyanidins. RDF suppressed NO production by 35.4% at 100 µg/mL. Proanthocyanidins have been reported to inhibit inducible NO synthase [29]. Therefore, RDF is thought to inhibit NO production by inhibition of NO synthase.

TABLE 28.1
The Effect of Constituents Isolated from Red Ginger on LPS-Induced NO Production in RAW/264 Cells

		Upper: NO in supernatant (μM) Lower: Inhibition (%)		
LPS	−	+	+	+	+
Conc. (μg/mL)	0	0	10	30	100
[4]-gingerol (1)	1.17 ± 0.18**	4.77 ± 0.28	4.98 ± 0.22	5.03 ± 0.45	4.98 ± 0.26
[6]-gingerol (2)	0.96 ± 0.14**	3.21 ± 0.27	3.27 ± 0.26	3.11 ± 0.22 (4.3)	2.81 ± 0.47 (17.6)
[8]-gingerol (3)	0.72 ± 0.18**	4.34 ± 0.21	3.86 ± 0.32 (13.3)	3.59 ± 0.21** (20.7)	3.20 ± 0.17** (31.5)
[10]-gingerol (4)	1.12 ± 0.43**	4.20 ± 0.17	4.33 ± 0.50	4.28 ± 0.72	3.55 ± 0.08** (21.1)
[6]-shogaol (5)	0.98 ± 0.17**	3.56 ± 0.30	3.21 ± 0.31 (13.6)	2.79 ± 0.09 (29.8)	1.22 ± 0.04** (90.7)
3S,5S-[6]-gingerdiol (6)	0.76 ± 0.12**	3.57 ± 0.29	3.35 ± 0.14 (7.8)	2.98 ± 0.11 (21.0)	1.36 ± 0.13** (78.7)
3R,5S-[6]-gingerdiol (7)	0.88 ± 0.11**	3.71 ± 0.22	3.56 ± 0.35 (5.3)	3.43 ± 0.32 (9.9)	1.60 ± 0.11** (74.6)
[10]-shogaol (8)	1.21 ± 0.18**	3.26 ± 0.64	2.76 ± 0.10 (24.4)	2.68 ± 0.70 (28.3)	2.62 ± 0.71 (31.2)
RDF	1.12 ± 0.29**	4.18 ± 0.31	3.97 ± 0.32 (6.9)	3.85 ± 0.39 (10.9)	3.10 ± 0.37 (35.4)

Note: RAW264 cells (2×10^5 cells in 200 μL medium) were precultured for 24 h. The medium was replaced with FCS-free medium and each test sample solution and LPS (20 μg/mL) were added. The cells were cultured for 20 h and the supernatant was collected. Each value represents the mean with SE of six experiments. Asterisks denote significant differences from the control group (LPS [+]) at **$p < 0.01$.

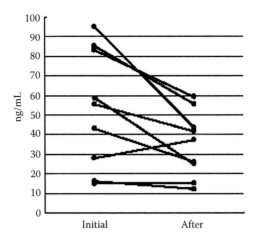

FIGURE 28.10 Blood hyaluronic acid changes in humans by 4 weeks of treatment with RGE.

CONCLUSIONS

As described earlier, RGE was found to suppress inflammation. The effect seemed to be stronger than common ginger. We conducted small-scale human trials in male volunteers, and gave RGE (50 mg/day) for 4 weeks. Blood hyaluronic acid was significantly reduced compared with the value before administration (Figure 28.10). RGE has been prescribed with chondroitin sulfate or glucosamine as a dietary supplement in Japan.

REFERENCES

1. Mazières B, Hucher M, Zaïm M, Garnero P. Effect of chondroitin sulphate in symptomatic knee osteoarthritis: a multicentre, randomised, double-blind, placebo-controlled study. Ann Rheum Dis 2007;66:639–645.
2. Herrero-Beaumont G, Ivorra JA, Del Carmen Trabado M, Blanco FJ, Benito P, Martín-Mola E, et al. Glucosamine sulfate in the treatment of knee osteoarthritis symptoms: a randomized, double-blind, placebo-controlled study using acetaminophen as a side comparator. Arthritis Rheum 2007;56:555–567.
3. Pham T, Hananff AL, Ravaud P, Dieppe P, Paolozzi L, Dougados M. Evaluation of the symptomatic and structural efficacy of a new hyaluronic acid compound, NRD101, in comparison with diacerein and placebo in a 1 year randomized controlled study in symptomatic knee osteoarthritis. Ann Rheum Dis 2004;63:1611–1617.
4. Altman RD, Marcussen KC. Effects of a ginger extract on knee pain in patients with osteoarthritis. Arthritis Rheum 2001;44:2531–2538.
5. Dedov VN, Tran VH, Duke CC, Connor M, Christie MJ, Mandadi S, Roufogalis BD. Gingerols: a novel class of vanilloid receptor (VR1) agonists. Br J Pharmacol 2002;137:793–798.
6. Kim SO, Kundu JK, Shin YK, Park JH, Cho MH, Kim TY, Surh YJ. [6]-Gingerol inhibits COX-2 expression by blocking the activation of p38 MAP kinase and NF-κB in phorbol ester-stimulated mouse skin. Oncogene 2005;24:2558–2567.
7. Ippoushi K, Azuma K, Ito H, Horie H, Higasio H. [6]-Gingerol inhibits nitric oxide synthesis in activated J774.1 mouse macrophages and prevents peroxynitrite-induced oxidation and nitration reactions. Life Sci 2003;73:3427–3437.
8. Young HY, Luo YL, Cheng HY, Hsieh WC, Liao JC, Peng WH. Analgesic and anti-inflammatory activities of [6]-gingerol. J Ethnopharmacol 2005;96:207–210.
9. De Guzman CC, Siemonsma JS. Ginger. In: De Guzman CC, Siemonsma JS, eds. The Prosea handbook. Plant resources of South-East Asia, Vol. 13. Spices. PROSEA, Bogor, Indonesia; 1999:241.
10. Lentera T. The health with ingredients. In: Utami P, ed. Traditional merit and benefit of red ginger. Jakarta, Indonesia: Agro Media Pustaka; 2002:12–13.

11. Shimoda H, Shan SJ, Tanaka J. Seki A, Seo JW, Kasajima N, Tamura S, Ke Y, Murakami N. Anti-inflammatory properties of red ginger (*Zingiber officinale* var. rubra) extract and its nitric oxide production inhibitory ingredients. J Med Food 2010;13:156–162.

12. Matsuda H, Li Y, Murakami T, Ninomiya K, Yamahara J, Yoshikawa M. Effects of escins Ia, Ib, IIa, and IIb from horse chestnut, the seeds of *Aesculus hippocastanum* L., on acute inflammation in animals. Biol Pharm Bull 1997;20:1092–1095.

13. Levy ASA, Simon O, Shelly J, Gardener M. 6-Shogaol reduced chronic inflammatory response in the knees of rats treated with complete Freund's adjuvant. BMC Pharmacol 2006;6(12). http://www.pubmedcentral.nih.gov/picrender.fcgi?artid=1599714&blobtype=pdf

14. Banerjee S, Haqqi TM, Luthra HS, Stuart JM, David CS. Possible role of V_β T cells receptor genes in susceptibility to collagen-induced arthritis in mice. J Exp Med 1988;167:832–839.

15. Tripathi S, Bruch D, Kittur DS. Ginger extract inhibits LPS induced macrophage activation and function. BMC Complement Altern Med 2008;8(1). http://www.pubmedcentral.nih.gov/picrender.fcgi?artid=2234390&blobtype=pdf

16. Zhuang JC, Wogan GN. Growth and viability of macrophages continuously stimulated to produce nitric oxide. Proc Natl Acad Sci U S A 1997;94:11875–11880.

17. Jolad SD, Lantz RC, Solyom AM, Chen GJ, Bates RB, Timmermann BN. Fresh organically grown ginger (*Zingiber officinale*): composition and effects on LPS-induced PGE_2 production. Phytochemistry 2004;65:1937–1954.

18. Jolad SD, Lantz RC, Chen GJ, Bates RB, Timmermann BN. Commercially processed dry ginger (*Zingiber officinale*): composition and effects on LPS-stimulated PGE_2 production. Phytochemistry 2005;66:1614–1635.

19. Lantz RC, Chen GJ, Sarihan M, Solyom AM, Jolad SD, Timmermann BN. The effect of extracts from ginger rhizome on inflammatory mediator production. Phytomedicine 2007;14:123–128.

20. Tjendraputra E, Tran VH, Liu-Brennan D, Roufogalis BD, Duke CC. Effect of ginger constituents and synthetic analogues on cyclooxygenase-2 enzyme in intact cells. Bioorg Chem 2001;29:156–163.

21. Nurtjahja-Tjendraputra E, Ammit AJ, Roufogalis BD, Tran VH, Duke CC. Effective anti-platelet and COX-1 enzyme inhibitors from pungent constituents of ginger. Thrombosis Res 2003; 111:259–265.

22. Kiuchi F, Iwakami S, Shibuya M, Hanaoka F, Sankawa U. Inhibition of prostaglandin and leukotriene biosynthesis by gingerols and diarylheptanoids. Chem Pharm Bull (Tokyo) 1992;40:387–391.

23. Flynn DL, Rafferty MF, Boctor AM. Inhibition of human neutrophil 5-lipoxygenase activity by gingerdione, shogaol, capsaicin and related pungent compounds. Prostaglandins Leukot Med 1986;24:195–198.

24. Oyanaggui Y. Nitric oxide and superoxide radical are involved in both initiation and development of adjuvant arthritis in rats. Life Sci 1994;54:PL285–289.

25. Stefanovic-Racic M, Meyers K, Meschter C, Coffey JW, Hoffman RA, Evans CH. *N*-monomethyl arginine, an inhibitor of nitric oxide synthase, suppresses the development of adjuvant arthritis in rats. Arthritis Rheum 1994;37:1062–1069.

26. Imanishi N, Mantani N, Sakai S, Sato M, Katada Y, Ueda K, Terasawa K, Ochiai H. Inducible activity of ginger rhizome (*Zingiber officinale* Rosc.) on the mRNA expression of macrophage-inducible nitric oxide (NO) synthase and NO production in a macrophage cell line, RAW264.7 cells. Am J Chin Med 2004;32:727–735.

27. Aktan F, Henness S, Tran VH, Duke CC, Roufogalis BD, Ammit AJ. Gingerol metabolite and a synthetic analogue Capsarol inhibit macrophage NF-κB-mediated iNOS gene expression and enzyme activity. Planta Med 2006;72:727–734.

28. Koh EM, Kim HJ, Kim S, Choi WH, Choi YH, Ryu SY, Kim YS, Koh WS, Park SY. Modulation of macrophage functions by compounds isolated from *Zingiber officinale*. Planta Med 2009;75:148–151.

29. Kolodziej H, Kayser O, Kiderlen AF, Ito H, Hatano T, Yoshida T, Foo LY. Proanthocyanidins and related compounds: antileishmanial activity and modulatory effects on nitric oxide and tumor necrosis factor-alpha-release in the murine macrophage-like cell line RAW 264.7. Biol Pharm Bull 2001;24,1016–1021.

29 Benefits of Radix *Tripterygium wilfordii* for Rheumatoid Arthritis

Xiaojuan He, Shaohua Xu, Miao Jiang, Na Lin, and Aiping Lu

CONTENTS

Rheumatoid arthritis (RA) is a severe, aggressive, and debilitating disease that has a high mortality rate. It affects nearly 1% of the world population, characterized by pain, swelling, and progressive destruction of synovial joints. Consequently, patients with severe disease face significant disability, deformity, and irreversible joint damage [1]. Even if there are many methods including physical treatment, chemical drug, surgery, and immune therapy, few patients have been cured. Until now, RA is still a refractory autoimmune disease.

Tripterygium wilfordii Hook F (TWHF), also called lei gong teng or thunder god vine, is a perennial vine growing in southern China. The herb has been used in Chinese medicine for treatment of immune inflammatory diseases including RA, systemic lupus erythematosus, nephritis, asthma, and ankylosing spondylitis for many years [2, 3]. The extracts of TWHF contain more than 70 compounds including diterpenoids, triterpenoids, sesquiterpenoids, β-sitosterol, dulcitol, and glycosides. Triptolide ($C_{20}H_{24}O_6$), a diterpene triepoxide, is a major component of TWHF extracts, which has been shown to possess potent anti-inflammatory and immunosuppressive properties [4]. Both phase I and phase II studies of the ethyl acetate (EA) extract of TWHF in patients with RA showed that it appeared to be safe and clinically beneficial [2, 5].

In recent years, many researches about the mechanism and application of TWHF have been done. In this chapter, we review the benefits of TWHF on the therapy of RA. The review includes two parts: the first part mainly describes the progress on mechanism research of TWHF in RA therapy, and the second part summarizes the clinic application of TWHF on RA therapy.

MECHANISM OF TWHF ON THERAPY OF RA

IMMUNOREGULATORY EFFECT OF TWHF

Effect on Immune Cells

T Lymphocytes

The immunopathogenesis of RA involves both the innate and the adaptive immune system. T lymphocyte, B lymphocyte, natural killer cell, dendritic cell (DC), macrophage, and so forth, are all involved in the occurrence and development of the disease.

Defects in the appropriate regulation of CD4+ T helper (Th) cell function have been implicated in the pathophysiology of many autoimmune diseases, including RA [6, 7]. Reports have demonstrated that the infiltration of activated T cells enhances osteoclastogenesis in the joint, coupled with the identification of elevated Th1-associated factors (macrophage colony-stimulating factor, interleukin-10 [IL-10], and tumor necrosis factor [TNF]) that induce osteoclastogenesis in synovial tissue [8–10]. Triptolide is found to inhibit mitogen- or antigen-induced proliferation of human peripheral blood T cells and expression of IL-1β, IL-6, TNF, interferon-γ (IFN-γ), monocyte chemotactic protein 1 (MCP-1), macrophage inflammatory protein 1α (MIP-1α), and MIP-1β [11, 12]. It also inhibits CD69 and CD25 expression of mouse CD3+ T cell [13]. Furthermore, triptolide induces T-cell apoptosis through activating caspases [14].

CD4+CD25+ regulatory T cells (Tregs), first proved by Sakaguchi, are a subset of CD4+ T cells with a critical role in the prevention of autoimmunity [15]. They account for approximately 5%–10% in peripheral CD4+ T cells. The role for Tregs in RA has been established in both patients and animal models [16]. A variety of approved and experimental drugs for RA have been proved to work, in part, by promoting the function or by increasing the numbers of Tregs [15]. The study by Zhang et al. [17] investigates the effect of triptolide on the differentiation of Tregs from CD4+ cells in rats, and they found that triptolide may promote the differentiation of CD4+ cells to FoxP3+ Tregs, which may be one of the pathways responsible for the immunosuppressive activity of triptolide.

T helper type 17 (Th17) cells represent a novel subset of CD4+ T cells and play an important role in the immunopathogenesis of autoimmune diseases. There is mounting evidence that inappropriate regulation of Th17 cells also participates in the pathogenesis of RA [18]. Recent study found that triptolide significantly inhibits the generation of Th17 cells from murine splenocytes and purified CD4+ T cells. Importantly, triptolide inhibits the transcription of IL-17 messenger RNA (mRNA) and IL-6-induced phosphorylation of STAT3, a key signaling molecule involved in the development of Th17 cells. The results of *in vivo* studies also demonstrate that the levels of collagen type II (CII)–specific IL-17 production and the percentages of CII-specific IL-17+ CD4+ T cells in the cells from draining lymph nodes and spleens are significantly reduced in collagen-induced arthritis (CIA) mice treated with triptolide [19].

B Lymphocytes

The critical role of B cells in the pathogenesis of RA has previously been investigated. Studies have proved that B-cell depletion treatment can improve this disease [20, 21]. B cells have different functions that may be relevant in the pathogenesis of RA, including antigen presentation, stimulation of T cells, production of cytokine, and autoantibodies [22]. An EA extract of TWHF can suppress proliferation of B lymphocytes [23]; another work shows that six compounds (T4, T7, T8, T9, T10, and L2) and component T1 from TWHF have significant inhibitory effects on the proliferation of B cells [24]. In addition, an alcohol extract of TWHF termed T2 inhibited antigen- and mitogen-stimulated proliferation of B cells and immunoglobulin production by B cells [25].

Dendritic Cells

Dendritic cells (DCs) are the professional antigen-presenting cells that play crucial roles in the regulation of immune response. The role of DCs has been extensively investigated in the pathogenesis of RA, and DCs have been regarded as one of the target for therapy of RA [26, 27]. Some studies have demonstrated that triptolide can affect the phenotype, maturation, function, and apoptosis of DCs [28–30]. Triptolide prevents the differentiation of immature human monocyte derived DC (MoDC) by inhibiting CD1a, CD40, CD80, CD86, and HLA-DR expression but upregulating CD14 expression as well as by reducing the capacity of MoDC to stimulate lymphocyte proliferation in the allergenic mixed lymphocyte reaction [29]. It also inhibits the production of IL-12 and the allostimulatory functions of DCs. Furthermore, the calcium mobilization and the chemotactic responses of LPS-stimulated DCs to secondary lymphoid tissue chemokine/CC chemokine ligand 21 (CCL21) are significantly lower in triptolide-treated than untreated DCs, in association with lower CC chemokine receptor 7 (CCR7) and higher CCR5 expression [31]. In addition, triptolide induces activation of p38, which preceded the activation of caspase-3, and then induces apoptosis of DCs [32].

Macrophages

Macrophages execute important functions in the immune system. Activated macrophages play a role in arthritis (a) by processing and presenting antigens to T cells; (b) by producing a variety of inflammatory mediators, including TNF-α, IL-1, IL-6, IL-12, nitric oxide (NO), and other free radicals (e.g., superoxide anion); and (c) by secreting tissue-degrading enzymes [33]. Moreover, the abundance and activation of macrophages in the inflamed synovial membrane/pannus significantly correlates with the severity of RA [34]. Studies have demonstrated that triptolide has an inhibitory effect on macrophages. Triptolide inhibits the production of superoxide anion, NO, and some key inflammation-related cytokines, such as TNF-α, IL-1, IL-6, and IFN-γ [35]. Triptolide is also found to suppress the activity of nuclear factor κB (NF-κB) and c-Jun NH2-terminal kinase, thus inhibiting transcription of the NO synthase (NOS) gene in macrophage cell line RAW 264.7 [36]. In addition, triptolide increases the generation of reactive oxygen species (ROS) and induced apoptosis of RAW 264.7 cells [37]. Triptolide impairs the antigen-presenting function of THP-1 cells by inhibiting CD80 and CD86 expressions [38].

Effect on Enteric Mucosal Immune System

Enteric mucosal membrane is the first barrier of preventing infection and plays an important role in regulating homeostasis of internal and external environment [39]. It consists of many immune cells and molecules scattered throughout the lamina propria and epithelium of the mucosa as well as organized lymphatic tissues such as Peyer's patches [40]. The enteric mucosal immune system is commonly divided into two parts: (i) inductive site, which includes intestinal lymph nodes (Peyer's patches) and mesenteric lymph nodes, and (ii) effector site, which mainly intraepithelial lymphocytes (IELs) and lamina propria lymphocytes (LPLs) [41, 42]. Enteric immune response might be actively involved in CIA pathogenesis [43]. The numbers of lymphocytes in enteric mucosal membrane have changed in CIA mice. Compared with the normal mice, more CD4+ and CD8+ T cells in Peyer's patches, less CD4+ and more CD8+ T cells in LPLs, and less CD8+ and more CD4+ T cells in IELs are, respectively, detected in CIA mice. Triptolide has an effect on enteric mucosal immune lymphocytes in Peyer's patch, IELs, and LPLs of CIA mice. Compared with the CIA mice, less CD8+ T cells in Peyer's patches and LPLs and more CD8+ T cells in IELs are, respectively, present in triptolide-treated mice [44].

Effect on Joint Cells

RA is a multifactorial disease characterized by chronic inflammation of the joints. Both genetic and environmental factors are involved in the pathogenesis of joint destruction and disability. In the inflamed RA joint, the synovium is highly infiltrated by CD4+ T cells, B cells, and macrophages [45]. These cells produce a number of cytokines such as TNF-α, IL-1, IL-6, IL-17, IFN-γ, and so forth. Besides these immune cells and cytokines, other cells including chondrocytes and synovial fibroblasts also participate in the progress of RA. Chondrocytes constitute the unique cellular component of articular cartilage [46]. Studies have shown that chondrocytes produce a number of inflammatory mediators, such as IL-1β and TNF-α, which are present in RA joint tissues and fluids. Chondrocytes respond to these proinflammatory cytokines by increasing the production of proteinases, prostaglandins, and NOs [47, 48]. Chondrocytes also express several chemokines as well as chemokine receptors that may participate in cartilage catabolism [49, 50]. Extracts of TWHF and triptolide inhibit cytokine-induced matrix metalloproteinase 3 (MMP-3) and MMP-13 gene expression in human chondrocytes, and they also suppress IL-1-, IL-17-, and TNF-α-induced expression of aggrecanases (a disintegrin and metalloprotease with thrombospondin motifs) in bovine chondrocytes. Thus, TWHF can protect cartilage from MMP- and aggrecanase-driven breakdown [51]. RA synovial fibroblasts are the effector cells of cartilage and bone destruction. These cells show an "intrinsically" activated and aggressive phenotype that result in the increased production of matrix-degrading enzymes and adhesion molecules [52]. TWHF has an antiproliferative effect on synovial fibroblast; it also reduces cyclooxygenase-2 (COX-2) and inducible NOS (iNOS) mRNA and protein expression and correspondingly reduces prostaglandin E$_2$ (PGE$_2$) and NO produced by synovial fibroblasts [53]. In addition, it suppress the production of pro-MMP-1 and pro-MMP-3 [54].

Effect on Vascular Endothelial Cells

Angiogenesis is the formation of new capillaries from preexisting vessels. A number of soluble and cell-bound factors may stimulate neovascularization, including growth factors, primarily vascular endothelial growth factor and hypoxia-inducible factors, as well as proinflammatory cytokines, various chemokines, matrix components, cell adhesion molecules, proteases, and others [55]. Neovascularization is another important feature in the development and maintenance of the disease state of RA. Angiogenesis aids in the delivery of inflammatory cells to the synovium and delivers blood borne elements to the pannus, which is an interdigitating folds of tissue resulting from synovial proliferation over articular surfaces.

Triptolide can function as a potent angiogenesis inhibitor [56]. It manifests the most potent anti-angiogenic activity against vessel formation. Further studies show that the angiopoietin (angpt)2/tie2 signaling pathway is involved in the antiangiogenic action of triptolide [57]. Celastrol, another major active component of TWHF, also inhibits angiogenesis both *in vitro* and *in vivo*. It inhibits the proliferation of vascular endothelial cells ECV-304. At the concentration of 0.2 mg/mL, it significantly inhibits cell migration and tube formation [58]. Tripterine, a chemical compound of TWHF, prominent inhibits the expression of E-selectin, vascular cell adhesion molecule 1, and intercellular adhesion molecule 1 in human umbilical vein endothelial cells in a dose-dependent manner. In addition, tripterine inhibits adhesion of human monocytes and T lymphocytes to TNF-α-stimulated human umbilical vein endothelial cells [59].

ANTI-INFLAMMATORY EFFECT OF TWHF

Inhibit the Production of Cytokine and Chemokine

In the past decade, many studies report that abnormal expression and regulation of some cytokines in patients are some of the important factors for the occurrence and development of RA. Cytokines are the major mediators of joint damage in chronic arthritis. High levels of IL-1β, IL-6, IL-10, IL-17, and TNF-α in the serum and synovial fluid are observed in patients with RA [60]. TWHF can relieve inflammatory responses by inhibiting the production of proinflammatory cytokines.

IL-1, TNF-α, and IL-6

IL-1 is a proinflammatory cytokine that has a pivotal role in the pathophysiology and clinical manifestations of RA. In patients with RA, there are increased amounts of IL-1 in the synovium [61]. Studies have shown that IL-1 stimulates the production of prostaglandins and other proinflammatory mediators such as NO, cytokines, chemokines, and adhesion molecules. Furthermore, IL-1 stimulates the synthesis and activity of MMPs and other enzymes involved in cartilage destruction in RA [62]. TNF-α, the primary mediator in RA, is secreted very early in the inflammatory process and joins in many immune reactions. TNF-α stimulates RA synovial cells to produce IL-1, IL-6, and granulocyte-macrophage colony-stimulating factor. TNF-α is also known to induce release of tissue degradative enzymes such as MMPs from neutrophils and various synoviocytes. In addition, TNF-α increases expression of iNOS in macrophages and vascular endothelial cells [63]. IL-6 is a mediator of host response to tissue injury. IL-6 can increase expression of pro-MMPs produced by IL-1-induced human synovial cells, thus increasing the damage of synovium.

Triptolide can suppress the gene expression of IL-1, TNF-α and IL-6 as well as the production of IL-1β and IL-6, the mechanism may be through the NF-κB inhibition [35, 54, 64, 65]. Moreover, triptolide also downregulates IL-6-induced phosphorylation of STAT3 [19].

IL-17

IL-17 family plays a key role in the regulation of inflammatory response and progression of autoimmune diseases. IL-17 can induce the production of proinflammatory cytokines, such as TNF-α and IL-1 [66]. In addition, IL-17 exerts synergistic effects with TNF-α and IL-1 in the induction of joint inflammation and cartilage and joint destruction [67].

Triptolide inhibits IL-17 production in a dose-dependent manner at the protein and mRNA levels. IL-17 production is almost completely inhibited at a concentration of 10 nM. Moreover, the production of IL-17 is still inhibited after removing triptolide from cell cultures [19].

IL-18

IL-18 is a representative proinflammatory factor and displays multiple biological functions. Study by Shao et al. [68] shows the expression levels of IL-18 and its receptor (IL-18R) in both serum and synovial fluid, and tissue of patients with RA are significantly increased compared with the samples from the control group. Triptolide effectively inhibits the bioactivity of IL-18 in PMA-stimulated RA synovial fibroblast. The expression of IL-18 and IL-18R at protein and gene levels is reduced by triptolide [69].

In addition, triptolide and its derivative (5R)-5-hydroxytriptolide (LLDT-8) also inhibit the expression of IL-2, IL-12, and IFN-γ [35, 38, 70, 71] and enhance the production of IL-10 and transforming growth factor β [28, 72].

Chemokines and their receptors are involved together in the development of inflammatory diseases, including RA [73, 74]. It has been reported that the expression of MCP-1, MIP-1α, RANTES, and CCR5 was upregulated in synovial tissue of rats with adjuvant-induced arthritis [75–77]. Triptolide can significantly inhibit overexpression of MCP-1, MIP-1α, RANTES, and CCR5 at both mRNA and protein levels in rats with adjuvant-induced arthritis [77, 78].

Inhibit the MMPs

RA is a chronic disease that causes progressive joint destruction. It is characterized by severe joint inflammation, synovial hyperplasia, and joint destruction [79, 80]. The cartilage destruction observed in RA is mostly caused by the activation of MMPs [81]. MMPs are a family of zinc-dependent endopeptidases involved in the degradation and remodeling of extracellular matrix. MMP-3 and MMP-13 are the two main enzymes involved in the erosion of cartilage extracellular matrix in the patients with arthritis. Triptolide directly suppresses the production of pro-MMP-1 and pro-MMP-3 and simultaneously upregulates tissue inhibitors of metalloproteinases in IL-1-treated human synovial fibroblasts [54]. Studies by Liacini et al. [51] also show that triptolide inhibits cytokine-induced MMP-3 and MMP-13 gene expression in many cells. Mechanistic studies reveal that TWHF partially inhibits DNA binding capacity of cytokine-stimulated activating protein 1 and NF-κB transcription factors.

Inhibit the NO

NO has been recognized as an important mediator of inflammation. It regulates T-cell function [82] and induces the production of cytokines, including IL-1 and TNF, and has been described as a cyto-toxic molecule with a pivotal role in apoptosis at the joints of patients with RA [83]. NO is synthe-sized within cells by an NOS. There are three NOS isoforms: neuronal NOS, endothelial NOS, and iNOS. The constitutive (neuronal and endothelial NOS) and inducible (iNOS) forms are responsible for regulating the physiological and pathological roles of NO, respectively [84]. Chronic inflamma-tion can lead to excessive production of NO. An increase in NO production has been found in patients with RA [82, 85, 86]. Administration of the EA extract of TWHF causes a reduction in production of NO in an animal model of arthritis [87]. Another study shows that treatment of mice with the EA extract inhibits NO production and iNOS mRNA expression both *in vivo* and *in vitro*. Triptolide sup-presses iNOS gene expression at the transcriptional level by inhibiting induction of the activity of Oct-1 [88]. NF-κB and JNK pathway might be involved in the inhibition of NO production and iNOS expression by triptolide [36]. In addition, triptolide can suppress the generation of superoxide anion, which is produced by activated macrophages and leads to tissue damage during inflammation [35].

Inhibit the PGE$_2$

PGE$_2$ is shown to be a potent immunoregulatory lipid mediator. COX-1 and inducible COX-2 are the rate-limiting enzymes for PGE$_2$ biosynthesis. Accumulating evidence has demonstrated that PGE$_2$ plays a pivotal role in the initiation and progression of various inflammatory diseases, including RA [89, 90]. It not only participates in IL-23-induced neutrophil migration in arthritis [91] but also promotes immune inflammation through Th1 differentiation and Th17 expansion [92]. In addition, it has regulatory effect on some cytokines, such as IL-17, TNF-α, IFN-γ, and so on [90, 93–95]. Recently, it has been reported that the EA extract of TWHF inhibits PGE$_2$ production in a variety of human cells [53, 96]. Further data show that triptolide inhibits the release of PGE$_2$ by suppressing COX-2 protein expression, and this suppression is mediated by modulating NF-κB transcriptional activity and JNK phosphorylation [97].

EFFECT ON APOPTOSIS

Apoptosis plays a pivotal role in tissue homoeostasis. Apoptosis disorders can lead to some serious diseases such as cancer and autoimmune diseases. Several reports suggest that triptolide or extract of TWHF induce apoptosis of many cells, including cancer cell lines, immune cells, and fibroblast-like synoviocytes [37, 98, 99].

Triptolide is found to induce apoptotic death of T-cell hybridomas and peripheral T cells. The triptolide-induced apoptosis is accompanied by the increase of DEVD-cleavable caspases activity and the degradation of caspase substrate poly(adenosine diphosphate ribose) polymerase. A specific inhibitor of caspases can prevent triptolide-induced poly(adenosine diphosphate ribose) polymerase degradation and DNA fragmentation [14]. Triptolide also induces apoptosis of RAW 264.7 cells through increasing the generation of ROS and NO. ROS initiates triptolide-induced apoptosis by the mitochondria signal pathway, whereas apoptotic cell death mediated by NO is not via mitochon-dria collapse and caspase-3 activation [37]. In addition, triptolide can dramatically induce apop-tosis of DCs, as demonstrated by phosphatidylserine exposure, mitochondria potential decrease, and nuclear DNA condensation. Triptolide induces activation of p38 in DCs, which precedes the activation of caspase-3 [32].

Several studies have shown that some characteristic changes in the composition and structure of the inflamed synovial membrane in RA are linked to an altered apoptotic response of synovial cells [100]. Triptolide can induce apoptosis of rheumatoid synovial fibroblasts (RSF). Triptolide induces DNA fragmentation in cultured RSF. When synovial cells are incubated with triptolide for 24 h, changes of cell morphology are observed, such as cellular rounding, shrinkage, and membrane blebbing, and the cells become separated from neighboring cells. Triptolide-induced apoptosis may be relevant with the caspases because the activation can be completely blocked by pan-caspase inhibitor Z-VAD-FMK. Data show that triptolide-induced DNA fragmentation in RSF is suppressed by Z-DEVD-FMK, ZIETD- FMK, and Z-LEHD-FMK, inhibitors of caspase-3, caspase-8, and caspase-9, respectively, in a concentration-dependent manner [101].

CLINICAL APPLICATION OF TWHF IN THE TREATMENT OF RA

RANDOMIZED, CONTROLLED CLINICAL STUDIES

A prospective, double-blind, placebo-controlled study was conducted to evaluate the efficacy and side effect of TWHF [102]. The patients involved in were long-standing RA in whom conventional therapy had failed. All patients were randomly assigned to receive a high dose (360 mg/day) of a TWHF ethanol/ethyl alcohol extracts, a low dose (180 mg/day), or a placebo. The therapeutic benefits according to American College of Rheumatology (ACR) criteria were evaluated at baseline and every 4 weeks. Thirty-five subjects were involved in the study; 8 of 11 patients in the high-dose group, 7 of 12 patients in the low-dose group, and 6 of 12 patients in the placebo group completed 20 weeks of treatment. Patients were withdrawing from the study because of adverse side effects; the withdrawing number was almost equal in the treatment and placebo groups. The significant improvements were seen in the group receiving 360 mg/day of the EA extract when compared with placebo ($p = 0.0001$). The effectiveness of the low-dose group was less than that of the high-dose group ($p = 0.027$) but greater than that of the placebo group ($p = 0.0287$). The results are similar to those reported previously in the mostly uncontrolled studies reported in the Chinese literature [103, 104] and consistent with the randomized, controlled trial conducted recently [105]. In the trial, 121 active patients with RA involved in the clinical study were randomly assigned to TWHF extract, 60 mg thrice daily, or sulfasalazine, 1 g twice daily, to compare the benefits and side effects of TWHF extract with those of sulfasalazine for the treatment of active RA. Patients could continue stable doses of oral prednisone or nonsteroidal anti-inflammatory drugs (NSAIDs) but had to stop taking disease-modifying antirheumatic drugs at least 28 days before randomization. Thirty-seven (62%) of 60 patients in the TWHF extract group and 25 (41%) of 61 patients in the sulfasalazine group completed 24 weeks of treatment. After 24 weeks, the improvement identified by ACR 20 were more noted in the TWHF group when compared with the sulfasalazine group ($p = 0.001$). Patients receiving TWHF also had significantly higher response rates for ACR 50 and ACR 70 in mixed-model analyses. Significant improvement was demonstrated in all individual components of the ACR response, including the Health Assessment Questionnaire disability score. IL-6 levels rapidly and significantly decreased in the TWHF group. Although not statistically significant, radiographic progression was lower in the TWHF group.

The extract of TWHF, specially the polyglycoside-enriched ingredients, has been widely used in China from 1980 to 1990 [106–109]. Patients enrolled into these trials had adult-onset RA of at least 6 months standing, had active symptoms, and had been nonresponsive to NSAID treatment of 2 months or longer. In these studies, patients were treated with *T. wilfordii* polyglycoside (60 mg/day) with therapeutic duration from 12 to 24 weeks. During the course, a stable dose of NSAID (ibuprofen 600 mg/day or indomethacin suppository 100 mg/day) was continued throughout the trial in all patients except those whose symptoms were markedly relieved. Various outcome measures were used to estimate the therapeutic effects, including tenderness score, swelling count, duration of morning stiffness, mean grip strength, 15 m walking time, erythrocyte sedimentation rate, C-reactive protein, IgG, IgM, IgA, physician and patient rated, and so forth. Results from most of the uncontrolled clinical trials of TWHF extracts have claimed significant therapeutic benefits, in which the responsive rates could reach as high as 80% and the frequencies of side effects ranged between 4% and 35%.

THERAPEUTIC EFFECT OF TWHF COMBINED WITH OTHER DRUGS IN RA

A clinical trial showed 70 patients with RA in the active stage treated with *T. wilfordii* polycoride tablets in combination with methotrexate [110]. In the trial, 70 patients were randomly divided into two groups, the one group (35 patients) taking *T. wilfordii* polyglycoside 30 mg orally within three times 1 day combined with methotrexate 7.5 mg orally once a week and the another group as control (35 patients) taking methotrexate 15 mg orally once a week. All the patients keep on taking NSAIDs for 3 months. The therapeutic efficacy showed no significant difference in statistic between the two groups ($p > 0.05$). There were significant differences in the clinical symptoms and signs, erythrocyte sedimentation rate, and rheumatoid factor between the treatment before and after in both groups. However, side effects came out in 20 cases in the methotrexate group and in 8 cases in the *T. wilfordii* polyglycoside treatment group. In addition, compared with methotrexate group, the frequency of adverse events was lower.

The outcome data suggested that the combination of *T. wilfordii* polycoride with methotrexate was favorable to treat acute RA with the definitely therapeutic effect. These results were similar to the results of the clinical trials [111, 112]. In addition, many similar randomized, controlled clinical trails were reported on the *T. wilfordii* polycoride combinations with small-dose cyclophosphamide for patients with treatment-refractory RA and *T. wilfordii* polycoride combinations with sulfasalazine for elderly patients with RA [113], and the results indicated that *T. wilfordii* polycoride combined with other drugs to treat RA could exert better therapeutic effects and cause fewer adverse events.

CONCLUSIONS

In recent years, great progresses have been made on the research and application of TWHF. It has been proved that TWHF is safe and effective as a drug for RA therapy. Mechanism researches show that TWHF can regulate various immune cells and cytokines, inhibit the production of inflammatory mediators, induce apoptosis, suppress the angiogenesis, and so forth. Nevertheless, there are still some questions need to be resolved, including the determination of active ingredients of TWHF, the exact receptor on cells recognized by TWHF, the effective dosage of TWHF in clinic application, the minimization of adverse effect of TWHF, the selection of effective people for TWHF therapy, and so forth. It is believed that further studies may improve the therapeutic success of TWHF on RA.

REFERENCES

1. American College of Rheumatology. Guidelines for the management of rheumatoid arthritis: 2002 Update. Arthritis Rheum 2002;46(2):328–346.
2. Tao X, Cush JJ, Garret M, Lipsky PE. A phase I study of ethyl acetate extract of the Chinese antirheumatic herb *Tripterygium wilfordii* Hook F in rheumatoid arthritis. J Rheumatol 2001;28(10):2160–2167.
3. Qiu D, Kao PN. Immunosuppressive and anti-inflammatory mechanisms of triptolide, the principal active diterpenoid from the Chinese medicinal herb *Tripterygium wilfordii* Hook. F. Drugs R D. 2003;4(1):1–18.
4. Chen BJ. Triptolide, a novel immunosuppressive and anti-inflammatory agent purified from a Chinese herb *Tripterygium wilfordii* Hook F. Leuk Lymphoma 2001;42(3):253–265.
5. Tao X, Younger J, Fan FZ, Wang B, Lipsky PE. Benefit of an extract of *Tripterygium wilfordii* Hook F in patients with rheumatoid arthritis: a double-blind, placebo-controlled study. Arthritis Rheum 2002;46(7):1735–1743.
6. Goodnow CC, Sprent J, de St Groth BF, Vinuesa CG. Cellular and genetic mechanisms of self tolerance and autoimmunity. Nature 2005;435(7042):590–597.

7. Goronzy JJ, Weyand CM. Rheumatoid arthritis. Immunol Rev 2005;204:55–73.
8. Kotake S, Udagawa N, Hakoda M, Mogi M, Yano K, Tsuda E, Takahashi K, et al. Activated human T cells directly induce osteoclastogenesis from human monocytes: possible role of T cells in bone destruction in rheumatoid arthritis patients. Arthritis Rheum 2001;44(5):1003–1012.
9. Yamada H, Nakashima Y, Okazaki K, Mawatari T, Fukushi JI, Kaibara N, Hori A, Iwamoto Y, Yoshikai Y. Th1 but not Th17 cells predominate in the joints of patients with rheumatoid arthritis. Ann Rheum Dis 2008;67(9):1299–1304.
10. Kotake S, Nanke Y, Mogi M, Kawamoto M, Furuya T, Yago T, Kobashigawa T, Togari A, Kamatani N. IFN-gamma-producing human T cells directly induce osteoclastogenesis from human monocytes via the expression of RANKL. Eur J Immunol 2005;35(11):3353–3363.
11. Tao X, Davis LS, Hashimoto K, Lipsky PE. The Chinese herbal remedy, T2, inhibits mitogen-induced cytokine gene transcription by T cells, but not initial signal transduction. J Pharmacol Exp Ther 1996;276(1):316–325.
12. Krakauer T, Chen X, Howard OM, Young HA. Triptolide attenuates endotoxin- and staphylococcal exotoxin-induced T-cell proliferation and production of cytokines and chemokines. Immunopharmacol Immunotoxicol 2005;27(1):53–66.
13. Yu Y, Zeng Y, Liu L, Ji Y, Zhao J. The effects of triptolide inhibition of mouse lymphocytes activated *in vitro*. Zhong Yao Cai 2005;28(6):499–502.
14. Yang Y, Liu Z, Tolosa E, Yang J, Li L. Triptolide induces apoptotic death of T lymphocyte. Immunopharmacology 1998;40(2):139–149.
15. Esensten JH, Wofsy D, Bluestone JA. Regulatory T cells as therapeutic targets in rheumatoid arthritis. Nat Rev Rheumatol 2009;5(10):560–565.
16. Boissier MC, Assier E, Biton J, Denys A, Falgarone G, Bessis N. Regulatory T cells (Treg) in rheumatoid arthritis. Joint Bone Spine 2009;76(1):10–14.
17. Zhang G, Liu Y, Guo H, Sun Z, Zhou YH. Triptolide promotes generation of FoxP3+ T regulatory cells in rats. J Ethnopharmacol 2009;125(1):41–46.
18. Pernis AB. Th17 cells in rheumatoid arthritis and systemic lupus erythematosus. J Intern Med 2009;265(6):644–652.
19. Wang Y, Jia L, Wu CY. Triptolide inhibits the differentiation of Th17 cells and suppresses collagen-induced arthritis. Scand J Immunol 2008;68(4):383–390.
20. Lemoine S, Morva A, Youinou P, Jamin C. Regulatory B cells in autoimmune diseases: how do they work? Ann N Y Acad Sci 2009;1173(1):260–267.
21. Renato GM. B cell depletion in early rheumatoid arthritis: a new concept in therapeutics. Ann N Y Acad Sci 2009;1173(1):729–735.
22. Boumans MJ, Tak PP. Rituximab treatment in rheumatoid arthritis: how does it work? Arthritis Res Ther 2009;11(6):134.
23. Tao X, Cai JJ, Lipsky PE. The identity of immunosuppressive components of the ethyl acetate extract and chloroform methanol extract (T2) of *Tripterygium wilfordii* Hook F. J Pharmacol Exp Ther 1995;272(3):1305–1312.
24. Zheng J, Feng K, Gu K. Screening of anti-inflammatory, immunosuppressive and antifertility components of *Tripterygium wilfordii* V. Effects of 7 diterpene lactone epoxide compounds on the proliferation of T and B lymphocytes *in vitro*. Zhongguo Yi Xue Ke Xue Yuan Xue Bao 1994;16(1):24–28.
25. Tao X, Davis LS, Lipsky PE. Effect of an extract of the Chinese herbal remedy *Tripterygium wilfordii* Hook F on human immune responsiveness. Arthritis Rheum 1991;34(10):1274–1281.
26. Khan S, Greenberg JD, Bhardwaj N. Dendritic cells as targets for therapy in rheumatoid arthritis. Nat Rev Rheumatol 2009;5(10):566–571.
27. Wenink MH, Han W, Toes RE, Radstake TR. Dendritic cells and their potential implication in pathology and treatment of rheumatoid arthritis. Handb Exp Pharmacol 2009;(188):81–98.
28. Liu Y, Chen Y, Lamb JR, Tam PK. Triptolide, a component of Chinese herbal medicine, modulates the functional phenotype of dendritic cells. Transplantation 2007;84(11):1517–1526.
29. Zhu KJ, Shen QY, Cheng H, Mao XH, Lao LM, Hao GL. Triptolide affects the differentiation, maturation and function of human dendritic cells. Int Immunopharmacol 2005;5(9):1415–1426.
30. Liu Y, Chen Y, Liu FQ, Lamb JR, Tam PK. Combined treatment with triptolide and rapamycin prolongs graft survival in a mouse model of cardiac transplantation. Transpl Int 2008;21(5):483–494.
31. Chen X, Murakami T, Oppenheim JJ, Howard OM. Triptolide, a constituent of immunosuppressive Chinese herbal medicine, is a potent suppressor of dendritic-cell maturation and trafficking. Blood 2005;106(7):2409–2416.

32. Liu Q, Chen T, Chen H, Zhang M, Li N, Lu Z, Ma P, Cao X. Triptolide (PG-490) induces apoptosis of dendritic cells through sequential p38 MAP kinase phosphorylation and caspase 3 activation. Biochem Biophys Res Commun 2004;319(3):980–986.

33. Jutta S, Ralf S, Gesa K, Peter KP, Steffen H, Raimund W, Rolf B. Systemic macrophage activation in locally-induced experimental arthritis. J Autoimmun 2001;17(2):127–136.

34. Kinne RW, Bräuer R, Stuhlmüller B, Palombo-Kinne E, Burmester GR. Macrophages in rheumatoid arthritis. Arthritis Res 2000;2(3):189–202.

35. Wu Y, Cui J, Bao X, Chan S, Young DO, Liu D, Shen P. Triptolide attenuates oxidative stress, NF-kappaB activation and multiple cytokine gene expression in murine peritoneal macrophage. Int J Mol Med 2006;17(1):141–150.

36. Kim YH, Lee SH, Lee JY, Choi SW, Park JW, Kwon TK. Triptolide inhibits murine-inducible nitric oxide synthase expression by down-regulating lipopolysaccharide-induced activity of nuclear factor-κB and c-Jun NH2-terminal kinase. Eur J Pharmacol 2004;494(1):1–9.

37. Bao X, Cui J, Wu Y, Han X, Gao C, Hua Z, Shen P. The roles of endogenous reactive oxygen species and nitric oxide in triptolide-induced apoptotic cell death in macrophages. J Mol Med 2007;85(1):85–98.

38. Liu J, Wu QL, Feng YH, Wang YF, Li XY, Zuo JP. Triptolide suppresses CD80 and CD86 expressions and IL-12 production in THP-1 cells. Acta Pharmacol Sin 2005;26(2):223–227.

39. Cao Y. Anti-tumor actions of gamma-delta T lymphocytes. Int J Immunol 2006;29(6):357–360.

40. Fan J. Intestinal mucosal immunity. Int J Immunol 2006;29(2):112–115.

41. Mowat AM, Viney JL. The anatomical basis of intestinal immunity. Immunol Rev 1997;156(1):145–166.

42. Bloom PD, Boedeker EC. Mucosal immune responses to intestinal bacterial pathogens. Semin Gastrointest Dis 1996;7(3):151–166.

43. Zhou J, Xiao C, Zhao L, Jia H, Zhao N, Lu C, Yang D, Tang JC, Chan AS, Lu AP. The effect of triptolide on CD4+ and CD8+ cells in Peyer's patch of SD rats with collagen induced arthritis. Int Immunopharmacol 2006;6(2):198–203.

44. Xiao C, Lu C, Zhao L, Liu Z, Zhang W, He Y, Chen S, Tang JC, Chan AS, Lu A. The effects of triptolide on enteric mucosal immune responses of DBA/1 mice with collagen-induced arthritis. Planta Med 2006;72(14):1268–1272.

45. Okamoto H, Hoshi D, Kiire A, Yamanaka H, Kamatani N. Molecular targets of rheumatoid arthritis. Inflamm Allergy Drug Targets 2008;7(1):53–66.

46. Goldring MB, Marcu KB. Cartilage homeostasis in health and rheumatic diseases. Arthritis Res Ther 2009;11(3):224.

47. Dayer JM. The process of identifying and understanding cytokines: from basic studies to treating rheumatic diseases. Best Pract Res Clin Rheumatol 2004;18(1):31–45.

48. Loeser RF. Molecular mechanisms of cartilage destruction: mechanics, inflammatory mediators, and aging collide. Arthritis Rheum 2006;54(5):1357–1360.

49. Borzi RM, Mazzetti I, Marcu KB, Facchini A. Chemokines in cartilage degradation. Clin Orthop Relat Res 2004;(427 Suppl):S53–S61.

50. Sandell LJ, Xing X, Franz C, Davies S, Chang LW, Patra D. Exuberant expression of chemokine genes by adult human articular chondrocytes in response to IL-1b. Osteoarthritis Cartilage 2008;16(12):1560–1571.

51. Liacini A, Sylvester J, Zafarullah M. Triptolide suppresses proinflammatory cytokine-induced matrix metalloproteinase and aggrecanase-1 gene expression in chondrocytes. Biochem Biophys Res Commun 2005;327(1):320–327.

52. Karouzakis E, Gay RE, Gay S, Neidhart M. Epigenetic control in rheumatoid arthritis synovial fibroblasts. Nat Rev Rheumatol 2009;5(5):266–272.

53. Yao H, Zhou J, Li D, Wu N, Bader A, Höxtermann S, Altmeyer P, Brockmeyer NH. FK506 enhances triptolide-induced down-regulation of cyclooxygenase-2, inducible nitric oxide synthase as well as their products PGE_2 and NO in TNF-alpha-stimulated synovial fibroblasts from rheumatoid arthritic patients. Eur J Med Res 2005;10(3):110–116.

54. Lin N, Sato T, Ito A. Triptolide, a novel diterpenoid triepoxide from *Tripterygium wilfordii* Hook. F., suppresses the production and gene expression of pro-matrix metalloproteinases 1 and 3 and augments those of tissue inhibitors of metalloproteinases 1 and 2 in human synovial fibroblasts. Arthritis Rheum 2001;44(9):2193–2200.

55. Szekanecz Z, Besenyei T, Paragh G, Koch AE. Angiogenesis in rheumatoid arthritis. Autoimmunity 2009;42(7):563–573.

56. He MF, Huang YH, Wu LW, Ge W, Shaw PC, But PP. Triptolide functions as a potent angiogenesis inhibitor. Int J Cancer 2010;126(1):266–278.
57. He MF, Liu L, Ge W, Shaw PC, Jiang R, Wu LW, But PP. Antiangiogenic activity of *Tripterygium wilfordii* and its terpenoids. J Ethnopharmacol 2009;121(1):61–68.
58. Zhou YX, Huang YL. Antiangiogenic effect of celastrol on the growth of human glioma: an *in vitro* and *in vivo* study. Chin Med J (Engl) 2009;122(14):1666–1673.
59. Zhang DH, Marconi A, Xu LM, Yang CX, Sun GW, Feng XL, Ling CQ, Qin WZ, Uzan G, d'Alessio P. Tripterine inhibits the expression of adhesion molecules in activated endothelial cells. J Leukoc Biol 2006;80(2):309–319.
60. Hussein MR, Fathi NA, El-Din AM, Hassan HI, Abdullah F, Al-Hakeem E, Backer EA. Alterations of the CD4(+), CD8(+) T cell subsets, interleukins-1beta, IL-10, IL-17, tumor necrosis factor-alpha and soluble intercellular adhesion molecule-1 in rheumatoid arthritis and osteoarthritis: preliminary observations. Pathol Oncol Res 2008;14(3):321–328.
61. Fong KY, Boey ML, Koh WH, Feng PH. Cytokine concentrations in the synovial fluid and plasma of rheumatoid arthritis patients: correlation with bony erosions. Clin Exp Rheumatol 1994;12:55–58.
62. Jacques C, Gosset M, Berenbaum F, Gabay C. The role of IL-1 and IL-1Ra in joint inflammation and cartilage degradation. Vitam Horm 2006;74:371–403.
63. Gonzalez-Gay MA, Garcia-Unzueta MT, Berja A, Vazquez-Rodriguez TR, Miranda-Filloy JA, Gonzalez-Juanatey C, de Matias JM, et al. Short-term effect of anti-TNF-alpha therapy on nitric oxide production in patients with severe rheumatoid arthritis. Clin Exp Rheumatol 2009;27(3):452–458.
64. Matta R, Wang X, Ge H, Ray W, Nelin LD, Liu Y. Triptolide induces anti-inflammatory cellular responses. Am J Transl Res 2009;1(3):267–282.
65. Xiao C, Zhou J, He Y, Jia H, Zhao L, Zhao N, Lu A. Effects of triptolide from Radix *Tripterygium wilfordii* (Leigongteng) on cartilage cytokines and transcription factor NF-kappaB: a study on induced arthritis in rats. Chin Med 2009;4:13–17.
66. Koenders MI, Joosten LA, van den Berg WB. Potential new targets in arthritis therapy: interleukin (IL)-17 and its relation to tumour necrosis factor and IL-1 in experimental arthritis. Ann Rheum Dis 2006;65(Suppl 3):iii29–iii33.
67. Paradowska A, Maśliński W, Grzybowska-Kowalczyk A, Łacki J. The function of interleukin 17 in the pathogenesis of rheumatoid arthritis. Arch Immunol Ther Exp (Warsz) 2007;55(5):329–334.
68. Shao XT, Feng L, Gu LJ, Wu LJ, Feng TT, Yang YM, Wu NP, Yao HP. Expression of interleukin-18, IL-18BP, and IL-18R in serum, synovial fluid, and synovial tissue in patients with rheumatoid arthritis. Clin Exp Med 2009;9(3):215–221.
69. Lu Y, Wang WJ, Leng JH, Cheng LF, Feng L, Yao HP. Inhibitory effect of triptolide on interleukin-18 and its receptor in rheumatoid arthritis synovial fibroblasts. Inflamm Res 2008;57(6):260–265.
70. Fu YF, Zhu YN, Ni J, Zhong XG, Tang W, Zhou R, Zhou Y, Dong JR, He PL, Wan H, et al. (5R)-5-hydroxytriptolide (LLDT-8), a novel triptolide derivative, prevents experimental autoimmune encephalomyelitis via inhibiting T cell activation. J Neuroimmunol 2006;175(1–2):142–151.
71. Brinker AM, Ma J, Lipsky PE, Raskin I. Medicinal chemistry and pharmacology of genus *Tripterygium* (Celastraceae). Phytochemistry 2007;68(6):732–766.
72. Xiao C, Zhao L, Liu Z, Lu C, Zhao N, Yang D, Chen S, Tang JC, Chan A, Lu AP. The effect of triptolide on CD4+ and CD8+ cells in the Peyer's patch of DA rats with collagen induced arthritis. Nat Prod Res 2009;23(18):1699–1706.
73. Haringman JJ, Kraan MC, Smeets TJM, Zwinderman KH, Tak PP. Chemokine blockade and chronic inflammatory disease: proof of concept in patients with rheumatoid arthritis. Ann Rheum Dis 2003;62(8):715–721.
74. Murdoch C, Finn A. Chemokine receptors and their role in inflammation and infectious diseases. Blood 2000;95(10),3032–3043.
75. Haas CS, Martinez RJ, Attia N, Haines GK 3rd, Campbel PL, Koch AE. Chemokine receptor expression in rat adjuvant-induced arthritis. Arthritis Rheum 2005;52(12),3718–3730.
76. Shahrara S, Amin MA, Woods JM, Haines GK, Koch AE. Chemokine receptor expression and *in vivo* signaling pathways in the joints of rats with adjuvant-induced arthritis. Arthritis Rheum 2003;48(12):3568–3583.
77. Wang Y, Wei D, Lai Z, Le Y. Triptolide inhibits CC chemokines expressed in rat adjuvant-induced arthritis. Int Immunopharmacol 2006;6(12):1825–1832.
78. Yifan W, Dengming W, Zheng L, Yanping L, Junkan S. Triptolide inhibits CCR5 expressed in synovial tissue of rat adjuvant-induced arthritis. Pharmacol Rep 2007;59(6):795–799.

79. Pap T, Muller-Ladner U, Gay RE, Gay S. Fibroblast biology. Role of synovial fibroblasts in the pathogenesis of rheumatoid arthritis. Arthritis Res 2000;2:361–367.

80. Yoshihara Y, Nakamura H, Obata K, Yamada H, Hayakawa T, Fujikawa K, Okada Y. Matrix metalloproteinases and tissue inhibitors of metalloproteinases in synovial fluids from patients with rheumatoid arthritis or osteoarthritis. Ann Rheum Dis 2000;59(6):455–461.

81. Miller MC, Manning HB, Jain A, Troeberg L, Dudhia J, Essex D, Sandison A, Seiki M, Nanchahal J, Nagase H, et al. Membrane type 1 matrix metalloproteinase is a crucial promoter of synovial invasion in human rheumatoid arthritis. Arthritis Rheum 2009;60(3):686–697.

82. Nagy G, Clark JM, Buzas E, Gorman C, Pasztoi M, Koncz A, Falus A, Cope AP. Nitric oxide production of T lymphocytes is increased in rheumatoid arthritis. Immunol Lett 2008;118(1):55–58.

83. Varadé J, Lamas JR, Fernández-Arquero M, Jover JA, de la Concha EG, Martínez A, Fernández-Gutierrez B, Urcelay E. NO role of NOS2A susceptibility polymorphisms in rheumatoid arthritis. Nitric Oxide 2009;21(3–4):171–174.

84. Moncada S, Palmer RM, Higgs EA. Nitric oxide: physiology, pathophysiology, and pharmacology. Pharmacol Rev 1991;43(2):109–142.

85. Nagy G, Clark JM, Buzás EI, Gorman CL, Cope AP. Nitric oxide, chronic inflammation and autoimmunity. Immunol Lett 2007;111(1):1–5.

86. Ueki Y, Miyake S, Tominaga Y, Eguchi K. Increased nitric oxide levels in patients with rheumatoid arthritis. J Rheumatol 1996;23(2):230–236.

87. Tao X, Ma L, Cai J, Mao Y, Taurog J, Lipsky PE. Treatment with an ethyl acetate extract of *Tripterygium wilfordii* Hook F improves joint inflammation in HLA B27-transgenic rats. Arthritis Rheum 1996;39 (Suppl 9):S298.

88. Wang B, Ma L, Tao X, Lipsky PE. Triptolide, an active component of the Chinese herbal remedy *Tripterygium wilfordii* Hook F, inhibits production of nitric oxide by decreasing inducible nitric oxide synthase gene transcription. Arthritis Rheum 2004;50(9):2995–2303.

89. Kojima F, Kapoor M, Kawai S, Yang L, Aronoff DM, Crofford LJ. Prostaglandin E$_2$ activates Rap1 via EP2/EP4 receptors and cAMP-signaling in rheumatoid synovial fibroblasts: involvement of Epac1 and PKA. Prostaglandins Other Lipid Mediat 2009;89(1–2):26–33.

90. Akaogi J, Nozaki T, Satoh M, Yamada H. Role of PGE$_2$ and EP receptors in the pathogenesis of rheumatoid arthritis and as a novel therapeutic strategy. Endocr Metab Immune Disord Drug Targets 2006;6(4):383–394.

91. Lemos HP, Grespan R, Vieira SM, Cunha TM, Verri WA Jr, Fernandes KS, Souto FO, et al. Prostaglandin mediates IL-23/IL-17-induced neutrophil migration in inflammation by inhibiting IL-12 and IFN gamma production. Proc Natl Acad Sci U S A 2009;106(14):5954–5959.

92. Yao C, Sakata D, Esaki Y, Li Y, Matsuoka T, Kuroiwa K, Sugimoto Y, Narumiya S. Prostaglandin E$_2$-EP4 signaling promotes immune inflammation through Th1 cell differentiation and Th17 cell expansion. Nat Med 2009;15(6):633–640.

93. Mathieu MC, Lord-Dufour S, Bernier V, Boie Y, Burch JD, Clark P, Denis D, Han Y, Mortimer JR, Therien AG. Mutual antagonistic relationship between prostaglandin E(2) and IFN-gamma: implications for rheumatoid arthritis. Eur J Immunol 2008;38(7):1900–1912.

94. Sheibanie AF, Khayrullina T, Safadi FF, Ganea D. Prostaglandin E$_2$ exacerbates collagen-induced arthritis in mice through the inflammatory interleukin-23/interleukin-17 axis. Arthritis Rheum 2007;56(8):2608–2619.

95. Stafford JB, Marnett LJ. Prostaglandin E$_2$ inhibits tumor necrosis factor-alpha RNA through PKA type I. Biochem Biophys Res Commun 2008 Feb 1;366(1):104–109.

96. Tao X, Schulze-Koops H, Ma L, Cai J, Mao Y, Lipsky PE. Effects of *Tripterygium wilfordii* Hook F extracts on induction of cyclooxygenase 2 activity and prostaglandin E$_2$ production. Arthritis Rheum 1998;41(1):130–138.

97. Gong Y, Xue B, Jiao J, Jing L, Wang X. Triptolide inhibits COX-2 expression and PGE$_2$ release by suppressing the activity of NF-kappaB and JNK in LPS-treated microglia. J Neurochem 2008;107(3):779–788.

98. Soundararajan R, Sayat R, Robertson GS, Marignani PA. Triptolide: an inhibitor of a disintegrin and metalloproteinase 10 (ADAM10) in cancer cells. Cancer Biol Ther 2009;8(21):2054–2062.

99. Chen ZK, Wang N, Lu HS. Overexpression of programmed cell death 5 factor enhances triptolides-induced fibroblast-like synoviocytes apoptosis in rheumatoid arthritis. Beijing Da Xue Xue Bao 2008;40(6):567–571.

100. Korb A, Pavenstädt H, Pap T. Cell death in rheumatoid arthritis. Apoptosis 2009;14(4):447–454.

101. Kusunoki N, Yamazaki R, Kitasato H, Beppu M, Aoki H, Kawai S. Triptolide, an active compound identified in a traditional Chinese herb, induces apoptosis of rheumatoid synovial fibroblasts. BMC Pharmacol 2004;(1);4:2.

102. Tao X, Younger J, Fan FZ, Wang B, Lipsky PE. Benefit of an extract of *Tripterygium Wilfordii* Hook F in patients with rheumatoid arthritis: a double-blind, placebo-controlled study. Arthritis Rheum 2002;46(7):1735–1743.

103. Su DF, Li RL, Sun YJ. Report of 270 patients with rheumatoidarthritis treated with ethyl acetate extract of Tripterygium wilfordii Hook F. Zhong Yao Yao Li Yu Lin Chuang 1989;5:40–42.

104. Yu DY. Clinical observation of 144 cases of rheumatoid arthritis treated with glycoside of radix Tripterygium wilfordii. J Tradit Chin Med 1983;3:125–129.

105. Goldbach-Mansky R, Wilson M, Fleischmann R, Olsen N, Silverfield J, Kempf P, Kivitz A, et al. Comparison of *Tripterygium wilfordii* Hook F versus sulfasalazine in the treatment of rheumatoid arthritis: a randomized trial. Ann Intern Med 2009;151:229–240.

106. Su DF, Li RL, Sun YJ. Report of 270 patients with rheumatoid arthritis treated with ethyl acetate extract of *Tripterygium wilfordii* Hook F. Zhong Yao Yao Li Yu Lin Chuang 1989;5:40–42.

107. Tao XL, Sun Y, Dong Y, Xiao YL, Hu DW, Shi YP. A doubleblind, controlled trial of *Tripterygium wilfordii* glycosides in the treatment of rheumatoid arthritis [abstract]. Arthritis Rheum 1987;30 (Suppl 5):S59.

108. Huang CF, Wu CB, Shen ZK. Study on the treatment of rheumatoid arthritis with polyglycosides of *Tripterygium wilfordii* Hook F: a randomized, controlled, crossover clinical trial. Proceedings of the 3rd National Meeting of Rheumatology of China. Shijiazhuang, China, 1989. Beijing: Chinese Association of Medicine 1989;31–33.

109. Tao XL, Cush JJ, Garret M, Lipsky PE. A phase I study of the ethyl acetate extract of the Chinese anti-rheumatic herb, *Tripterygium wilfordii* Hook F in rheumatoid arthritis. J Rheumatol 2001;28:2160–2167.

110. Wu Ya-jun, Lao Zhi-ying, Zhang Zhi-li. Clinical Observation on Small Doses *Tripterygium Wilfordii* Polyglycoside Combined with Methotrexate in Treating Rheumatoid Arthritis. Zhongguo Zhong Xi Yi Jie He Za Zhi 2001;21(12):895–896.

111. Shen Jie, Zhang Zhili. Clinical Observation on the Treatment of Rheumatoid Arthritis with Tripterygium Glycosides and Low Dosage Methopterin. Zejiang Journal of Integrated Traditional and Western Medicine 2002;12(6):334–336.

112. Sun Donghong and Shi Qun. Clinical observation on slow acting antirheumatic drugs combination on rheumatoid arthritis. Chin Remedies Clin 2003;3:203–204.

113. Wu Min, Xie Wen, Ma Ying Chun. The Clinical observation of *Tripterygium wilfordii* polycoride combined with sulfasalazine for elderly patients with RA. J Clin Med Pract 2005;9(5):87–88.

30 Dehydroepiandrosterone (DHEA)

A Review of Its Preclinical Use in the Management of Osteoarthritis

Kai Huang, Hai-li-Cai, Chun Zhang, Xiao-wen Zhang, Li-dong Wu, Li-feng Shen, and Qiao-feng Guo

CONTENTS

INTRODUCTION

Osteoarthritis (OA), the syndrome of joint pain and dysfunction caused by cartilage degeneration, affects more people than any other joint disease. It is characterized by degradation and loss of articular cartilage, subchondral bone remodeling, and, at the clinical stage of the disease, inflammation of the synovial membrane. The main structural macromolecules in the cartilage matrix are type II collagen and aggrecan. In healthy tissue, there is a balance between anabolic and catabolic processes that allows matrix turnover, whereas in OA this balance shifts toward catabolism, leading to cartilage destruction. Currently, there are many treatments available for OA. Conservative measures begin with lifestyle modifications, such as weight loss and decreased activity. Current medications for OA, including nonsteroidal anti-inflammatory drugs (NSAIDs) [1] or steroids [2], provide only symptomatic improvements. In particular, NSAID intake might have a deleterious structural effect in cases of OA, and *ex vivo* and *in vivo* studies have shown that some NSAIDs inhibit the synthesis of cartilage proteoglycans [3, 4], leading to decreased use in clinical practice. A relatively new treatment, hyaluronan injection, improves joint lubrication and can decrease pain [5]. The major disadvantage of all current treatments is that they mainly target the symptoms of OA but do not address the fundamental mechanisms by which articular cartilage damage develops. Consequently, a novel treatment capable of protecting or regenerating cartilage extracellular matrix (ECM) is desirable.

Dehydroepiandrosterone (DHEA) and its sulfate are the most abundant steroids in human plasma, having serum concentrations of 10^{-8} and 10^{-6} M, respectively. The concentrations in serum reach a peak between the ages of 25 and 30 years and thereafter decline steadily, so that by age 70 years, serum concentrations are only 5% to 10% of the corresponding values in young adults [6, 7]. Because of its decline with age, DHEA is known as an "antidote for aging," and a number of studies have examined its role in atherosclerosis, cancer, diabetes, obesity, and aging [8–12] as well as inflammatory arthritis, such as rheumatoid arthritis (RA) [13]. Although RA shares some clinical aspects with OA, there is limited information about the effects of DHEA on OA. This article reviews recent findings with regard to some catabolic enzymes as critical ECM degraders and DHEA as a therapeutic agent in OA and further discusses the fundamental mechanisms by which DHEA plays a protective role toward cartilage in the progression of OA.

THE NOVEL PROTECTIVE MECHANISMS OF DHEA: REGULATING THE ANABOLIC/CATABOLIC BALANCE OF ARTICULAR CARTILAGE

Among the many factors leading to cartilage degradation, the proteolytic activity of a panel of enzymes seems to play a major role, leading to the cleavage of collagen and proteoglycans, the two main components of cartilaginous matrix. Although various proteases in articular cartilage have been described, current studies indicate that members of two families of metalloproteases—matrix metalloproteinases (MMPs) and a disintegrin and metalloproteinase with thrombospondin motifs (ADAMTS)—are responsible for the degradation of the major components of the cartilage matrix [14]. These enzymes degrade ECM macromolecules and modulate factors governing cell behavior. Other studies indicated that, like MMPs and ADAMTSs, some members of the cysteine protease family, such as cathepsins K, B, L, and S, play a critical role in the morphologic and molecular alterations in the development of OA. Previous data demonstrate that cysteine proteases degraded both type II collagen and aggrecan in articular cartilage in OA [15–18].

The proteolytic axis in any biological system relies on a delicate balance between proteinases and their endogenous inhibitors. *In vivo*, the most efficient factors modulating the activity of catabolic enzymes in the body are their endogenous inhibitors. The existence of these endogenous inhibitors plays a key role in maintaining the balance between synthesis and degradation in normal articular cartilage. In OA, however, this anabolic/catabolic balance is disrupted with the excessive cleavage of collagen II and aggrecan by various proteases, ultimately leading to the destruction of articular cartilage. Thus, maintaining the equilibrium of anabolic/catabolic factors should be an efficient strategy for OA therapy, and it is important to understand how the inhibitors function to oppose the proteolytic events that occur during the inflammatory response.

DHEA is a 19-carbon steroid hormone and classified as an adrenal androgen. It is synthesized from pregnenolone (derived from cholesterol) and is rapidly sulfated to its ester form, DHEA sulfate, the predominant form in circulating plasma. An increasing line of evidence has demonstrated that this hormone has a beneficial effect on osteoarthritic cartilage, influencing the balance between anabolic and catabolic factors [19–21]. However, data concerning exactly how DHEA exerts its protective role on OA are limited. Therefore, knowing the mechanism of action of this steroid hormone is of particular importance.

REGULATING THE BALANCE BETWEEN MMPS AND THE TISSUE INHIBITOR OF METALLOPROTEINASE-1: A DEFINITE PROTECTIVE MECHANISM OF DHEA FOR OSTEOARTHRITIC CARTILAGE

Degenerative joint diseases like OA are commonly characterized by cartilage ECM degradation, where the loss of proteoglycans and type II collagen are hallmarks of developing disease. Although various types of proteases participate in matrix turnover, one group of key enzymes, the matrix metalloproteases (MMPs), has specifically been related to articular tissues. The role of MMPs in OA has been investigated over the last two decades. Most MMPs, including MMP-1, MMP-3, and MMP-13, are expressed by chondrocytes and synovial cells in human OA and are thought to play a critical role in cartilage degeneration [22, 23]. MMP-3 is known to play an important role in proteoglycan cleavage and is crucial for cartilage proteoglycan homeostasis [24, 25], whereas MMP-13 and MMP-1, enzymes involved with the same family, preferentially cleave type II collagen [26, 27], the primary collagen in cartilage tissue (90%–98% of the total tissue collagen) [28]. MMP-2 and MMP-9, which are both gelatinases, play a significant role in matrix breakdown, and their elevated levels reflect the inflammatory condition of joints [29]. The tissue inhibitor of metalloproteinase-1 (TIMP-1) is a glycoprotein and inhibits all MMPs on a 1:1 basis by forming high-affinity complexes [30]. A balance between MMPs and TIMP-1 regulates cartilage ECM remodeling and degradation in the normal joint. However, a deregulation of this balance is found in pathological conditions, which is thought to be important in the progression of OA [31]. Thus, decreasing the effects of MMPs by suppressing their synthesis and activity could then account for the beneficial effects of DHEA administration.

Our recently published study has demonstrated that DHEA could inhibit the activity of MMPs, upregulate levels of TIMP-1, and counteract the proinflammatory effects of catabolic cytokines, like interleukin-1β (IL-1β) in a rabbit model of OA, suggesting that it has a protective effect on osteoarthritic cartilage [32]. Similarly, in an earlier study, Jo et al. [19] analyzed the effects of DHEA on gene expression and protein synthesis of catabolic enzymes, such as MMP-1, MMP-3, and inhibitors of MMPs, for example, TIMP-1, which is known to play important roles in the progression of OA. Results showed that treatment of chondrocytes isolated from human osteoarthritic knee cartilage with DHEA significantly suppressed gene expression and protein synthesis of MMP-1 but increased gene expression and protein synthesis of TIMP-1, indicating that DHEA has an anticatabolic action, not only via suppression of MMPs but also via TIMP-1 induction. This study was the first to demonstrate the *in vitro* effects of DHEA on osteoarthritic chondrocytes and provided important evidence that DHEA has the ability to modulate the imbalance between MMPs and TIMP-1 during OA at the transcription level. Later, the same group of researchers [20] investigated the *in vivo* effects of intra-articular injections of DHEA on the maintenance of the cartilage matrix and on the gene expression of various inflammatory mediators during the development of OA in a rabbit anterior cruciate ligament transection (ACLT) model. Histomorphometric and gene expression analyses quantitatively demonstrated that exogenously administered DHEA has beneficial effects on the maintenance of articular cartilage matrix integrity, which is in agreement with the findings of the previous *in vitro* study. The results of the abovementioned studies indicate that DHEA may contribute to the prevention of cartilage destruction by modulating MMPs/TIMP-1 equilibrium in the progression of OA.

ADJUSTING CYSTEINE PROTEINASES/CYSTATIN C ENZYME EXPRESSION: A NOVEL MECHANISM OF DHEA ON CARTILAGE IN DIFFERENT STAGES OF OA

Cysteine proteases are lysosomal enzymes of the papain family, among which cathepsins K, B, L, and S are regarded as the most relevant to the development of OA. Cathepsin K is a cysteine protease of the papain family that cleaves triple-helical type II collagen and aggrecan, the major structural component of the extracellular matrix of articular cartilage [33]. Cathepsin B may act as an antagonist of cartilage repair because some studies find it is involved in the pathogenesis of human OA by demonstrating high extracellular enzyme activity around clefts and in zones of hypercellularity in OA [34–36]. Cathepsin L also contributes to the matrix destruction seen in articular cartilage affected by OA. Ariga et al. [37]. found that marked expression of cathepsin L was observed at the site of degeneration in the degenerative intervertebral disc, suggesting cathepsin L also has collagenolytic activity and degrades the ECM in cartilage. Cathepsin S is a potent cysteine protease that degrades a number of ECM molecules at a neutral pH [38], suggesting that cathepsin

S is an important player in degenerative disorders. Cystatin C, which is a small protein (13.3 kDa), is known as the specific endogenous inhibitor of cysteine proteinase. Increasing evidence demonstrates that cysteine proteinase activity increases as collagen and aggrecan are broken down in the process of OA, and the endogenous inhibitor (cystatin C), the most abundant extracellular inhibitor of cysteine proteases, is overwhelmed [39–41], implying that an imbalance of the cysteine proteinase/cystatin C system could be an important contributing factor in the development of OA [42, 43].

In our newly published study [44], we demonstrated that variation patterns of messenger RNA levels of the cysteine proteinase/cystatin C enzyme system were related to the progressive degeneration of articular cartilage. The upregulation of cathepsin K and cathepsin B expression coincided with the onset of articular cartilage damage in the differential stage of OA. In addition, we found increased levels of cysteine proteinases, including cathepsin K, B, L, and S, with downregulation of cystatin C during the early to medium stages of OA. The ratio of cystatin C to cysteine proteinases declined as OA progressed. Through intra-articular administration of DHEA in a rabbit model, we found that the ratio of cystatin C to cysteine proteinases in the DHEA group was much higher than that in the OA group. These data implied that DHEA had a role in protecting articular cartilage in the early and medium stages of OA by influencing the balance between cysteine proteinases and cystatin C enzymes.

DOWNREGULATING THE EXPRESSION OF THE UROKINASE PLASMINOGEN ACTIVATOR/PLASMINOGEN ACTIVATOR INHIBITOR-1 ENZYME SYSTEM: A NEWLY DISCOVERED MECHANISM OF DHEA ON OSTEOARTHRITIC CARTILAGE

Plasmin is formed upon cleavage of plasminogen by highly specific serine proteases, urokinase (u-PA) and plasminogen activators (PAs). The latter can have a direct role in the degradation of extracellular matrix glycoproteins [45] and can degrade connective tissue components, including proteoglycans [46, 47]. Both plasmin, the cleavage product of plasminogen, and u-PA can produce active forms of MMPs to accelerate the destruction of articular cartilage, such as gelatinases [48] and stromelysins [49]. PA inhibitor-1 (PAI-1), the major circulating PAI bound to extracellular matrix where it may regulate matrix breakdown [50], controls the rate of plasmin generation by forming irreversible inhibitory complexes with u-PA [51]. Martel et al. [52] found that the content and activity of u-PA increased in osteoarthritic cartilage whereas PAI-1 was significantly decreased, revealing that the deregulation of the u-PA/PAI-1 enzyme system probably contributes to the progressive turnover of extracellular components in OA pathophysiology. More recently, Chu et al. [53, 54] pointed out that some NSAIDs played a cartilage-protective role dependent on the downregulation of both u-PA and PAI-1, the upstream enzymes of MMP-2 and MMP-9. Likewise, the same authors reported that the therapeutic effects of using hyaluronic acid to treat early OA may partially depend on the downregulation of the u-PA/PAI-1 enzyme system and gelatinase expression, which delay the structural progression of the disease [55]. The above-presented evidence suggests that inhibition of the u-PA/PAI-1 enzyme system may be a strategy for OA therapy.

In our more recent study [44], we surgically induced OA in rabbits by ACLT to verify the *in vivo* effects of DHEA on the expression of u-PA and PAI-1 at different stages of knee OA. The use of experimental ACLT models is of particular clinical relevance because rupture of the ACL occurs in humans and also leads to the development of OA [56]. In addition, this OA model demonstrates biochemical and pathological changes identical to those found in human OA [57]. Encouragingly, our data demonstrated that DHEA could suppress the expression of both u-PA and PAI-1 in articular cartilage in the OA model, which is a new mechanism by which DHEA may protect against OA.

MODULATING THE BALANCE BETWEEN AGGRECANASES AND THE TIMP-3: A SPECULATED MECHANISM OF DHEA BY WHICH THIS AGENT EXERTS ITS PROTECTIVE ROLE IN OA

Of particular importance in cartilage degradation are members of a recently discovered family of zinc metalloproteases designated the "a disintegrin and metalloproteinase with thrombospondin motif" (ADAMTS) gene family [58]. Several members of ADAMTS proteases have been shown to cleave aggrecan at a specific cleavage site: the Glu373-Ala374 bond in the interglobular domain of aggrecan [59–61]. Of these, ADAMTS-4 (also known as aggrecanase-1) and ADAMTS-5 (also known as aggrecanase-2) are the most efficient aggrecanases [62]. Increasing evidence is accumulating for the significance of these two aggrecanases in cartilage turnover in OA, and recent work from a number of laboratories has begun to provide insight into the regulation of the secretion and activity of these proteins and the molecular basis of their role in aggrecan catabolism [63]. Although MMPs contribute to aggrecanolysis in degenerative joint diseases, more recent studies have showed that most aggrecan fragments detected in the synovial fluid and cartilage of patients with OA are derived from aggrecanase activity, suggesting that the predominant proteinase responsible for aggrecan degradation is aggrecanase [64, 65]. Moreover, evidence from a considerable amount of research has found that aggrecanases are the most likely candidates to play a role in the pathogenesis of OA [66–68]. Recent knockout mouse studies have shown that the deletion of ADAMTS-5 provided significant protection against proteoglycan degradation and decreased the severity of OA [69–71]. To investigate the importance and effects of a complete absence of ADAMTS-4 and ADAMTS-5 aggrecanase activity on the progression of OA, Majumdar et al. [72] generated mice with dual deletion of both genes. When the DAMTS-4/5 double-knockout mice were surgically induced with joint instability, it was encouraging to note that these mice were physiologically normal and showed a decrease in the progression of OA. The abovementioned studies with genetically modified mice show convincingly that targeting ADAMTS enzyme activity might efficiently protect against the development of early cartilage lesions in experimental OA because suppression of aggrecan degradation is regarded as a major goal in the prevention of cartilage destruction and loss of function in OA [73].

To date, there are four identified TIMP proteins (TIMP-1 to TIMP-4) that share many similarities [74]. Of the four TIMPs, TIMP-3 has a number of unique features. It binds tightly to the extracellular matrix through its N-terminal domain, which is rich in lysine and arginine residues, facilitating interaction with heparan and chondroitin sulfate [75]. Furthermore, evidence indicated that TIMP-3 is the most significant endogenous inhibitor of aggrecanases identified thus far [76, 77]; other TIMP members possess a limited inhibitory capacity [78]. Thus, it is possible that the ability of TIMP-3 to suppress aggrecanase activity might be relative to its unique ECM-binding capacity as cartilage ECM is the main substrate of aggrecanases. Although the suppressive effect of DHEA on some members of the MMP family in OA has been well demonstrated, the effect of DHEA on aggrecanase, which plays a more important role in aggrecan depletion in osteoarthritic cartilage, remains unknown. Does DHEA increase levels of TIMP-3, the endogenous inhibitor of ADAMTS-4 and ADAMTS-5? Could DHEA contribute to the prevention of cartilage destruction through modulating aggrecanases/TIMP-3 equilibrium in the progression of OA? All the uncertain mechanisms of this agent still need to be explored in further research. In our recent review, we hypothesize that DHEA plays a favorable role for osteoarthritic cartilage by inhibiting the expression of aggrecanases. We established this speculation on the basis of several studies. First, now that DHEA has been proven to delay the degeneration of cartilage via MMP inhibition, it is possible that DHEA also suppresses the activity of aggrecanases, which leads to the same result (cartilage ECM protection), because MMPs and aggrecanases are both members of the broader family of metalloproteinases, which cleave ECM proteins. Second, DHEA has been found to counteract proinflammatory effects of catabolic cytokines, such as IL-1β, tumor necrosis factor, and IL-6 [79, 80]. On the other hand, considerable studies have demonstrated that aggrecanase activity is induced in the presence of these proinflammatory factors [81–84]. Therefore, it is a reasonable prediction that DHEA has a favorable effect on cartilage by blocking proinflammatory pathways, which in turn suppresses the expression of aggrecanases. Third, as TIMP-3 is the most efficient endogenous inhibitor of aggrecanases, DHEA probably exerts its inhibitory role on these catabolic enzymes via upregulating TIMP-3 gene expression, that is, the steroid may have the ability to modulate the balance of aggrecanases/TIMP-3 gene expression.

PERSPECTIVES

Abundant evidence on the efficacy of DHEA administration for the treatment of cartilage ECM degeneration in OA can be found in preclinical animal studies as described above. This is especially true in the case of structural modification. However, the effects of DHEA on pain generation are not well understood and can only be obtained from the clinical data of patients rather than animal models. Although the results discussed above showed some evidence of the cartilage-protective effect of DHEA on different species of animal models, there are significant limitations to applying the results to humans. The experimental model produced chondral changes induced after an acute traumatic event (ACLT), and the pathology in this model may develop rapidly compared with OA in humans; human OA progression is slow and may occur over a period of 15–30 years. Therefore, the effect of DHEA in our animal models may not be completely generalizable to the slowly progressive damage in the degenerative arthritis of humans. To date, no clear data are available for the effects of DHEA on human OA cartilage; hence, further quantitative studies concerning the effects of DHEA on patients with OA are needed.

REFERENCES

1. Pincus T, Koch GG, Sokka T, Lefkowith J, Wolfe F, Jordan JM, Luta G, et al. A randomized, double-blind, crossover clinical trial of diclofenac plus misoprostol versus acetaminophen in patients with osteoarthritis of the hip or knee. Arthritis Rheum 2001;44:1587–1598.
2. Ravaud P, Moulinier L, Giraudeau B, Ayral X, Guerin C, Noel E, Thomas P, Fautrel B, Mazieres B, Dougados M. Effects of joint lavage and steroid injection in patients with osteoarthritis of the knee: results of a multicenter, randomized, controlled trial. Arthritis Rheum 1999;42:475–482.
3. Rainsford KD, Ying C, Smith FC. Effects of meloxicam, compared with other NSAIDs, on cartilage proteoglycan metabolism, synovial prostaglandin E$_2$, and production of interleukins 1, 6 and 8, in human and porcine explants in organ culture. J Pharm Pharmacol 1997;49:991–998.
4. Ding C, Cicuttini F, Jones G. Do NSAIDs affect longitudinal changes in knee cartilage volume and knee cartilage defects in older adults? Am J Med 2009;22:836–842.
5. Puhl W, Bernau A, Greiling H, Köpcke W, Pförringer W, Steck KJ, Zacher J, Scharf HP. Intra-articular sodium hyaluronate in osteoarthritis of the knee: a multicenter, double-blind study. Osteoarthritis Cartilage 1993;1:233–241.
6. Orentreich N, Brind JL, Rizer RL, Vogelman JH. Age changes and sex differences in serum dehydroepiandrosterone sulfate concentrations throughout adulthood. J Clin Endocrinol Metab 1984; 59:551–555.
7. Bélanger A, Candas B, Dupont A, Cusan L, Diamond P, Gomez JL, Labrie F. Changes in serum concentrations of conjugated and unconjugated steroids in 40- to 80-year-old men. J Clin Endocrinol Metab 1994;79:1086–1090.
8. Michos ED, Vaidya D, Gapstur SM, Schreiner PJ, Golden SH, Wong ND, Criqui MH, Ouyang P. Sex hormones, sex hormone binding globulin, and abdominal aortic calcification in women and men in the multi-ethnic study of atherosclerosis (MESA). Atherosclerosis 2008;200:432–438.
9. Arnold JT, Gray NE, Jacobowitz K, Viswanathan L, Cheung PW, McFann KK, Le H, Blackman MR. Human prostate stromal cells stimulate increased PSA production in DHEA-treated prostate cancer epithelial cells. J Steroid Biochem Mol Biol 2008;111:240–246.
10. Kanazawa I, Yamaguchi T, Yamamoto M, Yamauchi M, Kurioka S, Yano S, Sugimoto T. Serum DHEA-S level is associated with the presence of atherosclerosis in postmenopausal women with type 2 diabetes mellitus. Endocr J 2008;55:667–675.
11. Enomoto M, Adachi H, Fukami A, Furuki K, Satoh A, Otsuka M, Kumagae S, et al. Serum dehydroepiandrosterone sulfate levels predict longevity in men: 27-year follow-up study in a community-based cohort (Tanushimaru study). J Am Geriatr Soc 2008;56:994–998.
12. Watson RR, Huls A, Araghinikuam M, Chung S. Dehydroepiandrosterone and diseases of aging. Drugs Aging 1996;9:274–291.
13. Weitoft T, Larsson A, Rönnblom L. Serum levels of sex steroid hormones and matrix metalloproteinases after intra-articular glucocorticoid treatment in female patients with rheumatoid arthritis. Ann Rheum Dis 2008;67:422–424.

14. Robertson CM, Pennock AT, Harwood FL, Pomerleau AC, Allen RT, Amiel D. Characterization of pro-apoptotic and matrix-degradative gene expression following induction of osteoarthritis in mature and aged rabbits. Osteoarthritis Cartilage 2006;14:471–476.

15. Baici A, Lang A, Zwicky R, Müntener K. Cathepsin B in osteoarthritis: uncontrolled proteolysis in the wrong place. Semin Arthritis Rheum 2005;34:24–28.

16. Vinardell T, Dejica V, Poole AR, Mort JS, Richard H, Laverty S. Evidence to suggest that cathepsin K degrades articular cartilage in naturally occurring equine osteoarthritis. Osteoarthritis Cartilage 2009;17:375–383.

17. Keyszer GM, Heer AH, Kriegsmann J, Geiler T, Trabandt A, Keysser M, Gay RE, Gay S. Comparative analysis of cathepsin L, cathepsin D, and collagenase messenger RNA expression in synovial tissues of patients with rheumatoid arthritis and osteoarthritis, by in situ hybridization. Arthritis Rheum 1995;38:976–984.

18. Hou WS, Li W, Keyszer G, Weber E, Levy R, Klein MJ, Gravallese EM, Goldring SR, Brömme D. Comparison of cathepsins K and S expression within the rheumatoid and osteoarthritic synovium. Arthritis Rheum 2002;46:663–674.

19. Jo H, Park JS, Kim EM, Jung MY, Lee SH, Seong SC, Park SC, Kim HJ, Lee MC. The in vitro effects of dehydroepiandrosterone on human osteoarthritic chondrocytes. Osteoarthritis Cartilage 2003;11:585–594.

20. Jo H, Ahn HJ, Kim EM, Kim HJ, Seong SC, Lee I, Lee MC. Effects of dehydroepiandrosterone on articular cartilage during the development of osteoarthritis. Arthritis Rheum 2004;50:2531–2538.

21. Wu LD, Yu HC, Xiong Y, Feng J. Effect of dehydroepiandrosterone on cartilage and synovium of knee joints with osteoarthritis in rabbits. Rheumatol Int 2006;27:79–85.

22. Takaishi H, Kimura T, Dalal S, Okada Y, D'Armiento J. Joint diseases and matrix metalloproteinases: a role for MMP-13. Curr Pharm Biotechnol 2008;9:47–54.

23. Cawston TE, Wilson AJ. 2006. Understanding the role of tissue degrading enzymes and their inhibitors in development and disease. Best Pract Res Clin Rheumatol 2006;20:983–1002.

24. Nagase H, Enghild JJ, Suzuki K, Salvesen G. Stepwise activation mechanisms of the precursor of matrix metalloproteinase 3 (stromelysin) by proteinases and (4-aminophenyl)mercuric acetate. Biochemistry 1990;29:5783–5789.

25. Suzuki K, Enghild JJ, Morodomi T, Salvesen G, Nagase H. Mechanisms of activation of tissue procollagenase by matrix metalloproteinase 3 (stromelysin). Biochemistry 1990;29:10261–10270.

26. Nagase H, Suzuki K, Enghild JJ, Salvesen G. Stepwise activation mechanisms of the precursors of matrix metalloproteinases 1 (tissue collagenase) and 3 (stromelysin). Biomed Biochim Acta 1991;50:749–754.

27. Monfort J, Pelletier JP, Garcia-Giralt N, Martel-Pelletier J. Biochemical basis of the effect of chondroitin sulphate on osteoarthritis articular tissues. Ann Rheum Dis 2008;67:735–740.

28. Martel-Pelletier J, Boileau C, Pelletier JP, Roughley PJ. Cartilage in normal and osteoarthritis conditions. Best Pract Res Clin Rheumatol 2008;22:351–384.

29. Chu SC, Yang SF, Lue KH, Hsieh YS, Wu CL, Lu KH. Regulation of gelatinases expression by cytokines, endotoxin, and pharmacological agents in the human osteoarthritic knee. Connect Tissue Res 2004;45:142–150.

30. Dean DD, Woessner JF Jr. 1984. Extracts of human articular cartilage contain an inhibitor of tissue metalloproteinases. Biochem J 1984;218:277–280.

31. Martel-Pelletier J, McCollum R, Fujimoto N, Obata K, Cloutier JM, Pelletier JP. Excess of metalloproteases over tissue inhibitor of metalloprotease may contribute to cartilage degradation in osteoarthritis and rheumatoid arthritis. Lab Invest 1994;70:807–815.

32. Wu LD, Yu HC, Xiong Y, Feng J. Effect of dehydroepiandrosterone on cartilage and synovium of knee joints with osteoarthritis in rabbits. Rheumatol Int 2006;27:79–85.

33. Dejica VM, Mort JS, Laverty S, Percival MD, Antoniou J, Zukor DJ, Poole AR. Cleavage of type II collagen by cathepsin K in human osteoarthritic cartilage. Am J Pathol 2008;173:161–169.

34. Baici A, Hörler D, Lang A, Merlin C, Kissling R. Cathepsin B in osteoarthritis: zonal variation of enzyme activity in human femoral head cartilage. Ann Rheum Dis 1995;54:281–288.

35. Baici A, Lang A, Hörler D, Kissling R, Merlin C. Cathepsin B in osteoarthritis: cytochemical and histochemical analysis of human femoral head cartilage. Ann Rheum Dis 1995;54:289–297.

36. Berardi S, Lang A, Kostoulas G, Horler D, Vilei EM, Baici A. Alternative messenger RNA splicing and enzyme forms of cathepsin B in human osteoarthritic cartilage and cultured chondrocytes. Arthritis Rheum 2001;44:1819–18131.

37. Ariga K, Yonenobu K, Nakase T, Kaneko M, Okuda S, Uchiyama Y, Yoshikawa H. Localization of cathepsins D, K, and L in degenerated human intervertebral discs. Spine (Phila Pa 1976) 2001;26:2666–2672.

38. Petanceska S, Canoll P, Devi LA. Expression of rat cathepsin S in phagocytic cells. J Biol Chem 1996;271:4403–4409.

39. Ma J, Tanaka KF, Yamada G, Ikenaka K. Induced expression of cathepsins and cystatin C in a murine model of demyelination. Neurochem Res 2007;32:311–320.

40. Lenarcic B, Krasovec M, Ritonja A, Olafsson I, Turk V. Inactivation of human cystatin C and kininogen by human cathepsin D. FEBS Lett 1991;280:211–215.

41. Chapman HA, Riese RJ, Shi GP. Emerging roles for cysteine proteases in human biology. Annu Rev Physiol 1997;59:63–88.

42. Lecaille F, Brömme D, Lalmanach G. Biochemical properties and regulation of cathepsin K activity. Biochimie 2008;90:208–226.

43. Martel-Pelletier J, Cloutier JM, Pelletier JP. Cathepsin B and cysteine protease inhibitors in human osteoarthritis. J Orthop Res 1990;8:336–344.

44. Bao JP, Chen WP, Feng J, Zhao J, Shi ZL, Huang K, Wu LD. Variation patterns of two degradation enzyme systems in articular cartilage in different stages of osteoarthritis: regulation by dehydroepiandrosterone. Clin Chim Acta 2009;408:1–7.

45. Fairbairn S, Gilbert R, Ojakian G, Schwimmer R, Quigley J. The extracellular matrix of normal chick embryo fibroblasts: its effect on transformed chick fibroblasts and its proteolytic degradation by transformants. J Cell Biol 1985;101:1790–1798.

46. Mochan E, Keler T. Plasmin degradation of cartilage proteoglycan. Biochim Biophys Acta 1984;800:312–315.

47. Belcher C, Fawthrop F, Bunning R, Doherty M. Plasminogen activators and their inhibitors in synovial fluids from normal, osteoarthritis, and rheumatoid arthritis knees. Ann Rheum Dis 1996; 55:230–236.

48. Mazzieri R, Masiero L, Zanetta L, Monea S, Onisto M, Garbisa S, Mignatti P. Control of type IV collagenase activity by components of the urokinase plasmin system: a regulatory mechanism with cell-bound reactants. EMBO J 1997;16:2319–2332.

49. Ramos-DeSimone N, Hahn-Dantona E, Sipley J, Nagase H, French DL, Quigley JP. Activation of matrix metalloproteinase-9 (MMP-9) via a converging plasmin/stromelysin-1 cascade enhances tumor cell invasion. J Biol Chem 1999;274:13066–13076.

50. Knudsen BS, Harpel PC, Nachman RL. Plasminogen activator inhibitor is associated with the extracellular matrix of cultured bovine smooth muscle cells. J Clin Invest 1987;80:1082–1089.

51. Andreasen PA, Georg B, Lund LR, Riccio A, Stacey SN. Plasminogen activator inhibitors: hormonally regulated serpins. Mol Cell Endocrinol 1990;68:1–19.

52. Martel-Pelletier J, Faure MP, McCollum R, Mineau F, Cloutier JM, Pelletier JP. Plasmin, plasminogen activators and inhibitor in human osteoarthritic cartilage. J Rheumatol 1991;18:1863–1871.

53. Chu SC, Yang SF, Lue KH, Hsieh YS, Li TJ, Lu KH. Naproxen, meloxicam and methylprednisolone inhibit urokinase plasminogen activator and inhibitor and gelatinases expression during the early stage of osteoarthritis. Clin Chim Acta 2008;387:90–96.

54. Yang SF, Hsieh YS, Lue KH, Chu SC, Chang IC, Lu KH. Effects of nonsteroidal anti-inflammatory drugs on the expression of urokinase plasminogen activator and inhibitor and gelatinases in the early osteoarthritic knee of humans. Clin Biochem 2008;41:109–116.

55. Hsieh YS, Yang SF, Lue KH, Chu SC, Lu KH. Effects of different molecular weight hyaluronan products on the expression of urokinase plasminogen activator and inhibitor and gelatinases during the early stage of osteoarthritis. J Orthop Res 2008;26:475–484.

56. McDaniel WJ Jr, Dameron TB Jr. The untreated anterior cruciate ligament rupture. Clin Orthop 1983;172:158–163.

57. Brandt KD, Braunstein EM, Visco DM, O'Connor B, Heck D, Albrecht M. Anterior (cranial) cruciate ligament transection in the dog: a bona fide model of osteoarthritis, not merely of cartilage injury and repair. J Rheumatol 1991;18:436–446.

58. Mort JS, Billington CJ. Articular cartilage and changes in arthritis: matrix degradation. Arthritis Res 2001;3:337–341.

59. Sandy JD, Neame PJ, Boynton RE, Flannery CR. Catabolism of aggrecan in cartilage explants. Identification of a major cleavage site within the interglobular domain. J Biol Chem 1991;266: 8683–8685.

60. Ilic MZ, Handley CJ, Robinson HC, Mok MT. Mechanism of catabolism of aggrecan by articular cartilage. Arch Biochem Biophys 1992;294:115–122.

61. Loulakis P, Shrikhande A, Davis G, Maniglia CA. N-terminal sequence of proteoglycan fragments isolated from medium of interleukin-1-treated articular-cartilage cultures. Putative site(s) of enzymic cleavage. Biochem J 1992;284:589–593.

62. Tortorella MD, Malfait AM. 2008. Will the real aggrecanase(s) step up: evaluating the criteria that define aggrecanase activity in osteoarthritis. Curr Pharm Biotechnol 2008;9:16–23.

63. Arner EC. Aggrecanase-mediated cartilage degradation. Curr Opin Pharmacol 2002;2:322–329.

64. Struglics A, Larsson S, Pratta MA, Kumar S, Lark MW, Lohmander LS. Human osteoarthritis synovial fluid and joint cartilage contain both aggrecanase and matrix metalloproteinase-generated aggrecan fragments. Osteoarthritis Cartilage 2006;14:101–113.

65. Maehara H, Suzuki K, Sasaki T, Oshita H, Wada E, Inoue T, Shimizu K. G1-G2 aggrecan product that can be generated by M-calpain on truncation at Ala709-Ala710 is present abundantly in human articular cartilage. J Biochem (Tokyo) 2007;141:469–477.

66. Tortorella MD, Burn TC, Pratta MA, Abbaszade I, Hollis JM, Liu R, Rosenfeld SA, et al. Purification and cloning of aggrecanase-1: a member of the ADAMTS family of proteins. Science 1999;284:1664–1666.

67. Zeng W, Corcoran C, Collins-Racie LA, Lavallie ER, Morris EA, Flannery CR. Glycosaminoglycan-binding properties and aggrecanase activities of truncated ADAMTSs: comparative analyses with ADAMTS-5, -9, -16 and -18. Biochim Biophys Acta 2006;1760:517–524.

68. Fushimi K, Troeberg L, Nakamura H, Lim NH, Nagase H. 2008. Functional differences of the catalytic and non-catalytic domains in human ADAMTS-4 and ADAMTS-5 in aggrecanolytic activity. J Biol Chem 2008;283:6706–6716.

69. Glasson SS, Askew R, Sheppard B, Carito B, Blanchet T, Ma HL, Flannery CR, et al. Deletion of active ADAMTS5 prevents cartilage degradation in a murine model of osteoarthritis. Nature 2005;434:644–648.

70. Stanton H, Rogerson FM, East CJ, Golub SB, Lawlor KE, Meeker CT, Little CB, et al. ADAMTS5 is the major aggrecanase in mouse cartilage in vivo and in vitro. Nature 2005;434:648–652.

71. Little CB, MeekerCT, Golub SB, Lawlor KE, Farmer PJ, Smith SM, Fosang AJ. Blocking aggrecanase cleavage in the aggrecan interglobular domain abrogates cartilage erosion and promotes cartilage repair. J Clin Invest 2007;117:1627–1636.

72. Majumdar MK, Askew R, Schelling S, Stedman N, Blanchet T, Hopkins B, Morris EA, Glasson SS. Double-knockout of ADAMTS-4 and ADAMTS-5 in mice results in physiologically normal animals and prevents the progression of osteoarthritis. Arthritis Rheum 2007;56:3670–3674.

73. Gavrilovic J. Fibroblast growth factor 2. A new key player in osteoarthritis. Arthritis Rheum 2009;60:1869–1872.

74. Brew K, Dinakarpandian D, Nagase H. Tissue inhibitors of metalloproteinases: evolution, structure and function. Biochim Biophys Acta 2000;1477:267–283.

75. Sahebjam S, Khokha R, Mort JS. Increased collagen and aggrecan degradation with age in the joints of Timp3(–/–) mice. Arthritis Rheum 2007;56:905–909.

76. Kashiwagi M, Tortorella M, Nagase H, Brew K. TIMP-3 is a potent inhibitor of aggrecanase 1 (ADAM-TS4) and aggrecanase 2 (ADAM-TS5). J Biol Chem 2001;276:12501–12504.

77. Wayne GJ, Deng SJ, Amour A, Borman S, Matico R, Carter HL, Murphy G. TIMP-3 inhibition of ADAMTS-4 (Aggrecanase-1) is modulated by interactions between aggrecan and the C-terminal domain of ADAMTS-4. J Biol Chem 2007;282:20991–20998.

78. Hashimoto G, Aoki T, Nakamura H, Tanzawa K, Okada Y. Inhibition of ADAMTS4 (aggrecanase-1) by tissue inhibitors of metalloproteinases (TIMP-1, 2, 3 and 4). FEBS Lett 2001;494:192–195.

79. Straub RH, Konecna L, Hrach S, Rothe G, Kreutz M, Schölmerich J, Falk W, Lang B. Serum dehydroepiandrosterone (DHEA) and DHEA sulfate are negatively correlated with serum interleukin-6 (IL-6), and DHEA inhibits IL-6 secretion from mononuclear cells in man in vitro: possible link between endocrinosenescence and immunosenescence. J Clin Endocrinol Metab 1998;83:2012–2017.

80. Ramírez JA, Bruttomesso AC, Michelini FM, Acebedo SL, AlchéLE, Galagovsky LR. 2007. Syntheses of immunomodulating androstanes and stigmastanes: comparison of their TNF-alpha inhibitory activity. Bioorg Med Chem 2007;15:7538–7544.

81. Little CB, Hughes CE, Curtis CL, Jones SA, Caterson B, Flannery CR. Cyclosporin A inhibition of aggrecanase-mediated proteoglycan catabolism in articular cartilage. Arthritis Rheum 2002;46:124–129.

82. Koshy PJ, Lundy CJ, Rowan AD, Porter S, Edwards DR, Hogan A, Clark IM, Cawston TE. 2002. The modulation of matrix metalloproteinase and ADAM gene expression in human chondrocytes by interleukin-1 and oncostatin M: a time-course study using real-time quantitative reverse transcription-polymerase chain reaction. Arthritis Rheum 2002;46:961–967.
83. Bondeson J, Wainwright SD, Lauder S, Amos N, Hughes CE. The role of synovial macrophages and macrophage-produced cytokines in driving aggrecanases, matrix metalloproteinases, and other destructive and inflammatory responses in osteoarthritis. Arthritis Res Ther 2006;8:R187.
84. Werina J, Redlich K, Polzer K, Joosten L, KrönkeG, Distler J, Hess A, et al. TNF-induced structural joint damage is mediated by IL-1. Proc Natl Acad Sci U S A 2007;104:11742–11747.

31 Antiarthritic Potential of Green-Lipped Mussel and Other Marine-Based Nutraceuticals

Wendy Pearson and Michael I. Lindinger

CONTENTS

INTRODUCTION

Plant- and animal-based nutraceuticals are becoming increasingly important in the management of osteoarthritis and other articular arthropathies because there is a long history of some level of efficacy in various Australasian and Asian cultures and because there is no effective, conventional drug "cure." As with most nutraceuticals, those that are being used for the treatment of osteoarthritis have yet to be well characterized with respect to safety and efficacy in people and domestic animals.

The seas, particularly the nutrient-rich coastal areas, are an exciting and important resource for prospecting antiarthritic compounds. Rich in macro- and micronutrients known to participate in chondrocyte metabolism and/or matrix turnover, several sea-faring creatures have become unwitting participants in our fight against the pain and debilitation of arthritis. Ethnopharmacology provides a wealth of historical data on many marine animals as anti-inflammatory compounds. Coastal cultures across the globe have relied on natural medicines from the ocean to manage their arthritis symptoms. Such an example is the Maori from New Zealand, who have historically relied on abalone (AB; *Haliotis* sp.), New Zealand green-lipped mussel (NZGLM; *Perna canaliculus*) and cartilage from shark (SKC; *Galorhinus galeus*) to manage symptoms of arthritis. Each of these animals is easily harvested in the rich littoral areas surrounding the coastline. Admittedly, the native peoples had no scientific evidence to guide their choice of species. Rather, they were directed by advice from their community elders—advice gleaned for many generations of historical use.

In our contemporary culture that demands empirical evidence-based research results and clinical trials, "historical use" is a not the most influential reference letter for modern arthritis treatments.

It is thus somewhat surprising that it has only been in the last 25 years that the scientific literature has begun to report evidence for the effectiveness of nutraceuticals and traditional "medicines" as arthritis treatments. Some species such as *P. canaliculus* have accumulated a substantive scientific basis for use in arthritis, whereas others such as *G. galeus* and *Haliotis* sp. are relative strangers to the contemporary arthritis laboratory. The purpose of this chapter is to review the current scientific basis for the use of NZGLM, SKC, and AB for the treatment of osteoarthritis. Papers captured in this review include *in vitro* and *in vivo* studies that investigated raw, dried, and extracted portions or combinations of these three marine species as treatments for inflammatory conditions with relevance to osteoarthritis, and for safety.

NEW ZEALAND GREEN-LIPPED MUSSEL

NZGLM is a bivalve mollusk native to all coastal areas of mainland New Zealand (Figure 31.1). It is an economically important species to New Zealand, primarily as a food, and increasingly as a functional food/nutraceutical. The unique chemical and nutrient composition of NZGLM makes it interesting as a potential antiarthritis treatment. NZGLM is very high (~45% dry weight) in polyunsaturated fatty acids (PUFA), and almost 41% of this is composed of fatty acids (FA) of the omega-3 class (primarily docohexaenoic acid and eicosapentaenoic acid; Murphy et al., 2003). Other candidate bioactive chemicals include glycosaminoglycans (GAG) and specialized proteins.

PUFAs in NZGLM

PUFAs are composed of a hydrocarbon chain of variable length with several double bonds; the position of the first double bond, that is, the "omega," is what differentiates omega-3 and omega-6 FAs. Omega-3 and omega-6 FAs cannot be synthesized by the body, but are required for optimal health,

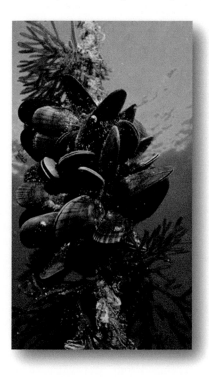

FIGURE 31.1 New Zealand green-lipped mussel. (From http://morporc.files.wordpress.com/2009/10/mglm1.jpg.)

and are thus termed "essential fatty acids" (EFAs). One of the most important roles of EFAs is their contribution to the structure and fluidity of the phospholipid bilayer of biological membranes. The fluidity of membranes is dependent on its lipid composition, with fluidity increasing with increasing number of double bonds (Grammatikos et al., 1994).

Once incorporated into cell membranes, FAs are vulnerable to peroxidation and catabolism, leading to their release from cell membranes and enzymatic renovation to eicosanoids (notably prostaglandins of the "E" series, prostacyclin, leukotrienes of the "B" series, and thromboxanes). The character of eicosanoids produced is dependent upon the type of FA that is liberated from cell membranes; omega-6 FAs are metabolized to proinflammatory PGE_2, whereas omega-3 FAs are metabolized to noninflammatory PGE_1 and PGE_3 (Maroon and Bost, 2006; Dobryniewski et al., 2007).

There have been a number of novel anti-inflammatory omega-3 PUFAs isolated from supercritical-CO_2 lipid extracts of tartaric acid–stabilized freeze-dried powdered NZGLM that have been found in bioactive fractions (Treschow et al., 2007). It appears that these omega-3 PUFAs competitively inhibit the formation of several proinflammatory molecules, including the proinflammatory interleukins (IL), 1, 6, and 12 (Mani and Lawson, 2006; Simopoulos, 2006), as well as inhibiting COX-1 and COX-2 activities (Mani and Lawson, 2006; McPhee et al., 2007) and immunoglobulin G (IgG) production *in vitro* (Mani and Lawson, 2006). Thus, it can be hypothesized that increasing the proportion of omega-3 FAs in the diet should impart an anti-inflammatory effect, and perhaps an immunomodulatory effect (Mani and Lawson, 2006). These hypothesis have been tested within the context of joint disease (Curtis et al., 2000, 2002, 2004; Halpern, 2000; Cho et al., 2003; Pollard et al., 2006; Lee et al., 2008, 2009; Pearson et al., 2009). For example, the eicosapentaenoic acid (20:5, *n*-3) is incorporated into cell membranes, from whence it can compete with arachidonic acid for the peroxidase catalytic site on the membrane-bound COX enzymes. Because of incomplete binding of this substrate to the enzyme, there results a 750-fold reduction in efficiency of the enzyme to oxidize arachidonic acid (Malkowski et al., 2001). This may account for the observed benefit of supplementation with *n*-3 fats in the treatment of inflammatory disorders (Navarro et al., 2000; Curtis et al., 2004), and may explain, at least in part, the anti-inflammatory activity of NZGLM.

GAGS IN NZGLM

In addition to a high percentage of omega-3 PUFAs, NZGLM is also a good source of dietary GAGs. GAGs are elongated, unbranched polysaccharide molecules that play important structural roles in cartilage. The major GAGs present in NZGLM include chondroitin sulfate, heparin sulfate, dermatan sulfate, and hyaluronic acid. There is an abundance of literature describing the effects of chondroitin sulfate and other GAGs on arthritis. Whereas a thorough analysis of the literature on GAGs for arthritis is beyond the scope of this chapter, the reader is directed to Chapter 21 in this book for a complete discussion of this topic, and although the quality of studies reporting the efficacy of dietary GAGs varies greatly (as do their results; Pearson and Lindinger, 2009), there prevails an ever-increasing demand for dietary GAG products to treat pathology of arthritis. In general, two hypotheses are currently supported, with scientific evidence, which rationalize a use for GAGs in arthritis. The first is the "substrate" hypothesis, in which dietary GAGs are predicted to find their way—intact—to the target tissue, that is, articulating cartilage, and provide substrate for the formation of new GAGs within the cartilage structure (Sobal et al., 2009). The second is a direct anti-inflammatory hypothesis, in which GAGs and related molecules (e.g., the hexosamine "glucosamine sulfate") impart a direct inhibitory effect on translation of inflammatory gene products and/or catabolic enzymes (Campo et al., 2009).

EXPERIMENTAL ANIMAL STUDIES ON NZGLM

Thus, a theoretical basis has been established for the anti-inflammatory potential of NZGLM. However, research which directly investigates the anti-inflammatory and/or anticatabolic effects of

NZGLM is somewhat limited. Two early papers reported on the anti-inflammatory activity of a crude extract of NZGLM administered to rats challenged with carrageenan in a hind footpad (Miller and Ormrod, 1980; Couch et al., 1982). The first provided NZGLM both i.p. and p.o. to rats at decreasing doses to detect a treatment and prophylactic effect of the test product on foot pad edema (Miller and Ormrod, 1980). There was no significant benefit of NZGLM p.o., but i.p. injections at a minimum dose of 500 mg/kg body weight significantly reduced swelling associated with carrageenan injections. The second study undertook to fractionate the crude extract of NZGLM to identify a candidate bioactive compound(s) and concluded that a proteinaceous fraction of NZGLM was responsible for the observed anti-inflammatory activity (Couch et al., 1982). Similar extracts were made from related bivalves, and anti-inflammatory activity was not observed with these extracts (Couch et al., 1982), indicating that this was a novel characteristic of NZGLM. In a later study, these investigators extracted a glycoprotein from NZGLM and demonstrated its ability to reduce edema and neutrophil infiltration in carrageenan-induced inflammation in the rat (Miller et al., 1993), providing evidence for an anti-inflammatory contribution of GAGs present in NZGLM. Other researchers have also demonstrated weak anti-inflammatory activity of a freeze-dried fraction of NZGLM on paw edema in rats (Rainsford and Whitehouse, 1980). Although the data on anti-inflammatory activity in this study were decidedly unspectacular, what was of interest was a marked gastroprotective activity of NZGLM against ulcers induced by nonsteroidal anti-inflammatory drugs aspirin and indomethacin. These data provide support for using NZGLM as an integral part of conventional drug treatments for articular inflammation.

CLINICAL EVIDENCE FOR EFFICACY OF NZGLM

The findings of Ormrod's research group sparked considerable interest and resulted in research aimed at purifying and identifying the anti-inflammatory components of NZGLM and to determine anti-inflammatory efficacy in various inflammatory disorders including joint disease. Well-designed and well-conducted clinical studies with NZGLM are few, but a group of scientists from Waltham have reported significant improvement in clinical signs of arthritis in dogs fed a diet containing NZGLM (Bui and Bierer, 2001, 2003; Bierer and Bui, 2002). For each study, 31 dogs were scored for mobility (average of individual scores for lameness in walking, trotting, and climbing stairs) and individual joints (carpus, elbow and shoulder or tarsus, stifle, and hip) of each limb were individually scored for degree of pain, swelling, crepitus, and reduction in range of movement. Summation of the mobility score and all individual joint scores for each dog comprised their total arthritic score. In all three studies, the authors reported that NZGLM added to the diet at an inclusion rate of 0.3% improved total arthritis score compared with controls. Other authors have also investigated the effect of NZGLM in 81 dogs with mild to moderate osteoarthritis (Pollard et al., 2006). Daily treatment with NZGLM (three to nine tablets depending on body weight; each tablet contained 125 mg NZGLM) for 56 days reduced subjective, owner-defined clinical signs of arthritis as well as objective veterinarian-defined musculoskeletal indicators of arthritis. Clinical evidence for efficacy of NZGLM for treating the symptoms of arthritis in humans has recently been reviewed (Brien et al., 2008). Four randomized controlled trials were included in the review, all of which reported some benefit of including NZGLM in the diet of arthritic humans. The review authors concluded that NZGLM is superior to placebo as a treatment of osteoarthritis and further trials are needed to determine optimum dose.

BRAND-SPECIFIC NZGLM-BASED PRODUCTS

The most extensively researched NZGLM-based product is Lyprinol (also known as Seatone; Lyprinol Ltd. Pharmalink, New Zealand). Lyprinol is a lipid-rich, supercritical fluid (CO_2) extraction of freeze-dried stabilized NZGLM. A search of the PubMed database (http://www.ncbi.nlm.nih. gov/pubmed?term=lyprinol) using the search term "Lyprinol" returned a listing of 26 research papers dating from 1997 to 2009. Systematic reviews of these papers have recently been published (Cobb and Ernst, 2006; Brien et al., 2008; Doggrell, 2009). In brief, some studies showed significant improvement of joint function and pain relief when receiving 1040 mg/day for 2 months (Cho et al., 2003), whereas other studies report no effect compared with placebo. Using rat tissues *in vitro*, Halpern (2000) demonstrated that Lyprinol subfractions inhibited LTB_4 biosynthesis by polymorphonuclear cells, and PGE_2 production by activated macrophages, and that this anti-inflammatory activity was largely associated with omega-3 PUFAs and natural antioxidants (e.g., carotenoids). When rats with adjuvant-induced arthritis were fed Lyprinol, they exhibited a transient analgesic effect (9–14 days of decreased pain; Lee et al., 2009) and the decreases in the inflammatory cytokines TNF-α and IFN-γ exceeded those of the (positive control) Naproxen, sham, and negative controls (Lee et al., 2008, 2009).

The main conclusions of the comprehensive reviews were that the literature showed mixed outcome measures and, at best, the evidence for clinical efficacy in inflammatory joint disease is weak, primarily because of methodological limitations (notably lack of stabilization of the PUFAs) of the research experiments. When used at the recommended doses, the product is probably not associated with adverse side effects (see next section).

Another NZGLM-based product [Sasha's EQ; (SEQ) Interpath Pty. Ltd., Australia] has recently been evaluated for anti-inflammatory and anticatabolic effects in cartilage explants (Pearson et al., 2007, 2008) as well as in a large animal model of early-stage arthritis (Pearson et al., 2009). These studies used a simulated digest of the product, and of each of its separate constituents, which mimicked upper gastrointestinal digestion and ultrafiltration across biological membranes (Pearson et al., 2008). When the extract of only NZGLM was applied to cartilage explants stimulated to an inflammatory state with IL-1, the explants showed reduced IL-1–induced PGE_2, as well as reduced IL-1–induced breakdown of proteoglycan structure of cartilage, compared with controls. When NZGLM was combined with other marine-based nutraceuticals (including abalone and cartilage from shark; NZGLM 50% w/w), the extract inhibited the inflammatory and catabolic consequences of IL-1 in cartilage explants, including inhibition of IL-1–induced PGE_2, NO, and GAG, to an even greater degree than any of the individual constituents alone (Pearson et al., 2008). Subsequent studies of the complex mixture (SEQ) fed to horses (15 g/day for 28 days) challenged with intra-articular IL-1 (on day 14) corroborated the *in vitro* findings, with the exception of NO which was not elevated in the synovial fluid of challenged horses either with or without SEQ feeding. A clinical trial with this product has since been completed, data from which further support a role for SEQ in inhibiting elevated PGE_2 associated with mild to moderate arthritis in horses (Pearson et al., unpublished).

The distinct contribution of NZGLM to overall bioactivity of SEQ is not known. However, *in vitro* studies using simulated digests of each individual ingredient on IL-1–stimulated cartilage explants demonstrated that NZGLM extract at a concentration of 0.06 mg/mL was more effective at reducing IL-1–induced PGE_2 and GAG release than any of the other single ingredients (Pearson et al., 2007). The main contributions of AB appear to be an inhibitory effect on IL-1–induced NO and GAG release; to our knowledge, these are the first data which substantiate the historical use of AB as an ethnopharmacological agent for arthritis. Similarly, SKC is often touted as a treatment for arthritis, primarily because of its mucopolysaccharide content (Volpi, 2003), and there is increasing objective science to support this claim in people (Monfort et al., 2008; Uebelhart, 2008). A single paper (written in Russian, with an English abstract) describes a beneficial effect of an SKC preparation on general condition of affected joints and immunopathology of infectious arthritis in rabbits (Pivnenko et al., 2005). The SEQ research supports these data by demonstrating that a simulated digest of SKC inhibited IL-1–induced PGE_2 and NO production at a concentration of 0.06 mg/mL (Pearson et al., 2007).

SAFETY OF INGESTING NZGLM AND ITS EXTRACTS

NZGLM and its extracts appear to be well-tolerated and reasonably safe. A number of safety-type studies have been performed on Lyprinol, a patented NZGLM extract with described 5-lipoxygenase

(5-LOX) inhibition characteristics. A recent study of 17 elderly individuals with advanced prostrate or breast cancer, received doses of Lyprinol, in 260 mg capsules twice daily, ranging between 1560 and 4160 mg/day, over a 76- to 306-day period (Sukumaran et al., 2010). The authors reported that a maximum tolerated dose was not reached; however, three patients showed evidence of dose-limiting toxicity including grade 4 hepatic dysfunction in two patients receiving 1040 or 1300 mg/day. The two most common adverse events were dyspepsia and anemia. In a multicenter study of 60 patients with knee or hip osteoarthritis receiving two capsules of Lyprinol twice daily, there were no adverse effects reported over a 2-month period (Cho et al., 2003). Similarly, there were no adverse effects of high dosages of SEQ fed to horses for a 3-month period (Pearson et al., 2009). Supplementation of SKC alone also appears to be well tolerated, with minimal adverse effects (Miller et al., 1998; Möller et al., 2010; Sawitzke et al., 2010). AB has been consumed as a food for millennia and there is no evidence in the literature which implicates AB in any systemic toxicity.

Mollusk (e.g., AB and NZGLM) allergies are well known (mild rashes to life-threatening anaphylactic shock) but rare (Taylor, 2008). In individuals with shellfish allergies, the consumption of shellfish-based nutraceuticals may be contraindicated. Other concerns regarding the consumption of shellfish include their ability to concentrate heavy metals and other in-shore contaminants (Whyte et al., 2009). Therefore, as with any food or nutraceutical, the quality of the product is important to the health and safety of the consumer.

CONCLUSIONS

NZGLM is an ethnopharmacological agent with considerable promise for preventing and treating the clinical signs and pathophysiology of osteoarthritis. Owing to its high content of omega-3 fatty acids and mucopolysaccharides, and a growing body of evidence for efficacy and safety, NZGLM should be considered a relevant and important therapeutic agent that must be investigated further within the context of contemporary science. Products built upon NZGLM such as Lyprinol and SEQ have been studied for their effect(s) on arthritis, but more research is needed to clearly establish dose, mode-of-action, and species-specific differences in bioactivity.

REFERENCES

Bierer TL, Bui LM. Improvement of arthritic signs in dogs fed green-lipped mussel (*Perna canaliculus*). J Nutr 2002;132(6 Suppl 2):1634S–1636S.

Brien S, Prescott P, Coghlan B, Bashir N, Lewith G. Systematic review of the nutritional supplement *Perna canaliculus* (green-lipped mussel) in the treatment of osteoarthritis. QJM 2008;101(3):167–179.

Bui LM, Bierer RL. Influence of green lipped mussels (*Perna canaliculus*) in alleviating signs of arthritis in dogs. Vet Ther 2001;2(2):101–111.

Bui LM, Bierer TL. Influence of green lipped mussels (*Perna canaliculus*) in alleviating signs of arthritis in dogs. Vet Ther 2003;4(4):397–407.

Campo GM, Avenoso A, Campo S, Traina P, D'Ascola A, Calatroni A. Glycosaminoglycans reduced inflammatory response by modulating toll-like receptor-4 in LPS-stimulated chondrocytes. Arch Biochem Biophys 2009;491(1–2):7–15.

Cho SH, Jung YB, Seong SC, Park HB, Byun KY, Lee DC, Song EK, Son JH. Clinical efficacy and safety of Lyprinol, a patented extract from New Zealand green-lipped mussel (*Perna canaliculus*) in patients with osteoarthritis of the hip and knee: a multicenter 2-month clinical trial. Eur Ann Allergy Clin Immunol 2003;35(6):212–216.

Cobb CS, Ernst E. Systematic review of a marine nutriceutical supplement in clinical trials for arthritis: the effectiveness of the New Zealand green-lipped mussel *Perna canaliculus*. Clin Rheumatol 2006;25(3):275–284.

Couch RA, Ormrod DJ, Miller TE, Watkins WB. Anti-inflammatory activity in fractionated extracts of the green-lipped mussel. N Z Med J 1982;95(720):803–806.

Curtis CL, Hughes CE, Flannery CR, Little CB, Harwood JL, Caterson B. n-3 fatty acids specifically modulate catabolic factors involved in articular cartilage degradation. J Biol Chem 2000;275(2):721–724.

Curtis CL, Rees SG, Little CB, Flannery CR, Hughes CE, Wilson C, Dent CM, Otterness IG, Harwood JL, Caterson B. Pathologic indicators of degradation and inflammation in human osteoarthritic cartilage are abrogated by exposure to n-3 fatty acids. Arthritis Rheum 2002;46(6):1544–1553.

Curtis CL, Harwood JL, Dent CM, Caterson B. Biological basis for the benefit of nutraceutical supplementation in arthritis. Drug Discov Today 2004;9(4):165–172.

Dobryniewski J, Szajda SD, Waszkiewicz N, Zwierz K. Biology of essential fatty acids (EFA). Przegl Lek 2007;64(2):91–99.

Doggrell SA. Lyprinol—is it a useful anti-inflammatory agent? Evid Based Complement Alternat Med 2009. [Epub ahead of print].

Grammatikos SI, Subbaiah PV, Victor TA, Miller WM. Diverse effects of essential (n-6 and n-3) fatty acids on cultured cells. Cytotechnology 1994;15(1–3):31–50.

Halpern GM. Anti-inflammatory effects of a stabilized lipid extract of *Perna canaliculus* (Lyprinol). Allerg Immunol (Paris) 2000;32(7):272–278.

Lee CH, Butt YK, Wong MS, Lo SC. A lipid extract of *Perna canaliculus* affects the expression of pro-inflammatory cytokines in a rat adjuvant-induced arthritis model. Eur Ann Allergy Clin Immunol 2008;40(4):148–153.

Lee CH, Lum JH, Ng CK, McKay J, Butt YK, Wong MS, Lo SC. Pain controlling and cytokine-regulating effects of lyprinol, a lipid extract of *Perna canaliculus*, in a rat adjuvant-induced arthritis model. Evid Based Complement Alternat Med 2009;6(2):239–245.

Malkowski MG, Thuresson ED, Lakkides KM, Rieke CJ, Micielli R, Smith WL, Garavito RM. Structure of eicosapentaenoic and linoleic acids in the cyclooxygenase site of prostaglandin endoperoxide H synthase-1. J Biol Chem 2001;276(40):37547–37555.

Mani S, Lawson JW. In vitro modulation of inflammatory cytokine and IgG levels by extracts of *Perna canaliculus*. BMC Complement Altern Med 2006;6:1.

Maroon JC, Bost JW. Omega-3 fatty acids (fish oil) as an anti-inflammatory: an alternative to nonsteroidal anti-inflammatory drugs for discogenic pain. Surg Neurol 2006;65(4):326–331.

McPhee S, Hodges LD, Wright PF, Wynne PM, Kalafatis N, Harney DW, Macrides TA. Anti-cyclooxygenase effects of lipid extracts from the New Zealand green-lipped mussel, *Perna canaliculus*. Comp Biochem Physiol B Biochem Mol Biol 2007;146(3):346–356.

Miller DR, Anderson GT, Stark JJ, Granick JL, Richardson D. Phase I/II trial of the safety and efficacy of shark cartilage in the treatment of advanced cancer. J Clin Oncol 1998;16(11):3649–3955.

Miller TE, Dodd J, Ormrod DJ, Geddes R. Anti-inflammatory activity of glycogen extracted from *Perna canaliculus* (NZ green-lipped mussel). Agents Actions 1993;38 Spec No:C139–C142.

Miller TE, Ormrod D. The anti-inflammatory activity of *Perna canaliculus* (NZ green lipped mussel). N Z Med J 1980;92(667):187–193.

Möller I, Pérez M, Monfort J, Benito P, Cuevas J, Perna C, Doménech G, Herrero M, Montell E, Vergés J. Effectiveness of chondroitin sulphate in patients with concomitant knee osteoarthritis and psoriasis: a randomized, double-blind, placebo-controlled study. Osteoarthritis Cartilage 2010;18(suppl 1):S32–S40. Epub May 10, 2010.

Monfort J, Martel-Pelletier J, Pelletier JP. Chondroitin sulphate for symptomatic osteoarthritis: critical appraisal of meta-analyses. Curr Med Res Opin 2008;24(5):1303–1308.

Murphy KJ, Mann NJ, Sinclair AJ. Fatty acid and sterol composition of frozen and freeze-dried New Zealand Green Lipped Mussel (*Perna canaliculus*) from three sites in New Zealand. Asia Pac J Clin Nutr 2003;12(1):50–60.

Navarro E, Esteve M, Olivé A, Klaassen J, Cabré E, Tena X, Fernández-Bañares F, Pastor C, Gassull MA. Abnormal fatty acid pattern in rheumatoid arthritis. A rationale for treatment with marine and botanical lipids. J Rheumatol 2000;27(2):298–303.

Pearson W, Cote N, Dejardins M, Hurtig MB. (*unpublished*) A dietary nutraceutical 'Sasha's EQ™ reduces synovial fluid PGE$_2$ in horses with osteoarthritis: a clinical study.

Pearson W, Lindinger MI. Low quality of experimental evidence for glucosamine-based nutraceuticals in equine lameness: a review of *in vivo* studies. Equine Vet J 2009;41:706–712.

Pearson W, Orth MW, Karrow NA, Lindinger MI. Effects of simulated digests of Biota orientalis and a dietary nutraceutical on interleukin-1- induced inflammatory responses in cartilage explants. Am J Vet Res 2008;69(12):1560–1568.

Pearson W, Orth MW, Karrow NA, Maclusky NJ, Lindinger MI. Anti-inflammatory and chondroprotective effects of nutraceuticals from Sasha's Blend in a cartilage explant model of inflammation. Mol Nutr Food Res 2007;51(8):1020–1030.

Pearson W, Orth MW, Lindinger MI. Evaluation of inflammatory responses induced via intra-articular injection of interleukin-1 in horses receiving a dietary nutraceutical and assessment of the clinical effects of long-term nutraceutical administration. Am J Vet Res 2009;70(7):848–861.

Pivnenko TN, Sukhoverkhova GIu, Epshteĭn LM, Somova-Isachkova LM, Timchenko NF, Besednova NN. Experimental morphological study of the therapeutic effect of shark cartilage preparation in a model of infective allergic arthritis [article in Russian]. Antibiot Khimioter 2005;50(5–6):20–23.

Pollard B, Guilford WG, Ankenbauer-Perkins KL, Hedderley D. Clinical efficacy and tolerance of an extract of green-lipped mussel (*Perna canaliculus*) in dogs presumptively diagnosed with degenerative joint disease. N Z Vet J 2006;54(3):114–118.

Rainsford KD, Whitehouse MW. Gastroprotective and anti-inflammatory properties of green lipped mussel (*Perna canaliculus*) preparation. Arzneimittelforschung 1980;30(12):2128–2132.

Sawitzke AD, Shi H, Finco MF, Dunlop DD, Harris CL, Singer NG, Bradley JD. Clinical efficacy and safety of glucosamine, chondroitin sulphate, their combination, celecoxib or placebo taken to treat osteoarthritis of the knee: 2-year results from GAIT. Ann Rheum Dis 2010;69(8):1459–1464. Epub Jun 4, 2010.

Simopoulos AP. Evolutionary aspects of diet, the omega-6/omega-3 ratio and genetic variation: nutritional implications for chronic diseases. Biomed Pharmacother 2006;60(9):502–507.

Sobal G, Menzel J, Sinzinger H. Uptake of 99mTc-labeled chondroitin sulfate by chondrocytes and cartilage: a promising agent for imaging of cartilage degeneration? Nucl Med Biol 2009;36(1):65–71.

Sukumaran S, Pittman KB, Patterson WK, Dickson J, Yeend S, Townsend A, Broadbridge V, Price TJ. A phase I study to determine the safety, tolerability and maximum tolerated dose of green-lipped mussel (*Perna canaliculus*) lipid extract, in patients with advanced prostate and breast cancer. Ann Oncol 2010;21(5):1089–1093.

Taylor SL. Molluscan shellfish allergy. Adv Food Nutr Res 2008;54:139–177.

Treschow AP, Hodges LD, Wright PF, Wynne PM, Kalafatis N, Macrides TA. Novel anti-inflammatory omega-3 PUFAs from the New Zealand green-lipped mussel, *Perna canaliculus*. Comp Biochem Physiol B Biochem Mol Biol 2007;147(4):645–656.

Uebelhart D. Clinical review of chondroitin sulfate in osteoarthritis. Osteoarthritis Cartilage 2008;16 (Suppl 3):S19-S21.

Volpi N. Oral absorption and bioavailability of ichthyic origin chondroitin sulfate in healthy male volunteers. Osteoarthritis Cartilage 2003;11(6):433–441.

Whyte AL, Hook GR, Greening GE, Gibbs-Smith E, Gardner JP. Human dietary exposure to heavy metals via the consumption of greenshell mussels (*Perna canaliculus* Gmelin 1791) from the Bay of Islands, northern New Zealand. Sci Total Environ 2009;407(14):4348–43455.

32 Antioxidant, Anti-Inflammatory, and Anticatabolic Potential of Rosmarinic Acid and High-Rosmarinic Acid Mint (*Mentha Spicata*) in Osteoarthritis

Wendy Pearson and Michael I. Lindinger

CONTENTS

INTRODUCTION

Rosmarinic acid (RA; $C_{18}H_{16}O_8$; Figure 32.1) is a polyphenolic carboxylic acid found in hornworts, in the fern family Blechnaceae, and in species of several orders of mono- and dicotyledonous angiosperms (Petersen et al., 2009). The mint herbs (family Lamiaceae) appear to be the most commonly used and studied sources. These include rosemary (*Rosmarinus officinalis*), basil (*Ocimum basilicum*), sage (*Salvia officinalis*), thyme (*Thymus vulgaris*), *Perilla frutescens* (a popular garnish in Japan), and mint (*Mentha X piperita*, *Mentha spicata*, and *Mentha aquatica*).

Historically, these plants have been ingested in various forms for millennia in middle eastern, far eastern, and western cultures. The most common forms ingested include a tea made from dried leaves and as a fresh or dried garnish on prepared foods. RA is well absorbed from gastrointestinal tract and through the skin. With respect to this chapter, these plants are of phytochemical and pharmacological interest because of their antioxidant activities (Chapado et al., 2010; Lamien-Meda et al., 2010; Pérez-Fons et al., 2010), anti-inflammatory activities (Takano et al., 2004), and anticatabolic activities in inflammatory conditions (Huang et al., 2009; Jiang et al., 2009). Plants that contain RA have also been investigated for other activities, including allergic dermatitis (Lee et al.,

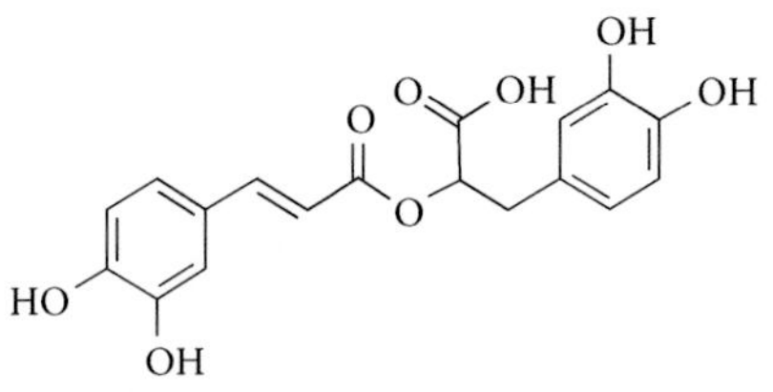

FIGURE 32.1   Chemical structure of RA. (Petersen M, Abdullah Y, Benner J, Eberle D, Gehlen K, Hücherig S, Janiak V, et al. Evolution of rosmarinic acid biosynthesis. Phytochemistry 2009;70(15–16):1663–1679.)

2008), treatment and prevention of bronchial asthma (Sanbongi et al., 2004), spasmogenic disorders, peptic ulcer, inflammatory diseases, hepatotoxicity, atherosclerosis, ischemic heart disease, cataract, cancer, and poor sperm motility (al-Sereiti et al., 1999).

RA is typically found in appreciable concentrations within the leaves, where it is synthesized. Structurally, RA obtains one of its phenolic rings from phenylalanine via caffeic acid and the other from tyrosine via dihydroxyphenyl-lactic acid. The biosynthesis of RA is initially similar to that of caffeoylshikimate and chlorogenic acid in the use of 4-coumaroyl-coenzyme A from the general phenylpropanoid pathway as a hydroxycinnamoyl donor. The hydroxycinnamoyl acceptor substrate comes from the shikimate pathway, with shikimic acid, quinic acid, and hydroxyphenyllactic acid all derived from L-tyrosine. The subsequent transfer of the 4-coumaroyl moiety to an acceptor molecule by hydroxycinnamoyl transferase is followed by the meta-hydroxylation of the 4-coumaroyl moiety in the ester by a cytochrome P450 monooxygenase (Petersen et al., 2009).

The main purpose of this review is to highlight the recent literature investigating the anti-inflammatory activity of RA and of dried plant leaves that contain RA in articular cartilage *in vitro and in vivo*. We will provide an overview of the inflammatory cascade in cartilage that is associated with osteoarthritis. This is followed by summarizing the roles of reactive oxygen species (ROS) in the inflammatory process, the anti-inflammatory, and the anticatabolic activities of RA. We briefly describe a new cultivar of *M. spicata* that has been shown to have anti-inflammatory activity *in vitro* that is likely not limited to the action of RA. Finally, we briefly summarize studies that have examined safety of *Mentha* sp. in animals.

THE INFLAMMATION OF OSTEOARTHRITIS

Osteoarthritis is a major degenerative disease of weight-bearing joint(s) that contributes to lameness and other movement disabilities in humans (Goldring and Goldring, 2007), horses (Goodrich and Nixon, 2006), and other domestic animals (Goldring and Goldring, 2007; Wu et al., 2010). The most affected joints are the highly mobile joints, including knees and lumbar vertebrae, ankles, and wrists. At the cellular and tissue level, osteoarthritis is characterized by accelerated articular chondrocyte maturation and extracellular matrix degradation (Wu et al., 2010). Although there are numerous causes of osteoarthritis, the majority of these can be classified as either acute or chronic (repetitive) trauma to the affects joint(s) and supporting structures (bones, tendons, muscles). As such, it may be difficult if not impossible to prevent the occurrence of osteoarthritis, even with ingestion of functional foods that have anti-inflammatory and related activities. Therefore, there is a strong emphasis using both pharmacological and nutraceutical approaches to treatment of the condition, with the goals of reducing pain, reducing inflammation, and slowing or stopping the progression of cartilage and joint degeneration. An ultimate goal is the development or discovery of compounds, which regenerate damaged cartilage and reverse the osteoarthritic condition within the affected joint.

Acute or repetitive trauma to a joint set into motion series of biochemical reactions within proinflammatory cells, resulting in cell–cell communication via a variety of signaling molecules that result in the inflammatory response (Figure 32.2). When the trauma is acute and severe, or

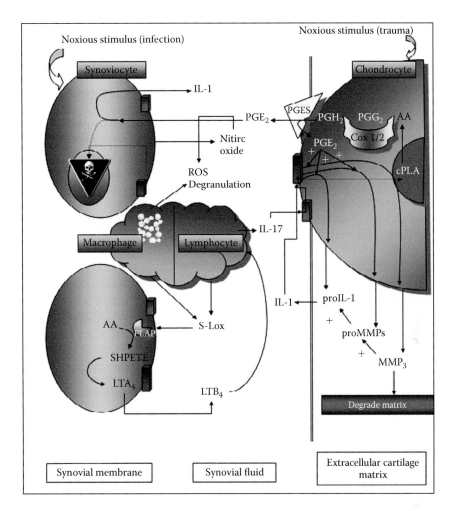

FIGURE 32.2 **(See color insert.)** Cellular response to injury within the joint capsule. (Pearson W. Development of in vitro and in vivo methods to evaluate putative dietary nutraceuticals. PhD Thesis. University of Guelph; 2007.) 5HPETE, 5-hydroperoxyeicosatetraenoic acid; 5-Lox, 5-lipoxygenase; AA, arachidonic acid; Cox-1/2, cyclooxygenase-1 and -2; cPLA, cytosolic phospholipase A; FLAP, 5-Lox activating protein; IL-1 and IL-17, interleukin-1 and interleukin-17; LTA_4 and LTB_4, leukotrienes A_4 and B_4; MMPs, matrix metalloproteinases; PGE_2, PGH_2, and PGG_2, prostaglandins E_2, H_2, and G_2; PGES, prostaglandin E synthase; proIL-1, pro-interleukin-1; proMMPs, pro-matrix metalloproteinases; ROS, reactive oxygen species.

excessively repetitive, a normal healing response to the inflammation cannot be achieved, resulting in a prolonged inflammatory state and degeneration of joint cartilage and bursa. Because the inflammation is a multifactorial process, there are several potential sites at which the inflammatory cascade can be influenced if not truly inhibited (Figure 32.2).

THE ROLES OF ROS IN OSTEOARTHRITIS

Cartilage is essentially avascular, aneural, and alymphatic and thus functions ostensibly as a hypoxic tissue (Falchuk et al., 1970). In comparison with other tissues, articular chondrocytes have relatively few mitochondria, and ATP production occurs primarily via substrate-level phosphorylation in glycolysis (Henrotin et al., 2005). Thus, chondrocytes have low metabolic activity and low oxygen requirements, consistent with the low PO_2 (7–35 mmHg depending on thickness of cartilage from the surface of the synovial fluid) typical of this avascular tissue. The mitochondria of chondrocytes are metabolically active and produce ATP in the usual manner. In chondrocytes, as in other tissues, ROS are produced within mitochondria as a normal product of electron transfer along the respiratory chain enzymes. Accordingly, the production of ROS is normally low in healthy articular cartilage. At low (normal physiological) concentrations, ROS appear to be required as intracellular signaling molecules for the normal, healthy functioning of articular cartilage (Gibson et al., 2008; White and Gibson, 2010).

With injury to a joint and consequent inflammation, there occurs an increased blood flow to the joint and an increase in permeability of the joint capsule, both of which results in the infiltration of proinflammatory cells into the synovium. This is often associated with increased production of ROS, which may result in abnormal catabolic events defined by pathological changes in the functional, structural, or metabolic processes of chondrocytes and/or their cartilage matrix (Loeser, 2008). This oxidative stress may result from increased ROS production, decreased ROS degradation, or a combination of the two. This had led to the suggestion that strong and consistent antioxidant compounds can be decisive interventions for mitigation of focal catabolism and pain (Sutipornpalangkul et al., 2009). A well-defined biochemical model for the precise and temporal contributions of ROS to joint destruction in OA has not yet been postulated. However, it has been hypothesized that ROS inhibit both the downregulation of catabolic events, which serve to remove damaged proteins, and the upregulation of the anabolic events of resynthesis and restoration (Loeser, 2008).

One of the primary enzymes responsible for the scavenging of ROS is superoxide dismutase (SOD), isoforms of which are found within the mitochondria and cytoplasm of chondrocytes and within extracellular fluid of cartilage (Regan et al., 2008). These researchers have reported that the extracellular SOD activity is greatly reduced in human osteoarthritic cartilage (Regan et al., 2005). Glutathione and ascorbic acid, other naturally occurring antioxidants normally found in relatively high concentration within synovial fluid of healthy joints, are also significantly decreased in joint fluid obtained from patients with severe osteoarthritis (Regan et al., 2008). These authors postulate that the resultant decrease in ROS degradation accelerates the detrimental oxidant effects on the extracellular matrix. Thus, in late-stage osteoarthritis, the typical upregulation of extracellular SOD seen in other tissues is suppressed or absent (Regan et al., 2008). Within the matrix, collagen proteoglycans are particularly susceptible to oxidative damage, resulting in impaired mechanical properties, water-holding capacity, and matrix stability (McCord, 1974; Monboisse and Borel, 1992). Damaged collagen fibrils and matrix deterioration render the cartilage vulnerable to mechanical failure under normal loads. The damaged collagen fibrils closely associated with chondrocytes are exposed to oxidant stress (Hollander et al., 1995), together with impaired localized, extracellular deficiency of oxidant scavenging.

The primary pathological consequences of elevated ROS in cartilage include chondrocyte activation resulting in production of inflammatory cellular products and chondrocyte death. Inflammatory cellular products resulting from elevated ROS in cartilage include catabolic enzymes (especially matrix metalloproteinases [MMPs] and aggrecanases; Cook-Mills, 2006), inflammatory cytokines (including interleukin-1α [IL-1α], IL-6, and IL-8; Li et al., 2007), and adhesion molecules including vascular cell adhesion molecule 1 (Cook-Mills, 2006). These inflammatory products, either directly or indirectly, upregulate other biomarkers for inflammation, including classical and alternative pathways of "complement" (Sjöberg et al., 2005) and prostaglandin E_2 (PGE$_2$). PGE$_2$ is a fatty acid–derived eicosanoid participating in nociception and is the pharmacological target for many nonsteroidal anti-inflammatory drugs (de Boer et al., 2009). Thus, there is support for a hypothesis that antioxidant interventions for elevated ROS in cartilage can downregulate inflammatory biomarkers and consequently reduce the catabolism and pain that defines the arthritic joint.

EVIDENCE FOR ANTIOXIDANT ACTIVITY OF RA

There is abundant evidence for direct and indirect antioxidant effects of RA. Direct free radical scavenging of RA can be assessed using an online HPLC method that selectively quantifies compounds with free radical scavenging activity (Raudonis et al., 2009). These authors reported that RA was the most active of all phytochemical compounds tested (including the flavonoids quercetin, rutin, and vitexin), with an antiradical activity equivalent >10 mg/g. RA also has a direct free radical scavenging effect on superoxide free radicals while inhibiting linoleic acid oxidation and reducing plasmid DNA damage by hydroxyl radicals (Zhang and Wang, 2009). In addition to scavenging existing free radicals, RA also reduces the production of ROS under conditions of oxidative stress and prevents depletion of endogenous cellular antioxidant enzymes (Zdarilová et al., 2009). This is consistent with other reports of strong antioxidant activity of RA in a variety of tests, including antioxidant partitioning and antioxidant capacity (CAT method) (Laguerre et al., 2010).

EVIDENCE FOR ANTI-INFLAMMATORY/ANTICATABOLIC ACTIVITIES OF RA

The well-documented antioxidant effect of RA is hypothesized to have downstream inhibitory effects on inflammatory biomarkers that are, at least in part, dependent on conditions of oxidative stress. These include various chondrocyte-derived catabolic enzymes (Roman-Blas et al., 2009), proinflammatory cytokines (Poveda et al., 2009), and PGE_2 (Roman-Blas et al., 2009). In support of this hypothesis, RA has shown an inhibitory effect on the activity of MMP-2 *in vitro* at an IC_{50} of 27.2 μM (Murata et al., 2009). MMP-2 is a chondrocyte-derived catabolic gelatinase enzyme, which is overexpressed in patients with rheumatoid (Chang et al., 2008) and osteoarthritis (Sánchez-Sabaté et al., 2009). Thus, inhibition of this enzyme may explain reports of reduced proteoglycan degradation in cartilage explants incubated in the presence of RA (Pearson et al., 2010). Other authors report RA-dependent inhibition of lipopolysaccharide (LPS)-induced production of various proinflammatory cytokines, including IL-6 (Vostálová et al., 2010), IL-1, and tumor necrosis factor α (Zdarilová et al., 2009). Other proinflammatory biomarkers with sensitivity to RA include monocyte chemoattractant protein 1 and macrophage inflammatory protein 1α (Kim et al., 2008).

Data describing the effect of RA on PGE_2 are equivocal and appear to be dependent on dose and on the cell type in which it is tested. One research group has reported an inhibitory effect of RA on LPS-induced PGE_2 production and an associated inhibitory effect on cyclooxygenase-2 expression in macrophages at an *in vitro* concentration of 30 μg/mL (Kim et al., 2008); for an average 78-kg person, this amounts to a dose of 12.5 g of pure RA. Lower doses of RA (0.64 μg/mL and 10 μM) do not inhibit LPS-induced PGE_2 production by cartilage explants (Pearson et al., 2010) or lung carcinoma cells *in vitro* (Koeberle et al., 2009).

The effects of RA on clinical presentation of arthritic signs or symptoms have not been well described and require further research. However, a single study reported that RA (50 mg/kg/day for 15 days) significantly reduced clinical signs of collagen-induced arthritis in mice as well as reduced expression of cyclooxygenase-2 (Youn et al., 2003).

Although several anti-inflammatory consequences of exposing cells to RA have been discussed, the cellular and molecular mechanisms by which these consequences are derived is not known. Experiments conducted in our laboratory suggest a mechanism that is, at least in part, independent of the hallmark proinflammatory cytokine IL-1, as we did not observe a significant inhibitory effect of RA on LPS-induced IL-1 production (Pearson et al., 2010). This is consistent with other reports. For example, RA induces an inhibition of chemokine recruitment of macrophages via the macrophage-activated protein kinase cell signaling pathway (Kim et al., 2008). Furthermore, RA appears to have an ability to inhibit phosphorylation of an inhibitor protein on nuclear factor κB (Iκ-Bα), which prevents binding of this nuclear transcription factor to DNA encoding inflammatory proteins (Lee et al., 2006; Kim et al., 2008; Moon et al., 2010). Taken together, these data suggest a primary effect of RA upstream of IL-1. The accumulating evidence supports a hypothesis that RA may be involved in downregulation of the complement cascade. The complement cascade is a complex series of zymogens that are dependent on a primary inflammatory signal for their cleavage (Englberger et al., 1988). There are three known pathways by which complement can be activated, and all three converge at C3 (Figure 32.3). Complement activation is important process in the amplification of signals involved in both inflammatory and immune responses to pathogens and pyrogens. Furthermore, genes encoding complement proteins are markedly increased in immune-mediated cartilage inflammation (Proctor et al., 2006). Complement is also an activator of calcium-independent phospholipase A_2 (Cohen et al., 2008), an enzyme that functions to liberate arachidonic acid from nuclear membranes. Arachidonic acid is the biological parent to inflammatory eicosanoids including PGE_2 and leukotriene B_4 (Figure 32.2); the production of both of these eicosanoids has been inhibited by RA in human polymorphonucleocytes (Kimura et al., 1987) and mouse macrophages (Huang et al., 2009). PGE_2, once formed, can stimulate chondrocyte secretion of MMPs (particularly MMP-13) and aggrecanases (notably ADAMTS-4), both of which process intact proteoglycans to smaller, less functional glycosaminoglycan fragments. Thus, it is tempting to propose that an inhibitory effect of RA on complement activation may afford protection of cartilage against eicosanoid-dependent inflammation and degradation and may account for some of the biological effects of RA on inflammatory compounds.

The first evidence that RA may be a complement activation inhibitor came more than two decades ago when investigators reported a strong, dose-dependent inhibitory effect of RA on immunohemolysis of antibody-coated erythrocytes by guinea pig serum (Englberger et al., 1988). They found that this biological effect resulted from inhibition of the C3-convertase enzyme of the classical complement pathway (Figure 32.3). A few years later, other scientists corroborated these findings,

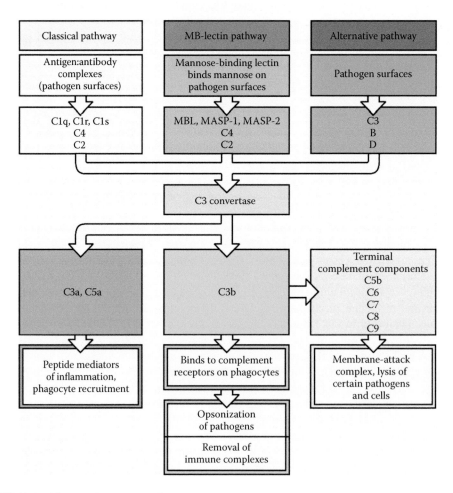

FIGURE 32.3 The complement cascade.

reporting a strong effect of RA on the classical pathway activation specifically via inhibition of C5-convertase (Peake et al., 1991). Since then, there has been vigorous research that has attempted to more clearly define the effect of RA on complement activation. *In vitro*, anticomplement activity (IC_{50}) via the classical pathway occurs at a concentration of 182 μM (Sahu et al., 1999; Si et al., 2008) and by the alternative pathway at 160 μM (Sahu et al., 1999). *In vivo* studies also support a hypothesis of complement inhibition; rats challenged with cobra venom to induce complement activation were protected from many inflammatory consequences by receiving RA (10 mg/kg) intravenously (Proctor et al., 2006). Of course, the million dollar question is "can a mechanism of inhibition of complement activation explain other anti-inflammatory effects of RA"? This is a question that must be examined in future research, but we do know that there is a dose-dependent inhibitory effect of RA on prostacyclin (a prostanoid related to PGE_2); prostacyclin has been shown to be upregulated by a complement activation assay (Rampart et al., 1986). Furthermore, there is evidence that endogenous (Basiglio et al., 2009) and exogenous (Ciocoiu et al., 2007) antioxidant compounds are capable of interfering with activation of the classical complement pathway, which further implicates the antioxidant actions of RA as a fundamental explanation for its inhibitory effect on complement activation.

DEVELOPMENT AND EFFECTS OF HIGH-RA MINT

Recent efforts have focused on spearmint (*M. spicata* L.), a herbaceous perennial plant with aerial leafy stolons found in many parts of the world and used in many cultures (Arumugan and Ramesh, 2009). The leaves are used for making chutney, and medicinally the leaves are used as a stimulant, a carminative, a mouthwash, an antispasmodic, a diuretic, and a relief from gastrointestinal gas pain, rheumatism, and muscle pain (Shaiq Ali et al., 2006). Oil extracts of the leaves have appreciable concentrations of monoterpenes such as menthol, menthone, carvone, and pulegone, all of which have a variety of biological properties (Choudhury et al., 2006). Plant extract had been found to have antioxidant and antiperoxidant properties due to the presence of eugenol, caffeic acid, RA, and α-tocopherol (Arumugam et al., 2006).

Mint (commonly *M. spicata, M. X piperita, M. aquatica*) is a common natural source for RA. Like pure RA, oil extracts of mint leaves also inhibit the inflammatory consequences of LPS and include inhibiting the production of IL-1, PGE_2, and leukotriene B_4 by LPS-stimulated human monocytes (Juergens et al., 1998). As these biological actions are considered to be related to the RA content of the plant (as opposed to other potential bioactive compounds within the leaves), considerable effort has been invested in developing strategies to upregulate biosynthesis of RA by genetically modified (GMO) plant tissues (Grzegorczyk et al., 2006; Tepe and Sokmen, 2007). These efforts have successfully resulted in RA accumulation of up to 45 mg/g plant leaf (dry weight). However, widespread commercialization of these technologies has lagged because of varying degrees to technical difficulties, low capacity for production of biomass, and complex regulatory environment for GMO products. Thus, although research into the biological effects of RA is illuminating a promising natural product, a frustrating limitation occurs at the level of the plant.

In an effort to encourage natural bioaccumulation of RA in higher plants, selective breeding of *M. spicata* clones under agronomically favorable conditions has generated plants that naturally overproduce RA, resulting in tissue concentrations of up to 122 mg/g dry weight (Fletcher et al., 2005, 2010)—more than double the content of high-RA-producing control clones and three times higher than GMO *Salvia* sp. (Grzegorczyk et al., 2006).

The high-RA *M. spicata* (HRAM) resulting from these experiments showed marked antioxidant activity *in vitro* (Fletcher et al., 2005), which led to further studies in cartilage. Cartilage explants cultured in the presence of a simulated digest of HRAM were decisively protected against the inflammatory consequences of LPS, most notably by virtual abbrogation of LPS-induced PGE_2 production (Pearson et al., 2010). There also resulted sharp declines in LPS-induced nitric oxide formation and LPS-induced catabolism of cartilage proteoglycan. Curiously, and of great interest,

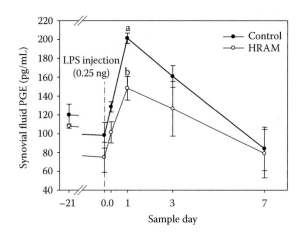

FIGURE 32.4 Synovial fluid PGE_2 concentration after intra-articular injection of LPS (0.25 ng) in healthy horses (preliminary results; $n = 2$ per group). Horses were fed a diet containing HRAM (0.05 g/kg body weight/day) or a control diet containing no HRAM for 21 days before and 7 days after intra-articular challenge with LPS. Synovial fluid was taken by aseptic arthrocentesis at baseline (Day –21), immediately before LPS injection (Day 0), then 6 h (Day 1.3), 1, 3, and 7 days after injection. Synovial fluid was analyzed for PGE_2 (ELISA). Letters represent significant differences between diets at given time point.

with the exception of the observed anticatabolic effect on cartilage, these actions of HRAM were independent of RA and three hepatic metabolites of RA (caffeic acid, ferulic acid, and coumaric acid). Upon the strength of these persuasive data, pilot studies testing a hypothesis of anti-inflammatory activity in large animals have since been initiated. HRAM was fed (0.05 g/kg body weight/day) for 21 days to horses that were challenged with low-dose intra-articular injections of LPS to detect a potential prophylactic effect of dietary HRAM (Pearson W, Fletcher RS, Kott LS, Hurtig MB. unpublished). Preliminary data suggest a decisive inhibitory effect of dietary HRAM on LPS-induced PGE_2 production in synovial fluid (Figure 32.4). Although still preliminary, these data encourage vigorous research into the anti-inflammatory effects of this plant. Questions remain as to the relative contributions of RA and its downstream hepatic metabolites, and these will be investigated in our future research.

A NOTE ON SAFETY

Peppermint has a long history of safe use, both in medicinal preparations and as a flavoring agent (Rodriguez-Fragoso et al., 2008). Peppermint is used as a remedy for the common cold, inflammatory processes of the mouth, pharynx, sinuses, liver, gallbladder, and bowel as well as gastrointestinal tract ailments such as nausea, vomiting, diarrhea, cramps, flatulence, and dyspepsia. Also it is used for headache, morning sickness, and dysmenorrhea. Peppermint leaf and oil contain acetaldehyde, amyl alcohol, menthyl esters, limone, pinene, phellandrene, cadinene, pugelone, and dimethyl sulfide. Trace constituents include alpha-pinene, sabinene, terpinolene, ocimene, gamma-terpinene, fenchene, alpha- and beta-thujone, citronellol, and other compounds (Nair, 2001; Inoue et al., 2002).

Peppermint (*M. piperita*) and peppermint oil are permitted flavoring agents for livestock feed in Canada (IFN# 8–17-854 and 8–17-850, respectively), which allow them to be included in livestock feed up to a maximum inclusion rate of 100 ppm (i.e., 100 mg/kg feed). Approximating an equivalent human dose from this would yield 50–100 mg of peppermint per day. However, traditional recommendations on the use of peppermint tea for treatment of various human ailments are three to four cups between meals (Akdogan et al., 2004a–c), with each cup made by pouring 250 mL of boiling water into a cup containing 5 g (one heaped teaspoon) of dried leaves and steeping for 5–10 min. Humans could thus consume aqueous extracts obtained from as much as 30–50 g of dried leaves per day.

In a series of articles, Akdogan et al. (2004a–c) reported the effects of ingesting tea made from dried peppermint (*M. spicata*) leaves in adult male rats. Adult rats that consumed 2.2 or 4.4 g/kg body weight *M. piperita* tea showed decreased serum iron and ferritin concentrations and an increase in unsaturated iron binding capacity, whereas *M. spicata* tea caused no significant change in serum iron, ferritin levels, and unsaturated iron binding capacity. Both herbal teas inhibited Fe absorption, and the inhibition caused by *M. spicata* tea was dose dependent (Akdogan et al., 2004a). Rats that consumed 2.2 or 4.4 g/kg body weight of *M. spicata* tea also showed increased serum concentrations of the liver enzymes aspartate aminotransferase and alanine aminotransferase. The 2.2-mg/kg dosage resulted in increased serum activities of SOD and glutathione peroxidase, but at the higher 4.4-g/kg dosage, these activities were significantly decreased compared with controls (Akdogan et al., 2004b). Both dosages also resulted in significant decreases in serum catalase activity and significant increases in the TBARS levels. Histopathology revealed mild (2.2 g/kg *M. piperita*) to severe (2.2 g/kg *M. spicata* and 4.4 g/kg of both teas) hepatic damage when compared with the control group. Importantly, *M. spicata* consumption was associated with granular or ballooning hepatocyte degeneration and necrosis and sinusoidal and central vein dilatation. The authors concluded that lipid peroxidation and hepatic damage resulting from consumption of teas made from *M. piperita* and *M. spicata* appears to be dose dependent. The authors went on to report that, in male rats, serum concentrations of follicle-stimulating hormone and luteinizing hormone increased and total testosterone decreased as a result of tea consumption as both dosages. Within testicular tissue, *M. piperita* resulted in segmental maturation arrest in the seminiferous tubules, whereas in addition, *M. spicata* also resulted in diffuse germ cell aplasia (Akdogan et al., 2004c). Irritable bowel syndrome, associated with inhibition of spontaneous peristaltic activity, reduced gastric emptying and total gastrointestinal transit, and decreased the basal tone in the gastrointestinal tract, has also been reported in humans (Mizuno et al., 2006). Taken together, the results of these studies suggest that *M. piperita* appears to be safer than *M. spicata* and that toxic effects of the herbs may occur when they are not used in the recommended fashion or at the recommended dose.

Safety of these and other *Mentha* species at higher inclusion rates is not known. Of particular interest and potential toxicity concern is a possible pro-oxidant effect of HRAM (or other RA-containing plants) at higher doses; a pro-oxidant effect has been reported in other studies testing high doses of traditionally antioxidant herbs (Pearson et al., 2005).

CONCLUSIONS

There is an ample body of literature implicating RA as a multifactorial anti-inflammatory compound, most likely owing to its antioxidant activity. RA has shown an inhibitory effect on inflammatory cytokines, prostanoids, MMPs, tissue edema, and ROS. However, widespread use of this natural compound in treating human cases of arthritis is limited by the ability of higher plants to accumulate RA in significant amounts. Thus, research is continuing, which seeks to enhance bioaccumulation of RA in plants that naturally produce this chemical. HRAM is one such plant, which has showed marked anticatabolic and anti-inflammatory activity in cartilage explants *in vitro*. Although preliminary *in vivo* data in horses has corroborated *in vitro* studies, it appears that RA is not the only bioactive chemical in HRAM and the search continues for other candidate chemicals.

REFERENCES

Akdogan M, Gultekin F, Yontem M. Effect of *Mentha piperita* (Labiatae) and *Mentha spicata* (Labiatae) on iron absorption in rats. Toxicol Ind Health 2004a;20(6–10):119–122.

Akdogan M, Ozguner M, Aydin G, Gokalp O. Investigation of biochemical and histopathological effects of *Mentha piperita* Labiatae and *Mentha spicata* Labiatae on liver tissue in rats. Hum Exp Toxicol 2004b;23(1):21–28.

Akdogan M, Ozguner M, Kocak A, Oncu M, Cicek E. Effects of peppermint teas on plasma testosterone, follicle-stimulating hormone, and luteinizing hormone levels and testicular tissue in rats. Urology 2004c;64(2):394–398.

al-Sereiti MR, Abu-Amer KM, Sen P. Pharmacology of rosemary (*Rosmarinus officinalis* Linn.) and its therapeutic potentials. Indian J Exp Biol 1999;37(2):124–130.

Arumugam P, Ramamurthy P, Santhiya ST, Ramesh A. Antioxidant activity measured in different solvent fractions obtained from Mentha spicata Linn.: an analysis by ABTS*+ decolorization assay. Asia Pac J Clin Nutr 2006;15(1):119–124.

Arumugam P, Ramesh A. Antigenotoxic and antioxidant potential of aqueous fraction of ethanol extract of Mentha spicata (L.) against 4-nitroquinoline-1-oxide-induced chromosome damage in mice. Drug Chem Toxicol 2009;32(4):411–416.

Basiglio CL, Arriaga SM, Pelusa F, Almará AM, Kapitulnik J, Mottino AD. Complement activation and disease: protective effects of hyperbilirubinaemia. Clin Sci (Lond) 2009;118(2):99–113.

Chang YH, Lin IL, Tsay GJ, Yang SC, Yang TP, Ho KT, Hsu TC, Shiau MY. Elevated circulatory MMP-2 and MMP-9 levels and activities in patients with rheumatoid arthritis and systemic lupus erythematosus. Clin Biochem 2008;41(12):955–959.

Chapado L, Linares-Palomino PJ, Salido S, Altarejos J, Rosado JA, Salido GM. Synthesis and evaluation of the platelet antiaggregant properties of phenolic antioxidants structurally related to rosmarinic acid. Bioorg Chem 2010;38(3):108–114.

Choudhury RP, Kumar A, Garg AN. Analysis of Indian mint (Mentha spicata) for essential, trace and toxic elements and its antioxidant behaviour. J Pharm Biomed Anal 2006;41(3):825–832. Epub 2006 Feb 28.

Ciocoiu M, Badescu MM, Lupusoru EC. The intervention of antioxidant therapy on platelet adhesion and immunomodulation in experimental physical stress. Free Radic Res 2007;41(7):829–838.

Cohen D, Papillon J, Aoudjit L, Li H, Cybulsky AV, Takano T. Role of calcium-independent phospholipase A2 in complement-mediated glomerular epithelial cell injury. Am J Physiol (Renal Physiology) 2008;294:F469–479.

de Boer TN, Huisman AM, Polak AA, Niehoff AG, van Rinsum AC, Saris D, Bijlsma JW, Lafeber FJ, Mastbergen SC. The chondroprotective effect of selective COX-2 inhibition in osteoarthritis: ex vivo evaluation of human cartilage tissue after in vivo treatment. Osteoarthritis Cartilage 2009;17(4):482–488.

Englberger W, Hadding U, Etschenberg E, Graf E, Leyck S, Winkelmann J, Parnham MJ. Rosmarinic acid: a new inhibitor of complement C3-convertase with anti-inflammatory activity. Int J Immunopharmacol 1988;10(6):729–737.

Falchuk KH, Goetzl EJ, Kulka JP. Respiratory gases of synovial fluids. An approach to synovial tissue circulatory-metabolic imbalance in rheumatoid arthritis. Am J Med 1970;49:223e31.

Fletcher RS, McAuley C, Kott L. (2005). Novel Mentha spicatum clones with enhanced rosmarinic acid and antioxidant activity. A Proceedings of WOCMAP III: The Third world Congress on Medical and Aromatic Plants Traditional Medicine and Nutraceuticals. Chiang Mai, Thailand. Feb 3–7, 2003. Acta Horticulturae Vol 6 no. 680: 31–40.

Fletcher RS, Slimmon T, Kott LS. Environmental factors affecting the accumulation of rosmarinic acid in spearmint (*Mentha spicata* L.) and peppermint (*Mentha piperita* L.). The Open Agriculture Journal 2010;4:10–16.

Gibson JS, Milner PI, White R, Fairfax TP, Wilkins RJ. Oxygen and reactive oxygen species in articular cartilage: modulators of ionic homeostasis. Pflugers Arch 2008;455(4):563–573.

Goldring MB, Goldring SR. Osteoarthritis. J Cell Physiol 2007;213(3):626–634.

Goodrich LR, Nixon AJ. Medical treatment of osteoarthritis in the horse—a review. Vet J 2006;171(1):51–69.

Grzegorczyk I, Królicka A, Wysokińska H. Establishment of *Salvia officinalis* L. hairy root cultures for the production of rosmarinic acid. Z Naturforsch C 2006, 61:351–356.

Henrotin Y, Kurz B, Aigner T. Oxygen and reactive oxygen species in cartilage degradation: friends or foes? Osteoarthritis Cartilage 2005;13(8):643–654.

Hollander AP, Pidoux I, Reiner A, Rorabeck C, Bourne R, Poole AR. Damage to type II collagen in aging and osteoarthritis starts at the articular surface, originates around chondrocytes, and extends into the cartilage with progressive degeneration. J Clin Invest 1995;96:2859–2869.

Huang N, Hauck C, Yum MY, Rizshsky L, Widrlechner MP, McCoy JA, Murphy PA, Dixon PM, Nikolau BJ, Birt DF. Rosmarinic acid in *Prunella vulgaris* ethanol extract inhibits lipopolysaccharide-induced prostaglandin E_2 and nitric oxide in RAW 264.7 mouse macrophages. J Agric Food Chem 2009;57(22):10579–10589.

Inoue T, Sugimoto Y, Masuda H, Kamei C. Antiallergic effect of flavonoid glycosides obtained from Mentha piperita L. Biol Pharm Bull 2002;25(2):256–259.

Jiang WL, Chen XG, Qu GW, Yue XD, Zhu HB, Tian JW, Fu FH. Rosmarinic acid protects against experimental sepsis by inhibiting proinflammatory factor release and ameliorating hemodynamics. Shock 2009;32(6):608–613.

Juergens UR, Stöber M, Vetter H. The anti-inflammatory activity of L-menthol compared to mint oil in human monocytes in vitro: a novel perspective for its therapeutic use in inflammatory diseases. Eur J Med Res 1998;3(12):539–545.

Kim HK, Lee JJ, Lee JS, Park YM, Yoon TR. Rosmarinic acid down-regulates the LPS-induced production of monocyte chemoattractant protein-1 (MCP-1) and macrophage inflammatory protein-1alpha (MIP-1alpha) via the MAPK pathway in bone-marrow derived dendritic cells. Mol Cells 2008;26(6):583–589.

Kimura Y, Okuda H, Okuda T, Hatano T, Arichi S. Studies on the activities of tannins and related compounds, X. Effects of caffeetannins and related compounds on arachidonate metabolism in human polymorphonuclear leukocytes. J Nat Prod 1987;50(3):392–399.

Koeberle A, Northoff H, Werz O. Curcumin blocks prostaglandin E_2 biosynthesis through direct inhibition of the microsomal prostaglandin E_2 synthase-1. Mol Cancer Ther 2009;8(8):2348–2355.

Laguerre M, López Giraldo LJ, Lecomte J, Figueroa-Espinoza MC, Baréa B, Weiss J, Decker EA, Villeneuve P. Relationship between hydrophobicity and antioxidant ability of "phenolipids" in emulsion: a parabolic effect of the chain length of rosmarinate esters. J Agric Food Chem 2010;58(5):2869–2876.

Lamien-Meda A, Nell M, Lohwasser U, Börner A, Franz C, Novak J. Investigation of antioxidant and rosmarinic acid variation in the sage collection of the genebank in Gatersleben. J Agric Food Chem 2010;58(6):3813–3819.

Lee J, Jung E, Kim Y, Lee J, Park J, Hong S, Hyun CG, Park D, Kim YS. Rosmarinic acid as a downstream inhibitor of IKK-beta in TNF-alpha-induced upregulation of CCL11 and CCR3. Br J Pharmacol 2006;148(3):366–375.

Lee J, Jung E, Koh J, Kim YS, Park D. Effect of rosmarinic acid on atopic dermatitis. J Dermatol 2008;35(12):768–771.

Li G, Luna C, Liton PB, Navarro I, Epstein DL, Gonzalez P. Sustained stress response after oxidative stress in trabecular meshwork cells. Mol Vis 2007;13:2282–2288.

Loeser RF. Molecular mechanisms of cartilage destruction in osteoarthritis. J Musculoskelet Neuronal Interact 2008;8(4):303–306.

McCord JM. Free radicals and inflammation: protection of synovial fluid by superoxide dismutase. Science 1974;185:529–531.

Mizuno S, Kato K, Ono Y, Yano K, Kurosaka H, Takahashi A, Abeta H, et al. Oral peppermint oil is a useful antispasmodic for double-contrast barium meal examination. J Gastroenterol Hepatol 2006;21(8):1297–1301.

Monboisse JC, Borel JP. Oxidative damage to collagen. EXS 1992;62:323–327.

Moon DO, Kim MO, Lee JD, Choi YH, Kim GY. Rosmarinic acid sensitizes cell death through suppression of TNF-alpha-induced NF-kappaB activation and ROS generation in human leukemia U937 cells. Cancer Lett 2010;288(2):183–191.

Murata T, Sasaki K, Sato K, Yoshizaki F, Yamada H, Mutoh H, Umehara K, et al. Matrix metalloproteinase-2 inhibitors from Clinopodium chinense var. parviflorum. J Nat Prod 2009;72(8):1379–1384.

Nair B. Final report on the safety assessment of mentha piperita (peppermint) oil, mentha piperita (peppermint) leaf extract, mentha piperita (peppermint) leaf, and mentha piperita (peppermint) leaf water. Int J Toxicol 2001;20 Suppl 3:61–73.

Peake PW, Pussell BA, Martyn P, Timmermans V, Charlesworth JA. The inhibitory effect of rosmarinic acid on complement involves the C5 convertase. Int J Immunopharmacol 1991;13(7):853–857.

Pearson W. Development of in vitro and in vivo methods to evaluate putative dietary nutraceuticals. PhD Thesis. University of Guelph. 2007.

Pearson W, Boermans HJ, Bettger WJ, McBride BW, Lindinger MI. Association of maximum voluntary dietary intake of freeze-dried garlic with Heinz body anemia in horses. Am J Vet Res. 2005;66(3):457–465.

Pearson W, Fletcher RS, Kott LS, Hurtig MB. Protection against LPS-induced cartilage inflammation and degradation provided by a biological extract of *Mentha spicata*. BMC Complement Altern Med 2010; 10(1):19.

Pérez-Fons L, Garzón MT, Micol V. Relationship between the antioxidant capacity and effect of rosemary (*Rosmarinus officinalis* L.) polyphenols on membrane phospholipid order. J Agric Food Chem 2010;58(1):161–171.

Petersen M, Abdullah Y, Benner J, Eberle D, Gehlen K, Hücherig S, Janiak V, et al. Evolution of rosmarinic acid biosynthesis. Phytochemistry 2009;70(15–16):1663–1679.

Poveda L, Hottiger M, Boos N, Wuertz K. Peroxynitrite induces gene expression in intervertebral disc cells. Spine (Phila Pa 1976) 2009;34(11):1127–1133.

Proctor LM, Strachan AJ, Woodruff TM, Mahadevan IB, Williams HM, Shiels IA, Taylor SM. Complement inhibitors selectively attenuate injury following administration of cobra venom factor to rats. Int Immunopharmacol 2006;6(8):1224–1232.

Rampart M, Beetens JR, Bult H, Herman AG, Parnham MJ, Winkelmann J. Complement-dependent stimulation of prostacyclin biosynthesis: inhibition by rosmarinic acid. Biochem Pharmacol 1986;35(8):1397–1400.

Raudonis R, Jakstas V, Burdulis D, Benetis R, Janulis V. Investigation of contribution of individual constituents to antioxidant activity in herbal drugs using postcolumn HPLC method. Medicina (Kaunas) 2009;45(5):382–394.

Regan EA, Bowler RP, Crapo JD. Joint fluid antioxidants are decreased in osteoarthritic joints compared to joints with macroscopically intact cartilage and subacute injury. Osteoarthritis Cartilage 2008;16(4):515–521.

Regan E, Flannelly J, Bowler R, Tran K, Nicks M, Carbone BD, Glueck D, Heijnen H, Mason R, Crapo J. Extracellular superoxide dismutase and oxidant damage in osteoarthritis. Arthritis Rheum 2005;52(11):3479–3491.

Rodriguez-Fragoso L, Reyes-Esparza J, Burchiel SW, Herrera-Ruiz D, Torres E. Risks and benefits of commonly used herbal medicines in Mexico. Toxicol Appl Pharmacol 2008;227(1):125–135. Epub 2007 Oct 12.

Roman-Blas JA, Contreras-Blasco MA, Largo R, Alvarez-Soria MA, Castañeda S, Herrero-Beaumont G. Differential effects of the antioxidant n-acetylcysteine on the production of catabolic mediators in IL-1beta-stimulated human osteoarthritic synoviocytes and chondrocytes. Eur J Pharmacol 2009;623(1–3):125–131.

Sahu A, Rawal N, Pangburn MK. Inhibition of complement by covalent attachment of rosmarinic acid to activated C3b. Biochem Pharmacol 1999;57(12):1439–1446.

Sanbongi C, Takano H, Osakabe N, Sasa N, Natsume M, Yanagisawa R, Inoue KI, et al. Rosmarinic acid in perilla extract inhibits allergic inflammation induced by mite allergen, in a mouse model. Clin Exp Allergy 2004;34(6):971–977.

Sánchez-Sabaté E, Alvarez L, Gil-Garay E, Munuera L, Vilaboa N. Identification of differentially expressed genes in trabecular bone from the iliac crest of osteoarthritic patients. Osteoarthritis Cartilage 2009;17(8):1106–1114.

Shaiq Ali M, Ahmed W, Saleem M, Khan T. Longifoamide-A and B: Two new ceramides from Mentha longifolia (Lamiaceae). Nat Prod Res 2006;20(10):953–960.

Si CL, Deng XJ, Liu Z, Kim JK, Bae YS. Studies on the phenylethanoid glycosides with anti-complement activity from Paulownia tomentosa var. tomentosa wood. J Asian Nat Prod Res 2008;10(11–12):1003–1008.

Sjöberg A, Onnerfjord P, Mörgelin M, Heinegård D, Blom AM. The extracellular matrix and inflammation: fibromodulin activates the classical pathway of complement by directly binding C1q. J Biol Chem 2005;280(37):32301–32308.

Sutipornpalangkul W, Morales NP, Harnroongroj T. Free radicals in primary knee osteoarthritis. J Med Assoc Thai 2009;92(Suppl 6):S268–274.

Takano H, Osakabe N, Sanbongi C, Yanagisawa R, Inoue K, Yasuda A, Natsume M, Baba S, Ichiishi E, Yoshikawa T. Extract of Perilla frutescens enriched for rosmarinic acid, a polyphenolic phytochemical, inhibits seasonal allergic rhinoconjunctivitis in humans. Exp Biol Med (Maywood) 2004;229(3):247–254.

Tepe B, Sokmen A. Production and optimisation of rosmarinic acid by Satureja hortensis L. callus cultures. Nat Prod Res 2007;21:1133–1144.

Vostálová J, Zdarilová A, Svobodová A. Prunella vulgaris extract and rosmarinic acid prevent UVB-induced DNA damage and oxidative stress in HaCaT keratinocytes. Arch Dermatol Res 2010;302(3):171–181.

White R, Gibson JS. The effect of oxygen tension on calcium homeostasis in bovine articular chondrocytes. J Orthop Surg Res 2010;5:27.

Wu Q, Zhu M, Rosier RN, Zuscik MJ, O'Keefe RJ, Chen D. Beta-catenin, cartilage, and osteoarthritis. Ann N Y Acad Sci 2010;1192(1):344–350.

Youn J, Lee KH, Won J, Huh SJ, Yun HS, Cho WG, Paik DJ. Beneficial effects of rosmarinic acid on suppression of collagen induced arthritis. J Rheumatol 2003;30(6):1203–1207.

Zdarilová A, Svobodová A, Simánek V, Ulrichová J. Prunella vulgaris extract and rosmarinic acid suppress lipopolysaccharide-induced alteration in human gingival fibroblasts. Toxicol In Vitro 2009;23(3):386–392.

Zhang Y, Wang ZZ. Phenolic composition and antioxidant activities of two Phlomis species: A correlation study. C R Biol 2009;332(9):816–826.

33 Potential Health Benefits of Orally Administered Hyaluronan in Alleviating Knee Joint Pain

Tomoyuki Kanemitsu and Akira Asari

CONTENTS

INTRODUCTION

Occurrence frequencies of osteoarthritis involving knee joint pain and inflammation are rapidly increasing with a growing population of elderly in the United States and Japan. In the United States, it is reported that approximately 40% of the population 60 years and older has such symptoms, and approximately 10% of them have problems in their daily life [1].

Articular cartilages consist of proteoglycans, type II collagen, and hyaluronan and joint fluid, which fills articular cavities and contains hyaluronan secreted from synovial membranes [2]. In particular, it has been determined that the concentration of hyaluronan in the joint fluid decreases with advancing age [3]. In general, hyaluronan is a macromolecular polysaccharide with a molecular weight from tens of thousands to millions and is composed of two types of sugars, *N*-acetylglucosamine

463

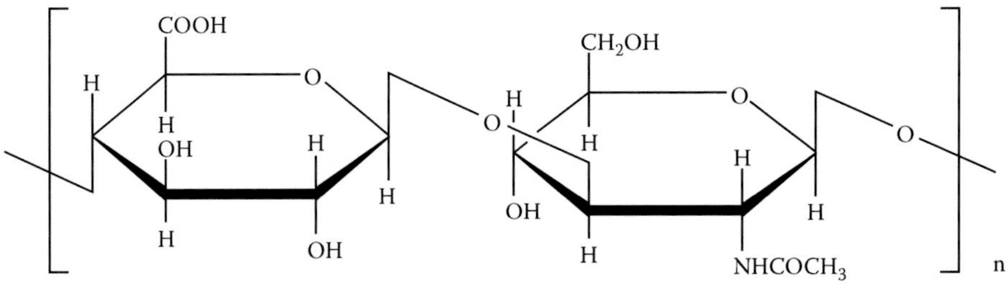

FIGURE 33.1 Chemical structure of hyaluronan.

TABLE 33.1
Results of Acute Toxicity

Animal Type	Dosage (mg/kg)	Number of Animals	Observation Period (days)	Fatal Number
Mouse	2400	20	8	0
Rat	800	20	8	0
Rabbit	1000	10	7	0

and D-glucuronic acid, linearly and alternately linked together (Figure 33.1). Because it has been confirmed that hyaluronan improves the symptoms of osteoarthritis by injection into the articular cavity, it is widely used as an intra-articular injection.

However, there are many elderly patients with knee joint pain who have not yet been diagnosed with osteoarthritis. For these patients, methods to prevent and relieve their knee joint pain are desired, especially those methods which are practicable at home. An example of such measures includes oral ingestion of dietary constituents to relieve knee joint pain. Verification of such improvement effect against knee joint pain through oral ingestion has been reported in glucosamine [4], chondroitin sulfate [5], type II collagen [6], and so forth. We have also previously reported that oral ingestion of 200–240 mg/day of hyaluronan (Hyabest (J), manufactured by Kewpie Corporation, Tokyo, Japan) was effective to improve knee joint pain in humans in oral ingestion tests conducted in Japan and the United States [7, 8]. In this chapter, the effects and mechanisms of orally administered hyaluronan for the improvement of the knee joint pain were described.

SAFETY STUDIES

Hyaluronan can be found in vertebrates and some microorganisms and is contained in tissues and organs such as the skin, blood vessels, cartilages, and internal organs in the body. In particular, chicken combs contain approximately 1% of hyaluronan and is used as a raw material for the industrial production of hyaluronan. In addition, chicken combs have been used as a cooking ingredient in France, China, and Japan; in other words, the history of eating hyaluronan is long. Therefore, the safety of orally ingested hyaluronan has empirically been indicated in addition to safety tests described in the following sections.

ACUTE TOXICITY TEST

As a result of acute toxicity tests, no abnormality was observed in oral administration of hyaluronan [9]. LD_{50} was >800 or 2400 mg/kg (Table 33.1). However, accurate LD_{50} would be a higher dosage because there were no fatal cases in any given dose in these animal studies.

Twenty-eight-day Oral Repeated Administration Toxicity Test

Twenty-eight-day repeated administration test for hyaluronan using rats resulted in no observed adverse effect level of approximately 3500 mg/kg/day [10].

Other Toxicity Tests

Reproductive and developmental toxicity, mutagenicity, and antigenicity tests were conducted and no toxicity was confirmed in these tests (Table 33.2).

HUMAN CLINICAL TRIAL

An oral administration test of hyaluronan in humans conducted in the United States is described in the next section.

Subjects

Men and women older than 40 years living in the United States, who were determined as grade II or III osteoarthritis according to the Kellgren–Lawrence grading scale on the basis of radiographs at the time of examinations, were included as subjects in this trial study. The protocol of this trial study was approved by the institutional review board, and the study was conducted after obtaining informed consent from the subjects.

Test Methods

Trial Food

Hard capsules containing 98% purity of hyaluronan produced by microbial fermentation and cornstarch were prepared. The daily dose was three capsules containing the total amount of 200 mg of hyaluronan. The capsules were administered after breakfast.

Administered Period

The test was a placebo-controlled double-blind test, and the administered period was for 8 weeks.

Evaluation Method

The subjects were evaluated using Western Ontario McMaster Universities Osteoarthritis Index (WOMAC). Question items in WOMAC consist of 5 items about "pain," 2 items about "stiffness," and 20 items about "activities of daily living." Each item was rated on a 0 to 4 points basis

---

TABLE 33.2
Other Toxicity

Test	Animal or Cell Type	Result
Reproductive and	Rat (50 mg/kg)	NOAEL 50 mg/kg/da
developmental toxicity	Rabbit (50 mg/kg)	NOAEL 50 mg/kg/day
Mutagenicity	Bacteria	Negative
	Mammalian cell	Negative
	Mouse	Negative
Antigenicity	Mouse	Negative

Abbreviation: NOAEL, no observed adverse effect level.

---

corresponding from the mildest to the most sever symptoms. When all symptoms were rated as the most severe, a total score of "pain," "stiffness," "activities of daily living," and their total score would be 20, 8, 68, and 96 points, respectively. In other words, the scores of each item and the total would decrease with the improvement of symptoms. Differences of the scores between before and 4 and 8 weeks after administration were evaluated.

Statistical Analysis

The Wilcoxon signed rank test (multiple comparisons were conducted using Bonferroni's inequality) was used for within-groups comparison of each WOMAC score and the total score, and the Mann–Whitney U test was used for comparison between groups. Significance level was set at <5% in both tests.

Results

The ingestion trial was started with 40 subjects; afterward, 3 subjects aborted the administration of their own reasons. Eventually, 37 subjects (8 men and 29 women) were included; 20 subjects were assigned to a hyaluronan-administered group, and 17 subjects were assigned to a control group (Table 33.3).

Transition of the scores of the evaluation items on the basis of WOMAC is shown in Table 33.4. Significant decreases were determined in the hyaluronan-administered and control groups from 4 weeks after the administration. Although there was no statistically significant difference in comparison between the groups, average scores of the evaluation items at 8 weeks after the administration became lower values in the hyaluronan-administered group.

TABLE 33.3
Background of Subjects

	Hyabest (J)	Placebo
Number	20	17
Age	65.6 ± 11.3	56.0 ± 7.6
Male	4	4
Female	16	13

TABLE 33.4
Transition of the Score of Evaluation Items Based on the Western Ontario McMaster Universities Osteoarthritis Index

	Group	Before Administration	After 4 weeks	After 8 weeks
Pain	Hyabest (J)	10.7 ± 1.1	8.3 ± 1.0*	6.2 ± 1.0*
	Placebo	10.6 ± 0.8	7.1 ± 0.9*	6.5 ± 1.0*
Stiffness	Hyabest (J)	4.8 ± 0.4	3.3 ± 0.4*	2.8 ± 0.5*
	Placebo	4.7 ± 0.4	3.2 ± 0.4*	3.2 ± 0.5*
ADL	Hyabest (J)	40.3 ± 3.5	28.8 ± 3.1*	22.4 ± 3.6*
	Placebo	38.5 ± 2.2	26.3 ± 3.1*	24.6 ± 3.1*
Total	Hyabest (J)	55.7 ± 4.9	40.4 ± 4.4*	31.3 ± 5.1*
	Placebo	53.0 ± 3.1	36.5 ± 4.3*	34.4 ± 4.5*

Abbreviation: ADL, activities of daily living.
*$p < 0.05$ versus before administration.

Discussion

In the hyaluronan-administered group, significant improvement of the scores was indicated from 4 weeks after the administration as compared with the scores before the administration. On the other hand, the placebo group also indicated significant improvement of the scores from 4 weeks after the administration; therefore, no significant difference was determined between the placebo and the hyaluronan-administered groups. However, average scores at 8 weeks after the administration became lower values in the hyaluronan-administered group compared with that of the placebo group.

The National Institutes of Health has conducted a study to evaluate the efficacy of orally administered glucosamine and chondroitin sulfate against knee osteoarthritis on the basis of WOMAC as an index. The study reported that the results of a stratified analysis between patient groups with low pain scores and high pain scores indicated that ingestion of glucosamine and chondroitin sulfate have efficacy for mitigation of the symptoms of osteoarthritis in the patient groups with high pain scores, although no significance was determined in a difference with a placebo group in this study [11]. Therefore, we conducted a stratified analysis using results from our trial study by defining the patients who had total pain scores on the basis of WOMAC of 10 and above as patients with high pain scores.

Evaluated subjects were 13 patients for a hyaluronan-administered group and 12 patients for a placebo group. Differences between "before the administration and 4 weeks after the administration" and "4 and 8 weeks after the administration" were evaluated because the placebo effect is expected to be strong until 4 weeks after the administration (Figure 33.2). If the difference of the

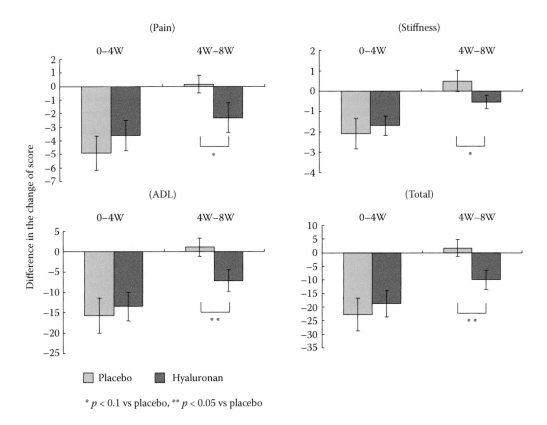

FIGURE 33.2 Difference in the change of score for each category of the subjects with a score of 10 or higher for "pain."

scores was minus, this means that the symptoms improved. As a result of the Mann–Whitney U test comparing both groups, there were no significant differences between "before the administration and 4 weeks after the administration" in either group; however, in the hyaluronan-administered group, a significant improvement was determined between "4 and 8 weeks after the administration" in activities of daily living scores and the total scores as compared with the placebo group. At the same time, the symptoms in the hyaluronan-administered group also showed a trend of improvement in scores of pain and stiffness as compared with the placebo group.

On the basis of the abovementioned results of the stratified analysis, it is suggested that the placebo effect has influence until 4 weeks after the administration and there is no significant difference between the groups; however, after that, administration of hyaluronan is effective in the improvement of knee joint pain.

ANIMAL AND CELL MODEL STUDIES

On the basis of the above test results, it has been determined that oral administration of hyaluronan could possibly relieve knee joint pain. It has been shown that hyaluronan may contribute to water retention and maintenance of tissue structures in the living body as well as immunity and inflammation mechanisms [12]. In accordance with such findings, the mechanisms of relieving knee joint pain with hyaluronan were examined in the following sections.

CHANGES IN GENE EXPRESSION CAUSED BY ORAL ADMINISTRATION OF HYALURONAN

To comprehensively identify changes in the living body caused by the oral administration of hyaluronan, changes in gene expression were examined with a DNA array using large intestine tissue derived from MRL-*lpr/lpr* mice orally administered 200 mg/kg/day of hyaluronan for 4 weeks (Table 33.5). As a result, it was clarified that the expression of SOCS3 (suppressor of cytokine signaling 3) gene was increased, whereas expression of the pleiotrophin gene was decreased. Consequently, we especially focused our attention on increasing SOCS3 because it was reported that the symptoms of osteoarthritis improved in an animal model of osteoarthritis when SOCS3 expression was enhanced [13]. We confirmed that the expression of SOCS3 also increased protein levels in Western blotting method using HT29 cells, which are model cells derived from the large intestine (Figure 33.3). In particular, SOCS3 is a cytokine regulator that has a role as a suppressor of anti-inflammatory cytokine. Therefore, changes in cytokines after the oral administration of hyaluronan were examined.

CHANGES IN CYTOKINE EXPRESSION AFTER THE ORAL ADMINISTRATION OF HYALURONAN

To test changes in cytokine expression after the oral administration of hyaluronan, serum obtained from the same mouse used for DNA array was analyzed with a cytokine array. As a result, changes in expression level were determined in some cytokines and chemokines, and an especially noticeable change was the increase of interleukin-10 (IL-10) (Figure 33.4). IL-10 is an anti-inflammatory cytokine that suppresses inflammatory cytokines. On the basis of these results, it has been suggested

TABLE 33.5
DNA Array of Large Intestine

	DNA Expression Ratio of Hyabest (J)/DW
SOCS3	2.0
Pleiotrophin	0.5

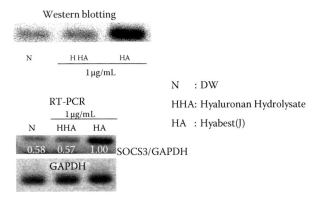

FIGURE 33.3   SOCS3 expression analyzed by Western blotting and RT-PCR.

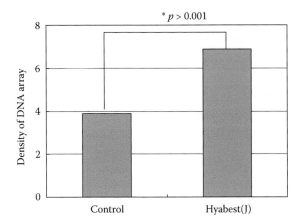

FIGURE 33.4   The change of expression of IL-10 hyaluronan administration.

that the mechanism by which orally administrated hyaluronan suppresses knee joint pain is attributable to the suppression of inflammatory cytokines.

HYALURONAN RECEPTOR IN THE LARGE INTESTINE TRACT

We hypothesized that a pathway in which orally administrated hyaluronan is absorbed from the digestive system and exerts its function and another pathway through signals mediated by receptors existing in the digestive system could be responsible for the mechanism of action of orally administrated hyaluronan relieving knee joint pain. The latter pathway mediated by receptors is described in the next paragraph.

Examples of the receptors existing in the digestive system that recognizes macromolecules derived from bacterial bodies include toll-like receptor 4 (TLR-4). We presupposed that this macromolecules' specific receptor is a receptor for hyaluronan; therefore, we conducted a double staining of TLR-4 and hyaluronan using large intestine tissue from mice administered hyaluronan (Figure 33.5). As a result, both stained areas were almost similar, and it is suggested that TLR-4 and hyaluronan could bind each other.

To verify these results, TLR-4 knockdown cells were prepared using HT29 cells, and binding of hyaluronan to the cell and expression of SOCS3 was examined using anti-SOCS3 antibody, anti-TLR-4 antibody, and biotinylated hyaluronan-binding protein (Figure 33.6). As a result, binding to

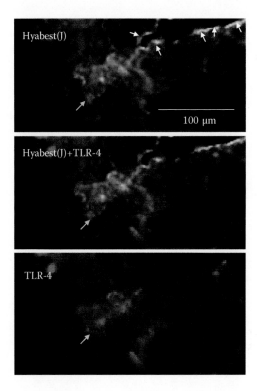

FIGURE 33.5 Double staining of hyaluronan and TLR-4.

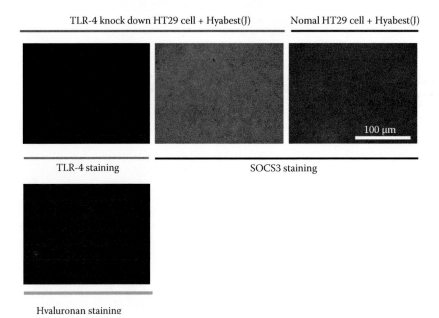

FIGURE 33.6 Suppression of hyaluronan binding and SOCS3 expression by knockdown of TLR-4.

the cells was lost and SOCS3 expression was also not increased in the TLR-4 knockdown cells as compared with normal cells.

On the basis of these results, it is suggested that orally ingested hyaluronan improves knee joint pain by binding with TLR-4, stimulating SOCS3 expression and then facilitating the production of IL-10.

CONCLUSIONS

There are many food products supplemented with hyaluronan appealing to patients with knee joint pain. However, the effect and the mechanisms of hyaluronan have not been scientifically elucidated. Findings in this study described relief of knee joint pain with hyaluronan for the first time, and it is expected that further elucidation of the function of hyaluronan would contribute to the improvement of the quality of life in patients suffering from knee joint pain in the future. It is anticipated that elucidation of the effect and mechanisms of action of the components, such as glucosamine and chondroitin sulfate, which are also expected to improve knee joint pain as well as hyaluronan, would promote studies using the characteristics of these constituents, for example, studies on synergetic effects, in years to come.

REFERENCES

1. Loeser RF Jr. Aging and the etiopathogenesis and treatment of osteoarthritis. Rheum Dis Clin North Am 2000;26(3):547–567.
2. "Arthritis" Edit Committe of Biochemistry on the disease: Vol. 4. Major symptom IV [in Japanese]. Tokyo: Nakayama Syoten Co., Ltd.; 1968:276–278.
3. Kondoh H. Research on viscosity of normal and diseased human joint fluid [in Japanese]. Kitazato-Igaku 1980;10:485–498.
4. Reginster JY, Deroisy R, Rovati LC, Lee RL, Lejeune E, Bruyere O, Giacovelli G, Henrotin Y, Dacre JE, Gosset C. Long-term effects of glucosamine sulphate on osteoarthritis progression: a randomized, placebo-controlled clinical trial. Lancet 2001;357:251–256.
5. Mazieres B, Combe B, Phan Van A, Tondut J, Grynfeltt M. Chondroitin sulfate in osteoarthritis of the knee: a prospective, double blind, placebo controlled muticenter clinical study. J Rheumatol 2001;28(1):173–181.
6. Trentham DE, Dynesius-Trentham RA, Orav EJ, Combitchi, Lorenzo C, Sewell KL, Hafler DA, Weiner HL. Effects of oral administration of type II collagen on rheumatoid arthritis. Science 1993;261:1727–1730.
7. Sato T, Iwaso H. An effectiveness study of hyaluronic acid [Hyabest (J)] in the treatment of osteoarthritis of the knee. J New Rem Clin 2008;57(2):128–137.
8. Sato T, Iwaso H. Examination of the efficacy and safety of oral administration of Hyabest (J) highly pure hyaluronic acid for knee joint pain. J Japanese Society of Clinical Sports Medicine 2009;17(3):566–572.
9. Nagao K, Goto Y. Acute toxicity test on sodium hyaluronate (SHP). Jpn Pharmacol Ther 1984;12(12):37–45.
10. Yoshida T. 28 day Oral repeated administration toxicity test of HA-LF. Company data in Kewpie corporation; 2006.
11. Daniel O, Domenic JR, Crystal LH, Marguerite AK, James RO, Michele MH, John DB, et al. Glucosamine, chondroitin sulfate, and the two in combination for painful knee osteoarthritis. N Engl J Med 2006;354(8):795–808.
12. Bollyky PL, Lord JD, Masewicz SA, Eyanko SP, Buckner JH, Wight TN, Nepon GT. High molecular weight hyaluronan promotes the suppressive effects of $CD4^+CD25^+$T-REG. J Immunol 2007;179(2):744–747.
13. Shouda T, Yoshida T, Hanada T, Yoshimura A. Induction of the cytokine signal regulator SOCS3/CIS3 as a therapeutic strategy for treating inflammatory arthritis. J Clin Invest 2001;108(12):1781–1788.

34 Pycnogenol—A Nutraceutical for Osteoarthritis

Om P. Gulati

CONTENTS

INTRODUCTION

Osteoarthritis (OA) is one of the most frequent diseases associated with pain and disability. In western population, it is one of the most frequent causes of pain, loss of function, and disability in adults. Radiographic evidence of OA occurs in the majority of people by 65 years of age and in approximately 80% of those older than 75 years. In the United States, it is second only to ischemic heart disease as a cause of work disability in men older than 50 years and accounts for more hospitalizations than rheumatoid arthritis each year [1, 2].

The pathogenesis of OA is a complex process involving inflammatory mediators and biomechanical and metabolic factors that alter the tissue homeostasis of articular cartilage and subchondral bone. Healthy cartilage is in a state of balance between matrix synthesis and matrix degradation. In OA cartilage, matrix degrading enzymes are overexpressed, shifting the balance in favor of net degradation of collagen proteoglycans from the matrix. The disease process affects the entire joint structure, including the cartilage, the subchondral bone, the ligaments, the capsule, the synovial membrane, and the periarticular muscles. Clinical features include joint pain, tenderness, and limitation of movements, crepitus, occasional effusions, and variable degree of inflammation [3]. Cytokines play an important role in the pathophysiology of OA [4]. The process involves imbalance of destructive cytokines over regulatory factors. Interleukin-1β (IL-1β), IL-17, tumor necrosis factor α (TNF-α), and other procatabolic cytokines activate the enzymatic degradation of cartilage matrix. The main enzymes involved in extracellular matrix (ECM) breakdown are matrix metalloproteinases (MMPs), which are sequentially activated by an amplifying cascade.

OA is characterized mainly by degenerative changes in joint cartilage, ultimately resulting in loss of cartilage and alterations in the subchondral bone. Osteoblasts in OA show a number of metabolic alterations that may interfere with normal cell metabolism and signaling, possibly leading to altered extracellular matrix composition [5]. Once cartilage degradation has begun, the synovial membrane phagocytoses the breakdown products released into the synovial fluid. Consequently, the membrane becomes hypertrophic and hyperplasic [6].

The present review provides an update of the multifaceted biological profile of the botanical nutraceutical Pycnogenol using a target oriented approach in light of pathophysiology of OA.

PYCNOGENOL®

Pycnogenol is French maritime pine bark extract produced by extraction of the outer bark of *Pinus pinaster Ait.* ssp. *atlantica*. Pycnogenol® is a trademark of Horphag Research. Its specifications are described in the U.S. Pharmacopeia 30–Dietary supplements [7]. On safety aspects, it is generally recognized as safe in the United States [8]. Pycnogenol has strong antioxidant and anti-inflammatory profiles proven by *in vitro* and *in vivo* studies in animals and further confirmed in clinical trials [9]. The historical development of Pycnogenol and the utilization of the pine bark as a health-promoting botanical [10] and its role relieving edema in chronic venous insufficiency are reviewed earlier [11]. The concept of orally administered Pycnogenol, either as "stand alone product" or in combination with other food ingredients, was developed during last two decades. Numerous clinical trials have investigated the efficacy of oral Pycnogenol in individuals with OA [12–15]. Most of the clinical research data on Pycnogenol are reviewed in different monographs and reviews [16–19].

PATHOPHYSIOGY OF OA

ROLE OF INFLAMMATION

Articular cartilage is a tissue in which chondrocytes and ECM interact reciprocally; that is, chondrocytes synthesize the proteins and proteoglycans of the matrix that, in turn, regulates chondrocyte metabolism [20]. Adhesion molecules send intracellular signals toward the external environment

[21]. Hence, these molecules do not solely take part in cell adhesion but actually play a key role in modulating an array of signals directed toward both intracellular and extracellular space [22]. Osteoarthritic chondrocytes lose their ability to perceive biomechanical signals from ECM and send biochemical signals to ECM and to modulate the synthesis of matrix components and metalloproteinases together with growth factors and cytokines. This abnormality in chondrocyte/ECM signaling may be an early, crucial event in activating the metabolic processes leading to OA. OA is characterized by progressive loss of cartilage, the main components of which are collagen and proteoglycan [23]. A series of biochemical and inflammatory mediators participate in the pathogenesis of OA. There is disturbance in the normal balance of degradation and repair in articular cartilage, synovial membrane, and subchondral bone [24]. Once cartilage degradation has begun, the synovial membrane phagocytoses the breakdown products released into the synovial fluid; consequently, the membrane gets hypertrophy and hyperplasia [6]. There is an increased number of lining cells and also an infiltration of the sublining tissue with a mixed population of inflammatory cells [25]. Some degree of synovitis develops even in the early stages of OA [26].

INFLAMMATORY MEDIATORS

The association between OA progression, the signs and symptoms of inflammation, is well documented. There are a number of biological markers to be associated with OA. These are cytokines, nitric oxide (NO), prostaglandins (PGs), leukotrienes (LTs), cartilage oligomeric proteins (COMPs) [27–29], C-reactive protein (CRP) [30, 31], and hyaluronic acid (HA) [32].

CYTOKINES AND GROWTH FACTORS

Cytokines and growth factors play an important role in the pathophysiology of OA. Cytokines are produced in the synovial membrane and are diffused into the cartilage through synovial fluid. They activate chondrocytes, which in turn produce catabolic factors such as proteases and proinflammatory cytokines. The major cytokines (proinflammatory and anti-inflammatory) involved in the pathophysiology of OA are IL-1α, IL-1β, IL-4, IL-6, IL-8, IL-10, IL-11, IL-13, IL-17, leukocytic inhibitory facto, and TNF-α. Proinflammatory cytokines play a pivotal role in the initiation and development of OA disease process, among which IL-1β and TNF-α appear prominent. IL-1β is important to cartilage destruction, whereas TNF-α appears to drive the inflammatory process [33, 34]. They activate synovial cells and chondrocytes and produce other cytokines such as IL-6, IL-8, leukocytic inhibitory facto, and their own production. They stimulate production proteases and prostaglandin E$_2$ (PGE$_2$). IL-1β and TNF-α also have been shown to increase osteoclastic bone resorption *in vitro* [35]. TNF-α also appears to be an important mediator of matrix degradation and a pivotal cytokine in synovial membrane inflammation.

The critical event which activates MMPs in OA is increased production of catabolic cytokines, such as IL-1β and tumor TNF-α [33]. These cytokines stimulate the metabolic activity of chondrocytes with activation of the mechanisms of matrix degradation. The relevance of IL-1β and TNF-α in the physiopathology of cartilage is further corroborated by the observation that the administration of IL-10, an inhibitor of IL-1β and TNF-α, in an experimental model of rheumatoid arthritis greatly reduces cartilage damage [36]. It is still unclear whether IL-1β and TNF-α act synergistically or independently in inducing osteoarthritic damage, or whether a functional hierarchy exists between the two cytokines. In animal models, it has been shown that blocking IL-1 or its activity prevents cartilage damage, whereas blocking TNF-α results in decreased inflammation [33, 34, 37], suggesting that IL-1 is the key cytokine causing cartilage lesions. IL-1 and TNF-α are produced in inflamed synovial membrane, by chondrocytes and osteoblasts, and act in an autocrine-paracrine manner. These cytokines not only increase the synthesis of MMPs and plasminogen activator, essential to convert pro-MMPs into MMPs, but also regulate the constitution of the ECM by enhancing the production of minor collagens, normally not present in cartilage, such as collagen types I and III, and decreasing the synthesis of proteoglycans and collagen types II and IX, which represent the "scaffolding" of cartilage. The local increase in IL-1β represents the key pathway in the cascade of events leading to tissue damage because it alters the MMP/TIMP (tissue inhibitor of MMP) balance by increasing MMP production and reducing TIMP synthesis [38].

IL-17 has similar functions to IL-1β because it increases the production of MMPs and NO by chondrocytes [39]. These cytokines enhance the expression of inducible NO synthase (iNOS) by chondrocytes and synoviocytes. Cytokines such as IL-1β and TNF-α produced by activated synoviocytes, mononuclear cells, or articular cartilage itself significantly upregulate MMP gene expression. Cytokines also blunt chondrocyte compensatory synthesis pathways required to restore the integrity of the degraded ECM. Moreover, in OA synovium, a relative deficit in the production of natural antagonists of the IL-1 receptor antagonist (IL-1Ra) has been demonstrated and could possibly be related to an excess production of NO in OA tissues. This, coupled with an upregulation in the receptor level, has been shown to be an additional enhancer of the catabolic effect of IL-1 in this disease.

IL-1β and TNF-α significantly upregulate the MMP-3 steady-state messenger ribonucleic acid (mRNA) derived from human synovium and chondrocytes. The neutralization of IL-1β and/or TNF-α upregulation of MMP gene expression appears to be a logical development in the potential medical therapy of OA. Indeed, recombinant IL-1Ra and soluble IL-1 receptor proteins have been tested in both animal models of OA for modification of OA progression. Soluble IL-1Ra suppressed MMP-3 transcription in the rabbit synovial cell line HIG-82. Experimental evidence showing that neutralizing TNF-α-suppressed cartilage degradation in arthritis also supports such strategy. The important role of TNF-α in OA may emerge from the fact that human articular chondrocytes from OA cartilage expressed a significantly higher number of the p55 TNF-α receptor, which could make OA cartilage particularly susceptible to TNF-α-degradative stimuli. In addition, OA cartilage produces more TNF-α and TNF-α convertase enzyme (TACE) and mRNA than normal cartilage. Because TACE is the regulator of TNF-α activity, limiting the activity of TACE might also prove efficacious in OA. IL-1β and TNF-α inhibition of chondrocyte compensatory biosynthesis pathways, which further compromise cartilage repair, must also be dealt with, perhaps by using stimulatory agents such as transforming growth factor β or insulin-like growth factor I.

Modulation of cytokines that control MMP gene upregulation would appear to be fertile targets for product development for OA. Several studies illustrate the potential importance of modulating IL-1β activity as a means to reduce the progression of the structural changes in OA. In the experimental dog and rabbit models of OA, it was demonstrated that *in vivo* intra-articular injections of the IL-Ra gene can prevent the progression of structural changes in OA.

MATRIX METALLOPROTEINASES

Chondrocytes act as a source of MMPs and inflammatory mediator production. There is a strong evidence for major involvement of MMPs in early cartilage structural changes [40]. Chondrocytes actively produce NO, PGs, IL-1β, TNF-α, IL-6, and IL-8. There is evidence that these molecules act within cartilage in an autocrine or paracrine manner to promote a catabolic state, which leads to progressive cartilage damage. MMPs produced by chondrocytes play an important role in the development of cartilage destruction and agents that can target on this biomarker may produce beneficial effects in OA [41]. MMPs are synthesized and secreted by chondrocytes in response to stimulants like IL-1 and TNF-α [42], which have been identified as OA biomarkers. Damage to collagen happens either by degradation of collagen or inhibition of collagen regeneration by disturbed enzymes metabolism involved in the biosynthesis of collagen. Reactive oxygen species (ROS) activate matrix degradation enzymes MMPs [43] and thus play a significant role as signaling molecules to contribute to cell injury and collagen degradation. Exposed subendothelial collagen leads to adhesions of platelets, platelet activation, and aggregation. Thromboplastin converts prothrombin to thrombin, which in turn converts fibrinogen to fibrin. The resulting fibrin network entraps RBCs and WBCs leading to further damage to articular cartilage.

NITRIC OXIDE

NO is another potential factor in the promotion of cartilage catabolism in OA [44]. Cartilage produces large amounts of NO, both under spontaneous and proinflammatory cytokine-stimulated conditions [45]. A high level of NO has been found in the synovial fluid and serum of patients with OA [46]. This is caused by increased levels of inducible form of NO synthase (iNOS), the enzyme responsible for NO production [46]. NO inhibits the synthesis of cartilage matrix and enhances MMP activity [47, 48]. Interestingly, a selective inhibitor of iNOS administered *in vivo* proved to exert positive therapeutic effects on the progression of lesions in an experimental canine OA model [49].

C-REACTIVE PROTEIN

CRP has been shown to be elevated and is related with radiographic progression of long-term knee OA [30, 31]. A small elevation in CRP levels was of a predictive value in women with mild to moderately severe knee OA, whose disease either progressed or showed no progression [31].

OTHER RISK FACTORS AND BIOMARKERS IN OA

There are enough published data demonstrating the correlation between the biological markers of inflammation and the appearance, progression, and risk factor involved in OA [24]. HA is another identified biomarker of inflammation. HA has been reported to be elevated in OA, and plasma HA levels were found to correlate with an objective functional capacity score and with articular index based on the total amount of cartilage in the involved joints [32]. COMP is a component of the ECM of articular cartilage and is found in high concentrations. COMP is formed by activated synovial cells; it is safe to speculate that elevated COMP may reflect synovitis [28, 29]. The expression of the inducible cyclooxygenase (COX), COX-2, is increased in OA chondrocytes that spontaneously produce PGE_2 *ex vivo* [50].

BIOLOGICAL PROFILE OF PYCNOGENOL

ANTIOXIDANT AND ANTI-INFLAMMATORY ACTIVITIES

Free radicals are produced as by-products during normal metabolism of nutrients and in the course of a large number of normal cellular responses, such as in the oxidative burst of activated neutrophils, in the course of cytochrome P450 activity, NO synthesis, and other activities. It has been calculated that approximately 2%–3% of oxygen is turned to free radicals and spinned off. Free radicals may attack different cellular and intracellular components. By attacking lipid, they lead to lipid peroxidation and may produce atherosclerosis. By attacking DNA, they cause mutation or cell death or disturb the normal cell cycle, leading to uncontrolled cell proliferation and cancer. By acting on proteins, they can cause enzyme malfunctions affecting in turn intracellular signaling and metabolic pathways, leading to cell defects and aging. As a potent antioxidant, Pycnogenol acts on these free radicals and neutralize them thus produce cell protection.

The antioxidant and anti-inflammatory profile of Pycnogenol has been reviewed [51–54]. These biological activities of Pycnogenol are shown *in vitro* and *in vivo* models and then have been confirmed in clinical studies. These include (1) antioxidant and free radical scavenging activity [55–59]; (2) antioxidant activity sparing vitamin C and recycling of vitamin E [60]; (3) inhibition of lipid peroxidation [61]; (4) protection of nerve cells against β-amyloid- or glutamate-induced toxicity [62];

(5) erythrocytes protection in G6PD-deficient human [63]; (6) inhibition of generation of inflammatory mediators in macrophages [64] and stimulation of antioxidative defense system [65]; (7) antierythema, antiedema, and anti-inflammatory [66–69]; (8) inhibition of proinflammatory cytokines [70]; (9) inhibition of matrix metalloproteases [71]; (10) inhibition of histamine release from mast cells [72]; and (11) wound-healing effects [73,74].

ANTIOXIDANT EFFECTS: *IN VITRO* STUDIES

Several studies made with Pycnogenol have been reported to demonstrate its free radical scavenging and/or antioxidant activity *in vitro*. Free radical (hydroxyl and superoxide) scavenging activity of Pycnogenol was measured using a highly sensitive electron spin resonance spectrometer and was compared with other bioactive free radical scavengers like *Ginkgo biloba* and green tea extract. An analog of vitamin C and vitamin E was used as reference standards for hydroxyl radicals. Superoxide dismutase (SOD) was used as the reference standard for superoxide anion scavenging activity. Macrophages were activated by the bacterial wall components and lipopolysaccharides (LPSs) and interferon-γ, which induces the expression of large amounts of the enzyme iNOS. Pycnogenol was found to be a potent free radical scavenger of hydroxyl, superoxide, and NO radicals [55, 56]. Pycnogenol participates in the cellular antioxidant network as indicated by its ability to regenerate the ascorbyl radical and to protect endogenous vitamin E and glutathione from oxidative stress. In addition, it was found to be resistant to the action of heat and ascorbate oxidase [60]. Pycnogenol protects DNA against Fenton reaction radicals, probably by chelating Fe. It also can induce SOD under oxidative stress [61]. In human umbilical vein endothelial cell cultures, Pycnogenol exhibited a dose-dependent suppression of TNF-α-induced activation of the transcriptional regulatory protein nuclear factor κB (NF-κB). Expression of cell surface molecules such as vascular cell adhesion molecule 1 (VCAM-1) and intercellular adhesion molecule 1 (ICAM-1) was reduced [62].

In two different *in vitro* studies, bovine vascular endothelial cells were treated with Pycnogenol before subjecting them to oxidative stress induced by t-butyl hydroperoxide (tBHP). Lactate dehydrogenase (LDH) release and malondialdehyde (MDA), respectively, were used as biological markers to assess cell death and lipid peroxidation. Preincubation of endothelial cells with Pycnogenol at concentrations 10–80 µg/mL for 16 h increased the cell viability after tBHP treatment and, in addition, caused a dose-dependent decline in MDA induced by tBHP [60, 61].

In another independent *in vitro* study model, bovine retina was used as the tissue substrate and lipid peroxidation as the target reaction action, giving rise to lipid hydroperoxide as the biological marker expressed as thiobarbituric acid reactive substances. Pycnogenol effectively inhibited lipid peroxidation at a concentration as low as 25 ng/mL. Lipid peroxidation was inhibited by Pycnogenol in a dose-dependent fashion and was completely absent at a concentration of 250 ng/mL. Pycnogenol was relatively more effective than grape seed extract, vitamin C, vitamin E, and lipoic acid [59].

Antioxidant activity of Pycnogenol was further confirmed in an independent laboratory using three different *in vitro* models addressing the oxidative burst, low-density lipoprotein (LDL) oxidation, and iron/ascorbic acid system as oxidant challenges on different substrates. Pycnogenol exhibited a concentration-dependent inhibition of oxidative burst triggered by zymosan in *J774* murine macrophages *in vitro*. Pycnogenol when coincubated with copper sulfate that is used to oxidize human plasma LDL cholesterol (formation of thiobarbituric acid reactive substances used as markers) resulted in inhibition of LDL oxidation in a concentration-dependent manner. Pycnogenol significantly minimized the cleavage of DNA caused by hydroxyl radical induced by exposure of pBR322 plasmid DNA to iron/ascorbic acid system and measured by agarose gel electrophoresis [58].

Pretreatment of murine macrophages (RAW 264.7) with LPS is associated with increased release of proinflammatory mediators like IL-1β and its mRNA. Incubation with Pycnogenol was associated with a dose-dependent decrease in the production of proinflammatory mediators. According to this report, Pycnogenol has been found to be able to block the activation of two major transcription factors NF-κB and activator protein 1 (AP-1) involved in the production of IL-1β. These results suggest the anti-inflammatory role of Pycnogenol on the basis of its free radical scavenging activity [58]. Pycnogenol enhances the endogenous antioxidant-enhancing activity, producing a concentration-dependent increase in intracellular GSH, GPX and GSSG-R, SOD, and chloramphenicol acetyl transferase (CAT) levels expressed as per milligrams of protein [65].

ANTIOXIDANT AND ANTI-INFLAMMATORY ACTIVITIES: *IN VIVO* ANIMAL STUDIES

Pycnogenol was shown to have remarkable free radical scavenging activity *in vitro* and anti-inflammatory activity *in vivo*. These activities bear close correlation indicating the involvement of free radicals in inflammation and the anti-inflammatory action of Pycnogenol at least partly because of its free radical scavenging effect [55]. Anti-inflammatory and wound-healing effects were demonstrated subsequently by the same group of authors [68, 69, 73].

There is enough experimental evidence that oxidative stress is involved in the pathophysiology of diabetes and its complications. In streptozotocin-induced diabetic rats, the glutathione-to-glutathione disulfide ratio and the activities of endogenous antioxidant enzymes SOD, CAT, glutathione peroxidase, glutathione reductase, and γ-glutamyl transpeptidase were significantly increased after Pycnogenol administration [75]. Another study from the same laboratory further showed that Pycnogenol administered alone or in combination with β-carotene once again increased glutathione reductase activities [76].

The experiments were repeated focusing on diabetic retinopathy. Decreased retinal γ-glutamyl transferase activity of diabetic rats was normalized by administration of Pycnogenol alone or in combination with β-carotene. Elevated activity of SOD in diabetic retina was normalized by Pycnogenol and β-carotene combination [77]. The results obtained from the above three studies reported from the same laboratory lead to conclude that Pycnogenol alters intracellular antioxidant defense mechanisms in streptozotocin-induced diabetic rats.

ANTIOXIDANT EFFECTS: CLINICAL STUDIES

Clinical research data on Pycnogenol are provided on the basis of its antioxidant activity in healthy volunteers. The effect of Pycnogenol on human antioxidant defenses was demonstrated by a significant ($p < 0.05$) decrease of oxygen radical absorbance capacity in plasma throughout the Pycnogenol supplementation period of 3 weeks. In addition to its ability to enhance plasma antioxidant capacity, Pycnogenol significantly reduced LDL cholesterol levels and increased high-density lipoprotein cholesterol levels in the blood [78]. In another independent double-blind study, Pycnogenol significantly increased plasma antioxidant activity ($p < 0.01$) [79].

Oxidative stress is also involved in the pathogenesis of other clinical conditions like skin aging, erythema, melasma abnormal sperm morphology, and gingival bleeding and plaque formation. The effects of Pycnogenol were studied independently in these conditions. Supplementation with Pycnogenol along with other micronutrients in a formulation Evelle improved visible signs of skin aging, increased skin elasticity, and decreased skin roughness [80]. Pycnogenol supplementation provided relief from erythema and melasma [66, 81]. The average melasma area and the intensity of pigmentation were found to be significantly reduced after supplementation [81]. In addition, Pycnogenol by virtue of its antioxidant profile has improved abnormal sperm morphology and functions [82], provided relief from pain in dysmenorrhea [83], and minimized gingival bleeding and plaque formation [84].

INHIBITION OF MMPs

After oral application of Pycnogenol, two major metabolites are formed *in vivo*, δ-(3,4-dihydroxyphenyl)-γ-valerolactone (M1) and δ-(3-methoxy-4-hydroxyphenyl)-γ-valerolactone (M2).

Both metabolites exert strong inhibitory effects on MMPs types 1, 2, and 9. M1 is also reported to have superoxide scavenger activities [71].

INHIBITION OF CYTOKINES

An acute exposure to ultraviolet radiation (UVR) leads to inflammatory response, skin erythema. Oxidative stress by releasing ROS and reactive nitrogen species is involved in producing this biological effect. UVR stimulates expression of many proinflammatory genes such as TNF-α, IL-1α, IL-1β, IL-6, and IL-8. All these cytokines/chemokines contain NF-κB binding sites in the 5⊠-flanking region of the gene. As oxidative stress through ROS and reactive nitrogen species is involved in the inflammation produced by UVR, antioxidants may counteract the damaging effects of UVR.

The preventive effects of orally supplemented Pycnogenol against UVR-induced skin erythema were studied. In addition, the inhibitory effects of Pycnogenol were shown on NF-κB-dependent gene expression, chosen as a marker of proinflammatory response induced in HaCaT cells after UV exposure.

Pycnogenol produced a significant increase in the dose of UVR necessary to achieve standardized erythema response (minimum erythema dose) of human skin. The activation of the proinflammatory transcription factor (NF-κB) plays a major role in the UVR-induced erythema. Pycnogenol inhibited UVR-induced NF-κB-dependent gene expression in a concentration-dependent manner; this may contribute to its antierythema effect [66].

CLINICAL RESEARCH IN OA

EFFICACY DATA

Four clinical studies have been performed in 2007–2008 on 343 patients with OA. The results of the clinical studies show the efficacy of Pycnogenol in patients with OA. They confirm that oxidative stress and inflammatory mediators such as cytokines, PGs, and CRPs play an important role in OA. The antioxidant and anti-inflammatory dietary supplement Pycnogenol may influence the healthy outcome of OA. The results are consistent with the proposed mechanism of action of Pycnogenol, the reduction of inflammation, the global Western Ontario and MacMaster Universities Osteoarthritis Index (WOMAC), and the individual parameters such as pain, stiffness, and mobility indices.

These studies are conducted making objective evaluation of various parameters involved in OA. These are individually reviewed.

A double-blind placebo-controlled clinical study was performed [12] to investigate the efficacy of Pycnogenol in 37 patients of either sex with age range between 25 and 65 years with OA. This was a randomized, parallel group, double-blind, placebo-controlled study. Pycnogenol was supplemented at a dose of 50 mg three times a day or a placebo for 3 months. The effects were evaluated by measuring WOMAC comprising joint pain, stiffness, physical function, and composite. A questionnaire containing a total of 24 visual analog scales (VASs) and frequency of and dosage of use of nonsteroidal anti-inflammatory drugs (NSAIDs) and COX-2 inhibitors was used.

After 2 months of supplementation, significant reduction in WOMAC pain physical function scores and composite WOMAC were observed in the Pycnogenol group compared with the baseline values as well as with the placebo group ($p < 0.05$). In addition, subjects receiving Pycnogenol showed a significant reduction in the monthly intake of NSAIDs and COX-2 inhibitor pills in both number of pills ($p < 0.01$) and number of days (<0.05) compared with baseline, whereas a marked increase in number of days was observed in the placebo group ($p < 0.001$).

At 90 days, supplementation resulted in a relevant improvement of the WOMAC composite index as well as each WOMAC subscale, with exception of stiffness compared with the placebo group ($p < 0.001$). A significant reduction of 43%, 35%, 52%, and 49% in pain, stiffness, physical function subscale, and composite WOMAC score, respectively, was reported in the Pycnogenol group, whereas the placebo group showed no significant changes as compared with the baseline values. Moreover, further reduction in the number of NSAIDs and COX-2 inhibitor pills ($p < 0.001$) and number of days ($p < 0.001$) was noted in the Pycnogenol group compared with the baseline. In contrast, in the placebo group, a significant increase in the number of pills ($p < 0.05$) and number of days ($p < 0.001$) was observed.

To conclude, the results of this randomized, double-blind, placebo-controlled trial with parallel group design indicate the efficacy of Pycnogenol in alleviating OA symptoms and in reducing the need of NSAIDs or COX-2 inhibitor pills in terms of both number of pills and days per month.

Another randomized, double-blind, placebo-controlled clinical study was performed [13] to investigate the efficacy of Pycnogenol in OA. One hundred patients of either sex with an age range between 25 and 65 years with mild OA and corresponding clinical symptoms were included. Pycnogenol was supplemented at a dose of 50 mg three times a day or a placebo for 3 months. The effects were evaluated by measuring WOMAC comprising joint pain, stiffness, and daily activities. VAS scores were also determined. The frequency of and dosage of use of NSAIDs and COX-2 inhibitors was recorded.

- The WOMAC score summarizing the scores of pain improved significantly in the Pycnogenol group ($p < 0.001$). The difference to baseline was statistically significant for the Pycnogenol group after 8, 12, and 14 weeks ($p < 0.001$).
- The WOMAC score summarizing the scores of stiffness improved in the Pycnogenol group versus baseline after 8, 12, and 14 weeks ($p < 0.01$). Statistically significant difference between Pycnogenol and placebo groups was observed at weeks 8 and 12 ($p < 0.05$).
- The WOMAC score summarizing the scores of daily activities improved significantly versus baseline after 8, 12, and 14 weeks ($p < 0.01$).
- The overall WOMAC score summarizing pain, stiffness, and daily activities improved significantly during the time of treatment in the Pycnogenol group versus baseline values after 8 weeks ($p < 005$). Statistically significant difference between Pycnogenol and placebo groups was observed at weeks 6, 8, and 12 ($p < 0.05$). The overall WOMAC score summarizing pain, stiffness, and daily activities of the placebo group was significantly different after weeks 12 and 14 ($p < 0.05$).
- The VAS pain scores were significantly decreased at 8, 12, and 14 weeks. The correlation of pain attenuation with time of treatment was statistically significant ($p < 0.05$), whereas the correlation was poor for placebo ($p = 0.17$).
- Patients in the Pycnogenol group could reduce the intake of analgesics or NSAIDs to a higher percentage (38%) than patients in the placebo group (8%). In contrast, in 10% of the patients in placebo group, the dose of analgesics was increased.

The results of this randomized, double-blind, placebo-controlled trial design indicate the efficacy of Pycnogenol in alleviating OA symptoms and in reducing the need of NSAIDs or COX-2 inhibitor pills. The basis for the observed positive effects of Pycnogenol in OA is the cascade of inhibitory actions by Pycnogenol on inflammation, starting from the inhibition of free radicals to the inhibition of transcription factors and proteases ending with inhibition of cytokines, adhesion factors, and COX-1 and COX-2. It is therefore concluded that Pycnogenol produces beneficial effects in OA because of its antioxidant and anti-inflammatory properties.

Another randomized, double-blind, placebo-controlled clinical study was performed to investigate the efficacy of Pycnogenol in OA [15]. One hundred fifty-six patients of either sex with a mean ± SD age of 48 ± 8 years with OA grade I and II in one or both knees had mild to moderate pain not adequately controlled with inflammatory drugs. Pycnogenol was supplemented at a dose of 50 mg two times a day or a placebo for 3 months. The effects were evaluated by measuring WOMAC comprising joint pain, stiffness, and daily activities. VAS scores were also determined. Frequency of and dosage of use of NSAIDs and COX-2 inhibitors were recorded.

- Scores for pain dropped significantly ($p < 0.05$) after Pycnogenol intake from 17.3 to 7.7; the placebo had no significant effect.
- The scores for stiffness were reduced significantly from 6.6 to 3.1 ($p < 0.05$); scores for the placebo remained unchanged after 3 months.
- The scores for physical function were more than halved; reducing from 55.3 at the start to 23.8 in the verum group ($p < 0.05$), the improvement under placebo was not significant.
- The global WOMAC score decreased after Pycnogenol treatment significantly from 79.2 to 34.6, with the placebo insignificantly from 76.9 to 69.5.
- Negative alterations of social functions by OA decreased significantly in the treatment group ($p > 0.05$) but not in the placebo group.
- The well-being of patients (emotional function) was significantly ($p < 0.05$) enhanced under Pycnogenol treatment; as reflected in scores for emotional function, the placebo produced a marginal improvement.
- In conclusion, all WOMAC scores improved significantly ($p < 0.05$) after 3 months of treatment relative to the start versus the placebo.
- The results of the exercise test on the treadmill demonstrated a convincing increase of performance of patients after the 3-month treatment with Pycnogenol. Patients could walk 68 m as mean distance at start but could go for a mean of 198 m after treatment versus only 65–88 m in the placebo group.
- The use of concomitant medication NSAIDs dropped by 58% in the Pycnogenol group versus 1% in the placebo group ($p < 0.05$).

The results of this randomized, double-blind, placebo-controlled trial design indicate the efficacy of Pycnogenol in alleviating OA symptoms and in reducing the need of NSAID pills. The basis for the observed positive effects of Pycnogenol in OA is the cascade of inhibitory actions by Pycnogenol on inflammation, starting from inhibition of free radicals to inhibition of transcription factors and proteases ending with inhibition of cytokines, adhesion factors, and COX-1 and COX-2. The judgment of patients was supported by the objective test of treadmill performance of patients with OA, showing that patients could walk more than twice the distance after Pycnogenol treatment compared with placebo.

MECHANISMS OF ACTION

It has been shown that Pycnogenol reduces NO production by activated macrophages, inhibits NF-κB-controlled iNOS expression, and lowers radical generation by activated macrophages during their oxidative burst [85]. Pycnogenol and its metabolites are potent inhibitors of MMPs [71].

Lowering of CRP, Free Radicals, and Fibrinogen Levels in Plasma

Elevated CRP levels have been suggested to be associated with disease progression in OA. The above study [14] was followed by reporting the values of biochemical markers (CRP, plasma free radicals, and fibrinogen) in selected 55 patients with OA, 29 treated with Pycnogenol and 26 treated with placebo. These patients had basal CRP levels higher than 3 mg/L. Comparison of blood specimens at baseline and after a 3-month supplementation with Pycnogenol showed that CRP levels were decreased from baseline values 3.9 to 1.1 mg/L (a decrease by 71.3%). Plasma free radicals were decreased by 29.9% and fibrinogen by 37.1%, respectively. In contrast, treatment with placebo had only marginal and nonsignificant effects on all three parameters. The reduction of all three biochemical parameters with Pycnogenol was statistically significant compared with the placebo controls ($p < 0.05$). The decrease of systemic inflammatory biomarkers suggests that Pycnogenol may exert anti-inflammatory activity in OA [15].

Ex Vivo Studies in Healthy Human Volunteers

Inhibition of NF-κB Activation and MMP-9 Secretion [71]

MMPs are matrix degrading enzymes significantly involved in the pathogenesis of OA. Pycnogenol has been shown to display a variety of anti-inflammatory effects *in vivo* [18]. It has been shown to reduce plasma or urine LT concentration in a double-blind, placebo-controlled, clinical study [54]. The aim of this study was to determine whether human plasma after oral intake of Pycnogenol contains sufficient concentration of active principles to inhibit key mediators of inflammation. Blood samples from seven healthy volunteers were obtained before and after 5 days of supplementation with Pycnogenol at a dose of 200 mg/day. Plasma samples significantly inhibited metalloproteinase-9 (MMP-9) release from human monocytes and NF-κB activation ($p < 0.05$). These findings provide evidence of bioavailability of Pycnogenol and support the evidence of its anti-inflammatory activity by inhibiting of proinflammatory gene expression, which is consistent with the documented clinical observations of relief of symptoms in OA.

PGs and LTs exert diverse modulatory roles in OA; PGs and leukotriene B_4 (LTB_4) have been shown to regulate proinflammatory cytokine and interstitial collagenase synthesis in human OA synovial membrane explants. OA osteoblasts produce variable levels of PGE_2 and LTB_4 compared with normal osteoblasts. PGE_2 levels can distinguish two types of patients with OA: osteoblasts from one group produce low levels of PGE_2 and IL-6 and the other shows an increase in production. In contrast, OA osteoblasts that produce high levels of PGE_2 produce low levels of LTB_4 and *vice versa*. This observation could be explained by the selective metabolism of arachidonic acid via the 5-lipoxygenase or COX pathways in OA osteoblasts [5].

Pycnogenol has been shown to display a variety of anti-inflammatory effects *in vivo* [18]. It has been shown to reduce plasma or urine LT concentration in a double-blind, placebo-controlled clinical study [54]. The aim of this study was to determine a possible inhibition of the enzymatic activity of COX-1 and COX-2 by human plasma after oral intake of Pycnogenol. Blood samples from seven healthy volunteers were obtained before and after 5 days of supplementation with Pycnogenol at a dose of 200 mg/day. Plasma samples significantly inhibited both COX-1 and COX-2 activities. In a second approach, 10 volunteers received a single dose of 300 mg of Pycnogenol. Only 30 min after ingestion of Pycnogenol, plasma samples induced a statistically significant inhibition of both COX-1 ($p < 0.02$) and COX-2 ($p < 0.002$) [86]. These findings provide evidence of strikingly rapid bioavailability of bioeffective compounds of Pycnogenol [87]. Pycnogenol was administered to healthy volunteers aged 35–50 years at a daily dose of 150 mg/day for 5 days. Before and after the final day of supplementation, blood was drawn and polymorphonuclear leukocytes were isolated. Polymorphonuclear leukocytes were primed with LPS and stimulated with the receptor-mediated agonist formyl-methionyl-leucil-phenylalanine to activate the arachidonic acid pathway and biosynthesis of LTs, thromboxane, and PGs. Pycnogenol supplementation inhibited 5-lipooxygensae 5-LOX and COX-2 gene expression and PLA2 activity. This effect was associated with a compensatory upregulation of COX-1 gene expression. Interestingly, Pycnogenol suspended the interdependency between 5-LOX and 5-lipoxygenase activating protein expression. Pycnogenol supplementation reduced LT production but did not leave PGs unaltered, which was attributed to the decline in COX-2 activity in favor of COX-1 [88].

Inhibition of MMPs and Free Radical Scavenging Activity of Metabolites of Pycnogenol

As already discussed after intake of Pycnogenol, two major metabolites are formed *in vivo*, δ-(3,4-dihydroxy phenyl)-γ-valerolactone (M1) and δ-(3-methoxy,4-hydroxyphenyl)-γ-valerolactone (M2). On cellular level, highly potent prevention of MMP-9 release was observed by both metabolites with 0.5 µM resulting in 50% inhibition of MMP-9 secretion. M1 was significantly more effective in superoxide scavenging than (+)-catechin, ascorbic acid, and trolox, whereas M2 displayed free radical scavenging activity. Both metabolites exhibited antioxidant activities in a redox-linked colorimetric assay, with M1 being significantly more potent than all other compounds tested in this model. These data contribute to the comprehension of Pycnogenol effect and provide a rationale for its use in prophylaxis and therapy of disorders relating to imbalance or excessive MMP activity such as in OA [71].

IN VIVO STUDIES IN ANIMALS

Antioxidant and Anti-inflammatory Activities

The experiments performed in rats showed that oral Pycnogenol enhances capillary resistance. The genetically induced capillary fragility of spontaneously hypertensive rats was reverted in a dose-dependent manner by oral administration of Pycnogenol 10–100 mg/kg. The effect was evident up to 8 h after oral administration, and it was higher or at least comparable with that observed with higher doses of O-(β-hydroxyethyl)-rutin and hesperidin-methyl-chalcone [89].

Blazso et al. [55] investigated the free radical scavenging activity of Pycnogenol: superoxide anion radicals activity was suppressed ($IC_{50} = 8.18$ μg/mL). In the same study, the anti-inflammatory activity of three different fractions of Pycnogenol was studied in the croton oil–induced ear edema in mice. The in vitro free radical scavenging and in vivo anti-inflammatory activities of Pycnogenol and its fractions were closely correlated ($r = 0.992$), indicating the involvement of free radicals in inflammation and that the anti-inflammatory action of Pycnogenol is related to its free radical scavenging effect.

In a subsequent study, Pycnogenol administered by intraperitoneal route significantly and dose-dependently decreased the carrageenan-induced inflammation in rats. When Pycnogenol was applied topically, a statistically significant and dose-dependent inhibition of UVB-induced erythema in rats was observed [68].

In another study performed and reported by the same group, the anti-inflammatory activity of Pycnogenol was confirmed in croton oil–induced ear edema in mice and compound 48/80–induced paw edema in rats. Pycnogenol was administered orally in liquid diet [69].

IN VITRO STUDIES

Antioxidant Activity and Inhibition of MMP-9 Secretion by Metabolites of Pycnogenol [71]

Pycnogenol has a well-documented antioxidant and anti-inflammatory activity [18]. After oral administration of Pycnogenol, two major metabolites are formed in vivo, δ-(3,4-dihydroxy phenyl)-γ-valerolactone (M1) and δ-(3-methoxy,4-hydroxyphenyl)-γ-valerolactone (M2). These metabolites possess antioxidant activity explaining their contribution to overall antioxidant effect of Pycnogenol. These metabolites have been shown to possess strong inhibitory effects toward the activity of MMP-1, MMP-2, and MMP-9. On the basis of micrograms per milliliter, both metabolites appeared to be more active than Pycnogenol. On a cellular level, highly potent prevention of MMP-9 release was observed in both metabolites, with a concentration of 0.5 μM, resulting in approximately 50% inhibition of MMP-9 secretion. M1 was significantly more effective in superoxide scavenging activity than (+)-catechin, ascorbic acid, and trolox, whereas M2 displayed no scavenging activity. Both metabolites exhibited antioxidant activities in a redox-linked colorimetric assay, with M1 being significantly more potent than all other compounds tested. These findings provide evidence of bioavailability of Pycnogenol and further provide rationale for its reducing the risk of inflammatory disorders such as OA related to imbalance or excessive MMP activity.

The effects of Pycnogenol on gene expression of proinflammatory cytokines IL-1β and IL-2 were investigated in murine cell lines of monocyte-macrophages RAW 264.7 cells and human

T lymphocytes Jurkat E6.1 (ATTCC TIB 152) cells, respectively. Pycnogenol exerted strong free radical scavenging activity against ROS generated by H_2O_2 in RAW 264.7 cells. Pretreatment of LPS (from *Escherichia coli* serotype 0127:B8) LPS-stimulated RAW 264.7 cells with Pycnogenol dose-dependently reduced both the production of IL-1β and its mRNA levels. Furthermore, in the same cells, Pycnogenol blocked the activation of NF-κB and AP-1, two major transcription factors centrally involved in IL-1β gene expression. Concordantly, pretreatment of the cells with Pycnogenol abolished the LPS-induced NK-κB degradation.

Pycnogenol inhibited the phorbol 12-myristate 13-acetate plus ionomycin–induced IL-2 mRNA expression. Pycnogenol inhibited both NF-AT and AP-1 CAT activities in transiently transfected Jurkat E6.1 but not NF-κB CAT activity. Pycnogenol also destabilized the phorbol 12-myristate 13-acetate plus ionomycin–induced IL-2 mRNA by posttranscriptional regulation [90].

The transcriptional regulatory protein NF-κB participates in the control of gene expression of many modulators of inflammatory and immune responses, including VCAM-1 and ICAM-1. The increased expressions of these molecules play a critical role in atherosclerosis and inflammation. Pretreatment with human umbilical vascular endothelial cells with Pycnogenol exhibited a concentration-dependent suppression of TNF-α-induced activation of NF-κB. Induction of VCAM-1 and ICAM-1 surface expression by TNF-α was dose-dependently reduced by Pycnogenol. TNF-α significantly increased the release of superoxide anion and H_2O_2 from human umbilical vascular endothelial cells. Pycnogenol dose-dependently inhibited their release [62]. All these findings support the therapeutic role of Pycnogenol in inflammatory conditions such as OA.

Inhibition of UVR-induced NF-κB-dependent Gene Expression

UVR-induced inflammatory response is one of the prevailing mechanisms involving proinflammatory cytokines and redox-regulated transcription factor NF-κB. NF-κB has been identified as the target biomarker during signal transduction initiated by UVR in human skin [91]. Because the activation of proinflammatory and redox-regulated transcription factor NF-κB is thought to play a major role in UVR-induced erythema, the effect of Pycnogenol was also investigated in human keratinocyte cell line HaCaT. Pycnogenol added to the cell culture medium inhibited UVER-induced NF-κB-dependent gene expression in a concentration-dependent manner [66]. These findings support the cause effect relationship of Pycnogenol in one of the identified biomarkers of OA.

Protection of Vascular Endothelium Against Oxidative Injury

Intact vascular endothelium is of paramount importance to keep capillary integrity and strength inhibiting vascular permeability and thus contributing to antiedema action.

Damage of endothelial cells may lead to increased vascular permeability resulting in edema. In an *in vitro* study, the antioxidant effect of Pycnogenol was investigated using vascular endothelial cells. Confluent monolayer of bovine pulmonary artery endothelial cells (PAECs) were preincubated with different concentrations of Pycnogenol for 16 h, washed, and then exposed to an organic oxidant tBHP for 3 or 4 h. Cellular injury was assessed by measuring cell viability with methylthiazol tetrazolium assay and by determining the release of intracellular LDH. Lipid peroxidation products of PAEC were monitored as MDA with a thiobarbituric acid fluorometric assay. Incubation of tBHP (75, 100, or 125 μM) with PAEC decreased cell viability, increased LDH release, and elevated MDH production. Preincubation of PAEC with Pycnogenol (10–80 μg/mL) before tBHP exposure significantly increased cell viability, decreased LDH release, and reduced MDA production. These results demonstrate that Pycnogenol can protect vascular endothelial cells from oxidant injury. The data thus suggest that Pycnogenol may be useful in conditions associated with oxidative damage [92].

CONCLUSIONS

In conclusion, Pycnogenol maintains or improves knee joint health by reducing the edema and inflammation and by improving the level of surrogate biomarkers of inflammation. Also, no

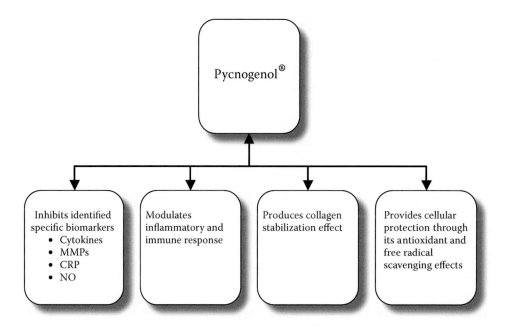

FIGURE 34.1   Proposed mechanisms of action of Pycnogenol in OA.

significant adverse events or toxicities were observed. The proposed mechanisms are shown in Figure 34.1 and are explained as follows:

- Inhibition/lowering of identified biomarkers: Pycnogenol inactivates NF-κB and gene expression of cytokines, inhibits release of MMPs, and decreases CRP levels in plasma.
- Modulation of inflammatory and immune response: Pycnogenol modulates inflammatory and immune responses working through inflammatory mediators including VCAM-1 and ICAM-1. Pycnogenol decreases capillary fragility, reduces vascular permeability, and increases capillary resistance contributing to reduction of inflammation and associated symptoms in OA.
- Protection of vascular endothelium: Pycnogenol protects vascular endothelium against oxidative injury through its antioxidant and/or free radical scavenging effects.
- Collagen stabilizing effect: Pycnogenol inhibits collagen degradation and increases its regeneration. It produces capillary sealing effect through its specific binding capacity with collagen.

REFERENCES

1. Arden N, Nevitt MC. Osteoarthritis: epidemiology. Best Pract Res Clin Rheumatol 2006;20(1):3–25.
2. Brooks P. Inflammation as an important feature of osteoarthritis. Bull World Health Organ 2003;81(9):689–690.
3. Martel-Pelletier J, Alaaeddine N, Pelletier JP. Cytokines and their role in the pathophysiology of osteoarthritis. Front Biosci 1999;4:D694-D703.
4. Fernandes JC, Martel-Pelletier J, Pelletier JP. The role of cytokines in osteoarthritis pathophysiology. Biorheology 2002;39(1–2):237–246.
5. Laufer S. Role of eicosanoids in structural degradation in osteoarthritis. Curr Opin Rheumatol 2003;15(5):623–627.
6. Myers SL, Brandt KD, Ehlich JW, Braunstein EM, Shelbourne KD, Heck DA, Kalasinski LA. Synovial inflammation in patients with early osteoarthritis of the knee. J Rheumatol 1990;17(12):1662–1669.

7. Maritime Pine Extract. United States Pharmacopoeia—National Formulary. Volume USP 30-NF 25. Rockville: United States Pharmacopeia Convention, Inc.; 2007:965–966.

8. Borzelleca JF, Burdock GA, Thomas JA. Opinion of an expert panel on the generally recognized as safe (GRAS) status of French maritime pine bark extract (Pycnogenol®) as a flavoring agent. Internal document; 2003.

9. Rohdewald PJ. Pycnogenol®, French Maritime Pine Bark Extract. Encyclopedia of Dietary Supplements. New York: Marcel Dekker Inc.; 2005:545–553.

10. Drehsen G. From ancient pine bark uses to Pycnogenol. In: Packer L, Hiramatsu M, Yoshikawa T, eds. Antioxidant Food Supplements in Human Health. New York: Academic Press; 1999:311–322.

11. Gulati OP. Pycnogenol®—a nutraceutical for venous health with a particular focus on chronic venous insufficiency. Biomed Rev 2009;19:1–12.

12. Farid R, Mirfeizi Z, Mirheidari M, Rezaieyazdi Z, Mansouri H, Esmaelli H, Zibadi S, Rohdewald P, Watson RR. Pycnogenol supplementation reduces pain and stiffness and improves physical function in adults with knee arthritis. Nutr Res 2007;27:692–697.

13. Cisar P, Jany R, Waczulikova I, Sumegova K, Muchova J, Vojtassak J, Durackova Z, Lisy M, Rohdewald P. Effect of pine bark extract (Pycnogenol®) on symptoms of knee osteoarthritis. Phytother Res 2008;22(8):1087–1092.

14. Belcaro G, Cesarone MR, Errichi S, Zulli C, Errichi BM, Vinciguerra G, Ledda A, et al. Variations in C-reactive protein, plasma free radicals and fibrinogen values in patients with osteoarthritis treated with Pycnogenol. Redox Rep 2008;13(6):271–276.

15. Belcaro G, Cesarone MR, Errichi S, Zulli C, Errichi BM, Vinciguerra G, Ledda A, et al. Treatment of osteoarthritis with Pycnogenol®. The SVOS (San Valentino Osteoarthritis Study). Evaluation of signs, symptoms, physical performance and vascular aspects. Phytother Res 2008;22(4):518–523

16. Gulati OP. The nutraceutical Pycnogenol: its role in cardiovascular health and blood glucose control. Biomed Rev 2005;16:49–57.

17. Gulati OP. Pycnogenol® in venous disorders: a review. Eur Bull Drug Res 1999;7(2):8–13.

18. Rohdewald P. A review of the French maritime pine bark extract (Pycnogenol), a herbal medication with a diverse clinical pharmacology. Int J Clin Pharmacol Ther 2002;40(4):158–168.

19. Blumenthal M. Pycnogenol (French maritime pine bark extract) *Pinus pinaster Aiton* subsp. Atlantica. The American Botanical Council guide to Herbs; 2003:369–373.

20. Poole AR, Billinghurst C, Nelson F. New perspectives in cartilage degeneration in osteoarthritis. Rheumatology in Europe 1995;24:57–65.

21. Damsky CH, Werb Z. Signal transduction by integrin receptors for extracellular matrix: cooperative processing of extracellular information. Curr Opin Cell Biol 1992;4(5):772–781.

22. Schlaepfer DD, Hanks SK, Hunter T, van der Geer P. Integrin-mediated signal transduction linked to Ras pathway by GRB2 binding to focal adhesion kinase. Nature 1994;372(6508):786–791.

23. Tanaka S, Hamanishi C, Kikuchi H, Fukuda K. Factors related to degradation of articular cartilage in osteoarthritis: a review. Semin Arthritis Rheum 1998;27(6):392–399.

24. Pelletier JP, Martel-Pelletier J, Abramson SB. Osteoarthritis, an inflammatory disease: potential implication for the selection of new therapeutic targets. Arthritis Rheum 2001;44(6):1237–1247.

25. Pelletier JP, Martel-Pelletier J, Howell DS. Etiopathogenesis of osteoarthritis. In: W.J. K, ed. Arthritis and allied conditions: a textbook of rheumatology. 14th ed. Baltimore: Williams and Wilkins; 2000:2195–2245.

26. Smith MD, Triantafillou S, Parker A, Youssef PP, Coleman M. Synovial membrane inflammation and cytokine production in patients with early osteoarthritis. J Rheumatol 1997;24(2):365–371.

27. Lohmander LS, Saxne T, Heinegard DK. Release of cartilage oligomeric matrix protein (COMP) into joint fluid after knee injury and in osteoarthritis. Ann Rheum Dis 1994;53(1):8–13.

28. Sharif M, Saxne T, Shepstone L, Kirwan JR, Elson CJ, Heinegard D, Dieppe PA. Relationship between serum cartilage oligomeric matrix protein levels and disease progression in osteoarthritis of the knee joint. Br J Rheumatol 1995;34(4):306–310.

29. Clark AG, Jordan JM, Vilim V, Renner JB, Dragomir AD, Luta G, Kraus VB. Serum cartilage oligomeric matrix protein reflects osteoarthritis presence and severity: the Johnston County Osteoarthritis Project. Arthritis Rheum 1999;42(11):2356–2364.

30. Sharif M, Shepstone L, Elson CJ, Dieppe PA, Kirwan JR. Increased serum C reactive protein may reflect events that precede radiographic progression in osteoarthritis of the knee. Ann Rheum Dis 2000;59(1):71–74.

31. Spector TD, Hart DJ, Nandra D, Doyle DV, Mackillop N, Gallimore JR, Pepys MB. Low-level increases in serum C-reactive protein are present in early osteoarthritis of the knee and predict progressive disease. Arthritis Rheum 1997;40(4):723–727.

32. Goldberg RL, Huff JP, Lenz ME, Glickman P, Katz R, Thonar EJ. Elevated plasma levels of hyaluronate in patients with osteoarthritis and rheumatoid arthritis. Arthritis Rheum 1991;34(7):799–807.

33. van de Loo FA, Joosten LA, van Lent PL, Arntz OJ, van den Berg WB. Role of interleukin-1, tumor necrosis factor alpha, and interleukin-6 in cartilage proteoglycan metabolism and destruction. Effect of in situ blocking in murine antigen- and zymosan-induced arthritis. Arthritis Rheum 1995;38(2):164–172.

34. Plows D, Probert L, Georgopoulos S, Alexopoulou L, Kollias G. The role of tumor necrosis factor (TNF) in arthritis: studies in transgenic mice. Rheumatol Eur 1995;2(Suppl 2):51–54.

35. Brennan FM, Chantry D, Jackson A, Maini R, Feldmann M. Inhibitory effect of TNF alpha antibodies on synovial cell interleukin-1 production in rheumatoid arthritis. Lancet 1989;2(8657):244–247.

36. Joosten LA, Lubberts E, Durez P, Helsen MM, Jacobs MJ, Goldman M, van den Berg WB. Role of interleukin-4 and interleukin-10 in murine collagen-induced arthritis. Protective effect of interleukin-4 and interleukin-10 treatment on cartilage destruction. Arthritis Rheum 1997;40(2):249–260.

37. Caron JP, Fernandes JC, Martel-Pelletier J, Tardif G, Mineau F, Geng C, Pelletier JP. Chondroprotective effect of intraarticular injections of interleukin-1 receptor antagonist in experimental osteoarthritis. Suppression of collagenase-1 expression. Arthritis Rheum 1996;39(9):1535–1544.

38. Martel-Pelletier J, McCollum R, Fujimoto N, Obata K, Cloutier JM, Pelletier JP. Excess of metalloproteases over tissue inhibitor of metalloprotease may contribute to cartilage degradation in osteoarthritis and rheumatoid arthritis. Lab Invest 1994;70(6):807–815.

39. Attur MG, Patel RN, Abramson SB, Amin AR. Interleukin-17 up-regulation of nitric oxide production in human osteoarthritis cartilage. Arthritis Rheum 1997;40(6):1050–1053.

40. Martel-Pelletier J, Tardif G, Fernandes JC, Pelletier JP. Metalloproteases and their modulation as treatment in osteoarthritis. In: Tsokos GC, ed. Principles of molecular rheumatology Totowa, NJ: Humana Press; 2000:499–514.

41. Wu YS, Hu YY, Yang RF, Wang Z, Wei YY. The matrix metalloproteinases as pharmacological target in osteoarthritis: statins may be of therapeutic benefit. Med Hypotheses 2007;69(3):557–559.

42. Mandelbaum B, Waddell D. Etiology and pathophysiology of osteoarthritis. Orthopedics 2005;28(Suppl 2):s207–s214.

43. Belkhiri A, Richards C, Whaley M, McQueen SA, Orr FW. Increased expression of activated matrix metalloproteinase-2 by human endothelial cells after sublethal H_2O_2 exposure. Lab Invest 1997;77(5):533–539.

44. Amin AR, Abramson SB. The role of nitric oxide in articular cartilage breakdown in osteoarthritis. Curr Opin Rheumatol 1998;10(3):263–268.

45. Pelletier JP, Mineau F, Ranger P, Tardif G, Martel-Pelletier J. The increased synthesis of inducible nitric oxide inhibits IL-1ra synthesis by human articular chondrocytes: possible role in osteoarthritic cartilage degradation. Osteoarthritis Cartilage 1996;4(1):77–84.

46. McInnes IB, Leung BP, Field M, Wei XQ, Huang FP, Sturrock RD, Kinninmonth A, Weidner J, Mumford R, Liew FY. Production of nitric oxide in the synovial membrane of rheumatoid and osteoarthritis patients. J Exp Med 1996;184(4):1519–1524.

47. Taskiran D, Stefanovic-Racic M, Georgescu H, Evans C. Nitric oxide mediates suppression of cartilage proteoglycan synthesis by interleukin-1. Biochem Biophys Res Commun 1994;200(1):142–148.

48. Murrell GA, Jang D, Williams RJ. Nitric oxide activates metalloprotease enzymes in articular cartilage. Biochem Biophys Res Commun 1995;206(1):15–21.

49. Pelletier JP, Jovanovic D, Fernandes JC, Manning P, Connor JR, Currie MG, Di Battista JA, Martel-Pelletier J. Reduced progression of experimental osteoarthritis in vivo by selective inhibition of inducible nitric oxide synthase. Arthritis Rheum 1998;41(7):1275–1286.

50. Amin AR, Attur M, Patel RN, Thakker GD, Marshall PJ, Rediske J, Stuchin SA, Patel IR, Abramson SB. Superinduction of cyclooxygenase-2 activity in human osteoarthritis-affected cartilage. Influence of nitric oxide. J Clin Invest 1997;99(6):1231–1237.

51. Virgili F, Kim D, Packer L. Procyanidins extracted from pine bark protect alpha-tocopherol in ECV 304 endothelial cells challenged by activated RAW 264.7 macrophages: role of nitric oxide and peroxynitrite. FEBS Lett 1998;431(3):315–318.

52. Packer L, Rimbach G, Virgili F. Antioxidant activity and biologic properties of a procyanidin-rich extract from pine (*Pinus maritima*) bark, Pycnogenol. Free Radic Biol Med 1999;27(5/6):704–724.

53. Virgili F, Kobuchi H, Noda Y, Cossins E, Packer L. Procyanidins from *Pinus maritima* bark: antioxidant activity, effects on the immune system and modulation of nitrogen monoxide metabolism. In: Packer L, Hiramatsu M, Yoshikawa T, eds. Antioxidant Food Supplements in Human Health. New York: Academic Press; 1999:323–342.

54. Lau BHS, Riesen SK, Truong KP, Lau EW, Rohdewald P, Barreta RA. Pycnogenol® as an adjunct in the management of childhood asthma. J Asthma 2004;41(8):825–832.

55. Blazso G, Gabor M, Sibbel R, Rohdewald P. Anti-inflammatory and superoxide radical scavenging activities of procyanidins containing extract from the bark of *Pinus pinaster* sol. and its fractions. Pharm Pharmacol Lett 1994;3:217–220.

56. Rong Y, Li L, Shah V, Lau BH. Pycnogenol protects vascular endothelial cells from t-butyl hydroperoxide induced oxidant injury. Biotechnol Ther 1995;5(3–4):117–126.

57. Noda Y, Anzai K, Mori A, Kohno M, Shinmei M, Packer L. Hydroxyl and superoxide anion radical scavenging activities of natural source antioxidants using the computerized JES-FR30 ESR spectrometer system. Biochem Mol Biol Int 1997;42(1):35–44.

58. Nelson AB, Lau BH, Ide N, Rong Y. Pycnogenol inhibits macrophage oxidative burst, lipoprotein oxidation, and hydroxyl radical-induced DNA damage. Drug Dev Ind Pharm 1998;24(2):139–144.

59. Chida M, Suzuki K, Nakanishi-Ueda T, Ueda T, Yasuhara H, Koide R, Armstrong D. In vitro testing of antioxidants and biochemical end-points in bovine retinal tissue. Ophthalmic Res 1999;31(6):407–415.

60. Cossins E, Lee R, Packer L. ESR studies of vitamin C regeneration, order of reactivity of natural source phytochemical preparations. Biochem Mol Biol Int 1998;45(3):583–597.

61. Kim J CJ, Pinnas JL, Mooradian AD. Effect of selected antioxidants on malondialdehyde modification of proteins. Nutrition 2000;16:1079–1081.

62. Peng Q, Wei Z, Lau BH. Pycnogenol inhibits tumor necrosis factor-alpha-induced nuclear factor kappa B activation and adhesion molecule expression in human vascular endothelial cells. Cell Mol Life Sci 2000;57(5):834–841.

63. Sharma SC, Sharma S, Gulati OP. Pycnogenol prevents haemolytic injury in G6PD deficient human erythrocytes. Phytother Res 2003;17(6):671–674.

64. Bayeta E BM, Lau HS. Pycnogenol inhibits generation of inflammatory mediators in macrophages. Nutr Res 2000;20(2):249–259.

65. Wei ZH, Peng Q, Lau B. Pycnogenol enhances endothelial cell antioxidant defenses. Redox Rep 1997;3(4):219–224.

66. Saliou C, Rimbach G, Moini H, McLaughlin L, Hosseini S, Lee J, Watson RR, Packer L. Solar ultraviolet-induced erythema in human skin and nuclear factor-kappa-B-dependent gene expression in keratinocytes are modulated by a French maritime pine bark extract. Free Radic Biol Med 2001;30(2):154–160.

67. Sime S, Reeve VE. Protection from inflammation, immunosuppression and carcinogenesis induced by UV radiation in mice by topical Pycnogenol. Photochem Photobiol 2004;79(2):193–198.

68. Blazso G, Rohdewald P, Sibbel R, Gabor M. Anti-inflammatory activities of procyanidin-containing extracts from *Pinus pinaster* sol. In: Antus S, Gabor M, Vetschera K, eds. Proc Int Bioflavonoid Symp. Budapest, Hungary: Akademieai Kiado; 1995 July 16–19:231–238.

69. Blazso G, Gabor M, Rohdewald P. Anti-inflammatory activities of procyanidin-containing extracts from *Pinus pinaster* Ait. after oral and cutaneous application. Pharmazie 1997;52(5):380–382.

70. Cho KJ, Yun CH, Packer L, Chung AS. Inhibition mechanisms of bioflavonoids extracted from the bark of *Pinus maritima* on the expression of proinflammatory cytokines. Ann N Y Acad Sci 2001;928:141–156.

71. Grimm T, Schafer A, Hogger P. Antioxidant activity and inhibition of matrix metalloproteinases by metabolites of maritime pine bark extract (Pycnogenol). Free Radic Biol Med 2004;36(6):811–822.

72. Sharma SC, Sharma S, Gulati OP. Pycnogenol inhibits the release of histamine from mast cells. Phytother Res 2003;17(1):66–69.

73. Blazso G, Gabor M, Schonlau F, Rohdewald P. Pycnogenol accelerates wound healing and reduces scar formation. Phytother Res 2004;18(7):579–581.

74. Belcaro G, Cesarone MR, Errichi BM, Ledda A, Di Renzo A, Stuard S, Dugall M, et al. Venous ulcers: microcirculatory improvement and faster healing with local use of Pycnogenol. Angiology 2005;56(6):699–705.

75. Maritim A, Dene BA, Sanders RA, Watkins JB, 3rd. Effects of Pycnogenol treatment on oxidative stress in streptozotocin-induced diabetic rats. J Biochem Mol Toxicol 2003;17(3):193–199.

76. Berryman AM, Maritim AC, Sanders RA, Watkins JB, 3rd. Influence of treatment of diabetic rats with combinations of Pycnogenol, beta-carotene, and alpha-lipoic acid on parameters of oxidative stress. J Biochem Mol Toxicol 2004;18(6):345–352.

77. Dene BA, Maritim AC, Sanders RA, Watkins JB, 3rd. Effects of antioxidant treatment on normal and diabetic rat retinal enzyme activities. J Ocul Pharmacol Ther 2005;21(1):28–35.

78. Devaraj S, Vega-Lopez S, Kaul N, Schonlau F, Rohdewald P, Jialal I. Supplementation with a pine bark extract rich in polyphenols increases plasma antioxidant capacity and alters the plasma lipoprotein profile. Lipids 2002;37(10):931–934.

79. Durackova Z, Trebaticky B, Novotny V, Zitnanova I, Breza J. Lipid metabolism and erectile function improvement by Pycnogenol®, extract from the bark of *Pinus pinaster* in patients suffering from erectile dysfunction—a pilot study. Nutr Res 2003;23:1189–1198.

80. Segger D, Schonlau F. Supplementation with Evelle improves skin smoothness and elasticity in a double-blind, placebo-controlled study with 62 women. J Dermatolog Treat 2004;15(4):222–226.

81. Ni Z, Mu Y, Gulati O. Treatment of melasma with Pycnogenol. Phytother Res 2002;16(6):567–571.

82. Roseff SJ. Improvement in sperm quality and function with French maritime pine tree bark extract. J Reprod Med 2002;47(10):821–824.

83. Kohama T, Suzuki N, Ohno S, Inoue M. Analgesic efficacy of French maritime pine bark extract in dysmenorrhea: an open clinical trial. J Reprod Med 2004;49(10):828–832.

84. Kimbrough C, Chun M, Dela Roca G, Lau BHS. Pycnogenol® chewing gum minimizes gingival bleeding and plaque formation. Phytomedicine 2002;9:410–413.

85. Bayeta E, Lau BHS. Pycnogenol inhibits generation of inflammatory mediators in macrophages. Nutr Res 2000;20(2):249–259.

86. Grimm T, Skrabala R, Chovanova Z, Muchova J, Sumegova K, Liptakova A, Durackova Z, Högger P. Single and multiple dose pharmacokinetics of maritime pine bark extract (Pycnogenol) after oral administration to healthy volunteers. BMC Clin Pharmacol 2006;6(4).

87. Schafer A, Chovanova Z, Muchova J, Sumegova K, Liptakova A, Durackova Z, Hogger P. Inhibition of COX-1 and COX-2 activity by plasma of human volunteers after ingestion of French maritime pine bark extract (Pycnogenol). Biomed Pharmacother 2005;60(1):5–9.

88. Canali R, Comitato R, Schonlau F, Virgili F. The anti-inflammatory pharmacology of Pycnogenol (R) in humans involves COX-2 and 5-LOX mRNA expression in leukocytes. Int Immunopharmacol 2009; 9:1145–1149. doi:10.1016/j.intimp.2009.06.001.

89. Gabor M, Engi E, Sonkodi S. Die Kapillarwandresistenz und ihre Beeinflussung durch wasserlösliche Flavonderivate bei spontan hypertonischen Ratten. Phlebologie 1993;22:178–182.

90. Cho KJ, Yun CH, Yoon DY, Cho YS, Rimbach G, Packer L, Chung AS. Effect of bioflavonoids extracted from the bark of *Pinus maritima* on proinflammatory cytokine interleukin-1 production in lipopolysaccharide-stimulated RAW 264.7. Toxicol Appl Pharmacol 2000;168(1):64–71.

91. Flohe L, Brigelius-Flohe R, Saliou C, Traber MG, Packer L. Redox regulation of NF-kappa B activation. Free Radic Biol Med 1997;22(6):1115–1126.

92. Rong Y, Li L, Shah V, Lau BH. Pycnogenol protects vascular endothelial cells from t-butyl hydroperoxide induced oxidant injury. Biotechnol Ther 1994–1995;5(3–4):117–126.

Section V

Orthopedic Approach

35 Total Knee Arthroplasty for Osteoarthritis

Shuichi Matsuda, Hiromasa Miura, and Yukihide Iwamoto

CONTENTS

The process of knee arthroplasty began its evolution in the 1960s. At that time, problems were early failures as a result of component loosening, infection, and metal synovitis. After modifications of design and implant materials, excellent long-term results were reported from late 1980s. Currently, predictable and sustainable pain relief and functional improvement are obtainable after total knee arthroplasty in more than 90% of patients for 10–15 years postoperatively [1]. The incidence of total knee arthroplasty varies between and within countries. More than 400,000 total knee arthroplasties are annually performed in the United States, and approximately 60,000 surgeries are done each year in Japan.

SURGICAL INDICATION

The primary indication for total knee arthroplasty is to relieve pain caused by severe arthritis in elder patients (usually older than 60 years). It should be considered when conservative treatments have been exhausted. The pain should be significant and disabling. Correction of significant contracture is rarely used as the primary indication for surgery because we cannot expect full range of motion after total knee arthroplasty. Radiographic findings must correlate with the clinical symptoms of knee arthritis (Figure 35.1).

IMPLANT DESIGN AND MATERIAL

In total knee arthroplasty, damaged articular cartilage and subchondral bone are removed and the joint surface is resurfaced with the implant (7–12 mm thickness). Design of the femoral component is largely replicating the anatomic profile of the femur, but the shape of the tibial component is slightly different to achieve knee stability because both menisci and anterior cruciate ligament are removed during surgery (Figure 35.2). In case of sacrificing the posterior cruciate ligament, many

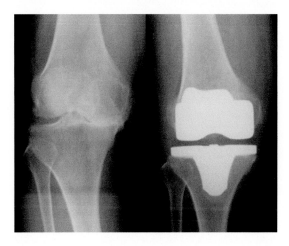

FIGURE 35.1   Preoperative (left) and postoperative (right) x-ray.

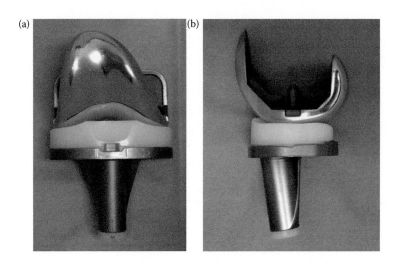

FIGURE 35.2   (a) Anterior view and (b) lateral view of a standard knee prosthesis.

knee prostheses have post-cam mechanism at the center of the knee joint to substitute function of the posterior cruciate ligament (Figure 35.3).

Cobalt chromium has been the material of choice as a bearing surface for the femoral component. Many prosthetic designs use modular tibial component that has polyethylene tibial insert and metal tibial tray (Figure 35.2). This modularity theoretically gives better stress distribution to bone–implant interface and allows surgeons to easily change the thickness of the tibial component during surgery. Tibial tray is made from cobalt chromium or titanium alloy.

SURGICAL TECHNIQUE

A standard skin incision is straight and about 10–15 cm long. A medial parapatellar arthrotomy (or subvastus, midvastus, or lateral parapatellar) is used to expose the knee joint (Figure 35.4). The distal femur and the proximal tibia are resected (Figures 35.5 and 35.6) using an intramedullary or extramedullary cutting guide so that the resected surface is perpendicular to the mechanical axis of the lower extremity (a line connecting the center of the hip joint and the center of the ankle joint)

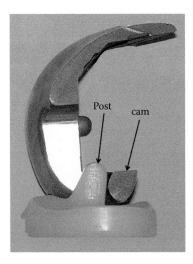

FIGURE 35.3 Sagittal view of the femoral component and polyethylene insert for posterior cruciate ligament-sacrificed total knee arthroplasty.

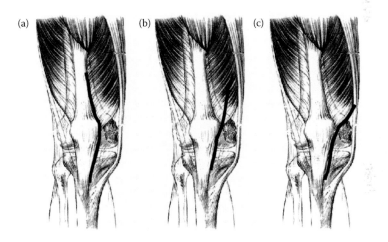

FIGURE 35.4 Surgical approach to the knee joint. (a) Parapatellar approach, (b) midvastus approach, and (c) subvastus approach.

(Figure 35.7). The anterior and posterior part of the femur was resected adjusting the anteroposterior dimension of the femur and the implant. The patella is resurfaced (Figure 35.8) or unresurfaced. Ligament balancing is performed after placement of trial component. Adequate joint gap should be achieved by releasing contracted structure and by adjusting thickness of tibial component. The components are fixed with cement or cementless manner. The cementless component has porous coating of the implant for bone ingrowth. Then the joint capsule and the skin are closed.

REHABILITATION

After surgery, the knee is placed in a continuous passive motion machine to maintain range of motion of the knee. This is started on the first or second day after surgery. Weight-bearing rehabilitation is started on the second or third day after surgery but protected with crutches or a walker.

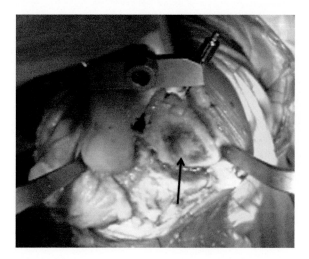

FIGURE 35.5   Distal femur is cut with bone saw. Articular cartilage is severely worn and subchondral bone is exposed at the medial femoral condyle (arrow).

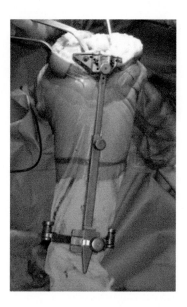

FIGURE 35.6   The proximal tibia is prepared to be cut with an extramedullary guide.

COMPLICATION

Most patients who undergo primary total knee arthroplasty achieve marked pain relief and improvement of function. A small percentage has continued pain, stiffness, or instability. The patients might have revision surgery because of loosening of the implants, wear of polyethylene, or instability of the knee joint. The estimated revision rate is less than 10% at 10 years after surgery. Many studies supported that proper surgical technique such as alignment or ligament balancing is important to decrease mechanical failure of the implant. Infection is another serious complication in total knee arthroplasty. The prevalence of deep infection after TKA is about 1%–2% [2].

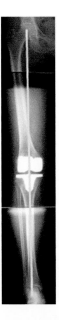

FIGURE 35.7   Postoperative full-length leg x-ray. The mechanical axis passes center of the knee joint.

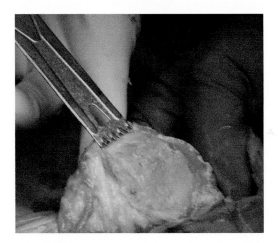

FIGURE 35.8   The patella is cut with an oscillating saw.

CURRENT TOPICS

POSTOPERATIVE ALIGNMENT AND COMPUTER-ASSISTED SURGERY

The clinical success of total knee arthroplasty depends on many factors, including the preoperative condition of the patient, the design and materials of the components, and the surgical techniques. It is important to position the femoral and tibial components accurately. Malpositioning of the component can lead to failures because of aseptic loosening, instability, polyethylene wear, and dislocation of the patella. Various surgical techniques and systems of instrumentation have been devised to obtain optimal postoperative alignment of the components. In the coronal plane, it is recommended that the femoral and tibial components be positioned with less than 3° of error, but such placement can only be achieved in 70%–80% of patients using intra- or extramedullary alignment guides.

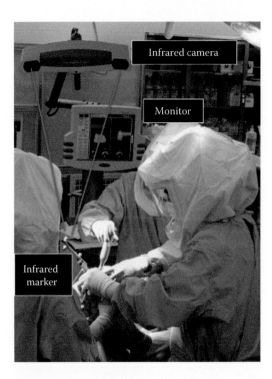

FIGURE 35.9   Computer-assisted total knee arthroplasty. Surgeon adjusts the position of the cutting guide according to information displayed on the monitor.

To improve postoperative alignment, navigation systems have been developed for total knee arthroplasty (Figure 35.9). Many clinical and experimental studies of these systems have shown that the accuracy of implanted components can be improved in spite of the increase in costs and operating time. With CT-based or image-free systems, more than 90% of the operated knees achieved alignment of the mechanical axis of the leg within 3° of neutral [3]. It is expected that the use of navigation would decrease wear problems and mechanical loosening by improved postoperative alignment.

Minimally Invasive Surgery

Although the long-term results have been excellent in standard total knee arthroplasty, recovery from the surgery is often long and painful for patients. The concept of minimally invasive total knee arthroplasty surgery evolved to reduce quadriceps muscle strength loss and to improve clinical outcome after total knee arthroplasty. The increasing interest in minimally invasive surgery among patients and orthopedic surgeons has been a driving force in the development of minimally invasive total knee arthroplasty. This surgery is less invasive for the extensor mechanism with minimal disruption of the quadriceps muscle and is performed without eversion of the patella. Minimally invasive surgery that avoids incision into the quadriceps tendon or the vastus medialis is reported to result in less pain postoperatively, a greater range of motion, and a shorter length of hospital stay than a standard total knee arthroplasty. Also, a mini-midvastus approach has been reported to lead to earlier improvement of range of motion and higher Knee Society scores than a standard technique. These reports suggest that techniques that avoid disruption of the extensor mechanism and eversion of the patella result in a more rapid recovery of knee function compared with traditional total knee arthroplasty exposures [4]. This technique leads to reduced access to surgical landmarks, and the average surgical time for minimally invasive technique is longer than for the standard technique, especially in early stage. A substantial learning curve may be required [5].

REFERENCES

1. Scott RD. Total Knee Arthroplasty. Philadelphia: Elsevier; 2006.
2. Wilson MG, Kelley K, Thornhill TS. Infection as a complication of total knee-replacement arthroplasty: risk factors and treatment in sixty-seven cases. J Bone Joint Surg Am 1990;72:878–883.
3. Mizu-uchi H, Matsuda S, Miura H, Okazaki K, Akasaki Y, Iwamoto Y. The evaluation of post-operative alignment in total knee replacement using a CT-based navigation system. J Bone Joint Surg Br 2008;90:1025–1031.
4. Tashiro Y, Miura H, Matsuda S, Okazaki K, Iwamoto Y. Minimally invasive versus standard approach in total knee arthroplasty. Clin Orthop Relat Res 2007;463:144–150.
5. King J, Stamper DL, Schaad DC, Leopold SS. Minimally invasive total knee arthroplasty compared with traditional total knee arthroplasty. Assessment of the learning curve and the postoperative recuperative period. J Bone Joint Surg Am 2007;89:1497–1503.

Section VI

Nonpharmacologic Interventions

36 Physical Exercise for Osteoarthritis of the Knee

Main Modality of Treatment and Possible Use for Prevention

Hisashi Kurosawa

CONTENTS

INTRODUCTION

Osteoarthritis (OA) of the knee is the most common source of morbidity, disability, and loss of function in elderly people. Knee OA causes knee pain, which limits daily activities such as getting in and out of chairs, walking comfortably, climbing stairs, performing personal care and household tasks, shopping, and doing errands in people older than 65 years old [1]. The resulting inactivity leads to physical deconditioning and may play an indirect role in the development of common chronic comorbidities (obesity, hypertension, cardiovascular and respiratory diseases, diabetes, depression, etc.) [2]. The large number of patients with knee OA results in significant health care expenditures [3, 4] and a socioeconomic burden [5] on society.

Disability caused by knee OA is influenced by a number of factors, many of which can be modified by exercise, which has an effect on strength, flexibility, body equilibrium, joint sense, endurance, cardiovascular fitness, respiratory function, obesity, and pain. For this reason, exercise for OA in the elderly has been intensively studied since the mid-1990s as a therapeutic measure primarily for pain and decreased function of the joint and secondarily for improvement of physical deconditioning and comorbidities.

In this article, the author intends to confirm the efficacy of exercise for knee OA by briefly reviewing preceding papers and considering how exercise reduces knee pain. He also considers the possibility of exercise as a preventive measure against progression of OA.

EFFICACY OF THERAPEUTIC EXERCISE FOR KNEE OA

Therapeutic measures for OA of the knee include pharmacological, nonpharmacological, and surgical measures. The primary complaint of knee OA patients is pain, which causes difficulty in getting in and out of chairs, walking, climbing up- and downstairs, going out of the home, and participating in social activities. For this reason, painkiller modalities have always been sought by patients. Acetaminophen or nonsteroidal anti-inflammatory drugs (NSAIDs) are the main drugs used to reduce pain from knee OA with or without other accompanying treatment measures. These drugs are used orally or topically, and oral use results in quick and effective pain reduction. However, long and continuous usage may lead to adverse effects on the stomach, kidney, or liver. Today, oral use is advised to be short and intermittent, and topical use of NSAIDs is a good substitute for a long-term use [6, 7]. Various nonpharmacological modalities have been used, including physical therapy, patient education, social support, psychoeducational therapy, irrigation of the joint, and surgical approaches. Among them, knowledge of and treatment with physical exercise has increased greatly during the past decade.

Physical exercise as a therapeutic measure for knee OA has been proven to be effective in reducing pain and disability in many randomized controlled trials (RCTs) performed since the mid-1990s. Some advantages over other therapeutic modalities can be expected from exercise. By continuing physical exercise, muscle strength and physical fitness can be increased in elderly people, who would otherwise become more weaker and frailer. Further, good effects on the depressed psychological state of arthritic patients have been observed [8, 9]. Recent guidelines for management of knee OA [6, 7] suggest that nonpharmacological treatment modalities, especially therapeutic physical exercise, should be applied as the treatments of choice.

In this section, reports on recent trials examining the effects of therapeutic physical exercise for OA of the knee are briefly reviewed, and the current status and limitations of exercise among the various therapeutic modalities are discussed.

EFFICACY OF EXERCISE ON KNEE OA

Since a report by Ettinger et al. in 1997 [10], the results of many RCTs on exercise for knee OA have been published. All have shown that exercise was effective in alleviating pain and functional impairment caused by knee OA, irrespective of the modalities adopted (Table 36.1).

Modality and Method of Exercise

Many trials have used aerobic exercise, such as walking [10, 12, 19, 25, 30, 31, 40, 49, 51] or cycling on cycle ergometers [22]. Muscle strengthening or resistance exercise was adopted in many trials, most of which used various types of isotonic muscle exercise or isometric exercise [10, 17, 20, 21, 25, 28, 29, 31, 33–36, 40]. Other studies reported use of training machines for isotonic or isokinetic exercise [15, 23, 36, 50]. Most of the therapeutic exercises described earlier were an assortment of multiple modes of exercise, for example, trunk and lower extremities, extensor and flexor muscles of the knee, or aerobic and anaerobic exercise. In this context, trials in which the effects of only one mode of muscle exercise, straight leg raising (SLR) exercise, were examined were unique and significant [11, 27, 54]. Exercise in water is popular in arthritic patients, and a few studies tried to compare the efficacy of land and aquatic exercise [49, 51].

In many of the trials, exercise was performed regularly at hospitals or other institutions under the supervision of physical therapists or fitness specialists [12, 15, 22–26, 29–31, 36].

There are some reports in which physical therapists regularly performed or guided the therapy of individual patients [20, 24, 26, 29]. There have also been many trials in which patients performed daily exercise at home after practice under physical therapists at hospitals [11, 13, 19, 21, 27, 28,

TABLE 36.1
Literature on Therapeutic Exercise for Knee OA

Year	Author	Trial	Time	Number of Participants	Method
1991	Shimizu et al. [11]	RCT	12 weeks	79	Compr SLR EX with NSAID cream. Assessed by the JOA score
1992	Kover et al. [12]	RCT	8 weeks	102	Compr walking directed by PT with health education. Assessed by the AIMS
1994	Fisher et al. [13]		12 weeks	9	
1995	Madsen et al. [14]	CCS		46	Measured quadriceps strength EX of 20 patients with knee OA
1996	Schilke et al. [15]	RCT	8 weeks	24	Compr maximal isokinetic EX of knee with control. Assessed by the 50-min walk time, muscle strength, Osteoarthritis Screening Index, and AIMS
1997	Slemenda et al. [16]	TS		462	Examine relationship between isokinetic strength EX of knee and presence of OA in community dwellers older than 65 years
	Ettinger [10]	RCT	18 months	439	Compr resistance EX, aerobic EX with health education. Assessed by the self-administered disability questionnaire
1998	O'Reilly et al. [17]	TS		600	Compr isometric strength EX of knee, disability in activities of daily living, and psychological status of patients with knee OA with control
	Rogind et al. [18]	RCT	3 months	25	Examine effect of balance, coordination, stretching, and isometric and isotonic muscle EX at 2/week on AFI, pain scale, and walking speed
	Toda et al. [19]	CCS	6 weeks	22	Examine effect of diet, appetite-suppression drug, and walking EX on body weight, fat rate, and Lequesne scale
	van Baar et al. [20]	RCT	12 weeks	201	Compr strength, motion, and coordination EX directed by PT with ordinary therapy by a home physician. Assessed by the pain and NSAID used
1999	O'Reilly et al. [21]	RCT	6 months	191	Compr isometric and isotonic EX with control. Assessed by the WOMAC and pain VAS
	Mangione et al. [22]	RCT	10 weeks	39	Compr high- with low-intensity cycle ergometer EX. Assessed by the AIMS, 6-min walking test, etc.
2000	Maurer et al. [23]	RCT	8 weeks	113	Compr isokinetic EX with health education. Assessed by the muscle strength test, VAS for pain and function, WOMAC, and SF-36
	Deyle et al. [24]	RCT	4 weeks	125	Compr manual therapy by PT and isometric and isotonic EX with low-dose US as control. Assessed by the 6-min walking test and WOMAC

continued

TABLE 36.1 (continued)
Literature on Therapeutic Exercise for Knee OA

Year	Author	Trial	Time	Number of Participants	Method
	Messier et al. [25]	RCT	24 weeks	24	Compr EX with EX + D. EX composed of isometric and isotonic EX of lower limb and upper body and walking. Assessed by the 6-min. walking test, etc.
	Hopman-Rock and Westhoff [26]	RCT	6 weeks	105	Compr EX of lower limb supervised by PT at 1/week with control. Assessed by pain, quality of life, BMI, activity scale, etc.
	Sakuraba et al. [27]	RCT	12 weeks	119	Compr SLR with stretching EX. Assessed by the JOA score and VAS for pain
	Petrella and Bartha [28]	RCT	8 weeks	177	Compr stretching, isometric, and isotonic EX having NSAID with NSAID alone. Assessed by the WOMAC, VAS for pain, and functional tests
2001	Fransen et al. [29]	RCT	8 weeks	126	Comp individual isometric and isotonic EX and cycle ergometer EX with the same EX in group. Assessed by the WOMAC, SF-36, and muscle and functional tests
	Halbert et al. [30]	RCT	12 months	299	Compr aerobic EX at 3/week or more with ordinary therapy. Assessed by frequency and time of walking, and symptom scores
	Penninx et al. [31]	RCT	3 months	250	Compr aerobic and isotonic EX of whole body at 3/week with control. Assessed by the ability in activities of daily living
	Mannienen et al. [32]	CCS	12 months	805	Examine activity between patients who have undergone TKR and control. Assessed by frequency and intensity of physical activities
	Baker et al. [33]	RCT	4 months	46	Compr H-EX of squat, step-up, and isotonic EX of lower limb with nutrition education. Assessed by the WOMAC and muscle test
2002	Topp et al. [34]	RCT	16 weeks	102	Compr isometric and isotonic EX with control. Assessed by the pain VAS and WOMAC
	Thomas et al. [35]	RCT	2 years	786	Compr among H-EX, H-EX + regular telephone call, telephone alone, and control. Assessed by the WOMAC, SF-36, and psychological and muscle tests
2003	Huang et al. [36]	RCT	8 weeks	132	Compr among isokinetic, isometric, isotonic, and control. Assessed by a dynamometer, VAS and Lequesne index
2004	McCarthy et al. [37]	RCT	8 weeks	214	Compr H-EX and H-EX with regular EX class. Assessed by the WOMAC and aggregated locomotor function
	Messier et al. [38]		18 months	316	Compr EX, D, EX + D, and healthy life as control. Assessed by the WOMAC, body weight, functional tests, and JSW on x-ray
	Rvaud et al. [39]	RCT	24 weeks	867	Compr regular assessment (RA), H-EX with video (EX), RA + EX, and ordinary treatment. Assessed by the WOMAC and VAS
2005	Kurosawa [40]	RCT	12 weeks	59	Compr isotonic extensor EX and walking. Assessed by the JOA, WOMAC, VAS, TUG, and self-paced walking test

TABLE 36.1 (continued)
Literature on Therapeutic Exercise for Knee OA

Year	Author	Trial	Time	Number of Participants	Method
	Focht et al. [41]	RCT	18 months	316	Compr H-EX after a 3-min EX class, D, D + EX and control. Assessed by the functional tests
	Thomas et al. [42]	RCT	2 years	759	Compr H-EX, H-EX + regular TC, TC alone, and control on overweight participants. Assessed by the WOMAC and fee used
2006	Kurosawa et al. [43]	CS	7 years	213	Examine survival rate of H-EX on outpatients who were instructed H-EX. Assessed by the life time table analysis
	Karatosum et al. [44]	RCT	18 months	105	Compr H-EX after EX class and three HA injections. Assessed by the Hospital for Special Surgery score
2007	Messier et al. [45]	RCT	12 months	89	First 6 months, GC and PLC group; second 6 months, GC + EX and PLC + EX. Assessed by the WOMAC, 6-min walking test, and muscle test
	Hurley et al. [46]	RCT	2 years	418	OT, OT + individual H-EX, and EX class. Assessed by the WOMAC
	Thornstensson et al. [47]	CCS	8 weeks	13	Measured varus moment during walking after 8 weeks of muscle strength, CKC, and neurocoordination EX
2008	Kawasaki et al. [48]	RCT	18 months	142	Compr H-EX, H-EX + glucosamine, and H-EX + risedronate. Assessed by the WOMAC, JOA score, and VAS
	Lund et al. [49]	RCT	8 weeks	79	Compr land EX and water EX of muscle strength and endurance. Assessed by the Knee Injury and Osteoarthritis Outcome Score, standing balance test, and muscle strength test
	Jan et al. [50]	RCT	8 weeks	102	Compr high-load (60% 1RM) and low-load (10% 1RM) leg press EX. Assessed by the WOMAC, walk test, and muscle strength test
	Silva et al. [51]	RCT	18 weeks	64	Compr land and water EX. Assessed by the VAS, WOMAC, and functional tests
	Lim et al. [52]	TS		107	Examine relationship between varus moment during walking and WOMAC, functional tests, and muscle strength test
	Lim et al. [53]	RCT	12 weeks	107	Assessed varus moment during walking in H-EX and control group
	Doi et al. [54]	RCT	8 weeks	142	Compr SLR EX and NSAID. Assessed by the JKOM, WOMAC, SF-36, and VAS
	Chua et al. [55]	RCT	18 months	193	Compr EX, D, EX + D, and control. Assessed by the serum cartilage oligometric matrix protein, HA, AgKS, and transforming growth factor β

Abbreviations: AFI, Algofunctional Index; AgKS, antigenic keratin sulfate; CKC, closed kinetic chain; Compr, compared; D, diet; EX, exercise; GC, glucosamine + chondroitin; H-EX, home exercise; OT, ordinary treatment; PLC, placebo; PT, physical therapist; TC, telephone contact; TKR, total knee replacement; TUG, timed up and go test; US, ultrasound.

33, 35, 37, 38]. Differences in the efficacy of home exercise and regular class exercise class were compared in a few trials [37, 46].

In a study by McCarthy et al. [37], 214 patients were randomly allocated to either home exercise or home supplemented with class-based exercise programs. Patients from the class-based group demonstrated significantly greater improvement in locomotor function and greater decrease in walking pain than the home-based group at the 12-month follow-up. However, Hurley et al. [46] reported that improvements because of exercise were similar whether participants received individual rehabilitation or group rehabilitation.

Methods to Evaluate Efficacy

For the evaluation of disease activity or progression or the effects of therapeutic intervention on a disease, some type of marker in the body fluid is usually used.

Changes in such markers are often simple, objective, and reliable indicators of disease status. For OA, a major problem is that such a marker does not currently exist. Serum cartilage oligometric matrix protein [56, 57], serum hyaluronate (HA) [58, 59], or urinary cross-linked telopeptide of type II collagen [59, 60] have been proposed as candidate markers; however, none of them are recognized as reliable and practical markers. Against this background, the effects of intervention on knee OA have usually been assessed by patient self-assessment. The following surveys have been used as primary outcome measures in RCTs for knee OA: Osteoarthritis Screening Index [15], Western Ontario and McMaster Universities Osteoarthritis Index (WOMAC) [61], AIMS [62], MOS Short-Form 36-Item Health Survey (SF-36) [63], Lequesne indices [64], Knee Injury and Osteoarthritis Outcome Score [65], Japanese Knee Osteoarthritis Measure (JKOM) [66], and Physical Activity Scale in Elderly [67]. These are self-administered questionnaires that take 10–15 min to complete. For assessment of pain, most of the trials have used the Visual Analog Scale (VAS), in which patients indicate their actual pain level using a 100-mm straight line as a scale.

As a secondary outcome measure, many studies used muscle strength measurement [11, 12, 18, 26, 29, 33, 35, 50]. Other functional tests, such as a self-paced walking test [28, 68], a 6-min walking test [10, 12, 22, 24], a self-paced stepping test [20], and a timed up-and-go test [28, 40, 69], have also been used as secondary or adjunctive assessment tools. Aggregated locomotor function is compounded with an 8-min walking test, a climbing- and descending-stair test, and the time to stand up from a chair [37]. Change in varus moment at the knee on walking was also used to assess intervention [47, 53].

Review of Exercise Trials

In the 1990s, many reports of RCTs were published on the effects of physical exercise on knee OA (Table 36.1). Almost all of the studies reported some beneficial effects on knee pain and disabilities, and none described negative results although the methods of assessment were diverse, as described earlier. The efficacy of therapeutic exercise on knee OA shown in these reports will be briefly discussed.

In 1991, Shimizu et al. [11] examined 79 knee OA patients for the efficacy of SLR exercise relative to a control group treated with topical indomethacin. After 4 weeks, the score for knee OA on the Japanese Orthopaedic Association (JOA) assessment significantly increased compared with that before the trial, and the improvement continued until the end of the trial at 12 weeks. The extensor muscle torque increased significantly on the signal joint side at 12 weeks, but not on the healthy joint side. In the control group, there was no significant increase in JOA score or extensor muscle torque at 4 or 12 weeks. In 1997, Ettinger et al. [10] recruited 439 knee OA patients and intervened randomly with aerobic exercise, resistance exercise, or a health education program for 18 months. Both exercise groups had lower self-reported disability scores, lower knee pain scores, and performed better on the 6-min walking test than the health education group. The authors concluded that exercise should be prescribed as part of the treatment for knee OA.

In 2003 and 2004, the JOA conducted an RCT of 142 knee OA patients to compare the effects of home-based SLR exercise with the effects of oral NSAID administration for 8 weeks [54]. Patients in both groups showed significant improvements from baseline in pain and activities of daily living, as assessed by WOMAC and JKOM. SLR exercise showed better improvement rates as assessed by JKOM than NSAID treatment. This study is unique in that the exercise was composed of a single mode of muscle contraction.

Karatosum et al. [44] examined the efficacy of intraarticular HA injection in comparison with exercise for 6 weeks on 105 patients. The two groups had similar improvement in the Hospital for Special Surgery score. In 2007, Hurley et al. [46] allocated 418 patients into three groups: ordinary outpatient treatment, outpatient treatment and home-based exercise, and outpatient treatment and exercise classes. After 18 months, they found that the exercise groups had significantly better WOMAC scores than the ordinary outpatient treatment group. There was no significant difference in the outcome of the two exercise groups. Kawasaki et al. [48] examined the additive effect of glucosamine or risedronate on home-based exercise for 18 months. Patients who took glucosamine or risedronate showed significantly greater improvement in the WOMAC pain subcategory than those in the exercise group. However, global WOMAC assessment did not show an additive effect of glucosamine or risedronate on exercise.

As briefly discussed earlier and including other reports that are not mentioned here, all of the published papers have confirmed the efficacy of any type of exercise on pain and disability in knee OA.

CONSIDERATION OF THE MECHANISMS OF THE EFFICACY OF THERAPEUTIC EXERCISE

As discussed earlier, the efficacy of exercise as a treatment for knee OA has been established. However, the mechanisms by which exercise helps pain or disability are not directly explained by such clinical trials. Pain, which is one of the most difficult issues in basic science, is the chief and central complaint in knee OA. Here, the author attempts to consider the mechanisms by which exercise is an effective treatment for knee joint OA by reviewing the published literature in details.

Mode of Exercise

Most of the published trials used multiple modes of exercise, and in such trials, it is not possible to determine which exercise was effective or most effective in alleviating pain and disability. Ettinger et al. [10] and Kurosawa [40] compared the effect of muscle training with that of walking, Topp et al. [34] compared the effect of isometric muscle training with that of isotonic one, and Huang et al. [36] compared the effect of isokinetic exercise with that of isotonic and isometric exercise. Such trials demonstrated that pain and disability were equally decreased by every mode of exercise. Thus, differences in type of muscle contraction, that is, isometric, isotonic, or isokinetic, and differences in type of energy consumption, that is, aerobic or anaerobic, do not influence the efficacy of exercise.

Exercise in the water has often been prescribed for knee OA patients, and two recently reported trials compared the effects of exercise on land or in the water [49, 51] with the rate and intensity of aerobic and anaerobic exercise set equally. One report concluded that both forms of exercise were equally beneficial for patients with knee OA when assessed by the global WOMAC score [51]. However, the second report concluded that exercise on the land decreased symptoms but that in the water did not [49].

Significance of Muscle Strengthening

For some time, it has been thought that the knee extensor muscle is a knee-stabilizing structure and that extensor strength reduces joint force during the stance phase of waking. Jefferson et al. [70] found that quadriceps force lightened the impact joint force at heel strike during walking. This suggested that extensor strength might be correlated with relief of knee symptoms in knee OA. Madsen et al. [14] found reduced isokinetic strength of the quadriceps muscle in painful OA knees, and O'Reilly et al. [17] demonstrated lower quadriceps strength in subjects with knee pain than in those without pain. Moreover, Slemenda et al. [16] demonstrated that women who had radiological knee OA without pain had weaker extensor isokinetic strength than those without radiological OA and pain. From these results, they concluded that quadriceps weakness was a primary risk factor for knee pain and OA progression. Most of the studies in which muscle strength was measured reported increased isometric, isotonic, or isokinetic strength of the quadriceps muscle with decreased symptoms and disability [11, 12, 17, 18, 23, 25, 26, 33, 35, 50]. These facts suggest that quadriceps muscle strength is correlated with pain and disability because of knee OA.

On the other hand, some studies have shown alleviation of pain and disability by walking alone or by aerobic exercise alone [10, 12, 19, 23, 30]. Studies comparing the effects of walking or strength exercise revealed that both modes of exercise were equally effective for diminishing symptoms [10, 31, 36]. From the theory of muscle physiology, walking or aerobic exercise is not expected to result in increased muscle strength. To carefully examine the effect of the intensity of exercise on symptoms, two studies set up different intensity therapeutic exercise [22, 50]. Mangione et al. [22] randomly allocated subjects into high-intensity (70% heart rate reserve) and low-intensity (40% heart rate reserve) groups using an ergometer bicycle. Jan et al. [50] allocated subjects into high-load (60% one-repetition maximum [1RM]) and low-load (10% 1RM) groups using a leg press machine. In both studies, the different intensity exercises gave rise to similar improvement in symptoms and disability, as assessed by VAS for pain and WOMAC or functional testing by a 6-min walking test or gait analysis. Interestingly, subjects in the low-load (10% 1RM) and high-load (60% 1RM) groups exhibited almost the same increment in muscle strength after completion of the study.

According to theories of muscle physiology, muscular strength increases through hypertrophy of muscle fibers after an overload of 60% of maximum load or more. It is unlikely that the applied load was more than 60% of the maximum in the therapeutic exercises for elderly patients with knee OA. These may suggest that the mechanism by which muscle strength increases after therapeutic exercise is different from theory and may also suggest that there is another pathway by which muscle exercise directly influences pain. Shimizu et al. [11] reported that symptoms and disability assessed by the JOA score significantly decreased after 1 month of SLR exercise for subjects with knee OA, whereas isometric muscle strength assessed significantly increased only after 3 months of exercise. This result also suggests the possibilities mentioned earlier.

It has been thought that in pathologic conditions, such as arthritis, inhibition might work from within the joint on the extensors of the knee to suppress contraction of the muscle. Indeed, it has been reported that afferent impulses from the joint capsule caused by arthritis or joint effusion can cause efferent impulses to suppress quadriceps contraction [71–74].

Most OA knees gradually exhibit varus deformity as the disease progresses. Lim et al. [53] noticed the possibility of changing varus moment by the increment of muscle force resulting from exercise. They measured varus moment during walking before and after therapeutic strengthening exercise of the quadriceps muscle using a three-dimensional gait analysis system. Although the strength of the quadriceps increased after 12 weeks of exercise, varus moment did not significantly change.

Effect of Reducing Body Weight

Obesity is one of the risk factors for OA of the knee [75, 76]. Many investigators have focused on the possibility that reducing weight might be an effective therapy for knee OA. Toda et al. [19] examined the effect of reducing weight on symptoms of knee OA for patients with a body mass index (BMI) of 26.1 or more using diet, appetite suppressants, and walking exercise. They found that reduction in percent body fat, but not reduction in body weight itself, and number of steps per day were strongly correlated with improvement in symptoms and disability, as assessed by the Lequesne index. Messier et al. [25] studied a muscle strength exercise plus diet (E + D) group and an exercise alone (E) group composed of patients with BMI of 28 or more for 24 weeks of therapy. The patients in the E + D group lost a mean of 8.5 kg of body weight, and the patients in the E group lost a mean of 1.8 kg of body weight after 24 weeks. Patients in both groups had equal improvement in symptoms and disability. Focht et al. [41] designed a study in which they allocated obese patients with knee OA into exercise alone (E), diet alone (D), E + D, and health education groups. After 18 months, patients in the E and E + D groups had equal and significant improvement in walking ability and in ascending and descending stairs. In summary, these studies showed that loss of weight alone did not directly lead to improvement of knee OA symptoms, but diet could improve disability in combination with exercise.

LIMITATIONS OF THE EFFICACY OF EXERCISE

It is now evident that some mode of exercise is beneficial for reducing the symptoms of knee OA. However, few studies have examined the severity of knee OA for which exercise was effective and time for which the therapy would continue to be effective. Fransen et al. [29] showed that patients with knees in which joint space width (JSW) was less than 1.9 mm at the baseline had inferior improvement than those in which JSW was 1.9 mm or more after 8 weeks of isokinetic and isotonic muscle exercise of the lower limbs.

From the results of our study, the rate of effectiveness of home exercise and improvement of symptoms and disability was different, depending on the progression of disease [43]. The degree of OA progression was classified as stage II when JSW was between 3 and 6 mm, as stage III when JSW was between 1 and 3 mm, and as stage IV when JSW was less than 1 mm as measured by x-ray. Since 1997, my colleagues and I have used home exercise as a treatment for every patient who has visited our hospital with painful OA of the knee. We retrospectively analyzed the time course of 297 patients who were prescribed home exercise at the first visit and continued home exercise for 2 years or more, with a mean follow-up term of 44 months [43]. The rate of effectiveness of home exercise according to x-ray stages was calculated using life timetable analysis with any surgery on the signal joint defined as an end point (Figure 36.1). The rate of effectiveness of home exercise was 91%, 52%, and 31% for patients with stage II, III, and IV knees at the baseline, respectively, at 78 months of home exercise. As demonstrated in the figure, the effectiveness of therapeutic exercise decreased with progression of OA, and only 31% of patients with stage IV knees experienced some efficacy from home exercise and continued to perform the regimen. The clinical symptoms and disability of patients who continued home exercise were assessed by the JOA score (Figure 36.2). Patients with stage II, III, and IV disease all showed statistically significant improvement in symptoms and disability in comparison with baseline. However, as the degree of OA advanced, the improvement reached was decreased.

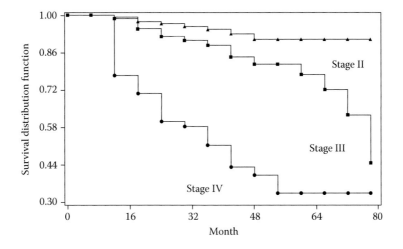

FIGURE 36.1 Survival rate of home-based exercise according to x-ray stages.

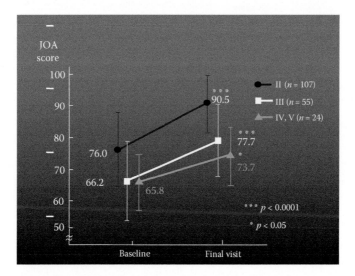

FIGURE 36.2 JOA scores according to x-ray stages.

Another of our studies, in which the efficacy of home exercise was compared with that of intra-articular HA injection [77] in 102 patients, confirmed that baseline JSW directly influenced the efficacy of home exercise or injection. Patients were divided into three groups according to baseline JSW (Figure 36.3). Patients with JSW in the upper third (3 mm or greater) had significantly more responders than those with JSW in the lower two-thirds as assessed by the Outcome Measures in Rheumatology Clinical Trials–Osteoarthritis Research Society International (OMERACT-OARSI) criteria [78]. These result showed that as OA progressed, the efficacy of exercise decreased. JSW of 3 mm may be a borderline that determines the prognosis of some treatments.

Age of a patient is also a factor that determines the prognosis of therapeutic exercise. We studied the possible additive effects of glucosamine or risedronate on therapeutic home exercise on 142 knee OA patients for 18 months [48]. Participants in the upper third in age (mean = 76.8 years, range = 73–84 years) had statistically inferior improvements after 18 months of exercise than those in the lower third (mean = 61.8 years, range = 52–67 years) by WOMAC or JOA score (Figure 36.4).

Thus, the efficacy of therapeutic exercise on OA of the knee was restricted by the degree of progression of OA and also by the age of the patient. Patients with severe OA (JSW < 3 mm) and patients 73 years or older had a tendency to show less efficacy of exercise than patients with less severe disease or who were younger.

SUMMARY AND PERSPECTIVE FOR EXERCISE

Exercise for OA of the knee is now an established therapeutic method shown to be effective by many trials. OARSI [6] and AAOS [7] now recommend that physicians encourage patients to try exercise before any passive therapy, such as administration of NSAID, or applying physical therapy. Most orthopedic surgeons in Japan have typically used pharmacological intervention, such as NSAID or intraarticular injection of HA from the early phases of treatment. In this context, however, ortho-pedic surgeons who treat patients with OA of the knee should change the paradigm of treatment. Further, in addition to the effects of exercise on symptoms of OA of the knee, exercise benefits general health.

As the fact that obesity and weakness of the lower limb muscles are risk factors for OA of the knee, this disease is lifestyle dependent. Regular exercise cannot only reduce pain and disability due to knee OA but also increase muscle strength, improve neuromuscular function, and increase daily activity; these improvements will, in turn, prevent further progression of OA and further gain

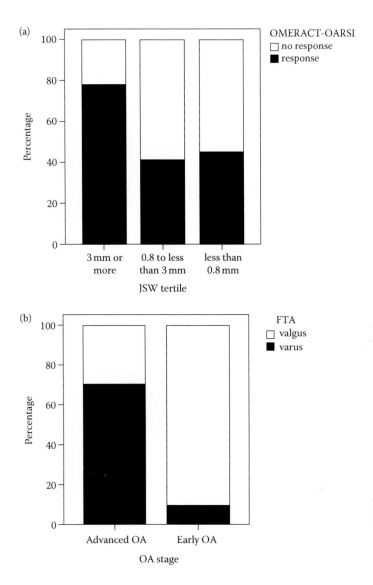

FIGURE 36.3   (a) Relation between the results of the OMERACT-OARSI and the JSW. There is a significant boundary at 3 mm of JSW. (b) Early OA exhibits valgus knee, whereas advanced OA shows a varus knee.

of body weight. Disability and poor health caused by knee OA are closely related to other musculoskeletal and cardiovascular morbidities. Most of the risk factors of disability and poor health can be prevented or reduced through regular physical activity and exercise. The American College of Sports Medicine and the Centers for Disease Control and Prevention have proposed recommendations for regular physical activity for all people [79]. As the Japanese population ages, the number of people with musculoskeletal and neuromuscular deficits has increased; this has now become a public health priority. Recommendations of exercise and regular physical activity should be used as goals for people with musculoskeletal disorders as therapeutic measures and also for healthy people older than 50 years as preventive measures.

Although there is much evidence that physical exercise is effective in reducing disability caused by knee OA, as described in this chapter, there are few studies examining whether exercise is also effective in preventing the occurrence and progression of musculoskeletal disorders in aged individuals. We must focus our study on this issue in the future.

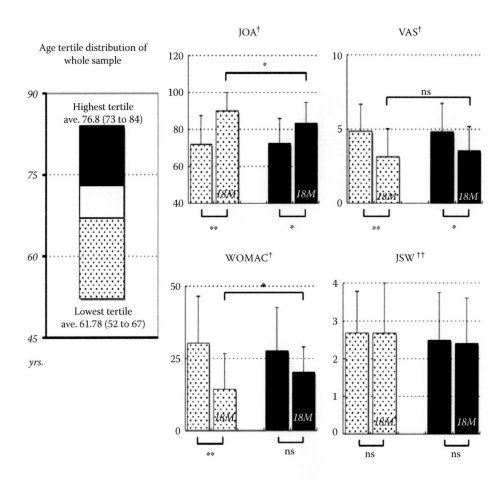

FIGURE 36.4 Factors effecting therapeutic effect. Black bar, highest age tertile; dotted bar, lowest age tertile; ns, not significant; $*p < 0.05$; $**p < 0.01$.

REFERENCES

1. Ettinger WH Jr. Physical activity, arthritis and disability in older people. Clin Geriatr Med 1998;12:633–640.
2. Dunlop DD, Lyons JS, Manheim LM, Song J, Chang RW. Arthritis and heart disease as risk factors for major depression: the role of functional limitation. Med Care 2004;42:502–511.
3. Gabriel SE, Crowson CS, Campion ME, O'Fallon WM. Indirect and non-medical costs among people with rheumatoid arthritis and osteoarthritis compared with nonarthritic controls. J Rheumatol 1997;24:43–48.
4. Leardini G, Salaffi F, Caporali R, Canesi B, Rovati L, Montanelli R, and the Italian Group for Study of the costs of Arthritis. Direct and indirect costs of osteoarthritis of the knee. Clin Exp Rheumatol 2004;22:699–706.
5. World Health Organization. The burden of musculoskeletal conditions at the start of the new millennium (Technical Report No. 919). Geneva: World Health Organization; 2003.
6. Zhang W, Moskowitz RW, Nuki G, Abramson S, Altman RD, Arden N, Bierma-Zeinstras, et al. OARSI recommendations for the management of hip and knee osteoarthritis: Part II, OARSI evidence-based, expert consensus guidelines. Osteoarthritis Cartilage 2008;16:137–162.
7. The American Academy of Orthopaedic Surgeons (ed.). Guideline on the treatment of osteoarthritis (OA) of the knee recommendation summary, Illinois, 2008. http://www.aaos.org/Research/guidelines/GuidelineOAKnee.asp. Accessed Nov. 11, 2009.
8. Stewart AL, Greenfield S, Hays RD, Wells K, Rogers WH, Berry S, McGlynn EA, Ware JE. Functional status and well being of patients with chronic conditions: results from medical outcomes study. JAMA 1989;262:907–913.

9. Maisiak R. Arthritis and the risk of depression: an epidemiological case control study. Arthritis Care Res 1990;Abstr 3:C36.

10. Ettinger WH, Burans R, Messier SP, Applegate W, Rejeski WJ, Morgan T, Shunmaker S, Berry MJ, O'Toole M, Monu J. A randomized trial comparing aerobic exercise and resistance exercise with a health education program in older adults with knee osteoarthritis. JAMA, 1997;27:25–31.

11. Shimizu N, Kurosawa H, Hoshikawa Y. Treatment of knee osteoarthritis by straight leg raising exercise [in Japanese]. Seikei Geka 1991;42:646–654.

12. Kover PA, Allegrante JP, Mackenzie CR, Peterson MGE, Cutin B, Charson ME. Supervised fitness walking in patients with osteoarthritis of the knee. Ann Inter Med 1992;116:529–534.

13. Fisher NM, Kane VD, Rouse L, Pendergast DR. Quantitative evaluation of a home exercise program on muscle and functional capacity of patients with osteoarthritis. Am J Phys Med Rehabil 1994;73:413–420.

14. Madsen OR, Bliddal H, Egsmose C, Sylvest J. Isometric and isokinetic quadriceps strength in gonarthrosis; inter-relations between quadriceps strength, walking ability, radiology, subchondral bone density and pain. Clin Rheumatol 1995;14:308–314.

15. Schilke JM, Johnson GO, Housh TJ, O'Dell JR. Effects of muscle-strength training on the functional status of patients with osteoarthritis of the knee joint. Nurs Res 1996;45:68–72.

16. Slemenda C, Brandt KD, Heilman K, Mazzuca S, Braunstein E, Katz BP, Wolinsky FD. Quadriceps weakness and osteoarthritis of the knee. Ann Intern Med 1997;127:97–104.

17. O'Reilly SC, Jones A, Muir KR, Doherty M. Quadriceps weakness in knee osteoarthritis: the effect on pain and disability. Ann Rheum Dis 1998;57:588–594.

18. Rogind H, Nielsen BB, Jensen B, Moller HC, Moller HF, Bliddal H. The effects of a physical training program on patients with osteoarthritis of the knee. Arch Phys Med Rehabil 1998;79:1421–1427.

19. Toda Y, Toda T, Takemura S, Wada T, Morimoto T, Ogawa R. Change in body fat, but not body weight or metabolic correlates of obesity, is related to symptomatic relief of obese patients with knee osteoarthritis after a weight control program. J Rheumatol 1998;25:2181–2186.

20. Van Baar ME, Dekker J, Oostendorp RAB, Bijl D, Voorn TB, Lemmmens JAM, Bijlsma WJ. The effectiveness of exercise therapy in patients with osteoarthritis of the hip or knee: a randomized clinical trial. J Rheumatol 1998;25:2432–2439.

21. O'Reilly SC, Muir KR, Doherty M. Effectiveness of home exercise on pain and disability from osteoarthritis of the knee: a randomized controlled trial. Ann Rheum Dis 1999;58:15–19.

22. Mangione KK, McCully K, Gloviak A, Lefebvre I, Hofmann M, Craik R. The effects of high-intensity and low-intensity cycle ergometry in older adults with knee osteoarthritis. J Gerontol 1999;54-A:191–196.

23. Maurer BT, Stern AG, Kinossian B, Cook KD, Schumacher HR. Osteoarthritis of the knee: isokinetic quadriceps exercise versus an educational intervention. Arch Phys Med Rehabil 1999;80:1293–1299.

24. Deyle GD, Henderson NE, Matekel RL, Ryder G, Garber MB, Allison SC. Effectiveness of manual physical therapy and exercise in osteoarthritis of the knee. Ann Intern Med 2000;132:173–181.

25. Messier SP, Loeser RF, Mitchell MN, Valle G, Morgan TP, Rejeski WJ, Ettinger W. Exercise and weight loss in obese older adults with knee osteoarthritis: a preliminary study. JAGS 2000;48:1062–1072.

26. Hopman-Rock M, Westhoff MH. The effects of a health educational and exercise program for older adults with osteoarthritis of the hip or knee. J Rheumatol 2000;27:1947–1954.

27. Sakuraba K, Kurosawa H, Ikeda H. Efficacy of therapeutic exercise for knee osteoarthritis [in Japanese]. Clin J Sport Med 2000;17:143–150.

28. Petrella RJ, Bartha C. Home based exercise therapy for older patients with knee osteoarthritis: a randomized clinical trial. J Rheumatol 2000;27:2215–2221.

29. Fransen M, Crosbie J, Edmonds J. Physical therapy is effective for patients with osteoarthritis of the knee: a randomized controlled clinical trial. J Rheumatol 2001;28:156–164.

30. Halbert J, Crotty M, Weller D, Ahern M, Silagy A. Primary care-based physical activity program: effectiveness in sedentary older patients with osteoarthritis symptoms. Arthritis Care Res 2001;45:228–234.

31. Penninx B, Messier SP, Rejeski WJ, Williamson JD, DiBari M, Cavazzini C, Applegate WB, Pahor M. Physical exercise and the prevention of disability in activities of daily living in older persons with osteoarthritis. Arch Intern Med 2001;161:2309–2316.

32. Manninen P, Riihimaki H, Heliovaara M, Suomalainen O. Physical exercise and risk of severe knee osteoarthritis requiring arthroplasty. Rheumatology 2001;40:432–437.

33. Baker KR, Nelson ME, Felson DT, Layne JE, Sarno R, Roubenoff R. The efficacy of home based progressive strength training in older adults with osteoarthritis: a randomized controlled trial. J Rheumatol 2001;28:1655–1665.

34. Topp R, Wooley S, Hornyak J, Khuder S, Kahaleh B. The effect of dynamic versus isometric resistance training on pain and functioning among adults with osteoarthritis of the knee. Arch Phys Med Rehabil 2002;83:1187–1195.

35. Thomas KS, Muir KR, Doherty M, Jones AC, O'Reilly SC, Bassey EJ. Home based exercise programme for knee pain and knee osteoarthritis: randomised controlled trial. BMJ 2002;325:752.

36. Huang MH, Lin YS, Yang RC, Lee CL. A comparison on various therapeutic exercises on the functional status of patients with knee osteoarthritis. Semin Arthritis Rheum 2003;32:398–406.

37. McCarthy CJ, Mills PM, Pullen R, Roberts R, Silman A, Oldham JA. Supplementing a home exercise programme with a class-based exercise programme is more effective than home exercise alone in the treatment of knee osteoarthritis. Rheumatology 2004;43:880–886.

38. Messier SP, Loeser RF, Miller GD, Morgan TM, Rejeski WJ, Sevick MA, Ettinger WH, Pahor M, Williamson JD. Exercise and dietary weight loss in overweight and obese older adults with knee osteoarthritis. Arthritis Rheum 2004;50:1501–1510.

39. Ravaud R, Giraudeau B, Logeart I, Larguier JS, Rolland D, Treves R, Euller-Ziegler L, Bannwarth B, Dougados N. Management of osteoarthritis (OA) with an unsupervised home based exercise programme and/or patient administered assessment tools. A cluster randomized controlled trial with a 2*2 factorial design. Ann Rheum Dis 2004;63:703–708.

40. Kurosawa H. Conservative treatment of knee osteoarthritis by home-based exercise [in Japanese]. J Jpn Orthop Ass 2005;79:793–805.

41. Focht BC, Rejeski WJ, Ambrosius WT, Katula JA, Messier SP. Exercise, self-efficacy, and mobility performance in overweight and obese older adults with knee osteoarthritis. Arthritis Rheum 2005;53:659–665.

42. Thomas KS, Miller P, Doherty M, Muir KR, Jones AC, O'Reilly SC. Cost effectiveness of a two-year home exercise program for the treatment of knee pain. Arthritis Rheum 2005;53:388–394.

43. Kurosawa H, Ikeda H, Kim SG, Ohsawa A, Seto H, Takazawa Y. Conservative treatment of knee osteoarthritis: efficacy rate of home-based exercise [in Japanese]. J Jpn Orthop Ass 2006;80:933–941.

44. Karatosum V, Unver B, Gocen Z, Sen A, Gunal I. Intra-articular hyaluronic acid compared with progressive knee exercises in osteoarthritis of the knee: a prospective randomized trial with long-term follow-up. Rheumatol Int 2006;26:277–284.

45. Messier SP, Mihalko S, Loeser RF, Lagault C, Jolla J, Pfruender J, Prosser B, Adrian A, Williamson JD. Glucosamine/chondroitin combined with exercise for the treatment of knee osteoarthritis: a preliminary study. Osteoarthritis Cartilage 2007;15:1256–1266.

46. Hurley MV, Walsh NE, Mitchell HL, Patel A, Williamson E, Jones RH, Dieppe PA, Reeves BC. Clinical effectiveness of a rehabilitation program integrating exercise, self-management, and active coping strategies for chronic knee pain: a cluster randomial trial. Arthritis Rheum 2007;57:13211–13219.

47. Thornstensson CA, Henriksson M, von Porat A, Sjoedahl C, Roos EM. The effect of eight weeks exercise on knee adduction moment in early knee osteoarthritis—a pilot study. Osteoarthritis cartilage 2007;15:1163–1170.

48. Kawasaki T, Kurosawa H, Ikeda H, Kim SG, Osawa A, Takazawa Y, Kubota M, Ishijima M. Additive effects of glucosamine or risedronate for the treatment of osteoarthritis of the knee combined with home exercise: a prospective randomized 18-month trial. J Bone Miner Metab 2008;26:279–287.

49. Lund H, Weile U, Christensen R, Rostock B, Downey A, Bartels EM, Danneskiold-Samsoe B, Bliddal H. A randomized controlled trial of aquatic and land-based exercise in patients with knee osteoarthritis. J Rehabil Med 2008;40:137–144.

50. Jan MH, Lin JJ, Liau JJ, Lin YF, Lin DH. Investigation of clinical effects of high- and low-resistance training for patients with knee osteoarthritis: a randomized controlled trial. Phys Ther 2008;88:427–436.

51. Silva LE, Valim V, Pessanha APC, Olivelira LM, Myamoto S, Jones A, Natour J. Hydrotherapy versus conventional land-based exercise for the management of patients with osteoarthritis of the knee: a randomized clinical trial. Phys Ther 2008;88:12–21.

52. Lim BW, Hinman RS, Bennel KL. Varus malalignment and its association with impairments and functional limitations in medial knee osteoarthritis. Arthritis Rheum 2008;59:935–942.

53. Lim BW, Hinman RS, Wrigley TV, Sharma L, Bennell KL. Does knee malalignment mediates the effects of quadriceps strengthening on knee adduction moment, pain, and function in medial knee osteoarthritis? A randomized controlled trial. Arthritis Rheum [Arthritis care & Research] 2008;59:943–951.

54. Doi T, Akai M, Fujino K, Iwaya T, Kurosawa H, Hayashi K, Marui E. Effect of home exercise of quadriceps on knee osteoarthritis compared with nonsteroidal antiinflamatory drugs: a randomized controlled trial. Am J Phys Med Rehabil 2008;87:258–269.

55. Chua SD, Messier SP, Legault C, Lenz ME, Thonar JMA, Loeser RF. Effect of an exercise and dietary intervention on serum biomarkers in overweight and obese adults with osteoarthritis of the knee. Osteoarthritis Cartilage 2008;16:1047–1053.

56. Sharif M, Saxne T, Shepstone L, Kirwan JR, Elson CJ, Heinegard D, Dieppe OA. Relationship between serum cartilage oligometric matrix protein levels and disease progression in osteoarthritis of the knee joint. Br J Rheumatol 1995;34:306–310.

57. Reijman M, Hazes J, Bierma-Zeinstra S, Koes B, Christgau S, Christiansen C, Uiterlinden A, Pols H. A new marker for osteoarthritis cross-sectional and longitudinal approach. Arthritis Rheum 2004;50:2471–2478.

58. Sharif M, George E, Shepstone L, Knudson W, Thonar EJ-MA, Cushnaghan J, Dieppe P. Serum hyaluronic acid level as a predictor of disease progression in osteoarthritis of the knee. Arthritis Rheum 1995;38:760–767.

59. Garnero P, Piperno M, Gineyts E, Delmas PD, Vignon E. Cross sectional evaluation of biochemical markers of bone, cartilage, and synovial tissue metabolism in disease activity and joint damage. Ann Rheum Dis 2001;60:619–626.

60. Mouritzen U, Christgau S, Lehmann H-J, Tanko LB, Christiansen C. Cartilage turnover assessed with a newly developed assay measuring collagen type degradation products: influence of age, sex, menopause, hormone replacement therapy, and body mass index. Ann Rheum Dis 2003;62:3–6.

61. Bellamy N, Buchanan WW, Goldsmith CH, Campbel J, Stitt LW. Validation study of WOMAC. J Rheumatol 1988;15:1833–1840.

62. Meenan RF, Gertman PM, Mason H. Measuring health status in arthritis. Arthritis Rheum 1980;23:146–152.

63. McHorney CA, Ware JE, Raczek AE. The MOS 36-item Short-Form Health Survey (SF-36): II. Med Care 1993;31:247–263.

64. Lequesne MG, Mery C, Samson M, Gerad P. Indexes of severity for osteoarthritis of the hip and knee. Scand J Rheumatol Suppl 1987;65:85–89.

65. Roos EM, Roos HP, Ekdahl C, Lohmander LS. Knee Injury and Osteoarthritis Outcome Score (KOOS)—validation of Swedish version. Scand J Med Sci Sports 1998;8:439–448.

66. Akai M, Doi T, Fujino K, Kurosawa H, Hoshino Y. An outcome measure for Japanese people with knee osteoarthritis. J Rheumatol 2005;32:1524–1532.

67. Washburn RA, Smith KW, Jette AM, Janney CA. The Physical Activity Scale for the Elderly (PASE): development and evaluation. J Clin Epidemiol 1993;46:153–162.

68. Cunningham DA, Rechnitzer PA, Pearce ME, Donner AP. Determination of self-paced walking pace across ages 19–66. J Gerontol 1982;37:560–564.

69. Podsiadlo D, Richardson S. The timed "Up & Go"; a test of basic functional mobility for frail elderly persons. J Am Geriatr Soc 1991;39:142–148.

70. Jefferson RJ, Collins JJ, Whittle MW, Radin EL, O'Conner JJ. The role of the quadriceps in controlling impulsive forces around the heel. J Engineer Med 1990;204:21–28.

71. Iles J, Roberts RC. Inhibition of monosynaptic reflexes in the human lower limb. J Physiol 1987; 385:69–87.

72. Fahrer H, Rentsch HU, Beyeler HW. Knee effusion and reflex inhibition of the quadriceps. J Bone Joint Surg 1988;70:635–638.

73. Hurley MV, Newham DJ. The influence of arthrogenous muscle inhibition on quadriceps rehabilitation of patients with early, unilateral osteoarthritic knees. Br J Rheumatol 1993;32:127–131.

74. Hopkins JT, Ingersoll JT, Krause BA, Edwards JE, Cordova ML. Effect of knee joint effusion on quadriceps and soleus motoneuron pool excitability. Med Sci Sports Exerc 2001;33:123–126.

75. Felson DT, Zhang Y, Anthony JM, Naimark A, Anderson JJ. Weight loss reduces the risk for symptomatic knee osteoarthritis in women. Ann Intern Med 1992;116:535–539.

76. Must A, Spadano J, Coakley EH, Field AE, Colditz G, Dietz WH. The disease burden associated with overweight and obesity. JAMA 1999;282:1523–1529.

77. Kawasaki T, Kurosawa H, Ikeda H, Takazawa Y, Ishijima M, Kubota M, Kajihara H, et al. Therapeutic home exercise versus intraarticular hyaluronate injection for osteoarthritis of the knee: 6-month prospective randomized open-labeled trial. J Orthopaedic Sci 2009;14:182–191.

78. Pham T, van der Heijde D, Altman RD, Anderson JJ, Bellamy N, Hochberg M, et al. OMERACT-OARSI initiative: Osteoarthritis Research Society International set of responder criteria for osteoarthritis clinical trials revised. Osteoarthritis Cartilage 2004;12:389–399.

79. Pate RR, Pratt M, Blair SN, Haskell WL, Macera A, Bouchard C, Buchner D, et al. Physical activity and public health. A recommendation from the Centers for Disease Control and Prevention and American College of Sports Medicine JAMA 1995;273:402–407.

37 Acupuncture for the Treatment of Arthritis

Hi-Joon Park and Hyangsook Lee

CONTENTS

INTRODUCTION

In recent years, there are rapid growths in demanding the improvement of medical service worldwide, which provides the human-centered medical service as well as reestablishes the concept of the health to improve the quality of life. Therefore, in the Western society, the demand of integrated health care that incorporates conventional and complementary therapies such as acupuncture has increased. In particular, it shows remarkable trend in chronic diseases such as osteoarthritis (OA) and rheumatoid arthritis (RA) as average geriatric population becomes extended.

Acupuncture is one of the most important therapeutic modalities in traditional East Asian medicine alongside herbal medicine. It involves stimulation of specific sites on the skin and underlying tissues, called *acupuncture points*, which are claimed to be more effective than other sites, by manually inserting and manipulating fine needles for therapeutic purposes and/or promoting health. Manual acupuncture is the most commonly used in practice, where fine, disposable stainless steel needles are inserted into (usually) individually selected acupuncture points and manipulated by rotating to elicit specific needle sensation called *de-qi*. Acupuncture treatment is based on the theory that the vital energy (qi) and blood flow throughout the body along the meridians/channels that cover all over the body in and out, and by acupuncture stimulation, we can control the flow of qi and spirit.

Several other methods are also used for stimulation of acupuncture points, for example, electrical currents, laser light, and moxibustion (burning herbal preparations containing *Artemisia vulgaris* or mugwort to deliver heat into acupuncture points). The choice of acupuncture points, stimulation

519

modalities, manipulation methods, and duration and number of treatment sessions mainly depends on the patient's characteristics, the practitioner's experience and preference, and the condition/disease and is often individualized.

Despite its long history, acupuncture has been a highly controversial subject. Since James Reston's article in the *New York Times* on his experience with acupuncture during recovery from emergency appendectomy in 1971 [1], acupuncture has been one of the most intensely researched areas of complementary and alternative medicine. Over the past three decades, we have also witnessed an unprecedented growth in the practice of acupuncture on the West. In East Asian countries including China, Korea, and Japan, acupuncture has been so far retained mostly in parallel with Western medicine. The landmark 1997 consensus development conference by the National Institutes of Health stated that acupuncture was supported by positive evidence for a range of conditions including adult postoperative and chemotherapy-induced nausea and vomiting and postoperative dental pain [2]. The consensus statement also suggested that there are other situations such as drug addiction, stroke rehabilitation, headache, menstrual cramps, tennis elbow, fibromyalgia, myofascial pain, OA, low back pain, carpal tunnel syndrome, and asthma, where acupuncture may be useful as an adjunct or an acceptable alternative treatment or be included in a comprehensive management program [2]. Then, 10 years after the consensus conference of the National Institutes of Health, accumulated biological and clinical research evidence was presented [3, 4], and the most recent evidence from the *Cochrane Database of Systematic Reviews* indicates a suggestion of benefit from acupuncture in chronic low back pain [5], postoperative nausea and vomiting [6], tension-type headache [7], migraine [8], assisted conception [9], neck pain [10], hip/knee OA [11], and chemotherapy-induced nausea or vomiting [12].

With or without solid evidence, acupuncture has been used for virtually any kind of diseases/conditions and is better known for the treatment of conditions associated with pain. In traditional East Asian medicine including Chinese medicine, all forms of arthritis are covered by the bi syndrome, also known as the painful obstruction syndrome, with further differentiation on the basis of the signs and symptoms. Unlike etiology in Western medicine, traditional East Asian medicine sees that arthritis is developed by external pathogens such as wind, cold, and dampness and exacerbated when vital energy and/or blood is deficient [13] (Figure 37.1). Wind-dominant pattern arthritis, usually affecting upper part of the body, is characterized by the sudden onset of the disease and variability in the manifestation of the symptoms. It is usually diagnosed as such in the early stage of the arthritis. In arthritis of cold-dominant pattern, symptoms get worse when the patient is exposed to cold and improve when heat is applied. The concept of "dampness" is associated with the weather or environment; rainy season or sleeping on wet ground may initiate or worsen the symptoms. All these factors usually come together to manifest the so-called *wind–cold–dampness mixed pattern* arthritis (Figure 37.1). The treatment is individualized with a focus on relieving symptoms, removing the root of the pathogen that originally caused the arthritis, and strengthening qi or blood

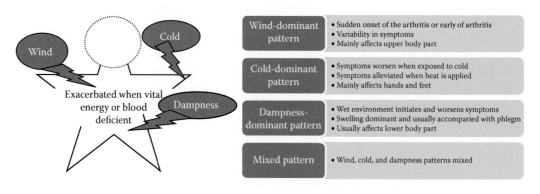

FIGURE 37.1   The concept of pathogenesis for arthritis in traditional East Asian medicine.

deficiency, if any. As the traditional East Asian medicine recognizes that the symptoms of arthritis occur when the flow of "qi" gets blocked or deviates from its way and thus formulates obstruction and pain, that is, bi syndrome, acupuncture stimulation on specific acupuncture points on the corresponding meridians mostly aims at removing the "qi" blockage. Acupuncture needles are manually stimulated, or electrical current is connected to maintain or strengthen analgesia.

Acupuncture has been widely used for painful conditions. Several hypotheses for the mechanisms of acupuncture's analgesic effects have been suggested on the basis of the findings from a number of neurophysiological studies [14]; acupuncture analgesia is mediated by activating afferent fibers and by releasing various endogenous opioids [15]. Hypothalamus–pituitary–adrenocortical axis is also known to be activated by acupuncture stimulation [16]. In addition, it has been demonstrated that acupuncture has anti-inflammatory effects. Acupuncture has been reported to increase levels of interferon-γ and interleukin (IL)-2, IL-4, and IL-6 while reducing level of tumor necrosis factor-α in peripheral blood of patients with asthma [17]. Acupuncture treatment is also shown to suppress inflammatory processes in RA patients [18]. In RA patients, acupuncture stimulation increased IL-2 level [18], and a number of studies have demonstrated anti-inflammatory effects of acupuncture in a range of animal models such as collagen-induced arthritic mice [19] and Freud's adjuvant-induced arthritic model [20, 21].

In this chapter, we investigate the current evidence on acupuncture for OA and RA. The focus is mainly on clinical studies where main diverse acupuncture interventions are compared with a range of controls including no treatment, wait-list control, sham acupuncture, and/or active medication, that is, usual or standard care. We stress the quality of the studies and also present limitations and unresolved questions in acupuncture research to offer a future perspective in this area. This chapter, therefore, is aimed at providing an unbiased evidence synthesis and thus helping doctors and patients make an informed decision.

THE EFFECT OF ACUPUNCTURE IN OA OF PERIPHERAL JOINTS

OA is the main cause of disability in older adults [22, 23], and an important burden in health care cost. The most commonly affected by OA is the knee and hip joints [24, 25]. Because there is no cure for OA, a multimodal pharmacological and nonpharmacological approach is recommended until replacement surgery is applied [26, 27]. Nonsteroidal anti-inflammatory drugs are the most commonly used to treat the symptoms of this disorder [28–30]. However, these drugs produce severe side effects, such as gastrointestinal bleeding [31]. The need for additional effective and safe therapies for OA is evident. Patients with chronic pain are increasingly using acupuncture for pain relief because it is safe treatment with a low risk for serious side effects [32–35].

In this section, we summarize the present status of randomized controlled trials (RCT) of acupuncture for OA and evaluate the evidence for the effectiveness of acupuncture. We included RCTs published within recent 10 years. To be included in the review, studies needed to meet the following three criteria: patients were randomly allocated to either acupuncture or a control group, patients were diagnosed as OA of the peripheral joints (i.e., knee and hip), and acupuncture treatment was given to the patients for at least 4 weeks or more than eight sessions of acupuncture treatments because trials with a shorter duration or lack of optimal dose were considered irrelevant for the question of whether acupuncture is properly given to elicit therapeutic effects in a chronic disease like OA. The acupuncture methods that are not traditional acupuncture (i.e., laser acupuncture, transcutaneous electrical nerve stimulation, and trigger point needling) were excluded. The data were extracted from the original article. We also referred to the recently published systematic reviews when the extractable data were missing. Finally, 10 RCTs were included representing 2994 randomized OA participants [36–45]. Six RCTs included only people with OA of the knee, three included only people with OA of the hip, and one included a mix of people with OA of the hip and/or that of the knee.

ACUPUNCTURE EFFECT ON KNEE OA

All studies had patients diagnosed as knee OA with mean pain duration (5–9.2 years) and mean age (61–67 years); two studies used manual acupuncture, three studies used electroacupuncture (EA), and two studies used manual acupuncture with EA. Most studies (8 of 10) used the Western Ontario and McMaster Universities Osteoarthritis Index (WOMAC). Other outcomes such as visual analog scale (VAS) for pain, 36-item Short-Form Health Survey (SF-36), SF-12, and global assessment were also used. The methodological quality of the included studies is high (average 4.4 of maximum 5 points). The control groups such as minimal acupuncture, nonpenetrating needling to nonacupuncture point, education, waiting list, or medication were used. The characteristics of included studies were presented in Table 37.1.

Acupuncture was compared with sham controls in five RCTs [36–40]. Overall results suggested that the short-term effects (within 2 or 3 months) of acupuncture for knee OA are clinically significant. When compared with the sham control group, acupuncture showed improvements in the pain and function (Figure 37.2). Three studies provided available long-term data. The analysis at long-term follow-up (around 6 months) indicated that the effect of acupuncture is slightly more significant than to the sham control group and function, but it is clinically irrelevant improvements in pain (Figure 37.3).

Three studies provided the data from the comparison between acupuncture and waiting list [40–42]. Acupuncture showed clinically relevant improvement of pain and function in knee OA at a short-term period (Figure 37.4).

Acupuncture was compared with other active treatments in two studies. Acupuncture was compared with the supervised education control [36] and physical consultation control [38], and it was associated with clinically meaningful short- and long-term improvements in pain and function.

ACUPUNCTURE EFFECTS ON HIP OA

Three RCTs regarding hip OA were analyzed. All studies had patients diagnosed as hip OA with mean pain duration (5.8–8 years) and mean age (61–67 years); three studies used manual acupuncture, and one study used EA. Two studies used the WOMAC. Other outcomes such as VAS for pain, Disability Rating Index, Lequesne scale, SF-36, and global assessment were also used. The methodological quality of the included studies is relatively high (average 3.4 of maximum 5 points). The control groups such as same needling to nonacupuncture point, advice and exercise, hydrotherapy, education, and waiting list were used. In Fink's [43] study, there were no significant differences of pain or function between the acupuncture and the sham control groups. In Haslam's [44] study, there were significant improvements in the acupuncture group compared with the supervised exercise group at 6 and 8 weeks, respectively. Trials where EA was compared with education alone found improvements in pain and function [45]. However, because the attrition rate was so high in the three studies mentioned (up to ~50%), the interpretation of the studies needs to be cautious. In Witt's [42] study, acupuncture was superior to waiting list control at the end of treatment (3 months) and at a 6-month follow-up period. On the basis of four studies so far, there is only limited evidence for the effectiveness of acupuncture for hip OA. The number and overall methodological quality of the primary data are limited to draw firm conclusions.

THE EFFECT OF ACUPUNCTURE FOR RA

Regarding current evidence on acupuncture for RA, we conducted an overview of published RCTs meeting the following criteria: patients were randomly allocated to acupuncture or control, patients were diagnosed as having an RA, and acupuncture intervention involved needle insertion. Studies comparing two or more different forms of acupuncture or where no clinical data were reported were excluded. The data were extracted from the original articles and relevant systematic reviews [46, 47]

TABLE 37.1
Summary of the RCTs for OA

Year	Author	RCT Design Quality Score,[a] Allocation Concealment (Adequate, Inadequate/ Unclear)	Participants (Diagnosis, Mean Disease Duration, Mean Age)	Acupuncture Group (No. of Randomized Patients)	Control (No. of Randomized Patients)	Main Outcome Measures	Intergroup Differences	Comments
2004	Berman [36]	Parallel, three arms $1+1+1+1+1=5$ Adequate	Patients with knee OA with mean pain duration of 50% more than 5 years, mean age = 65.5 years	MA + EA (formula), 20 min/session, 23 times for 26 weeks ($n = 190$)	(A) Combined insertion/ noninsertion procedure: penetrating needles at two nonpoint, two tapes, tube at true points, plus one noninserted needle: 20 min/ session, 23 times for 26 weeks ($n = 191$) (B) Education: 60 min/session, six times ($n = 189$)	(1) WOMAC pain at 4, 8, 14, and 26 weeks after baseline (2) WOMAC function at 4, 8, 14, and 26 weeks after baseline (3) Patient global assessment at 4, 8, 14, and 26 weeks after baseline (4) SF-36 Physical Health at 8 and 26 weeks after baseline	Acu vs A: (1) NS at 4 and 8 weeks, $p < 0.02$ at 14 weeks, $p < 0.01$ at 26 weeks (2) NS at 4 weeks, $p = 0.01$ at 8 weeks, $p = 0.04$ at 14 weeks, $p < 0.01$ at 26 weeks (3) NS at 4, 8, and 14 weeks, $p = 0.02$ at 26 weeks (4) NS at 8 and 26 weeks A vs B: (1) $p < 0.001$ at 4 and 8 weeks, $p = 0.001$ at 14 weeks, $p < 0.01$ at 26 weeks (2) $p = 0.05$ at 4 weeks, $p < 0.001$ at 8 and 14 weeks, $p = 0.01$ at 26 weeks (3) NS at 4 and 8 weeks, $p = 0.03$ at 14 weeks, NS at 26 weeks (4) $p = 0.02$ at 8 weeks, $p = 0.01$ at 26 weeks	Major AEs: no Minor AEs: NS

continued

TABLE 37.1 (continued)
Summary of the RCTs for OA

Year	Author	RCT Design Quality Score,[a] Allocation Concealment (Adequate, Inadequate/Unclear)	Participants (Diagnosis, Mean Disease Duration, Mean Age)	Acupuncture Group (No. of Randomized Patients)	Control (No. of Randomized Patients)	Main Outcome Measures	Intergroup Differences	Comments
2002	Sangdee [37]	Parallel, four arms $1+0+0+1+1=3$ Unclear	Patients with knee OA with mean pain duration of 5 years, mean age = 63 years	(A) EA, formula, 20 min/session, 12 times plus placebo diclofenac, t.i.d. for 4 weeks ($n=48$) (C) EA, 20 min/session, 12 times plus diclofenac, t.i.d. for 4 weeks ($n=49$)	(B) Sham patch electrodes on surface of acupuncture point, 20 min/session, 12 times plus placebo diclofenac, t.i.d. for 4 weeks ($n=48$) (D) Sham patch electrodes on surface of acupuncture point, 20 min/session, 12 times plus diclofenac, t.i.d. for 4 weeks ($n=47$)	(1) VAS at 4 weeks (2) WOMAC pain at 4 weeks (3) Lequesne at 4 weeks	A vs B: (1) $p<0.05$, (2) WOMAC, NS, (3) $p<0.05$ A vs D: (1) $p<0.05$, (2 and 3) NR B vs C: (1 and 3) NS, (2) $p<0.05$	Minor AEs: local contusions around the knee in the Acu and control groups
2006	Scharf [38]	Parallel, three arms $1+1+1+1+1=5$ Adequate	Patients with knee OA with mean pain duration of 5.4 years, mean age = 63 years	MA, flexible formula, 20–30 min/session, 10 times for 6 weeks ($n=330$)	(A) Sham acupuncture: minimal depth of needling, avoiding real acupoints, 20–30 min/session, 10 times for 6 weeks, ($n=367$)	(1) WOMAC pain at 13 weeks and at follow-up 26 weeks after randomization/start of treatment	(1–2) MA vs A: each $p<0.001$ (3) MA vs A: each $p<0.001$, A vs B: $p=0.003$ at 13 weeks, $p<0.001$ at 26 weeks, MA vs B: each NS (4) MA vs A, A vs B, MA vs B: each NS	A total of 285 patients had at least one AE (91 in the MA group, 97 in the A group, 97 in the B group) Major AEs: 50 events (23 in the MA group, 9 in the A group, 18 in the B group)

Year	Study	Design	Patients	Intervention	Outcomes	Results	Adverse events
				(B) Physician practitioner with consultation and a prescription: 10 times for 6 weeks ($n = 342$)	(2) WOMAC function (3) SF-12 physical subscale (4) SF-12 mental subscale (5) Global patient assessment	(5) MA vs A: each $p < 0.001$. A vs B: each $p < 0.001$, MA vs B: NS at 13 weeks, $p = 0.004$ at 26 weeks	Minor AEs: hematoma more often in the MA group and A groups than that in the B group. Syncope and stroke (one case in MA group), myocardial infarction (one case in A group), renal failure, melena, and deep venous thrombosis (one case each in the B group)
2004	Vas [39]	Parallel, two arms $1 + 1 + 0 + 1 + 1 = 4$ Adequate	Patients with knee OA with mean pain duration of 7.5 years, mean age = 67 years	EA (formula), 12 times for 12 weeks ($n = 48$). Noninsertion, placebo control, used which seems appropriate: 12 times ($n = 49$)	(1) WOMAC pain at 1 week after the end of the 12-week treatment period (2) WOMAC function (3) WOMAC total	(1–3) $p < 0.001$	Minor AEs: three cases with bruising at the acupuncture points
2005	Witt [40]	Parallel, three arms $1 + 1 + 1 + 1 + 1 = 5$ Adequate	Patients with knee OA with mean pain duration of 9.2 years, mean age = 64 years	MA (flexible formula), 30 min/session, 12 times for 8 weeks ($n = 150$). (A) Minimal sham insertion control at nonacupuncture points: 30 min/session, 12 times for 8 weeks ($n = 76$). (B) Waiting list ($n = 74$)	(1) WOMAC pain at 8 weeks, at follow-up 26 and 52 weeks later (2) WOMAC function (3) WOMAC total (4) SF-36 physical health	(1) Acu vs A: $p < 0.001$ at 8 weeks, $p = 0.137$ at 26 weeks, $p = 0.285$ at 52 weeks. Acu vs B: $p < 0.001$ at 8 weeks. Acu vs A: NS at 26 and 52 weeks. (2) Acu vs A: $p < 0.001$ at 8 weeks, $p = 0.053$ at 26 weeks, $p = 0.081$ at 52 weeks. Acu vs B: $p < 0.001$ at 8 weeks	Major AEs: 9 (3 in MA, 2 in A, and 4 in B group). Minor AEs: In MA group: small hematoma of bleeding (18 cases) and other side effects (6), such as needling pain. In A group: small hematoma or bleeding (9), local inflammation at the needling site (1), and other side effect (6)

continued

TABLE 37.1 (continued)
Summary of the RCTs for OA

Year	Author	RCT Design Quality Score,[a] Allocation Concealment (Adequate, Inadequate/Unclear)	Participants (Diagnosis, Mean Disease Duration, Mean Age)	Acupuncture Group (No. of Randomized Patients)	Control (No. of Randomized Patients)	Main Outcome Measures	Intergroup Differences	Comments
							Acu vs A: NS at 26 and 52 weeks	
							(3) Acu vs A: $p = 0.0002$ at 8 weeks	
							Acu vs B: $p < 0.0001$ at 8 weeks	
							Acu vs A: NS at 26 and 52 weeks	
							(4) Acu vs A: $p = 0.003$ at 8 weeks	
							Acu vs B: $p < 0.001$ at 8 weeks	
							Acu vs A: NS at 26 and 52 weeks	
2004	Tukmachi [41]	Open, three arms $1 + 1 + 0 + 1 + 1 = 4$ Adequate	Patients with knee OA with mean pain duration of 10 years, mean age = 62 years	(A) MA + EA, formula), 20–30 min/session, 10 times plus medication, for 5 weeks ($n = 9$) (B) MA + EA, (formula), 20–30 min/session, 10 times without medication, for 5 weeks ($n = 10$)	(C) Only medication for 5 weeks ($n = 10$)	(1) VAS pain at 5 weeks (2) WOMAC pain and stiffness at 5 weeks (3) Global assessment	(1) A vs C and B vs C: $p < 0.05$ at 5 weeks (2, 3) NA	No

Year	Study	Design	Patients	Intervention	Comparison	Outcomes	Results	Adverse events
2006	Witt [42]	Open, parallel, six arms; 1 + 1 + 0 + 0 + 1 = 3; Adequate	Patients with knee or hip OA with mean pain duration of 5.4 years, mean age = 61 years	Knee: MA (individualized), 30 min/session, 11 times for 13 weeks (n = 175); Hip: MA (individualized), 30 min/session, 11 times for 13 weeks (n = 51); Hip and knee: MA (individualized), 30 min/session, 11 times for 13 weeks (n = 96)	Hip: waiting list (n = 41); Knee: waiting list (n = 167); Hip and knee: waiting list (n = 102)	(1) WOMAC pain at 3 months, at follow-up 6 months later (2) WOMAC function (3) WOMAC total (4) SF-36 physical component (5) SF-36 mental component	(1–4) each $p < 0.001$ at 3 months, NS at 6 months (5) $p = 0.048$ at 3 months, NS at 6 months; (1–4) each $p < 0.001$ at 3 months, NS at 6 months (5) each NS; (1–4) each $p < 0.001$ at 3 months, NS at 6 months (5) $p = 0.024$ at 3 months, NS at 6 months	Minor AEs: minor local bleeding or hematoma (66%), pain at the site of needle insertion (5%), vegetative symptoms (4%), and other (25%) of total cases (219 cases)
2001	Fink [43]	Parallel, two arms; 1 + 1 + 1 + 1 + 1 = 5; Unclear	Patients with hip OA with mean pain duration of 5.2 years, mean age = 62 years	MA (formula), 20 min/session, 10 times for 6 weeks (n = 23)	Sham acupuncture: same needling methods with acupuncture group on nonacupuncture point (n = 34)	(1) VAS at 2 weeks, 6 and 6 months after the end of treatment (2) Lequesne (3) Overall assessment (4) Quality of life	(1, 2) NS at 2 and 6 weeks, NR at 6 months (3) NR at 2 weeks, NS at 6 weeks, NR at 6 months (4) NS at 2 and 6 weeks and 6 months	No
2001	Haslam [44]	Open, parallel, two arms; 1 + 1 + 0 + 0 + 1 = 3; Unclear	Patients with hip OA with mean pain duration of 8 years, mean age = 67 years	MA (formula), 10 min for the first session, and 25 min for subsequent sessions, six times for 6 weeks (n = 16)	Advice and exercise: 30 min/session, three times for 6 weeks (n = 16)	Modified WOMAC total at immediately, 8 weeks	$p = 0.02$ at immediately, $p = 0.03$ at 8 weeks	

continued

TABLE 37.1 (continued)
Summary of the RCTs for OA

Year	Author	RCT Design Quality Score,[a] Allocation Concealment (Adequate, Inadequate/ Unclear)	Participants (Diagnosis, Mean Disease Duration, Mean Age)	Acupuncture Group (No. of Randomized Patients)	Control (No. of Randomized Patients)	Main Outcome Measures	Intergroup Differences	Comments
2004	Stener-Victorin [45]	Open, parallel, three arms 1 + 1 + 0 + 0 + 1 = 3 Adequate	Patients with hip OA, mean age = 67 years	EA (flexible formula), 30 min/session, 10 times for 5 weeks (n = 15)	(A) Hydrotherapy: 30 min/session, 10 times for 5 weeks (n = 15) (B) Education and exercise: 120 min/session, two times (n = 15)	(1) VAS (2) DRI at 1 month, 3 months after the last treatment (3) The global self-rating index	(1) No differences between all three groups (2) A vs B: $p < 0.01$ at 1 month EA vs B: $p < 0.01$ at 3 months, A group vs B group: $p < 0.05$ at 3 months (3) EA vs A: $p < 0.05$ at 1 month, EA vs B: $p < 0.01$ at 1 month, EA vs B: $p < 0.05$ at 3 months	No

Abbreviations: Acu, acupuncture; AE, adverse event; DRI, Disability Rating Index; EA, electroacupuncture; MA, manual acupuncture; Med, medication; Moxa, moxibustion; NR, not reported; NS, not significant; OKS, Oxford Knee Score; t.i.d., three times a day.

[a] Modified Jadad score.

[Pain]

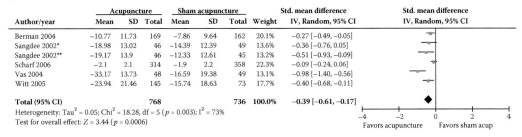

Author/year	Acupuncture			Sham acupuncture			Weight	Std. mean difference IV, Random, 95% CI
	Mean	SD	Total	Mean	SD	Total		
Berman 2004	−3.15	3.75	169	−2.66	3.28	162	20.3%	−0.14 [−0.35, 0.08]
Sangdee 2002*	−6.28	5.22	46	−4.9	3.71	49	13.5%	−0.30 [−0.71, 0.10]
Sangdee 2002**	−5.65	4	46	−3.31	4.58	45	13.1%	−0.54 [−0.96, −0.12]
Scharf 2006	−2.2	2.1	315	−1.9	2.3	358	22.5%	−0.14 [−0.29, 0.02]
Vas 2004	−10.71	3.96	48	−5.7	5.87	49	12.9%	−0.99 [−1.41, −0.57]
Witt 2005	−25.43	21.31	145	−17.59	20.42	73	17.7%	−0.37 [−0.66, −0.09]
Total (95% CI)			**769**			**736**	**100.0%**	**−0.36 [−0.58, −0.15]**

Heterogeneity: Tau^2 = 0.05; Chi^2 = 17.62, df = 5 (p = 0.003); I^2 = 72%
Test for overall effect: Z = 3.28 (p = 0.001)

[Function]

Author/year	Acupuncture			Sham acupuncture			Weight	Std. mean difference IV, Random, 95% CI
	Mean	SD	Total	Mean	SD	Total		
Berman 2004	−10.77	11.73	169	−7.86	9.64	162	20.1%	−0.27 [−0.49, −0.05]
Sangdee 2002*	−18.98	13.02	46	−14.39	12.39	49	13.6%	−0.36 [−0.76, 0.05]
Sangdee 2002**	−19.17	13.9	46	−12.33	12.61	45	13.2%	−0.51 [−0.93, −0.09]
Scharf 2006	−2.1	2.1	314	−1.9	2.2	358	22.3%	−0.09 [−0.24, 0.06]
Vas 2004	−33.17	13.73	48	−16.59	19.38	49	13.1%	−0.98 [−1.40, −0.56]
Witt 2005	−23.94	21.46	145	−15.74	18.63	73	17.7%	−0.40 [−0.68, −0.11]
Total (95% CI)			**768**			**736**	**100.0%**	**−0.39 [−0.61, −0.17]**

Heterogeneity: Tau^2 = 0.05; Chi^2 = 18.28, df = 5 (p = 0.003); I^2 = 73%
Test for overall effect: Z = 3.44 (p = 0.0006)

FIGURE 37.2 Effects of acupuncture versus sham acupuncture in knee OA at the short-term time point. *With a diclofenac cointervention; **with a placebo diclofenac co-intervention.

[Pain]

Author/year	Acupuncture			Sham acupuncture			Weight	Std. mean difference IV, Random, 95% CI
	Mean	SD	Total	Mean	SD	Total		
Berman 2004	−3.79	3.93	142	−2.92	3.61	141	24.5%	−0.23 [−0.46, 0.00]
Scharf 2006	−2.2	2.1	318	−2	2.3	360	58.8%	−0.09 [−0.24, 0.06]
Witt 2005	−20.59	22.37	146	−17.89	23.38	72	16.8%	−0.12 [−0.40, 0.16]
Total (95% CI)			**606**			**573**	**100.0%**	**−0.13 [−0.24, −0.01]**

Heterogeneity: Tau^2 = 0.00; Chi^2 = 0.97, df = 2 (p = 0.62); I^2 = 0%
Test for overall effect: Z = 2.19 (p = 0.03)

[Function]

Author/year	Acupuncture			Sham acupuncture			Weight	Std. mean difference IV, Random, 95% CI
	Mean	SD	Total	Mean	SD	Total		
Berman 2004	−12.42	13.29	142	−9.94	11.07	142	24.6%	−0.20 [−0.44, 0.03]
Scharf 2006	−2.1	2.2	318	−1.9	2.3	360	58.7%	−0.09 [−0.24, 0.06]
Witt 2005	−20.32	21.71	146	−15.34	19.89	72	16.7%	−0.23 [−0.52, 0.05]
Total (95% CI)			**606**			**574**	**100.0%**	**−0.14 [−0.26, −0.03]**

Heterogeneity: Tau^2 = 0.00; Chi^2 = 1.15, df = 2 (p = 0.56); I^2 = 0%
Test for overall effect: Z = 2.39 (p = 0.02)

FIGURE 37.3 Effects of acupuncture versus sham acupuncture in knee OA at the long-term time point.

and tabulated (Tables 37.2 and 37.3). In our overview, we included 11 RCTs involving 832 randomized RA participants [48–58].

ACUPUNCTURE VERSUS ACTIVE TREATMENT

Seven Chinese studies involving 636 patients (mean = 48 patients for acupuncture group versus 42 for control group) tested acupuncture against active treatment (Table 37.2). All studies had patients

[Pain]

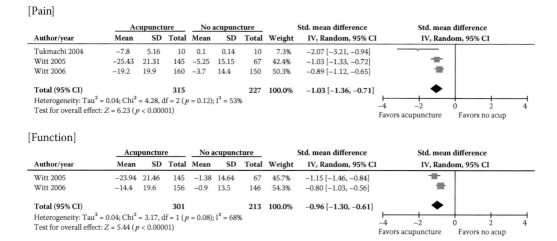

[Function]

FIGURE 37.4   Effects of acupuncture versus waiting list in knee OA at the short-term time point.

diagnosed according to the 1987 American College of Rheumatology (ACR) criteria, with a range of disease duration (<1–4.3 years) and a mean age (41.5–44.1 years); six of seven studies adopted manual acupuncture, but interventions greatly varied in terms of dosage of acupuncture treatment, number of sessions, duration of the whole treatment period, and acupuncture points used. Moxibustion was concomitantly given in five studies and warm needling in two studies, indicating that heat stimulation is often used in symptom management of RA patients in China. As an active treatment control, diclofenac with or without methotrexate and indomethacin were compared with acupuncture. Outcomes were assessed using a variety of measures, including clinical outcomes of total effectiveness rate, morning stiffness in minutes, pain intensity on VAS, tender joint count, and swollen joint count and hematological parameters such as erythrocyte sedimentation rate, C-reactive protein, and rheumatoid factor. In most studies, acupuncture improved symptoms but showed no significant difference compared with active medication (Table 37.2, Figure 37.5). It does not mean that acupuncture is equivalent to active treatment because these studies were not designed to answer such questions. Acupuncture or moxibustion-related adverse events were rare. The methodological quality is generally poor; thus, the results should be interpreted with great caution; six of seven trials reported they randomized patients without providing the methods or procedures they used. Blinding and reporting of withdrawals and dropouts are missing in their reports, which may lead to a bias. As inadequate or unclear allocation concealment is associated with overestimates of the intervention's effect [59], it is problematic that none of the reviewed studies described how they concealed group assignment.

From the findings of the trials in Table 37.2, we may develop the idea on adequate or practical acupuncture treatment for patients with RA. The current evidence, however, should not be judged either positive, that is, acupuncture is as effective as active medication, or just negative.

ACUPUNCTURE VERSUS SHAM/PLACEBO TREATMENT

To investigate specific effects of acupuncture treatment, sham/placebo-controlled trials are required. Four studies involving 196 patients tested acupuncture against sham/placebo-controlled treatment (Table 37.3). The results of probably the first sham-controlled trial comparing EA with sham EA by Man and Baragar in 1974 [58] are quite impressive. The RA patients suffering from bilateral knee pain received 5 mA of EA treatment on one knee and steroid injection on the other just once. For the control group, a single (probably identical) needling on nonacupuncture points was given and the

TABLE 37.2
Summary of the RCTs Comparing Acupuncture with Active Treatment for RA

Year	Author	RCT Design, Quality Score,[a] Allocation Concealment (Adequate/ Inadequate/ Unclear)	Participants (Diagnosis, Mean Disease Duration, Mean Age)	Acupuncture Group (No. of Randomized Patients)	Control Group (No. of Randomized Patients)	Main Outcome Measures	Intergroup Differences	Comments
2009	Chen [48]	Open, parallel, two arms $1 + 1 + 0 + 0 + 1 = 3$ Unclear	Patients with RA (1987 ACR criteria) with mean disease duration of 9.4 months, mean age = 43.1 years	MA, 30 min/session, q.d., for 3 months plus direct moxibustion at the 1st, 11th, and 21st day after MA, repeated three times ($n = 30$)	Diclofenac sodium, 25 mg, t.i.d. plus MTX, i.m., once weekly, (increasing dose of 5, 10, and 15 mg by week), for 3 months ($n = 30$)	Total effectiveness rate Morning stiffness (min) Pain intensity (VAS) at rest TJC SJC Hand grip strength (mmHg) ESR, RF 15-min walk (s)	(1–9) NS	Minor AEs including dizziness ($n = 2$) and infection ($n = 3$) after moxibustion 13 AEs including leukopenia ($n = 3$) and AST/ALT ↑ ($n = 4$) in the control group
2005	Xiang [49]	Open, parallel, two arms $1 + 0 + 0 + 0 + 0 = 1$ Unclear	Patients with RA (1987 ACR criteria) with mean disease duration of <1 year, mean age = 44.1 years	MA plus electronic moxibustion: three courses (one course consisting of 40 min/session of MA plus electronic moxibustion at 3–5 local acupuncture points for 10–20 min, q.d., for 15 days), 1 and 2 days of interval between courses ($n = 30$)	Diclofenac sodium tablet, b.i.d., for 7 weeks ($n = 30$)	Total effectiveness rate Morning stiffness (min) Pain intensity (VAS) at rest TJC SJC Hand grip strength (mmHg) 15-min walk (s) Joint function on four grades SOFI ESR, RF	(10) NS	Significantly different incidence of AEs between groups: feeling of faintness ($n = 1$) in the acupuncture group vs headache ($n = 1$), dizziness ($n = 1$), nausea ($n = 2$), and stomachache ($n = 4$) in the control group (incidence rate 3.3% vs 26.7%, $p < 0.05$)

continued

TABLE 37.2 (continued)
Summary of the RCTs Comparing Acupuncture with Active Treatment for RA

Year	Author	RCT Design, Quality Score,[a] Allocation Concealment (Adequate/ Inadequate/ Unclear)	Participants (Diagnosis, Mean Disease Duration, Mean Age)	Acupuncture Group (No. of Randomized Patients)	Control Group (No. of Randomized Patients)	Main Outcome Measures	Intergroup Differences	Comments
2003	Liu [50]	Open, parallel, two arms $1 + 0 + 0 + 0 + 0 = 1$ Unclear	Patients with RA (1987 ACR criteria) with mean disease duration of 3.6 years, mean age = 41.5 years	MA, 20 min/session, b.i.d. plus moxibustion on acupuncture point ST36 for 10 min, for 3 months ($n = 120$)	Diclofenac sodium, 25 mg, t.i.d. plus MTX, i.m., once weekly, (increasing dose of 5, 10, and 15 mg by week), for 3 months ($n = 120$)	Total effectiveness rate Morning stiffness (h) SJC Hand grip strength (mmHg) ESR, RF	(3) $p < 0.05$ (6) NS	No medication for the acupuncture group No AEs in the acupuncture group AEs in the control group including GI symptoms ($n = 14$), AST/ALT ↑ ($n = 3$), dizziness ($n = 2$), urine occult blood ($n = 1$), and skin eruption ($n = 1$)
2003	Jiang [51]	Open, parallel, two arms $1 + 0 + 0 + 0 + 0 = 1$ Unclear	Functional class 1 and 2 patients with RA (1987 ACR criteria) with mean disease duration of 4.3 years, mean age = 45.3 years	MA, 30 min/session, every other day for 1 month plus moxibustion ($n = 40$)	Indomethacin, 25 mg, t.i.d. ($n = 20$)	Total effectiveness rate SJC TJC Morning stiffness (h) Hand grip strength (mmHg) ESR, CRP RF	(2) NS, $p < 0.05$ (7) NS, $p < 0.05$	No AEs in the acupuncture group AEs in the control group including GI symptoms ($n = 3$) and headache ($n = 1$)

Year	Author [Ref]	Design, Jadad score	Patients	Intervention	Control	Outcomes	p	Adverse events
2002	Wang [52]	Open, parallel, two arms; 1 + 0 + 0 + 0 + 0 = 1; Unclear	Patients with RA (1987 ACR criteria) with disease duration of 45 days to 1 year, age of 24–58 years	MA, acute stage: b.i.d. for 7 days, recovery stage: once daily for 15 days (n = 61)	Indomethacin, 50 mg, t.i.d. plus *Tripterygium wilfordii* (triptolide) 20 mg, t.i.d. (n = 48)	Total effectiveness rate	p < 0.01	No medication for the acupuncture group; AEs were not reported
2001	Cui [53]	Open, parallel, two arms; 1 + 0 + 0 + 0 + 0 = 1; Unclear	Patients with RA (1987 ACR criteria), no information on disease duration or age	Warm needling, 20–30 min/session, q.d., for 1 month, repeated three times for 3 months with 5–7 days of intervals (n = 31)	Diclofenac sodium ointment, b.i.d., for 3 months (n = 31)	Tenderness index of joints; TJC; Morning stiffness	(1–3) NS	No AEs in the acupuncture group
2000	Zhou [54]	Open, parallel, two arms; 1 + 0 + 0 + 0 + 0 = 1; Unclear	Functional class 1 and 2 patients with RA (1987 ACR criteria) with mean disease duration of 3 years, mean age = 45 years	MA, 40 min/session, every other day plus warm needling and indirect moxibustion on the back for 1 month (n = 30)	Indomethacin, 25 mg, t.i.d., for 1 month (n = 15)	Total effectiveness rate; SJC; TJC; Morning stiffness (h); Hand grip strength (mmHg); ESR, CRP, RF	(8) NS	No medication for the acupuncture group; No AEs in the acupuncture group; Headache (n = 1) and GI symptoms (n = 2) in the control group

Abbreviations: ↑, increase; AE, adverse event; ALT, alanine aminotransferase; AST, aspartate aminotransferase; b.i.d., twice a day; CRP, C-reactive protein; ESR, erythrocyte sedimentation rate; GI, gastrointestinal; i.m., intramuscular injection; MA, manual acupuncture; MTX, methotrexate; NS, no significant difference; q.d., once a day; RF, rheumatoid factor; SJC, swollen joint count; SOFI, signs of functional impairment; t.i.d., three times a day; TJC, tender joint count.

a   Modified Jadad score [60].

TABLE 37.3
Summary of the RCTs Comparing Acupuncture with Sham/Placebo Treatment for RA

Year	Author	RCT Design, Quality Score,[a] Allocation Concealment (Adequate/ Inadequate/Unclear)	Participants (Diagnosis, Mean Disease Duration, Mean Age)	Acupuncture Group (No. of Randomized Patients)	Sham/Placebo Group (No. of Randomized Patients)	Main Outcome Measures	Intergroup Differences	Comments
2008	Zanette [55]	Parallel, two arms 1 + 1 + 1 + 1 = 5 Unclear	Patients with RA (1987 ACR criteria) with mean disease duration of 4.3 years, mean age = 45.3 years	MA, 40 min/ session, 10 sessions, twice weekly for 5 weeks ($n = 20$)	Sham acupuncture: superficial needling on nonacupuncture points, 20 min, 10 sessions, twice weekly for 5 weeks ($n = 20$)	Primary outcome: ACR 20 at 5th and 10th sessions and 1 month after the end of treatment Secondary outcomes: DAS Morning stiffness (min) Physician's global assessment of disease activity CRP	NS A, B, and D: NS, C: $p < 0.001$ at 10th session, $p = 0.011$ at 1 month after the end of treatment	Previous medications maintained and paracetamol allowed for both groups No formal testing of patient masking No major AEs in both groups
2007	Tam [56]	Parallel, three arms 1 + 1 + 1 + 1 = 5 Adequate	Patients with active RA (1987 ACR criteria), mean disease duration of 9.6 years, mean age = 52.3 years	(1) MA, 40 min/ session, 20 sessions, twice weekly for 10 weeks ($n = 12$) (2) EA, 40 min, 20 sessions, twice weekly for 10 weeks, 4/20 Hz ($n = 12$)	Sham EA: superficial needling and quickly withdrawn, no electrical current, 20 sessions, twice weekly for 10 weeks ($n = 12$)	(1) Primary outcome: pain intensity (VAS) at 10th week (2) Secondary outcomes: (A) ACR 20 (B) DAS28	(1, 2) NS	No medication for the acupuncture group For sham EA, withdrawn needles were mounted in a 2-cm cube of foam material adherent to the skin around the acupuncture point and connected to the inactive electrical current generator Minimal AEs

Year	Author	Study design / Jadad	Patients	Intervention	Comparison	Outcomes	Results	Comments
1999	David [57]	Crossover, two arms $1+1+1+1+1=5$ Adequate	Patients with RA (1987 ACR criteria), median disease duration of 8 and 12 years, median age = 61 and 57 years[b]	MA, 4 min/session, five sessions, once weekly for 5 weeks followed by 6 weeks of washout and sham acupuncture (n = 56)	Sham acupuncture: nonpenetrating sham on acupuncture point, patient's vision shielded, 4 min, five sessions, once weekly for 5 weeks followed by 6 weeks of washout and MA (n = 56)	(1) ESR, CRP (2) Pain intensity (VAS) (3) Patient global assessment (VAS) (4) SJC (5) TJC (6) DAS (7) GHQ (8) Analgesics	(1–8) NS	No AEs in both groups Medication allowed for both groups
1974	Man [58]	Parallel, two arms $1+0+0+0+1+0=2$ Unclear	Patients with seropositive RA for ≥5 years, for whom bilateral knee pain was a major problem	EA, 15 min/session, once, 5 mA, on one knee and steroid injection on the other knee (n = 10)	Sham acupuncture: (probably) identical needling on nonacupuncture points, 15 min/session, once, 5 mA, on one knee and steroid injection on the other knee (n = 10)	Pain reduction on a five-point Likert type scale	No patient improved in the sham acupuncture group 10 patients experienced improvement at 24 h, 7 patients at 1 month, 4 patients at 2 months, and 1 patient at 4 months after the end of treatment	The study knee was selected at random Medication maintained for both groups AEs were not reported

Abbreviations: ↑, increase; AE, adverse event; CRP, C-reactive protein; DAS, Disease Activity Score; ESR, erythrocyte sedimentation rate; GHQ, general health questionnaire; MA, manual acupuncture; NS, no significant difference; SJC, swollen joint count; TJC, tender joint count.

a Modified Jadad score [60].

b For the first and second sequences, respectively.

[Tender joint index]

Author/year	Acupuncture			Medication			Weight	Mean difference IV, Random, 95% CI	Mean difference IV, Random, 95% CI
	Mean	SD	Total	Mean	SD	Total			
Xiang 2005	5.17	2.55	30	4.37	2.87	30	68.3%	0.80 [−0.57, 2.17]	
Zhou 2000	7.1	7.35	30	4	3.07	15	31.7%	3.10 [0.05, 6.15]	
Total (95% CI)			**60**			**45**	**100.0%**	**1.53 [−0.57, 3.63]**	

Heterogeneity: Tau^2 = 1.18; Chi^2 = 1.81, df = 1 (p = 0.18); I^2 = 45%
Test for overall effect: Z = 1.43 (p = 0.15)

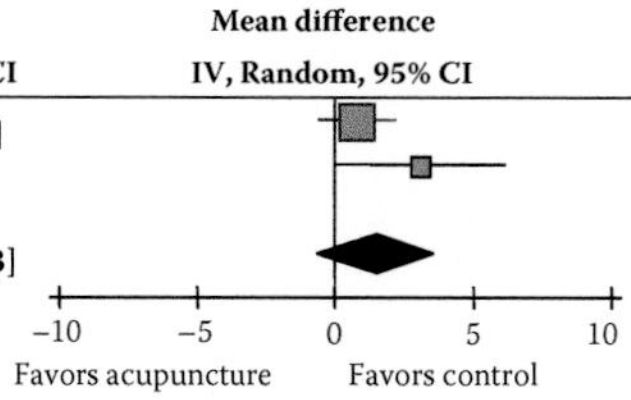

−10 −5 0 5 10
Favors acupuncture   Favors control

[Swollen joint index]

Author/year	Acupuncture			Medication l			Weight	Mean difference IV, Random, 95% CI	Mean difference IV, Random, 95% CI
	Mean	SD	Total	Mean	SD	Total			
Xiang 2005	6.03	3.01	30	6.33	3.71	30	67.4%	−0.30 [−2.01, 1.41]	
Zhou 2000	2.2	4.77	30	0.8	3.89	15	32.6%	1.40 [−1.21, 4.01]	
Total (95% CI)			**60**			**45**	**100.0%**	**0.25 [−1.31, 1.82]**	

Heterogeneity: Tau^2 = 0.18; Chi^2 = 1.14, df = 1 (p = 0.28); I^2 = 13%
Test for overall effect: Z = 0.32 (p = 0.75)

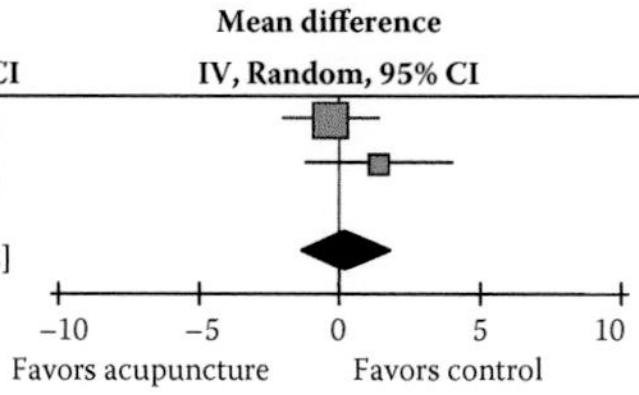

−10 −5 0 5 10
Favors acupuncture   Favors control

FIGURE 37.5   Acupuncture plus moxibustion versus active medication for symptom management of RA.

[Pain on a 100-mm visual analogue scale]

Author/year	Acupuncture			Sham acupuncture			Weight	Mean difference IV, Random, 95% CI	Mean difference IV, Random, 95% CI
	Mean	SD	Total	Mean	SD	Total			
Tam 2007	0.3	2.42	12	1.4	2.14	12	51.6%	−1.10 [−2.93, 0.73]	
Zanette 2009	2.24	3.72	20	1.46	2.4	20	48.4%	0.78 [−1.16, 2.72]	
Total (95% CI)			**32**			**32**	**100.0%**	**−0.19 [−2.03, 1.65]**	

Heterogeneity: Tau^2 = 0.84; Chi^2 = 1.91, df = 1 (p = 0.17); I^2 = 48%
Test for overall effect: Z = 0.20 (p = 0.84)

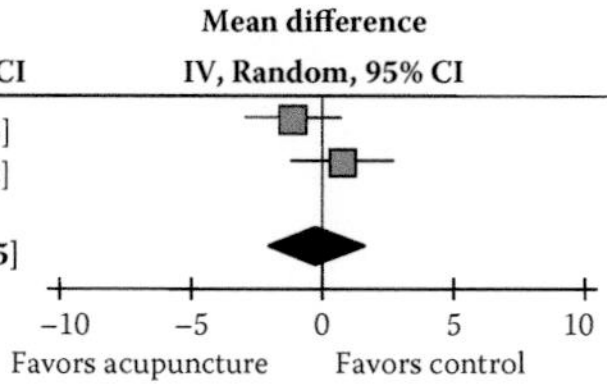

−10 −5 0 5 10
Favors acupuncture   Favors control

FIGURE 37.6   Acupuncture versus sham/placebo treatment for pain relief in RA.

needles were connected to a 5-mA electrical current on one knee and steroid injection on the other. In view of other trials of arthritis, it is rather surprising that pain relief from a single EA treatment sustained over a month.

In 1999, a crossover study was published in the United Kingdom [57]. It obtained a maximum 5 points on the modified Jadad scale [60, 61], its allocation concealment was assessed adequate, and it had the biggest sample size published ever (56 patients per arm is the largest so far). However, it was later criticized for its lack of validity in their acupuncture intervention, a 4-min long, once weekly treatment using a single distant acupuncture point [62, 63]. Not unexpectedly, this study resulted in no significant difference between real and sham acupuncture.

The other two trials, from Hong Kong [64] and Brazil [65], failed to find any significant difference compared with sham acupuncture in ACR 20 [65] and pain intensity change [64], and no clear anti-inflammatory effects were demonstrated (Figure 37.6). They were methodologically sound in terms of random sequence generation, patient and outcome assessor blinding, and reporting withdrawals and dropouts. Manual acupuncture or EA were given twice weekly for 5–10 weeks; thus, the intervention was considered intensive compared with the previous two trials [57, 58]. The outcome measures used were universal ones such as ACR 20 or Disease Activity Score.

The overall results suggest that acupuncture does not relieve pain or suppress inflammation in patients with RA. The trials, however, are small in number, and the evidence is limited because of various factors such as small sample size and inadequate acupuncture treatment and duration.

OTHER ACUPUNCTURE-RELATED TECHNIQUES FOR ARTHRITIS

MOXIBUSTION

Moxibustion uses thermal and chemical stimulants by burning herbal materials, including mugwort (*Artemisia vulgaris*, moxa), whereas acupuncture uses physical stimulation via insertion of needles. The therapeutic components of moxibustion are assumed as the combination of heat, tar (extract), aroma (fume), and psychological stress [66]. Recently, experimental studies suggested that moxibustion boosts the immune system [66, 67] and enhances physiological functions [68]. The moxibustion has been applied to chronic disease more frequently, and arthritis is one of the representative target disease for moxibustion. For the effects of indirect moxibustion ($n = 29$, moxa cone moxibustion, three times per week, total 20 times) improved the symptoms of OA compared with medication (sodium diclofenate, $n = 27$) at the 2-month follow-up period [69]. More rigorous clinical studies are required to confirm the efficacy of moxibustion for OA or RA.

BEE VENOM ACUPUNCTURE

Bee venom (BV) therapy has been used since ancient times, including administering honeybee stings, injection of BV, and BV acupuncture (BVA). BVA involves injecting purified and diluted BV into acupuncture points to intensify the therapeutic effects in clinical settings [70, 71]. BVA has been known to have pharmacological actions such as analgesic, antiarthritic, and anti-inflammatory effects through bioactive BV compounds, including peptides (melittin, adolapin, and apamin), enzymes (phospholipase A2), and amines. In some Asian countries including Korea, it is used for treating arthritis, reducing pain, and treating rheumatoid diseases. In clinical research, one RCT found that the pain associated with OA of the knee was controlled better by BVA ($n = 40$) than by classic acupuncture ($n = 20$) after eight sessions of treatment for 4 weeks [72, 73].

CONSTITUTIONAL APPROACH FOR THE ACUPUNCTURE TREATMENT

Pharmacogenetic knowledge indicates that genetic variations influence clinical treatment outcomes [74]. This concept of tailored medicine has been developed using an individualized and practical approach in traditional East Asian Medicine, and Korean constitutional medicine represented with "Sasang constitutional medicine" or "Four constitution medicine" takes the lead in this field. Constitution acupuncture method is that each person has a specific constitution, which determines the body's inherent strengths and weaknesses. In eight constitution acupuncture, each of the four constitutions is further divided into another two constitutions. Appearance, characteristics, body composition, and disease type together with the pulse diagnosis provide key information for discriminating the constitution.

In clinical trials, 20 sessions of eight constitution acupuncture treatment, which was prescribed differently according to patient's constitution ($n = 20$, three times per week, total 20 sessions), showed better improvement in pain VAS than classic acupuncture ($n = 20$) for knee OA at 7 weeks after randomization [75].

CONCLUSIONS

On the basis of the findings from sham-controlled trials, acupuncture seems to improve pain management and function in patients with knee OA for 2 or 3 months, but the effect is not maintained over a long-term period, and this requires further investigation. Acupuncture appears to be more effective than supervised education or physical consultation in both short- and long-term improvements in pain and function, but the evidence is rather limited. For hip OA, acupuncture showed statistically significant and clinically relevant benefit up to 6 months compared with waiting list control, but the cautious interpretation is needed due to the characteristics of the control group.

We have little convincing evidence that acupuncture helps patients with RA; that is, the results suggest that acupuncture does not relieve pain or suppress inflammation in patients with RA. The trials, however, are small in number, and the evidence is limited because of various factors such as small sample size and inadequate acupuncture treatment and duration.

It should be noted that the reviewed trials were clinically and methodologically heterogeneous to a large extent, for example, a range of controls including sham acupuncture that is still a controversial issue, various acupuncture interventions in terms of acupuncture point selection, manipulation and stimulation methods, and treatment frequency and period, and heterogeneous outcome measures that make data pooling and the interpretation difficult. All these complicated issues should be considered with caution in designing and conducting future research.

REFERENCES

1. Reston J. Now, about my operation in Peking. New York Times; July 26, 1971.
2. NIH Consensus Conference. Acupuncture. JAMA 1998;280(17):1518–1524.
3. Napadow V, Ahn A, Longhurst J, Lao L, Stener-Victorin E, Harris R, Langevin H. The status and future of acupuncture clinical research. J Altern Complement Med 2008;14(7):861–869.
4. Park J, Linde K, Manheimer E, Molsberger A, Sherman K, Smith C, Sung J, Vickers A, Schnyer R. The status and future of acupuncture clinical research. J Altern Complement Med 2008;14(7):871–881.
5. Furlan AD, van Tulder MW, Cherkin D, Tsukayama H, Lao L, Koes BW, Berman BM. Acupuncture and dry-needling for low back pain. Cochrane Database Syst Rev 2005;(1):CD001351.
6. Lee A, Fan L. Stimulation of the wrist acupuncture point P6 for preventing postoperative nausea and vomiting. Cochrane Database Syst Rev 2009;15(2):CD003281.
7. Linde K, Allais G, Brinkhaus B, Manheimer E, Vickers A, White AR. Acupuncture for tension-type headache. Cochrane Database Syst Rev 2009;(1):CD007587.
8. Linde K, Allais G, Brinkhaus B, Manheimer E, Vickers A, White AR. Acupuncture for migraine prophylaxis. Cochrane Database Syst Rev 2009;(1):CD001218.
9. Cheong YC, Hung YNE, Ledger WL. Acupuncture and assisted conception. Cochrane Database Syst Rev 2008;(4):CD006920.
10. Trinh K, Graham N, Gross A, Goldsmith CH, Wang E, Cameron ID, Kay TM; Cervical Overview Group, Acupuncture for neck disorders. Cochrane Database Syst Rev 2006;3:CD004870.
11. Manheimer E, Cheng K, Linde K, Lao L, Yoo J, Wieland S, van der Windt DAWM, Berman BM, Bouter LM. Acupuncture for peripheral joint osteoarthritis. Cochrane Database Syst Rev 2010;(1):CD001977.
12. Ezzo J, Richardson MA, Vickers A, Allen C, Dibble S, Issell BF, Lao L, et al. Acupuncture-point stimulation for chemotherapy-induced nausea or vomiting. Cochrane Database Syst Rev 2006;2:CD002285.
13. Bi syndromes. In: Shin H, Kim S, Lee J, Chung S, Lim H, Lee M, Lee I, et al., eds. Korean Medical Rehabilitation. Seoul: Seowondang; 1995:95–116.
14. Wang SM, Kain ZN, White P. Acupuncture analgesia: I. The scientific basis. Anesth Analg 2008;106:602–610.
15. Han JS. Acupuncture and endorphins. Neurosci Lett 2004;361(1–3):258–261.
16. Pan B, Castro-Lopes J, Coimbra A. Chemical sensory deafferentation abolishes hypothalamic pituitary activation induced by noxious stimulation or electroacupuncture but only decreases that caused by immobilization stress. A c-*fos* study. Neuroscience 1997;78(4):1059–1068.
17. Jeong HJ, Kim BS, Oh JG, Kim KS, Kim HM. Regulatory effect of cytokine production in asthma patients by SOOJI CHIM (Koryo Hand Acupuncture Therapy). Immunopharmacol Immunotoxicol 2002;24(2):265–274.
18. Xiao J, Liu X, Sun L, Ying S, Zhang Z, Li Q, Li H, et al. Experimental study on the influence of acupuncture and moxibustion on interleukin-2 in patients with rheumatoid arthritis. Zhen Ci Yan Jiu 1992;17(2):126–128, 132.
19. Yim YK, Lee H, Hong KE, Kim YI, Lee BR, Son CG, Kim JE. Electro-acupuncture at acupoint ST36 reduces inflammation and regulates immune activity in collagen-induced arthritic mice. Evid Based Complement Alternat Med 2007;4(1):51–57.
20. Kwon BY, Lee HJ, Han HJ, Mar WC, Kang SK, Yoon OB, Beitz AJ, Lee JH. The water-soluble fraction of bee venom produces antinociceptive and anti-inflammatory effects on rheumatoid arthritis in rats. Life Sci 2002;71(2):191–204.

21. Kwon YB, Lee JD, Lee HJ, Han HJ, Mar WC, Kang SK, Beitz AJ, Lee JH. Bee venom injection into an acupuncture point reduces arthritis associated edema and nociceptive responses. Pain 2001;90(3):271–280.

22. Peat G, McCarney R, Croft P. Knee pain and osteoarthritis in older adults: a review of community burden and current use of primary health care. Ann Rheum Dis 2001;60(2):91–97.

23. Prevalence of self-reported arthritis or chronic joint symptoms among adults—United States, 2001. MMWR Morb Mortal Wkly Rep 2002;51(42):948–950.

24. Felson DT, Zhang Y. An update on the epidemiology of knee and hip osteoarthritis with a view to prevention. Arthritis Rheum 1998;41(8):1343–1355.

25. Oliveria SA, Felson DT, Reed JI, Cirillo PA, Walker AM. Incidence of symptomatic hand, hip, and knee osteoarthritis among patients in a health maintenance organization. Arthritis Rheum 1995;38(8):1134–1141.

26. Recommendations for the medical management of osteoarthritis of the hip and knee: 2000 update. American College of Rheumatology Subcommittee on Osteoarthritis Guidelines. Arthritis Rheum 2000;43(9):1905–1915.

27. Pendleton A, Arden N, Dougados M, Doherty M, Bannwarth B, Bijlsma JW, Cluzeau F, et al. EULAR recommendations for the management of knee osteoarthritis: report of a task force of the Standing Committee for International Clinical Studies Including Therapeutic Trials (ESCISIT). Ann Rheum Dis 2000;59(12):936–944.

28. Wegman A, van der Windt D, van Tulder M, Stalman W, de Vries T. Nonsteroidal antiinflammatory drugs or acetaminophen for osteoarthritis of the hip or knee? A systematic review of evidence and guidelines. J Rheumatol 2004;31(2):344–354.

29. Ausiello JC, Stafford RS. Trends in medication use for osteoarthritis treatment. J Rheumatol 2002;29(5):999–1005.

30. Tramèr MR, Moore RA, Reynolds DJ, McQuay HJ. Quantitative estimation of rare adverse events which follow a biological progression: a new model applied to chronic NSAID use. Pain 2000;85(1–2):169–182.

31. Griffin MR, Piper JM, Daugherty JR, Snowden M, Ray WA. Nonsteroidal anti-inflammatory drug use and increased risk for peptic ulcer disease in elderly persons. Ann Intern Med 1991;114(4):257–263.

32. Cherkin DC, Sherman KJ, Deyo RA, Shekelle PG. A review of the evidence for the effectiveness, safety, and cost of acupuncture, massage therapy, and spinal manipulation for back pain. Ann Intern Med 2003;138(11):898–906.

33. White A, Hayhoe S, Hart A, Ernst E. Adverse events following acupuncture: prospective survey of 32 000 consultations with doctors and physiotherapists. BMJ 2001;323(7311):485–486.

34. MacPherson H, Thomas K, Walters S, Fitter M. The York acupuncture safety study: prospective survey of 34 000 treatments by traditional acupuncturists. BMJ 2001;323(7311):486–487.

35. Melchart D, Weidenhammer W, Streng A, Reitmayr S, Hoppe A, Ernst E, Linde K. Prospective investigation of adverse effects of acupuncture in 97 733 patients. Arch Intern Med 2004;164(1):104–105.

36. Berman BM, Lao L, Langenberg P, Lee WL, Gilpin AM, Hochberg MC. Effectiveness of acupuncture as adjunctive therapy in osteoarthritis of the knee: a randomized, controlled trial. Ann Intern Med 2004;141(12):901–910.

37. Sangdee C, Teekachunhatean S, Sananpanich K, Sugandhavesa N, Chiewchantanakit S, Pojchamarnwiputh S, Jayasvasti S. Electroacupuncture versus diclofenac in symptomatic treatment of osteoarthritis of the knee: a randomized controlled trial. BMC Complement Altern Med 2002;2:3.

38. Scharf H-P, Mansmann U, Streitberger K, Witte S, Kramer J, Maier C, Trampisch H-J, Victor N. Acupuncture and knee osteoarthritis: a three-armed randomized trial. Ann Intern Med 2006;145(1):12–20.

39. Vas J, Méndez C, Perea-Milla E, Vega E, Panadero MD, León JM, Borge MA, Gaspar O, Sánchez-Rodríguez F, Aguilar I, et al. Acupuncture as a complementary therapy to the pharmacological treatment of osteoarthritis of the knee: randomised controlled trial. BMJ 2004;329(7476):1216.

40. Witt C, Brinkhaus B, Jena S, Linde K, Streng A, Wagenpfeil S, Hummelsberger J, Walther HU, Melchart D, Willich SN. Acupuncture in patients with osteoarthritis of the knee: a randomised trial. Lancet 2005;366(9480):136–143.

41. Tukmachi E, Jubb R, Dempsey E, Jones P. The effect of acupuncture on the symptoms of knee osteoarthritis—an open randomised controlled study. Acupunct Med 2004;22(1):14–22.

42. Witt CM, Jena S, Brinkhaus B, Liecker B, Wegscheider K, Willich SN. Acupuncture in patients with osteoarthritis of the knee or hip: a randomized, controlled trial with an additional nonrandomized arm. Arthritis Rheum 2006;54(11):3485–3493.

43. Fink MG, Kunsebeck H, Wipperman B, Gehrke A. Non-specific effects of traditional Chinese acupuncture in osteoarthritis of the hip. Complement Ther Med 2001;9(2):82–89.

44. Haslam R. A comparison of acupuncture with advice and exercises on the symptomatic treatment of osteoarthritis of the hip—a randomised controlled trial. Acupunct Med 2001;19(1):19–26.

45. Stener-Victorin E, Kruse-Smidje C, Jung K. Comparison between electro-acupuncture and hydrotherapy, both in combination with patient education and patient education alone, on the symptomatic treatment of osteoarthritis of the hip. Clin J Pain 2004;20(3):179–185.

46. Lee MS, Shin BC, Ernst E. Acupuncture for rheumatoid arthritis: a systematic review. Rheumatology 2008;47(12):1747–1753.

47. Wang C, de Pablo P, Chen X, Schmid C, McAlindon T. Acupuncture for pain relief in patients with rheumatoid arthritis: a systematic review. Arthritis Rheum 2008;59(9):1249–1256.

48. Chen XH, Yao WM, Zou CP, Xu HB. Observation on therapeutic effect of muscular needling combined with scarring moxibustion on active stage of rheumatoid arthritis. Zhongguo Zhen Jiu 2009;29(11):884–886.

49. Xiang QX. Study of the early curative effect on rheumatoid arthritis by acupuncture combined with electronic moxibustion. Heilongjiang, China;Heilongjiang Traditional Chinese Medicine College. Master's thesis. 2005.

50. Liu W, Liu B, Wang Y, Chou YL, Zhang L, Shi XM. Observation on the therapeutic effect of acupuncture and moxibustion in 120 cases of rheumatoid arthritis. Zhongguo Zhen Jiu 2003;23(10):577–578.

51. Jiang S, Fan FY. Clinical observation on 40 cases of atrophic arthritis treated by acupuncture and moxibustion. Hunan Guiding J Trad Chin Med Pharmacol 2003;9(7):41–42.

52. Wang YJ. Combined acupuncture and west medication treating 109 cases of rheumatoid arthritis. Hunan Guiding J Trad Chin Med Pharmacol 2002;8(12):769–770.

53. Cui L, Guo RX, Gen W. Analgesic effect of warming needles in treating rheumatoid arthritis. Zhen Ci Yan Jiu 2001;26(3):185–186.

54. Zhou JL, Zhu Q. Effects of acupuncture on the rheumatoid arthritis. Chin J Rheumatol 2000;4(3):169–171.

55. Zanette S de A, Born IG, Brenol JC, Xavier RM. A pilot study of acupuncture as adjunctive treatment of rheumatoid arthritis. Clin Rheumatol 2008;27(5):627–635.

56. Tam LS, Leung PC, Li TK, Zhang L, Li EK. Acupuncture in the treatment of rheumatoid arthritis: a double-blind controlled pilot study. BMC Complement Altern Med 2007;7:35.

57. David J, Townsend S, Sathanathan R, Kriss S, Dore CJ. The effect of acupuncture on patients with rheumatoid arthritis: a randomized, placebo-controlled cross-over study. Rheumatology 1999;38(9):864–869.

58. Man S, Baragar F. Preliminary clinical study of acupuncture in rheumatoid arthritis. J Rheumatol 1974;1(1):126–129.

59. Pildal J, Hróbjartsson A, Jørgensen KJ, Hilden J, Altman DG, Gøtzsche PC. Impact of allocation concealment on conclusions drawn from meta-analyses of randomized trials. Int J Epidemiol 2007;36(4):847–857.

60. Jadad AR, Moore RA, Carroll D, Jenkinson C, Reynolds DJ, Gavaghan DJ, McQuay HJ. Assessing the quality of reports of randomized clinical trials: is blinding necessary? Control Clin Trials 1996;17:1–12.

61. White AR, Ernst E. A systematic review of randomized controlled trials of acupuncture for neck pain. Rheumatology 1999;38:143–147.

62. Tukmachi E. Acupuncture and rheumatoid arthritis. Rheumatology 2000;39(10):1153–1154.

63. Casimiro L, Barnsley L, Brosseau L, Milne S, Robinson VA, Tugwell P, Wells G, et al. Acupuncture and electroacupuncture for the treatment of rheumatoid arthritis. Cochrane Database Syst Rev 2005;(4):CD003788.

64. Tam LS, Leung PC, Li TK, Zhang L, Li EK. Acupuncture in the treatment of rheumatoid arthritis: a double-blind controlled pilot study. BMC Complement Altern Med 2007;7:35.

65. Zanette S de A, Born IG, Brenol JC, Xavier RM. A pilot study of acupuncture as adjunctive treatment of rheumatoid arthritis. Clin Rheumatol 2008;27(5):627–635.

66. Yamashita H, Ichiman Y, Tanno Y. Changes in peripheral lymphocyte subpopulations after direct moxibustion. Am J Chin Med 2001;29(2):227–235.

67. Kung YY, Chen FP, Hwang SJ. The different immunomodulation of indirect moxibustion on normal subjects and patients with systemic lupus erythematosus. Am J Chin Med 2006;34(1):47–56.

68. Shen X, Ding G, Wei J, Zhao L, Zhou Y, Deng H, Lao L. An infrared radiation study of the biophysical characteristics of traditional moxibustion. Complement Ther Med 2006;14(3):213–219.

69. Kim SY, Chae Y, Lee SM, Lee H, Park HJ. The effectiveness of moxibustion: an overview during 10 years. Evid Based Complement Alternat Med 2009;doi:10.1093/ecam/nep163.

70. Yin C, Park HJ, Chae Y, Ha E, Park HK, Lee HS, Koh H, et al. Korean acupuncture: the individualized and practical acupuncture. Neurol Res 2007;29(Suppl 1):S10–S15.

71. Lee JD, Park HJ, Chae Y, Lim S. An overview of bee venom acupuncture in the treatment of arthritis. Evid Based Complement Alternat Med 2005;2(1):79–84.

72. Ryu S, Lee JS, Kim SS, Jung SH. The effect of intraarticular bee venom injection on osteoarthritis of the knee. J Oriental Rehab Med 2004;14(1):35–52.

73. Won C, Choi E, Hong S. Efficacy of bee venom injection for osteoarthritis patients. J Korean Rheum Assoc 1999;6:218–226.

74. Lerman C, Shields PG, Wileyto EP, Audrain J, Pinto A, Hawk L, Krishnan S, Niaura R, Epstein L. Pharmacogenetic investigation of smoking cessation treatment. Pharmacogenetics 2002;12(8):627–634.

75. Chae S, Song H. The effect of 8 constitution acupuncture on degenerative arthritis of knee joint. J Korean Acupunct Moxibust Soc 2004;21:65–73.

38 Rehabilitative Strategies for Arthritis
Physical, Agents, Exercise, and Prosthesis Therapies

Nobuyuki Kawate, Mitsumasa Yoda, Naomi Yoshioka, and Masazumi Mizuma

CONTENTS

PHYSICAL AGENTS

Physical agents are a therapeutic system that uses physical energies such as heat, electricity, water pressure, magnetism, and acoustic waves to provoke a reaction in the body that in turn alleviates symptoms of diseases. It is a rehabilitation medicine that is often used for arthritis in conjunction with exercise therapy.

Physical agents has a long history, and there are records of therapies using heat or water regularly being used to treat arthropathy or respiratory diseases in the ancient Roman and the Greek eras [1]. In recent years, bathing in hot springs has been a popular folk remedy that promotes good health in general and relaxation. However, in today's medical care environment, physical agents are mostly used as a supplementary means to be used with exercise therapy, and it is rarely used alone as a core therapy.

Physical agents are classified into three major domains: thermotherapy, mechanotherapy, and electrotherapy (Table 38.1). Thermotherapy, in which thermal energy is used, is further classified into (1) therapies using conductive heat that is gradually transferred from the surface, (2) therapies using conductive heat generated deep in an object on the target tissue, and (3) therapies using converted heat. Thermotherapies are also classified as superficial heating or providing deep heating, which depend on the extent of heat penetration into the tissue. Traction, compression, and water are used in mechanotherapy, and low-frequency waves, transcutaneous electrostimulation, and magnetic stimulation are used in electrotherapy.

In this chapter, thermotherapy is described as it is often used in the treatment of arthritis. The expected effects of thermotherapy are as follows: (1) improved extension of collagen fibers, including those in contracted tendon and joint capsule [2]; (2) relaxation of muscle by reducing activity of γ-nerve fibers and, consequently, muscle [3]; (3) increased local blood flow, enhancing enzyme activity and metabolism in the tissue; (4) promotion of inflammatory reaction and tissue repair; and (5) analgesic effect by increasing the pain threshold.

THERMOTHERAPY

A hot pack is the most frequently used approach of thermotherapy because of its simplicity (Figure 38.1). A pack filled with hygroscopic material is placed in a thermostat bath at 80°C to maintain an optimal temperature for therapy. The pack should be wrapped with plastic cover and four to five towels before applying to the affected site.

To perform a paraffin bath (Figure 38.2), paraffin is heated in an automatic thermoregulated heating bath until it melts at around 50°C–55°C. The affected site is then dipped in the melted paraffin, or the melted paraffin is applied to the site. A few recommended methods by which paraffin bath

TABLE 38.1
Classification of Physical Agents

Thermotherapy
  Superficial heat
    Conduction heat: hot pack
      Paraffin bath
    Convect heat: Warm bath
    Radiant heat: Infrared ray
  Providing deep heating
    Conversive heat: Ultrashortwave therapy
      Microwave therapy
      Ultrasound therapy
Mechanotherapy
    Traction: Skeletal traction
      Indirect traction
    Compression: Elastic cartilage
    Water: Whirlpool bath
Electrotherapy
      Low-frequency current therapy
      Transcutaneous electrical nerve stimulation
      Functional electrical stimulation
      Magnetic stimulation

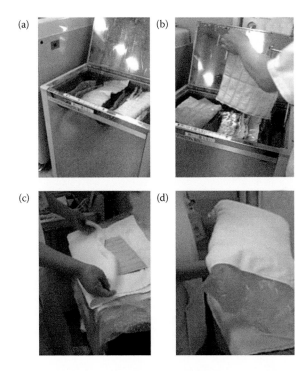

FIGURE 38.1 Hot pack. (a) A thermostat bath at 80°C. (b) The scene which picks up a pack from a thermostat bath. (c) The pack should be wrapped with plastic cover and four to five towels. (d) The completion of a hot pack. This is put on the affected part.

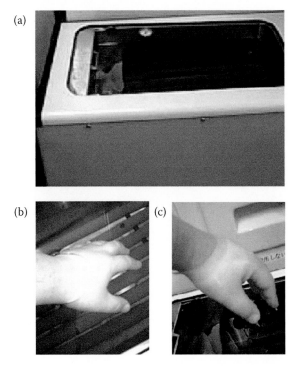

FIGURE 38.2 Paraffin bath. (a) An automatic thermoregulated heating bath at around 50°C–55°C. (b) The affected site is then dipped in the melted paraffin. (c) "Paraffin glove."

can be performed. One is the glove method, in which the affected hand, for example, is immersed into paraffin in bath for 2–3 s, then the hand is removed from the bath until the paraffin becomes hardened and is again re-placed in the bath. The aforementioned procedure is repeated approximately 10 times, thereby producing the so-called "paraffin glove."

Ultrashortwave and microwave therapies that belong to thermotherapies generate energies ranging from 30 to 300 MHz and from 300 to 3000 MHz for treatments, respectively (Figure 38.3). Ultrashortwave therapy is not a preferred choice in Japan because of large sizes of the equipment and accessories for storing at limited space. Frequency and output for a microwave therapy device are defined to be 2450 MHz and 200 W or lower, respectively. Irradiation should last approximately 20 min, and the applicator should be held approximately 10 cm from the skin.

Ultrasound therapy is a thermotherapy that uses acoustic waves of 1–3 MHz (Figure 38.4). It is used either by a direct method or underwater method. In the direct method, the applicator is directly applied to and moved around on the affected area, which is covered with ultrasound cream, whereas in

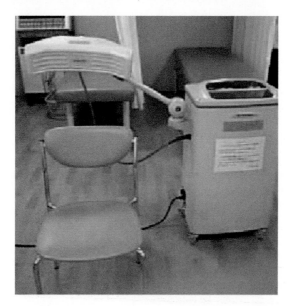

FIGURE 38.3   Microwave therapy.

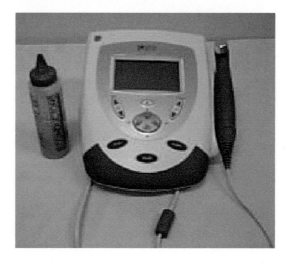

FIGURE 38.4   Ultrasound therapy.

TABLE 38.2
Contraindications for Thermotherapy

General contraindications

- Consciousness
- Sensory loss
- Severe circulatory impairment
- Acute phase inflammatory disease
- Malignant tumors
- Bleeding tendency
- Heart failure

Specific contraindications

Ultrashortwave therapy and microwave therapy
- Pacemakers
- Implanted metals (prostheses)
- Eye balls

Ultrasound therapy
- Malignant tumor
- Central nerves
- Deep vein thrombosis

---

the underwater method, the affected limb is placed in water and irradiated from a distance of approximately 1 cm. Thermal and nonthermal effects can be expected when using these methods. Irradiation is performed at 1.0–2.5 and 0.5–1.0 W/cm^2 to exert thermal and nonthermal effects, respectively. Microvibration can be expected to have massaging and other effects on the connective tissue [4].

Contraindications for Thermotherapy

Contraindications for thermotherapy [5, 6] including general contraindications and those specific to each treatment method are shown in Table 38.2. General contraindications are as follows: (1) patients with impaired consciousness or sensory loss who cannot complain of a burn risk; (2) severe circulatory impairment in which oxygen supply may become insufficient because of increases in localized metabolic activities caused by heat, possibly leading to tissue necrosis; (3) acute phase inflammatory disease with marked redness, swelling, and feeling hot; (4) malignant tumors; (5) bleeding tendency; and (6) heart failure. Specific contraindications are as follows: (1) pacemakers, implanted metals including prostheses; (2) the eyeballs for ultrashort and microwave therapies; (3) malignant tumors, irradiation of sites with central nerves exposed by laminectomy or other treatments; and (4) deep vein thrombosis for ultrasound therapy [7].

EXERCISE THERAPY

Arthritis causes arthralgia, joint contracture, and joint deformity as well as dysfunctions such as limited range of motion in joints and muscle weakness leading to disabilities including gait disturbance and activities of daily living impairment. Among exercise therapies for arthritis are approaches to treat dysfunction, including ranges of joint motion training and muscle strength training and approaches to treat disability, including gait training, basic movement training, and activities of daily living training. The basic ranges of joint motion training and muscle strength training are discussed in the next paragraph.

The aim of range of joint motion training is to move joints through their entire range of motion; it is effective for maintaining mobility. In addition, mobility can be improved by active or passive extension at the maximum range of motion, when the range is limited because of joint contracture or other factors. Several types of training for joints include as follows: (1) the active motion method, in which patients move their joints themselves; (2) the passive motion method, in which joints are moved solely by an external force such as that provided by therapists; and (3) the assisted active motion method, in which patients move their joints assisted by external force. When a patient undertakes training as treatment for arthritis, one of the above methods is selected on the basis of the severity of inflammation or presence of pain. Anti-inflammatory treatment should be prioritized in patients with a severe inflammatory condition such as redness and swelling. If inflammation is under control, thermotherapies such as the hot pack therapy can enhance the efficacy of range of motion training when provided before the onset of the training. Hence, thermotherapy is often conducted in combination with motion training. However, an excessive range of motion training can cause symptoms in other areas as a result of compensation by adjacent joints. Therefore, for example, the joints of the spine, the pelvis and the lower extremities must all be considered in range of motion training for lower extremities.

Muscle strength training is divided into isometric, isotonic, and isokinetic training based on the form of muscle contraction. Isometric training is preferred for active arthritis, for which overload on joints should be avoided. For stable arthritis, isotonic training, which is the physiological exercise of the joints, is used, and patients can also undertake progressive resistance exercise with increasing exercise load. Furthermore, hydro-training, including walking in a heated pool, is considered effective because of the reduction in weight bearing due to buoyancy, the exercise load created by fluid resistance, pain relief due to the heat, and increase in muscle blood flow.

OSTEOARTHRITIS

Osteoarthritis (OA) causes degenerative change in joint components such as the articular cartilage, and subsequent destruction and proliferative change in cartilages and bones, which may result in pain and dysfunctions such as limited range of motion and muscle weakness. In particular, OA of lower extremities such as the hip or knee joints can easily lead to decreased movement ability and activities of daily living. Previous reports conclude that exercise therapy is effective for pain relief of lower extremities and improvement of dysfunction [8–11].

In range of joint motion training, it should be noted that flexion contracture and limited abduction and medial rotation of the hip joints often develop at advanced to terminal stages of OA, especially hip OA in late middle age. Limited extension of the hip joints can exacerbate anterior inclination of the pelvis and lumbar lordosis. In addition, knee OA can be complicated by secondary synovitis or hydrarthrosis in its exacerbation period, which causes acute deterioration in range of motion in many cases. The presence of these complications should be investigated before undertaking thermotherapy prior to range of motion training. An intervention including arthrocentesis should be performed in patients with hydrarthrosis before any range of motion training, whereas training volume may have to be reduced if a severe inflammatory condition is observed.

As for muscle strength training, isometric training is often preferred for OA of lower extremities because of joint pain during exercise and limited range of motion. In hip OA, the progressive disease gradually causes the epiphysis to shift outward leading to decreased abductor muscle strength in the hip joints. Reinforcement of the joint hip abductor muscle, particularly the gluteus medius, is effective for inhibiting disease progression and alleviating pain (Figure 38.5). Patients with knee OA need to reinforce quadriceps strength (Figure 38.6) because a decrease in quadriceps strength is likely to accelerate disease progression due to exacerbation of symptoms as well as decrease in stability and impact absorption of the knee joints.

RHEUMATOID ARTHRITIS

RA causes decreased motor functions including joint pain, limited range of motion, joint deformation, and muscle weakness because of arthritis (mainly synovitis) and subsequent joint destruction,

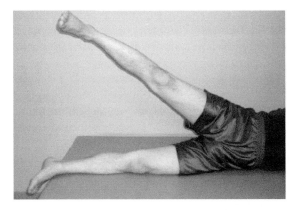

FIGURE 38.5 Reinforcement of the joint hip abductor muscle.

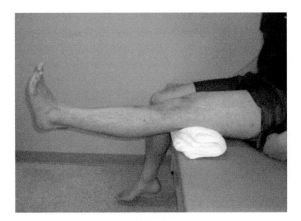

FIGURE 38.6 Reinforcement of quadriceps strength.

for which exercise therapies such as range of joint motion and muscle strength training are crucial. Adequate attention should be paid to exercise load during periods of active inflammation coinciding with a period of joint destruction progression; such cases basically require rest without overloading of the joints. However, measures should be taken to prevent progression of disuse even in this period. Aggressive exercise therapy should be carried out in a period of nonactive inflammation to improve dysfunctions that have occurred in the inflammation period. Joint protection, however, always has to be considered to prevent disease progression when performing training, even in this period.

In range of joint motion training, active motion, assisted active motion, or passive motion is used on the basis of the patient's ability to perform joint movements without assistance. In an acute inflammation period, active motion or assisted active motion can be used, while paying attention to not causing pain. However, for synovitis, which is highly active and accompanied by pain and muscle spasm, active motion causes hypertonia and increased compressive force on the joints. Therefore, gentle passive motion combined with muscle relaxation may be more effective. Extension (stretching) training is effective for the contracted joints. However, training must be performed carefully, as in an acute phase, pain from extension training elicits muscle spasm, adding load to a structure that is already maximally extended by joint swelling, which may lead to an enlarged injury area in the joints.

Muscle strength training is important as muscle weakness increases load to the joints, potentially leading to joint destruction. In an acute inflammation phase, joint movement can aggravate joint pain or destruction, therefore, isometric training without joint movement is used. When no inflammation is present, isotonic resistance exercise may enhance the effect.

The abductor muscle group strength can be reinforced to prevent deformation of the hip joints in adduction and medial rotation direction. In addition, because limitations easily occur in extension of the hip joints, exercise in extension direction should be performed in standing or supine position. Concerning the knee joints, quadriceps strength in particular should be particularly reinforced as their extension is limited in many cases. Pes planus often develops because of the collapse of the arch in the area surrounding the foot joints. When this occurs, body weight applied to the area under the metatarsophalangeal joints may cause callus, and pulling on the toe flexor tendon group may contribute to hammer toe. Effective exercises for prevention include those where the patient tries to lift the plantar arch while pulling a towel on the floor toward them (Figure 38.7). As an exercise of the foot joints to maintain range of motion, patients can perform low dorsiflexion or rotational motion in sitting position.

PROSTHESIS THERAPY FOR RA

Prostheses are used at various sites in RA patients. The purposes are as follows: (1) stabilization of the affected sites, (2) prevention of deformation, (3) alleviation of weight bearing, (4) relief of pain, and (5) support [12–17]. However, prostheses do not have the effect of correcting established deformities. Therefore, it is important to prevent deformity or contracture by applying a prosthesis when patients first complain of symptoms, in the early stage of the disease, of joint swelling, pain, or discomfort in their daily life. Prostheses should be selected depending on the joint deformity condition or pathology as well as requests from and the life style of the patients.

CERVICAL SPINE PROSTHESES

Patients with RA often develop cervical spine lesions in the upper cervical spine. Atlantoaxial subluxation is especially frequent in such patients and neurologic symptoms including paralysis in extremities and sensory disorder may develop in the advanced stage. Progression of dislocation should therefore be prevented with prosthetic fixation [12, 17].

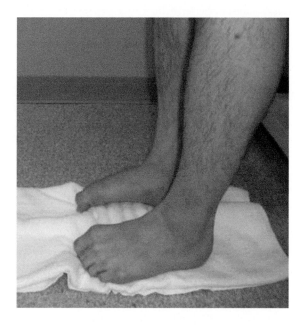

FIGURE 38.7 "Towel gathering" (pulling a towel on the floor).

There are soft, semirigid, and rigid types of cervical spine prostheses. Soft prostheses used in the early stage are effective for preventing hyperextension of the cervical spine, but their fixation strength is relatively weak. Semirigid or rigid prostheses limits movement of the cervical spine on the sagittal plane more strongly than soft prostheses, but their control on lateral flexion or rotation is weaker. A prosthesis that covers the cervical to thoracic region is necessary for a stronger fixation.

PROSTHESES FOR UPPER EXTREMITIES

Upper extremities prostheses, which stabilize the joints, are used to prevent pain or deformation, maintain and protect residual functions, and recover lost function [17]. Their applications should be considered when patients first complain of joint swelling or discomfort when moving, instead of considering it after any deformation has occurred. Ideal prostheses should not only have good stability and functionality but should also be compact, easy to apply/remove, comfortable when applied, and aesthetically satisfying.

Shoulder Joints

Supporters may be used to keep warm.

Elbow Joints

Supporters for providing rest in an inflammatory period and a prosthesis with a strut for reducing joint instability are used but are only indicated in a small number of cases.

Wrist Joints

Fixation of the wrist joints in dorsiflexion can maintain finger function, while reducing pain by giving rest to the affected joints. A prosthesis is also used for correcting ulnar deviation [12].

Fingers

A soft prosthesis or a plastic prosthesis is used for Z-deformity or swan-neck deformity of the thumb. Care should be taken not to put pressure on deformed or protruding bones or joints. A skeletal arch can be applied to the hand to allow smooth motions including grasping or antagonistic movements. When using a finger prosthesis, functional positioning is important [12, 18, 19].

PROSTHESES FOR THE LOWER EXTREMITIES

Prostheses should be made such that they relieve pain and prevent bone destruction, decreased weight-bearing strength, and deformation [17].

Hip Joints

Hip joint prostheses are used to help fixation and reduce weight bearing. However, their indications are limited because of their large size and resulting physical burden.

Knee Joints

Supporters are often applied to relieve pain and prevent hydrarthrosis. A knee prosthesis with struts may be used in patients with unstable weight-bearing property, bone destruction, genu valgum, or bowleg.

Foot Joints

For varus or valgus instability, a foot joint supporter or a short prosthesis to support bilateral malleoli are applied. A sole prosthesis is used to prevent pes planovalgus caused by talocalcaneal joint slippage.

Feet and Toes

RA patients may develop hallux valgus, buionette, hammer toe, or pes planus caused by plantar ligament laxity. These symptoms can be corrected using a hallux valgus corrective orthotic or a specific insole in the early stages. However, because advanced deformity can cause plantar callus or clavus, tailor-made shoes of specific size must be prepared. Such shoes must be devised using appropriate devices, such as a metatarsal bone pad, a plantar plate of soft material, or large toe box [12].

REFERENCES

1. Kunihiko Fukui. Hydrotherapy. In: Moichi Sunahara, ed. Physical Agents, 3rd ed. Tokyo: Ishiyaku Publishers, Inc.; 1991:177–179.
2. Lentell G, Hetherington T, Eagen J, Moragan M. The use of thermal agents to influence the effective of low load prolonged stretch. J Orhop Sport Phys Ther 1992;16(5):200–207.
3. Mense S. Effects of temperature on the discharges of muscle spindles and tendon organs. Plugers Arch 1978;374:159–166.
4. Lehmann JF. The biophysical basis of biologic ultrasonic reaction with special reference to ultrasonic therapy. Arch Phys Med Rehabil 1953;34:139–152.
5. Feucht BL, et al. Effect of implanted metals on tissue hyperthermia produced by microwaves. Arch Phys Med Rehabil 1949;30:164–169.
6. Yasutomo O. Physical therapy in modern textbook of rehabilitation medicine, 3rd ed. Edited by NaoichChino. Tokyo: KANAHARA Co., Ltd., 2007, 237–242.
7. Kouji Shomoto. Outline of ultrasound therapy. In: Kazuho Hosoda, ed. Physical Agents Text. Tokyo: Nankodo; 2008:103–114.
8. Thomas KS, Muir KR, Doherty M, Jones AC, O'Reilly SG. Home based exercise programme for knee pain and knee osteoarthritis: Randomised controlled trial. BMJ 2002;325:752–756.
9. Topp KR, Wolley S, Hornyak J III, Khuder S, Kahaleh B. The effects of dynamic versus isometric resistance training on pain and functioning among adults with osteoarthritis of the knee. Arch Phys Med Rehabil 2002;83:1187–1195.
10. Hoeksma HL, Dekker J, Ronday HK, Heering A, van der Lubbe N, Vel C, Breedveld FC, van den Ende CH. Comparison of manual therapy and exercise therapy in osteoarthritis of the hip: a randomized clinical trial. Arthritis Rheum 2004;51:722–729.
11. Weigl M, Angst F, Stucki G, Lehmann S, Aeschlimann A. Inpatient rehabilitation for hip or knee osteoarthritis: 2 year follow up study. Ann Reum Dis 2004;63:360–368.
12. Hsu J, Michael J, Fisk J. *AAOS* Atlas of Orthoses and Assistive Devices. 4th ed. Philadelphia: Elsevier Mosby.
13. Murasawa A. Conservative therapy. In: Takahiro Ochi, Shinichi Kikuchi, eds. New Book of Orthopaedics: I. Rheumatoid Arthritis. Tokyo: KANAHARA Co. Ltd; 1997:170–178.
14. Kawamura J, Takeuchi T. *Gishisougugaku*. 2nd ed. Igakushoin; 2000.
15. Clark H, Rome K. A critical review of foot orthoses in the rheumatoid arthritic foot. Rheumatology 2006;45:139–145.
16. Murasawa A. Rehabilitation to rheumatoid arthritis. MB Orthopaedics 2009;9:67–71.
17. Murasawa A. Rehabilitation to rheumatoid arthritis. MB Orthopaedics 2005;10:176–183.
18. Fukuda E. Occupational therapy for rheumatoid arthritis. Medical Rehabilitation 2006;71:47–53.
19. Nakaki U. Sprinting to hands and fingers. MB Medical Rehabilitation 2008;95:13–19.

39 Rehabilitation for Arthritis
Daily Life Guidelines

Fumihito Kasai and Masazumi Mizuma

CONTENTS

INTRODUCTION

Rheumatoid arthritis (RA) and osteoarthritis (OA) are complicated rheumatic diseases that require multifaceted support for treatment. To improve a normal lifestyle and to live comfortably, daily life guidance (DLG) is necessary in addition to surgical/medical therapy and exercise therapy. The purpose of DLG is to establish an exercise routine and lifestyle for preventing/improving functional disorders without applying excessive load on the joints.

REST AND EXERCISE

Despite the fact that there have been no randomized clinically controlled trials that adequately assess the value of rest in cases of RA and OA, various "rest therapies" have received attention and support mainly in the treatment of RA. In fact, in the past, hospitalization to allow for complete bed rest was recommended as a treatment method, and it had been well known that joint fixation with plaster and a splint could achieve noticeable inflammatory suppression and pain relief. Rest, in current arthritis treatments, refers to patients with arthritis discontinuing physical activities during exacerbations of the disease, taking regular rests during the day, and adjusting their physical surroundings to reduce fatigue and load onto the joints that are unavoidable in daily life.

The expected effects of rest as a treatment must be compared with the inevitable side effect of disuse syndrome caused thereby. Reduced physical strength is a complication that is always associated with forced rest even in case of healthy individuals, with more significant influence on patients who have already been weakened by chronic arthritis. Therefore, to obtain the original benefits of rest, it is essential to practice a rest program, taking into consideration the current physical ability of the patient and balancing the program with an appropriate exercise therapy.

To maintain and to improve activities of daily living (ADL), both joint range of motion and muscle strength training are important. For maintaining muscle strength, it is said that by exercising for around 15 min at a time, pain diminishes within 2 h or that by simply performing exercise that does not result in fatigue the next day three times a week. It is possible to maintain and improve endurance, and thus, it is also indispensable to provide guidance for exercise routines in daily life.

ACTUAL DLG

The basics of DLG are "joint protection" and "energy conservation." "Joint protection" refers to the avoidance of movements that promote inflammation and deformation of the joints, utilization of equipment, changing methods to those which put less loads on the joints, and usage of tools. "Energy conservation" includes checking posture during work and work descriptions to avoid excessive load on the joints, attempting various methods of rest, and arranging environments such that tasks can be performed safely and comfortably, for example.

Swezey [1] described four principles of joint protection: (1) joints protected by splints, rest, or during activities should be positioned to avoid deformities; (2) transferring skills (e.g., ability to arise from a chair or get in a car) must be instructed to provide optimal independence, joint protection, safety, and energy conservation; (3) the strongest joints should be used insofar as possible during activities (e.g., shoulder strap vs a handle on a purse); and (4) planning and pacing activities to minimize prolonged or excessive joint use and to conserve energy. In addition, Melvin [2] described the following 10 items as principles of joint protection: (1) respect for pain; (2) rest and work balance; (3) maintenance of muscle strength and joint range of motion; (4) reduction of effort; (5) avoidance of positions of deformity; (6) use of stronger/larger joints; (7) use of each joint in its most stable anatomical and functional plane; (8) avoidance of staying in one position; (9) avoidance of activities that cannot be stopped; and (10) use of assistive equipment and orthoses.

Next, we will list precautions when performing DLG. First, it is requisite to sufficiently understand the daily life and lifestyle of the patient. As a characteristic of the joint disease, symptoms will vary significantly during the day and depending on the day, and consequently, the condition of ADL is different depending on the time of day. In the case of prolonged progression, the family and the patient might have already attempted various methods that are not appropriate to alleviate the symptoms; therefore, it is needed to tailor guidance for each patient in consideration of what kind of care is insufficient in the life of the patient, what kind of guidance is important, and so forth. Second, it is necessary to respect self-determination. Because the patient and the family are the decision makers in terms of quality of life, it is inevitable that instructors be careful not to impose their own ideals. As a rule, instructors should respect the patients' independence and approach them with the attitude of assisting their own self-determination. As a particular guidance method, it is important to carefully evaluate the remaining ability in light of the psychological aspect and comfort and to provide minimal necessary assistance and environmental arrangement.

Because joint destruction and deformation frequently occur in delicate fingers, it is required to advise not to lift heavy objects and to protect the fingers in daily life. The load from daily life activities placed on the fingers causes ulnar side deflection, buttonhole deformation, swan-neck deformation, multilane deformation, and so forth. Subluxation due to RA deformation is a result of broken bones and is difficult to cure even by resetting with a brace. It is desirable to prevent this in the early stages through life guidance and wearing corrective/resting braces. Some biological pharmaceuticals require self-injection, and thus, it may be necessary to consider braces/self-help tools for the purpose of treatment of arthritis itself.

Destruction and deformation in the joint of the lower leg develop when muscle strength increasingly declines because of rest, and walking also becomes detrimental; however, when walking training is actively performed, destruction and deformation of the lower leg joint occur. To prevent deformation of the foot by RA and to correct deformation in the early phase, intensified joint range of motion and muscle strength training are encouraged in daily life. It is also advised not to walk on the floor barefoot and to choose a pair of shoes suitable for walking and the foot itself.

EVIDENCE OF DLG

Employing 311 cases of the intervention group selected from multiple facilities and 233 cases of a control group, Barlow et al. [3] conducted a 6-week arthritis self-management program for the intervention group once a week for 2 h a day. This program is a patient education method, with the aim of acquiring pain management techniques on the basis of behavior learning theory. The content to be passed on included providing information on arthritis, principles of self-management, appropriate exercise techniques, cognitive ethological management methods, methods for coping with depression, appropriate nutrition, and so forth, using *The Arthritis Helpbook* [4] as a textbook. In comparing effects after 4 months from the initiation of the intervention, significant improvement was observed in activity (Stanford Health Assessment Questionnaire), pain (Visual Analog Scale), self-awareness of arthritis, acquisition of the method of cognitive ethological pain management, fatigue, and depressive tendencies in the intervention group. Employing 65 cases of the intervention group and 62 cases of a control group selected from two facilities, Hammond et al. [5, 6] conducted a joint protection program on the basis of behavioral therapy and motor learning for groups of three to four individuals of the intervention group at four times for 2 h at a time, whereas for the control group, they provided a lecture only. It was described that when comparing the effects, significant improvement was noted after 6 and 12 months from the intervention in hand pain, stiffness in the morning, level of acquisition of the joint protection, and activity level shown by the Arthritis Impact Measurement Scale 2 in the intervention group, and that even after 4 years, the acquisition level of joint protection and ADL were significantly high. Solomon et al. [7] conducted a 6-week self-management program in 104 cases of the intervention group, including OA selected from multiple facilities once a week for 2 h at a time while providing *The Arthritis Helpbook*, [4] and in only 74 cases in the control group; then the two groups were compared. As a result of the study, no differences were observed between the tested groups according to the Stanford Health Assessment Questionnaire and the Medical Outcome Study 36-item Short-Form Health Survey after 4 months in pain, activity, level of mental health, physical activity, and self-awareness of pain, repudiating the effectiveness of patient education.

APPROACH TO PSYCHOLOGICAL ASPECTS

From the background of RA that frequently occurs in young to middle-aged women, a psychological approach is important, including esthetical issues as well as marriage and sex-related issues. In addition, personality change has also been pointed out in patients with RA; because it is known that the disease deteriorates attributed to stress, it is important to adjust living environment, for example, by maintaining a stable mood. To create such an environment in which the patient can live comfortably, involving only patient and medical staff is inadequate, and it is thus necessitous to obtain support from the family. It is very important for the patient to consider a daily life with as little stress as possible. Furthermore, a cohesive family environment is essential for mental support and a supportive environment that allows the solving of a wide variety of problems that the patient may possess.

REFERENCES

1. Swezey RL. Essential therapies for joint, soft tissue, and disc disorders. Philadelphia: Hanley & Belfus; 1998.
2. Melvin JL. Rheumatic disease in the adult and child: occupational therapy and rehabilitation. 3rd ed. Philadelphia: FA Davis Company; 1989:421–424.
3. Barlow JH, Turner AP, Wright CC. A randomized controlled study of the arthritis self management programme in the UK. Health Educ Res 2000;15:659–663.

4   Lorig K, Fries JF. The Arthritis Helpbook: A Tested Self-Management Program for Coping with Arthritis and Fibromyalgia, 6th Edition, Cambridge, MA, Da Capo Press, 2006.

5. Hammond A, Freeman K. One year outcomes of a randomized controlled trial of an educational–behavioral joint protection programme for the people with rheumatoid arthritis. Rheumatology 2001;40:1044–1051.

6. Hammond A, Freeman K. The long term outcomes from a randomized controlled trial of an educational behavioral joint protection programme for the people with rheumatoid arthritis. Clin Rehabil 2004; 18:520–528.

7. Solomon DH, Warsi A, Brown-Stevenson T, Farrell M, Gauthier S, Mikels D, Lee TH. Does self-management education benefit all populations with arthritis? A randomized controlled trial in a primary care physician network. J Rheumatol 2002;29:362–368.

Section VII

Commentary

40 Arthritis, Aging Society, Exercise, Nutrition, and Other Precautionary Measures

Siba P. Raychaudhuri, Hiroyoshi Moriyama, and Debasis Bagchi

CONTENTS

INTRODUCTION

Arthritis literally means "joint inflammation," which imposes debilitating and detrimental effects on human health. Arthritis is a leading cause of disability in the United States, which afflicts as many as one in five Americans or approximately 40 million Americans or 20% of the U.S. population. This number is going to rise to 60 million by the year 2020, and approximately two-thirds of all Americans living with arthritis are women. Approximately $15 billion is the direct annual costs of medical care, whereas lost wages account for some $50 billion in indirect costs related to arthritis. The population with arthritis divides almost evenly between those 65 years and older and the rest of population. More than half of those with arthritis are younger than 65 years, including almost 200,000 children. There are individuals who have arthritis who lead active, productive lives, whereas others need assistance to accomplish basic activities associated with daily living.

In arthritis, more than 100 different conditions exist that affect the joints as well as the muscles and other tissues. Osteoarthritis (OA) or degenerative arthritis, the most common form of arthritis, results from the breakdown of the cartilage inside the joints, whereas rheumatoid arthritis is characterized by inflammation of the synovial tissue. OA is a degenerative disease caused by continued wearing down of the structure and/or tissue in the joints, including cartilage and connective tissue. OA usually affects the major joints, especially those that bear the weight of the body, and may not affect the same joints on the opposite sides of the body.

ARTHRITIS AND AGING SOCIETY

Healthy aging has been defined as "the development and maintenance of optimal physical, mental, and social well-being and function in older adults," as defined by Healthy Aging Research Network (http://depts.washington.edu/hansite/drupal/overview.html), which is supported by the Centers for Disease Control and Prevention. It has been demonstrated that advancing age, food habits, genetic inheritance, and several other factors are associated with appropriate healthy aging phenomenon, and it is very difficult to maintain and manage the situation ideally because there are several variables/factors associated. Advancing age is known to have an increasing impact on the propensity of arthritis (Kimura, 2009). Physical and mental stresses are associated with a number of degenerative diseases including arthritis (Rao, 2009). Both physical and mental stresses increase with advancing age. Thus, there are several factors, and we need to handle the overall situation very carefully and delicately.

ARTHRITIS AND EXERCISE

Exercise is an integral tool in managing arthritis. One may consider walking a small distance on a regular basis or start a yoga class. Moderate exercise on a regular basis can provide the following significant benefits (Arthritis Foundation, 2010) to people suffering from arthritis:

1. Reduces joint pain and stiffness
2. Builds strong muscle around the joints and provides joint support
3. Increases flexibility and endurance
4. Reduces arthritis-induced inflammatory responses
5. Reduces the risk of other chronic conditions
6. Promotes overall health, helps better sleep, maintains healthy body weight, and improves self-esteem
7. Reduces the risks of osteoporosis and cardiovascular diseases

The Arthritis Foundation recommends to start the exercise slow and make it fun. It is ideal to start with flexibility and stretching exercises, which will improve the movements and daily activities. Once the subjects are accustomed, they can go for weight training and endurance exercises such as bicycling.

If the arthritic subjects are reluctant to exercise because of pain, then they might consider doing the water exercise. In the water, the body's buoyancy reduces stress on hips, knees, and spine while building strength and increasing movements (Arthritis Foundation, 2010). Water provides 12 times greater resistance as compared with air, so the individual can perform a great workout without the wear and tear of the joints (Arthritis Foundation, 2010). Indian traditional yoga (Garfinkel and Schumacher, 2000) and traditional Chinese martial art tai chi (Uhlig et al., 2010) have been extensively studied in arthritis. Thus, appropriate moderate exercise may help the arthritic subjects to a big extent.

OTHER PRECAUTIONARY MEASURES

There are several precautionary measures, and treatments have been extensively studied over the last several years. However, maintaining a state of ideal conditions in humans is basically impossible. Nobody accepts the facts or diseased conditions unless it happens to him or her. However, this mental strength declines with work pressure or advancing age. Mental stress is another major factor. Food or proper nutrition is another key factor.

A balanced diet and a healthy life style, which includes stress relaxation, regular exercise, and good sleep habits, are important measures to control arthritis as well as other diseases. Drinking one glass of freshly squeezed orange juice a day may minimize or reduce the risk of developing inflammatory forms of arthritis. Consumption of certain dietary carotenoids, including beta-cryptoxanthin, provitamin A carotenoid, and zeaxanthin, and vitamin C demonstrated lower risk of developing inflammatory arthritis. Peppers, pumpkins, winter squash, persimmons, tangerines, and papayas have the highest levels of beta-cryptoxanthin. However, lutein and lycopene exhibited no protective effect against arthritis (Pattison et al., 2005). Furthermore, bioactives as antioxidants, including EPA in fish oils, for example, were reported to play an adjunctive role in ameliorating inflammatory disorders, including rheumatoid arthritis and OA (Darlington and Stone, 2001).

CONCLUSIONS

It might be desirable to maintain a decent healthy lifestyle with moderate exercise in conjunction with novel, scientifically supported supplements/drugs, which may retard or prevent the onset of arthritis in humans. However, advancing age potentiates joint disorders in humans and animals, while appropriate therapies and treatments are the only indispensible options.

REFERENCES

Arthritis Foundation. http://www.arthritis.org/exercise-intro.php. 2010.

Darlington LG, Stone TW. Antioxidants and fatty acids in the amelioration of rheumatoid arthritis and related disorders. Brit J Nutr 2001;85:251–269.

Garfinkel M, Schumacher HR. Yoga. Rheum Dis Clin North Am 2000;26:125–132.

Kimura T. Progress of research in osteoarthritis. An overview of the recent knowledge on osteoarthritis: pathogenesis, evaluation and therapies. Clin Calcium 2009;19:1565–1571.

Pattison DJ, Symmons DP, Lunt M, Welch A, Bingham SA, Day NE, Silman AJ. Dietary beta-cryptoxanthin and inflammatory polyarthritis: results from a population-based prospective study. Amer J Clin Nutr 2005;82:451–455.

Rao K. Recent research in stress, coping and women's health. Curr Opin Psychiatry 2009;22:188–193.

Uhlig T, Fongen C, Steen E, Christie A, Odegard S. Exploring tai chi in rheumatoid arthritis: a quantitative and qualitative study. BMC Musculoskelet Disord 2010;11:43.

Index

Note: Page references followed by "*f*" and "*t*" denote figures and tables, respectively.